First published in the United Kingdom in 2003
by Martin Dunitz, an imprint of the Taylor & Francis Group plc, 11 New Fetter Lane, London EC4P 4EE

Tel.:   +44 (0) 20 7583 9855
Fax.:   +44 (0) 20 7842 2298
E-mail: info@dunitz.co.uk
Website: http://www.dunitz.co.uk

Although every effort has been made to ensure that drug doses and other information are presented
accurately in this publication, the ultimate responsibility rests with the prescribing physician. Neither the publishers
nor the authors can be held responsible for errors or for any consequences arising from the use of information contained
herein. For detailed prescribing information or instructions on the use of any product or procedure discussed herein,
please consult the prescribing information or instructional material issued by the manufacturer.

A CIP record for this book is available from the British Library.

ISBN 1 84184 202 8

Distributed in the USA by
Fulfilment Center
Taylor & Francis
10650 Toebben Drive
Independence, KY 41051, USA
Toll Free Tel.: +1 800 634 7064
E-mail: taylorandfrancis@thomsonlearning.com

Distributed in Canada by
Taylor & Francis
74 Rolark Drive
Scarborough, Ontario M1R 4G2, Canada
Toll Free Tel.: +1 877 226 2237
E-mail: tal_fran@istar.ca

Distributed in the rest of the world by
Thomson Publishing Services
Cheriton House
North Way
Andover, Hampshire SP10 5BE, UK
Tel.: +44 (0)1264 332424
E-mail: salesorder.tandf@thomsonpublishingservices.co.uk

Composition by EXPO Holdings, Malaysia
Printed in Spain by Grafos SA

Contents

Section VI   Emerging CMR applications

**Section VII   CMR clinical laboratory
and economics**

Contributors

Ergin Atalar PhD
Associate Professor of Radiology, BME and ECE
Johns Hopkins University
Baltimore, MD, USA

David A Bluemke MD PhD
Associate Professor
Clinical Director, MRI, Associate Professor of Radiology
Johns Hopkins University School of Medicine
Johns Hopkins Hospital
Baltimore, MD, USA

Christina M Bove MD
Fellow in Cardiovascular Disease
University of Virginia Health System
Charlottesville, VA, USA

James R Brookeman PhD
Professor of Radiology and Biomedical Engineering
Director of Magnetic Resonance Research
University of Virginia
Charlottesville, VA, USA

Peter Caravan MD
EPIX Medical, Inc.
Cambridge, MA, USA

James C Carr MD
Department of Radiology,
Northwestern Memorial Hospital,
Chicago, IL, USA

Shelton D Caruthers PhD
Senior MR Clinical Scientist, Philips Medical Systems
Associate Director, Cardiovascular MR Laboratories
Washington University School of Medicine
Department of Medicine
Division of Cardiology
St Louis, MO, USA

Robin P Choudhury MA DM MRCP
Clinical Lecturer
Oxford University Department of Cardiovascular Medicine
John Radcliffe Hospital
Oxford, UK

Cindy R Comeau BS RT (N)(MR)
Educational Director Cardiovascular MRI
Advanced Cardiovascular Imaging
Cardiovascular Research Foundation
New York, NY, USA

Vibhas Deshpande PhD
Siemens Medical Solutions
Los Angeles, CA, USA

Alexander J Dick MD FRCPC
Division of Cardiology
Sunnybrook & Women's College Health Sciences Centre
Toronto, Ontario, Canada

Timm Dickfeld MD
Fellow in Cardiology
Johns Hopkins School of Medicine
Johns Hopkins Hospital
Baltimore, MD, USA

Howard V Dinh
The Zena and Michael A Wiener Cardiovascular Institute
Mount Sinai School of Medicine
Mount Sinai Medical Center
New York, NY, USA

Frederick H Epstein PhD
Associate Professor of Radiology and Biomedical
Engineering
University of Virginia
Charlottesville, VA, USA

Zahi A Fayad PhD
Imaging Science Laboratories
Departments of Radiology and Medicine (Cardiology)
The Zena and Michael A. Wiener Cardiovascular Institute
The Marie-Josée and Henry R. Kravis Cardiovascular
Health Center
Mount Sinai School of Medicine
New York, NY, USA

Victor A Ferrari MD
Associate Professor of Medicine and Radiology
Cardiovascular Medicine Division
University of Pennsylvania School of Medicine
Associate Director, Noninvasive Imaging Laboratory
Hospital of the University of Pennsylvania
Philadelphia, PA, USA

J Paul Finn MD
Medical Director of MRI
Department of Radiology
Northwestern Memorial Hospital
Chicago, IL, USA

Mark A Fogel MD FACC FAAP
Associate Professor of Pediatrics, Cardiology and
Radiology
Director of Cardiac MRI and Cardiac MRI Research
The University of Pennsylvania School of Medicine
The Children's Hospital of Philadelphia
Philadelphia, PA, USA

Stephen Frohwein MD
Director of Cardiovascular Imaging
American Cardiovascular Research Institute
Atlanta, GA, USA

Valentin Fuster PhD
The Zena and Michael A. Wiener Cardiovascular Institute
The Marie-Josée and Henry R. Kravis Cardiovascular
Health Center
Mount Sinai School of Medicine
New York, NY, USA

Ling Gao ME
Research Associate, Department of Medicine
Research Project Manager
Dartmouth Advanced Imaging Center
Lebanon, NH, USA

Sandeep Gautam MD
Post-Doctoral Fellow
Department of Medicine-Cardiovascular,
School of Medicine,
Johns Hopkins University
Baltimore, MD, USA

Jeffrey P Goldman MD
Assistant Professor of Radiology
Clinical Director Cardiovascular
and Body MRI
Mount Sinai School of Medicine
New York, NY, USA

Michael A Guttman MS
Staff Scientist
Laboratory of Cardiac Energetics
Division of Intramural Research
National Heart, Lung and Blood Institute
National Institutes of Health
Bethesda, MD, USA

Henry Halperin MD MA
Professor or Medicine
Biomedical Engineering and Radiology
Division of Cardiology
Johns Hopkins Hospital
Baltimore, MD, USA

Randall Higashida MD
Clinical Professor
Department of Radiology
University of California at San Francisco
San Francisco, CA, USA

Charles B Higgins
Professor
Department of Radiology
UCSF
San Francisco, CA, USA

Robert M Judd PhD
Associate Professor of Medicine and Radiology
Duke Cardiovascular Magnetic Resonance Center
Duke University
Durham, NC, USA

Raymond JM Kim MD
Duke Cardiovascular Magnetic Resonance Center
Duke University
Durham, NC, USA

Michael C Knopp
Department of Radiology
The Ohio State University Hospitals
Columbus, OH, USA

Christopher M Kramer MD
Associate Professor of Radiology and Medicine
Director, Cardiac MRI
University of Virginia Health System
Charlottesville, VA, USA

Titus Kuehne MD
Department of Radiology
University of California at San Francisco
San Francisco, CA, USA

Gregory M Lanza MD PhD FACC
Assistant Professor of Medicine and Bioengineering
Washington University School of Medicine
Department of Medicine
Division of Cardiology
St Louis, MO, USA

Albert C Lardo PhD
Departments of Radiology, Medicine, Surgery and
Biomedical Engineering
Johns Hopkins University School of Medicine
Baltimore, MD, USA

Robert J Lederman MD
Investigator
Cardiovascular Branch
Division of Intramural Research
National Heart, Lung and Blood Institute
National Institutes of Health
Bethesda, MD, USA

Randall Lee MD PhD
Associate Clinical Professor
Department of Electrophysiology
University of California at San Francisco
San Francisco, CA, USA

Debiao Li PhD
Associate Professor of Radiology and Biomedical
Engineering
Director, Cardiovascular MR Research
Departments of Radiology and Biomedical Engineering
Northwestern University
Chicago, IL, USA

Joao AC Lima MD MBA
Associate Professor of Medicine, Radiology and
Epidemiology
Director Cardiovascular Imaging in Cardiology
Johns Hopkins University
Baltimore, MD, USA

Christine H Lorenz PhD
Senior Member Technical Staff
Imaging and Visualization
Siemens Corporate Research Inc
Siemens
Princeton, NJ, USA

Jeffrey Maki MD PhD
Department of Radiology
School of Medicine
Veteran's Administration Medical Center
Seattle, WA, USA

Heiko Marholdt MD
Duke Cardiovascular Magnetic Resonance Center
Duke University
Durham, NC, USA
and Robert-Bosch-Medical Center
Stuttgart, Germany

Alastair J Martin PhD
Department of Radiology
University of California at San Francisco
San Francisco, CA, USA
and
Philips Medical Systems
Best, the Netherlands

Elliot R McVeigh PhD
Investigator
Laboratory of Cardiac Energetics
Division of Intramural Research
National Heart, Lung and Blood Institute
National Institutes of Health
Bethesda, MD, USA

Phillip Moore MD
Associate Clinical Professor
Department of Pediatric Cardiology
University of California at San Francisco
San Francisco, CA, USA

Eike Nagel MD
Cardiology
Germany Heart Institute
Berlin, Germany

Stefan Neubauer MD MRCP
Professor of Cardiovascular Medicine
Director, University of Oxford Clinical Magnetic
Resonance Research Centre
Department of Cardiovascular Medicine
John Radcliffe Hospital
Oxford, UK

Nael F Osman PhD
Assistant Professor
Department of Radiology and Radiological Science
Johns Hopkins University
Baltimore, MD, USA

Justin D Pearlman MD ME PhD
Professsor of Medicine and Radiology, Dartmouth
Medical School
Adjuunct Professor MIT/HST
Thayrer School of Engineering and Computer Sciences
Director, Dartmouth Advanced Imaging Centre
Section of Cardiology and Departments of Medicine
Dartmouth-Hitchcock Medical Center
Lebanon, NH, USA

Dudley J Pennell MD
Cardiovascular Magnetic Resonance Unit
Royal Brompton Hospital
London, UK

Dana C Peters PhD
Postdoctoral Fellow
Laboratory of Cardiac Energetics
Division of Intramural Research
National Heart, Lung and Blood Institute
National Institutes of Health
Bethesda, MD, USA

Sanjay Prasad MD MRCP
Consultant Cardiologist.
CMR Unit
Royal Brompton Hospital
London, UK

Martin R Prince MD PhD
Chief of MRI, New York Hospital
Professor of Radiology, Weill Medical College of
Cornell University
Professor of Radiology, Columbia College of Physicians
and Surgeons
New York, NY, USA

Michael Poon MD FACC
Director, The Mount Sinai Pulmonary Hypertension
Program
Medical Director, The Cardiac MR/CT Imaging Program
The Zena and Michael A Wiener Cardiovascular Institute
Mount Sinai School of Medicine
New York, NY, USA

Venkatesh K Raman MD
Cardiovascular Branch
Division of Intramural Research
National Heart, Lung and Blood Institute
Bethesda, MD, USA

Tracy John Robertson
Executive Director, Performance Solutions
Global Solutions Division
Siemens Medical Solutions
Malvern, PA, USA

Maythem Saeed DVM PhD
Adjunct Professor
Department of Radiology
University of California at San Francisco
San Francisco, CA, USA

Jürg Schwitter MD
Associate Professor
Division of Cardiology
and Co-Director CardioVascular MR Center
University Hospital Zurich
Zurich, Switzerland

Simon Schalla MD
Department of Radiology
University of California at San Francisco
San Fransicci, CA, USA

Craig H Scott MD
Assistant Professor of Medicine
University of Pennsylvania
Philadelphia, PA, USA

Udo Sechtem MD FESC
Robert-Bosch-Medical Center
Stuttgart, Germany

Leslee J Shaw PhD
Director, Outcomes Research
Associate Professor of Medicine
Atlanta Cardiovascular Research Institute
Atlanta, GA, USA

Michael Simons MD
Anna Gundlach Huber Professor of Medicine
(Cardiology) and of Pharmacology and Toxicology
Chief, Section of Cardiology
Director, Angiogenesis Research Center
Departments of Medicine & Pharmacology
Dartmouth Medical School
Dartmouth Hitchcock Medical Center
Lebanon, NH, USA

Daniel K Sodickson MD PhD
Assistant Professor of Radiology and Medicine,
Harvard Medical School
Director, Laboratory for Biomedical Imaging Research
Beth Israel Deaconess Medical Center
Boston, MA, USA

Matthias Stuber PhD
Associate Professor
Department of Radiology
Johns Hopkins University Medical School
Baltimore, MD, USA

Gilberto Szarf MD
Post Doc Fellow
Associate Professor
Clinical Director, MRI, Associate Professor of Radiology
Johns Hopkins University School of Medicine
Johns Hopkins Hospital
Baltimore, MD, USA

Louise Thomson
Duke Cardiovascular Magnetic Resonance Center
Duke University
Durham, NC, USA

Anja Wagner MD
Visiting Assistant Professor of Medicine
Duke Cardiovascular Magnetic Resonance Center
Duke University
Durham, NC, USA
also at Robert-Bosch-Medical Center
Stuttgart, Germany

William P Warren MD
Cardiology Fellow,
Johns Hopkins University
Baltimore, MD, USA

Oliver M Weber PhD
Department of Radiology
University of California at San Francisco
505 Parnassus Avenue, Box 0628
San Francisco, CA, USA

Robert M Weisskoff PhD
Head of Imaging
EPIX Medical, Inc.
Cambridge, MA, USA

Samuel A Wickline MD FACC
Professor of Medicine, Biomedical Engineering,
and Physics
Washington University
Department of Medicine
Division of Cardiology
Barnes-Jewish Hospital
St Louis, MO, USA

Xiaoming Yang MD PhD
Associate Professor of Radiology
Co-Director, Center for Image-Guided Interventions
Johns Hopkins University School of Medicine
Baltimore, MD, USA

Aysegul Yegin MD
Lead Scientist and Clinical Program Manager
American Cardiovascular Research Institute
Atlanta, GA, USA

Preface

Cardiovascular magnetic resonance (CMR) has slowly evolved from a research tool to become a clinical mainstay of diagnostic imaging for several medical disciplines. CMR continues to play an increasingly important role in the understanding of cardiac disease progression and clinical management algorithms. The most recent advances in hardware and pulse sequence design now allow for a truly impressive range of cardiac and vascular imaging opportunities that have improved existing applications and have extended the utility of CMR well beyond anatomic diagnostic studies. Despite these advances and continued progress in clinical studies, however, CMR has yet to play a primary role in the clinical management of patients with cardiovascular disease. In part, the lack of complete clinical acceptance may be related to the often intimidating technical enigma of CMR and/or the dizzying array of new and evolving applications that appear in the literature on a weekly to monthly basis. Thus, concise dissemination of this new and rapidly evolving body of information is likely critical for widespread growth of CMR.

The purpose of *Cardiovascular Magnetic Resonance: Established and Emerging Applications* is to consolidate this wide and growing body of information into a single balanced source. This highly illustrated text is designed to provide the most recent and practical information on established foundational applications of CMR as well as to give the reader a look into the future through the presentation of state-of-the-art therapeutic applications in various stages of development. *Cardiovascular Magnetic Resonance* targets a broad readership as the editors include chapters authored by both academic and private practice clinicians, academic and industrial biomedical engineers and MR technologists.

Albert Lardo, Zahi Adel Fayad,
Nicolas AF Chronos, Valentin Fuster

1

Physics of MRI – Basic principles

Frederick H Epstein, James R Brookeman

Introduction

Magnetic resonance imaging (MRI) was developed in the early 1980s on the basis of the technique known as nuclear magnetic resonance (NMR), which had been employed since the 1940s to study the structure and dynamics of molecular systems. Not all atoms are suitable for NMR studies, but if the nucleus of an atom has an odd number of protons or an odd number of neutrons, such as hydrogen (1 odd proton) or carbon-13 (6 protons and 7 neutrons), then the entire nucleus will have a nuclear spin with an associated magnetic moment. This spin property causes the nucleus, such as the proton in hydrogen, to behave as a tiny bar magnet that, when placed in an external magnetic field, will tend to align itself with the direction of the applied field. Because of a quantum mechanical effect, this alignment is not complete. Instead, the nuclear magnet behaves much like a gyroscope that precesses around the axis of the applied external field with a frequency f_0 (Figure 1.1). This precession frequency f_0 is called the Larmor frequency and is proportional to the magnitude B_0 of the external magnetic field $\mathbf{B}_0$ and a unique property of each nucleus called the gyromagnetic ratio γ. For protons in the hydrogen nucleus of a water molecule in an applied magnetic field of 1.5 tesla (T) the Larmor precession frequency is approximately 64 million cycles per second (64 megahertz, MHz). The precession frequency f_0 can be determined at any other magnetic field strength B_0 from the Larmor equation:

$$f_0 = \frac{\gamma}{2\pi} B_0.$$

The hydrogen nucleus has a nuclear spin of $\frac{1}{2}$, and because of the quantum nature of the energy of the spin in a magnetic field, there are in fact only two allowed orientations of the precessing nuclear gyroscope. These are a *low-energy* orientation in which the nucleus precesses about an axis parallel to the applied field, and a *high-energy* position precessing with an orientation *antiparallel* to the applied magnetic field. Transitions between these

two energy states may be induced by an externally applied radiofrequency (RF) electromagnetic field from an RF coil, or by fluctuations of the local magnetic field at the nucleus. These local magnetic field fluctuations can be due to either other nearby nuclear spins or to paramagnetic substances such as dissolved oxygen or gadolinium (Gd)-DTPA, a well known MRI contrast agent. Substances such as oxygen and gadolinium, which have unpaired orbital electron spins, possess very large electronic magnetic moments and so can be very effective at inducing changes in nearby nuclear spin energy states.

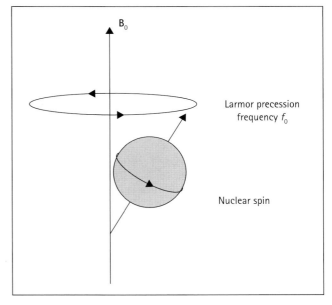

Figure 1.1
Precessing nuclear magnetic moment. When an atom with nuclear spin (i.e. an atom with an odd number of protons or neutrons) is placed in an applied static magnetic field $\mathbf{B}_0$, the magnetic moment associated with the nuclear spin will precess like a gyroscope about the applied field $\mathbf{B}_0$. The precession frequency f_0 is called the Larmor frequency and is proportional to the applied field strength.

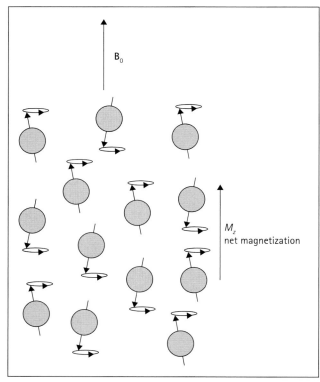

Figure 1.2
Generation of net magnetization M_z. Nuclear spins may align either parallel or antiparallel to the applied field $\mathbf{B}_0$. A slight excess tend to align in the low-energy state parallel to $\mathbf{B}_0$, and lead to a net magnetization M_z. The net magnetization leads to the detected NMR signal.

At room temperature and typical magnetic fields of 1.5 T, the equilibrium distribution of hydrogen proton spins in tissues between the low- and high-energy orientations is almost equal, with just a slight excess of spins in the low-energy parallel state. For every two million protons, there are on average just nine more protons aligned with the field than against, and these nine therefore provide a net macroscopic proton magnetization aligned with the applied field $\mathbf{B}_0$ (Figure 1.2). It is this net magnetization, known as M_z, that is key to the generation of the MR signal, since under the influence of an electromagnetic RF field, applied at the resonant Larmor frequency, transitions will be induced between the proton spin energy states. These transitions result in the net magnetization being caused to nutate or tip away from the direction of the main field $\mathbf{B}_0$. A burst of RF energy of just a few milliseconds duration from the coil surrounding the tissue is sufficient to tip the net magnetization away from alignment with $\mathbf{B}_0$. An RF pulse able to tip the magnetization by 90° is known as a 90° pulse, whereas a 180° pulse has sufficient energy to rotate the net magnetization by 180°.

Origin of the magnetic resonance signal

The proton density

In order to understand how the precessing nuclear spins in the hydrogen atoms of tissue water molecules are able to generate an MR signal, we need to consider the individual picture elements that make up an MR image. For an image with a section thickness of 5 mm and an in-plane resolution of 2 mm × 2 mm, each voxel will have a volume of 0.02 ml. The MR signal from this voxel will come from the net magnetization M_z of the proton spins within the voxel and is representative of the total *proton density* in that voxel picture element. The total number of protons in the hydrogen atoms of the water molecules in 0.02 ml can be determined from Avogadro's number to be approximately 1.3×10^{21}. At room temperature and in a magnetic field of 1.5 T approximately 6×10^{15} of these protons will therefore provide the net magnetization for this voxel. In response to a 90° RF pulse, this net magnetization M_z can be rotated away from alignment with $\mathbf{B}_0$, the z-axis or *longitudinal direction*, onto the x–y or *transverse plane*, which is perpendicular to the z-axis (Figure 1.3). In the laboratory frame of reference, this response appears as a nutation of M_z (Figure 1.3a), whereas in a frame of reference rotating at the Larmor frequency, this response appears as a simple rotation of M_z (Figure 1.3b). The continued precession of the net magnetization vector $\mathbf{M}_{xy}$ in the x–y plane will, by Faraday's law of electromagnetic induction, induce an electrical current, oscillating at the Larmor frequency, in an appropriately placed pick-up coil (Figure 1.4). This oscillating current in the pick-up coil, in the absence of any applied RF pulse, can persist for a duration of several tens of milliseconds, and is known as the *free induction decay* (FID). The actual duration of the FID signal for any particular voxel depends on a number of factors, such as the local homogeneity of the applied magnetic field $\mathbf{B}_0$, the interaction of the spins with nearby magnetic moments, and resonant fluctuations of the magnetic environment stimulating the return of the proton spin states to their equilibrium configuration, and thereby the realignment of the net magnetization with the projection of $\mathbf{B}_0$ on the z-axis. These factors together determine the rate of decay of the FID, which has an approximate exponential form, with a time constant known as the spin-phase memory time T2*, where T2* represents the time for the amplitude of the FID to decay by 63% of its initial value. T2* is the shortest of the three major time constants (T1, T2, T2*) used to describe the behavior of the spin magnetization. This is because T2* includes both the *extrinsic* factors that contribute to the signal decay, such as magnetic field inhomogeneities,

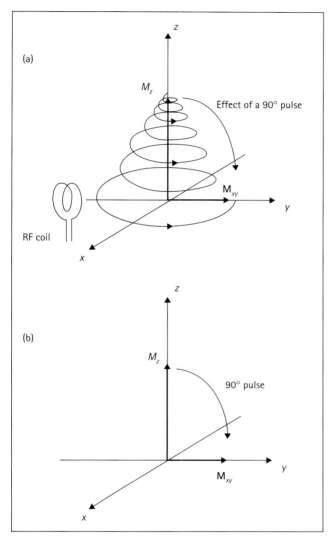

Figure 1.3
Generation of transverse magnetization M_{xy} by transmitting a radio-frequency (RF) electromagnetic pulse. In the laboratory frame of reference (a), application of a short RF pulse at the Larmor frequency causes M_z to nutate into the transverse plane, generating the transverse magnetization M_{xy}. In a frame of reference rotating at the Larmor frequency (b), M_z is simply tipped into the transverse x–y plane.

and the *intrinsic* factors, such as the nuclear spin–spin and spin–lattice interactions T2 and T1. Hence, for all tissues, $T1 \geq T2 \geq T2^*$.

Properties of the magnetization

T1 relaxation

The longitudinal relaxation time T1, also known as the spin–lattice relaxation time, is a measure of the time for

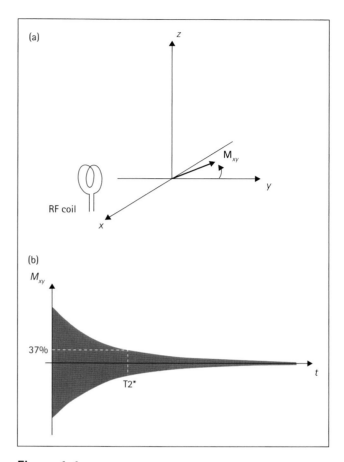

Figure 1.4
Signal reception using a receiver coil. By Faraday's law of induction, a precessing transverse magnetization M_{xy} that causes flux through the RF coil will induce a current in the coil with frequency f_0 (a). The signal detected immediately after application of a 90° RF pulse is called the free induction decay (FID), which decays exponentially with time constant $T2^*$ (b).

the spin system to return to equilibrium after a perturbation such as a 90° pulse. The return of M_z to equilibrium has an approximate exponential form, where T1 is the time for M_z to attain 63% of its equilibrium value M_0 (Figure 1.5). The regrowth of longitudinal relaxation requires a net transfer of energy from the nuclear spin system to the various molecular energy states of the surrounding tissue environment. In early NMR studies of materials, the surrounding environment was usually a crystalline lattice of molecules – hence the term 'spin–lattice relaxation'. However, in the biological systems common in MRI, this lattice is more often a fluid or soft tissue rather than a solid. Because T1 relaxation requires an energy exchange, it can occur only when a proton experiences another magnetic field fluctuating near the Larmor frequency. The source of this fluctuating field is typically another proton or an unpaired electron such as in Gd-DTPA. For a proton or electron to produce

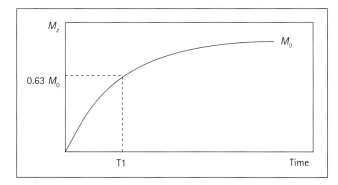

Figure 1.5
T1 relaxation. After a 90° RF pulse, the return of the longitudinal magnetization M_z toward its equilibrium value M_0 has an approximately exponential form, where T1 is the time for M_z to attain 63% of the equilibrium value.

a fluctuating magnetic field, the molecule in which it resides must be moving or tumbling. To be efficient at T1 relaxation, the molecule must be moving with a fluctuation rate at or near the Larmor frequency. Water, with its small molecular size, tumbles much too rapidly to be effective at T1 relaxation. The T1 value for free water is approximately 4 s and is longer than that of any other substance in the body. However, if the water is in a partially bound state exchanging between the bulk-water phase and the hydration shells that surround proteins or other macromolecules, its motion may be slowed to a rate closer to the Larmor frequency. The T1 value of water in this situation is therefore much shorter than that of free water. For example, a fluid such as blood, which contains various macromolecules, has a T1 of approximately 1 s. At the other extreme, the hydrogen protons in large macromolecules, which tumble quite slowly compared with the Larmor frequency, have relatively long T1 values.

The perfusion of a T1 contrast agent such as Gd-DTPA into a tissue will significantly reduce the T1 value of the tissue. Normal myocardium has a T1 of approximately 850 ms at 1.5 T, but with Gd-DTPA infusion this is reduced to about 300 ms. Similarly, intravenous injection of a bolus of Gd-DTPA will reduce the T1 of blood from 1 s to about 200–400 ms, depending on the Gd-DTPA concentration in the tissue.

T2 relaxation

The transverse relaxation time, also called the spin–spin relaxation time, is a measure of the phase coherence time for the individual spins to precess together. In contrast to T1 relaxation, where energy transfer from the spin system to the lattice occurs, T2 relaxation takes place either with or without energy exchange. Therefore, T2 is always less

than or equal to T1. For most biological tissues, T1 values are typically 10 times longer than T2 values.

T2 relaxation results from any intrinsic process that causes the spins to lose their phase coherence in the transverse plane. Most frequently, it results from static or slowly fluctuating local magnetic field variations within the tissue itself. If a spin temporarily experiences a change in its local static field due to an interaction with another spin, the spin will temporarily precess at a slightly different frequency and thereby gain or lose phase compared with the other spins. In large macromolecules, where molecular motions are extremely slow, T2 relaxation is extraordinarily efficient, and T2 values may be as short as 5–10 μs. These extremely short T2 values cause the signal to decay so rapidly that protons in most macromolecules are essentially invisible in an MRI experiment. However, a recently developed technique known as *magnetization transfer* is able to reveal the presence of some of these very short T2 protons by a process of spin exchange.[1] When molecular motion is very rapid, any local field inhomogeneity experienced by a proton averages to zero over a short period of time. Consequently, these protons experience no consistent changes in their local magnetic fields. In rapidly moving molecules, therefore, T2 relaxation processes are weak and T2 values are correspondingly long. Although the amount of bulk water present is a strong predictor of the T1 and T2 values for most tissues, the contribution to the MR signal from the protons bonded to carbon atoms in lipids must be considered in many tissues. In fats, many protons have short T1 values since fat molecules are intermediate in size and their motions are close to the Larmor frequencies of 42–64 MHz of conventional 1.0–1.5 T MR scanners. In adipose tissues, for example, nearly all the MR signal arises from such lipid protons. In other tissues, such as bone marrow, fat and water protons make almost equal contributions to the total signal and net relaxation times. The fat and water protons also precess at only slightly different frequencies in the same externally applied magnetic field. This is due to the different magnetic shielding effects of the hydrogen–oxygen versus the hydrogen– carbon bonding electrons at the nuclear sites. While this effect, which is called the *chemical shift*, is very small, just 3.5 parts per million (ppm), or 220 Hz, in 64 MHz at 1.5 T, it can nevertheless lead to some subtle *chemical shift artifacts* in the MR image. These artifacts are seen as a slight misregistration of the fat and water tissues in the frequency-encoding direction of the image.

MR image contrast

Immediately following an excitation RF pulse, such as a 90° pulse, each voxel will contain a certain amount of precessing net magnetization. This magnetization, rotating at the Larmor frequency in the transverse $x–y$ plane, will induce an oscillating current or signal in the RF receiver coil. The induced current or signal from each voxel will be in proportion to the instantaneous magnitude and coherence of the precessing magnetization in the voxel. In time, the signal from each voxel will decay under the influence of the various relaxation processes T1, T2 and T2* that pertain to that voxel, where T1 determines the loss of the transverse magnetization as it relaxes back to the longitudinal axis, and T2 and T2* characterize the phase coherence of the remaining net magnetization $\mathbf{M}_{xy}$ in the transverse plane. If adjacent voxels contain tissues with different relaxation properties, then a signal difference or contrast will develop that can be used to distinguish different voxels from each other and thereby also one tissue type from another. Therefore, an image reconstructed from the assembled signals from all the voxels at one particular time following the excitation pulse will show an image contrast that is based on the relaxation

properties of the different tissues. For example a T1-weighted image has a contrast that shows a high signal intensity for those voxels containing tissues with short T1 values (quick to recover) and a low signal for voxels with tissues having long T1 values, whereas a T2-weighted image will have a high signal for voxels containing tissues with long T2 values (slow to decay) and a low signal for voxels containing tissues with short T2 values. A proton-density weighted image, which is a measurement of $\mathbf{M}_{xy}$ before any of the relaxation processes have had a significant effect, has a high signal from voxels with a high equilibrium magnetization $\mathbf{M}_0$.

In the following sections, it can be seen that a great strength of MRI is the ability to create many different image contrasts by manipulating the image timing parameters, such as the repetition time of the RF excitation pulses (TR), the time to acquire the spin-echo signal (TE), and the time following a 180° pulse inverting the M_z magnetization (TI). These manipulations in the image timing parameters permit the operator to tease out various tissue properties to create a particular contrast in the image. Figure 1.6 indicates one method to distinguish normal myocardium (T1 = 850 ms) from Gd-enhanced infarcted myocardium (T1 = 300 ms).[2] Following a 180° inversion pulse, the tissue magnetization is allowed to recover until a significant difference in M_z values separates Gd-enhanced myocardium from normal myocardium. At this time, $t = 350$ ms, the image acquired shows high contrast between the two tissue types based on the differential spin–lattice recovery times, T1 = 300 ms versus 850 ms.

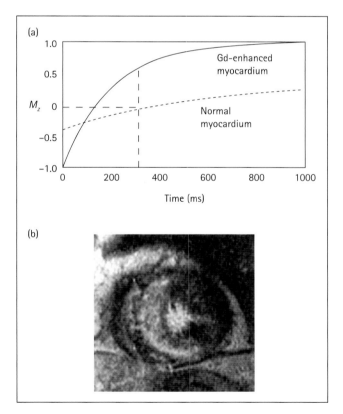

Figure 1.6
T1-weighted post-infarct short-axis image of the heart after infusion of Gd-DTPA (Gd), a T1-shortening contrast agent. Using a 180° inversion RF pulse applied at time $t = 0$ followed by a delay time sufficient to null normal myocardium (a), a heavily T1-weighted image is acquired where Gd-enhanced infarcted myocardium has high signal intensity and unenhanced normal myocardium has low signal intensity (b).

Slice selection, frequency encoding, and phase encoding

The previous section included a description of the origin of the MRI signal and how it can be detected using receiver coils. In this section, we describe how the signal can be localized in three-dimensional (3D) space for the purpose of creating images. Either two-dimensional (2D) images or 3D image volumes may be created by MRI. Signal localization is achieved for 2D MRI by processes called *slice selection*, *frequency encoding*, and *phase encoding*. For 3D MRI, frequency encoding is used for one dimension and phase encoding is used for the other two dimensions.

The common theme of the different spatial localization methods is the application of magnetic field gradients to equate the precession frequency or phase of magnetization to position in space. MRI scanners have three coils for producing linear magnetic field gradients in the x-, y-, and z-directions. The magnetic field gradients, which are produced by applying currents through the gradient coils, add to or subtract from the main $\mathbf{B}_0$ field linearly as a function of position. Since precession frequency is proportional to field strength, the precession frequency becomes a linear function of position when a magnetic field gradient is applied. For example, if a gradient pulse of strength G_x is applied in the x direction, then

$$f(x) = \frac{\gamma}{2\pi}\left(B_0 + G_x x\right),$$

where x is position and f is the precession frequency.

Slice selection

An MRI plane can be selected by a process called slice-selective excitation, or, more concisely, slice selection. Slice selection is performed by applying a magnetic field gradient G_{SS}, while a band-limited RF electromagnetic pulse $B_1(t)$ is simultaneously applied (Figure 1.7a). The time-varying RF pulse is chosen to have an approximately rectangular frequency spectrum, with an adjustable center frequency f_0 and bandwidth Δf (Figure 1.7b). The magnetic field gradient creates a linear dependence of the precession frequency on position z. Because the magnetic field gradient equates precession frequency with spatial position, the *center frequency* of the RF pulse corresponds to the *spatial center* of the imaging slice, z_0 (Figure 1.7c). Similarly, for a given bandwidth of the RF pulse, the value of G_{SS} determines the spatial slice thickness (Figure 1.7c). Based on these relationships, we see that the slice thickness can be readily adjusted by changing the gradient strength, and the slice position can be readily adjusted by changing the center frequency of the RF pulse. Because the magnetic field gradient can be applied in any arbitrary direction, imaging planes can be prescribed in any direction, including directions oblique to the principal axes of the magnet.

Using slice-selective excitation, only longitudinal magnetization with precession frequencies within the selected slice is exposed to a $\mathbf{B}_1$ field at the resonant frequency. The $\mathbf{B}_1$ field tips the longitudinal magnetization within the slice into the transverse plane, creating transverse magnetization only within the slice. By changing the power of the applied $\mathbf{B}_1$ field, the RF pulse flip angle can be adjusted. A flip angle of 90° tips all of the longitudinal magnetization into the transverse plane, whereas flip angles of less than 90° leave some magnetization aligned along the z-axis. A flip angle of 180° inverts the longitudinal magnetization. Although Figure 1.7 shows an exactly rectangular frequency profile, in practice the profile contains ripples both within and outside the desired slice as well as a transition band at the edges of the slice. Because of these effects, gaps of around 10–20% of the slice thickness are typically used in multislice imaging to avoid slice-to-slice crosstalk.

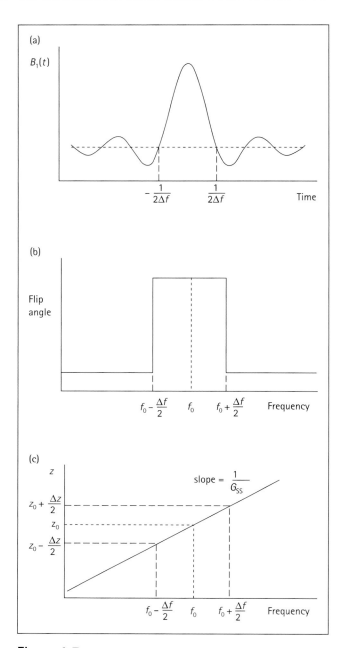

Figure 1.7
Slice-selective excitation. A time-varying radiofrequency (RF) electromagnetic pulse $B_1(t)$ is applied (a) simultaneously with a constant magnetic field gradient pulse with amplitude G_{SS} (not shown). The properly shaped RF pulse excites magnetization within a specific band of precession frequencies Δf centered at a specific frequency f_0 (b). The power of the RF pulse determines the flip angle. Since the gradient pulse equates precession frequency with spatial position z, the excited frequency band and the gradient amplitude determine the center z_0 and thickness Δz of the excited slice (c).

Frequency encoding

Following slice-selective excitation, additional magnetic field gradient pulses are used to spatially encode the transverse magnetization in the remaining two dimensions. In one in-plane direction, the *frequency-encoding* or *'readout'* *direction*, a frequency-encoding gradient pulse is applied while the signal is being sampled. Acquiring the signal while the gradient pulse is applied allows one to sample the spatial frequency spectrum of the image, and forms the basis of 'Fourier' encoding. This method can be explained as follows.

Consider the effect of applying a magnetic field gradient G_{FE} on the transverse magnetization $\mathbf{M}_{xy}(x, y, t)$ during data sampling. Because the magnetic field gradient causes a linear relationship between precession frequency and position, at each instance in time while the gradient is applied the phase (direction) of the transverse magnetization vectors is determined by their position in the frequency-encoding direction (Figure 1.8). At the center of the gradient pulse ($t = t_1$ in Figure 1.8), all of the transverse magnetization vectors have the same phase. As time progresses ($t = t_2$, t_3 in Figure 1.8), the amount of spatial phase warping of the transverse magnetization increases. The maximum amount of phase warping occurs just before the readout gradient is switched off, where a spatial frequency of 0.5 cycles/pixel occurs. At each instance in time, a given spatial frequency of $\mathbf{M}_{xy}(x, y, t)$ is described by the variable k_x, which has units of cycles/pixel.

At each spatial frequency k_x, the receiver coil detects the signal from the entire imaging plane. This aggregate signal is different for different values of k_x. By sampling the signal over the proper set of spatial frequencies ($k_x = -0.5$ to 0.5 cycles/pixel), the *spatial frequency spectrum* of the object being imaged is acquired. Fourier transformation of the spatial frequency spectrum can then be used to reconstruct a projection of the object in the frequency-encoding direction (Figure 1.9). This method is called frequency encoding because the precession frequency at each position x is directly proportional to x while the frequency-encoding gradient is applied.

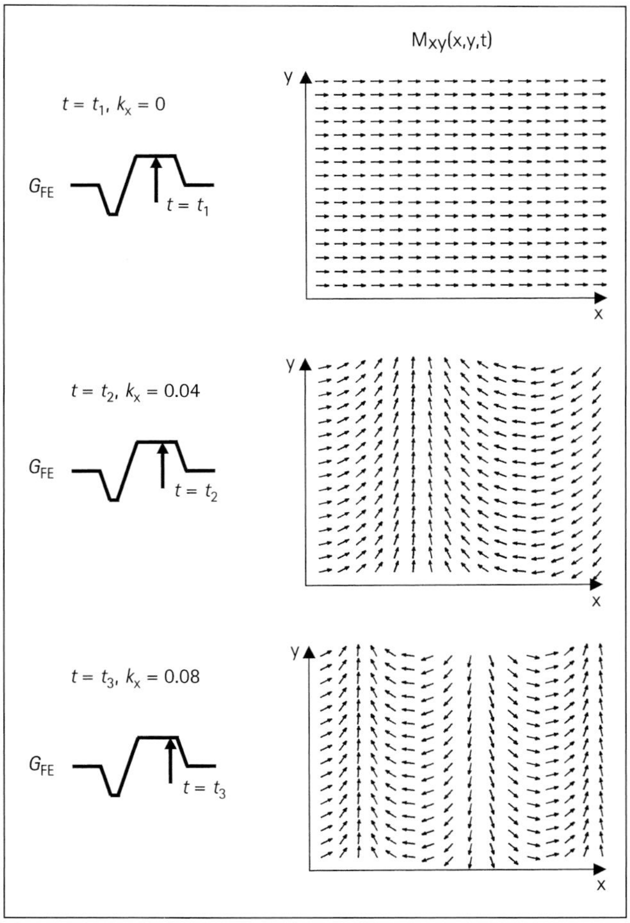

Figure 1.8

Frequency encoding. When a magnetic field gradient pulse is applied in the x-direction, the precession frequency of the transverse magnetization $M_{xy}(x,y,t)$ is proportional to position x. As time progresses ($t = t_1$, t_2, t_3 are shown), the spatial phase warping pattern in the frequency-encoding direction changes. At $t = t_1$, $k_x = 0$ cycles/pixel occur; at t = t_2, $k_x = 0.04$ cycles/pixel occur; and at $t = t_3$, $k_x = 0.08$ cycles/pixel occur. By sampling the signal over the spatial frequency spectrum of an object created by the frequency-encoding gradient ($k_x = -0.5$ to 0.5 cycles per pixel), a projection of the object onto the x-axis can be reconstructed by use of the Fourier transform.

Phase encoding

Spatial localization in the second in-plane direction is achieved using *phase encoding*, which, like frequency encoding, is based on the concept of sampling the spatial frequency spectrum of the image. Just as a range of spatial frequency states along the x-direction (described by different values of k_x) are required to reconstruct a projection of the object in the frequency-encoding direction, sampling the proper range of spatial frequencies along the y-direction (described by different values of k_y) is required for image reconstruction in the phase-encoding direction. Since k_x and k_y are independent, the full range of k_x values must be sampled for each value of k_y. In other words, the complete 2D **k**-space (k_x, k_y) must be sampled for 2D Fourier reconstruction.

To achieve a single spatial frequency state in the phase-encoding direction (a single value of k_y), a 'phase-

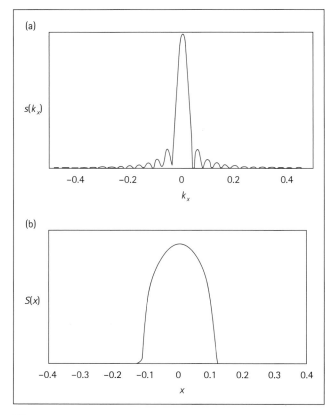

Figure 1.9
One-dimensional (1D) reconstruction by Fourier transform. After sampling the 1D spatial frequency spectrum of an object (a), Fourier transformation of the sampled signal $s(k_x)$ yields a projection of the object in the x-direction, $S(x)$ (b). In this example, a transverse slice of a water-filled cylinder was excited by slice-selective excitation, and the signal was localized in one dimension using a frequency-encoding gradient pulse.

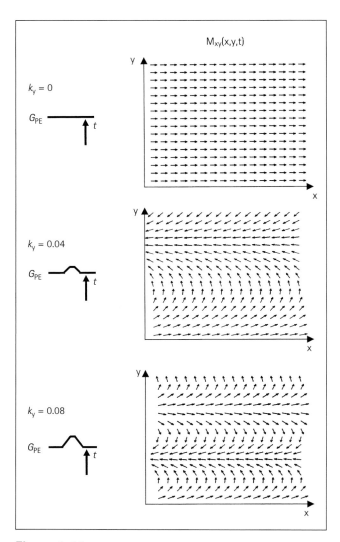

Figure 1.10
Phase encoding. After each phase-encoding gradient pulse is applied, the phase of the transverse magnetization $M_{xy}(x,y,t)$ is proportional to its spatial position y and the area of the phase-encoding gradient G_{PE}. The spatial phase warping pattern in the phase-encoding direction is different for each phase-encoding pulse. Examples are shown for k_y = 0, 0.04, and 0.08 cycles/pixel. By sampling the spatial frequency spectrum (k_y = −0.5 to 0.5 cycles/pixel) of an object, a projection of the object onto the y-axis can be reconstructed by use of the Fourier transform.

encoding' gradient pulse G_{PE} is applied in the y-direction and then switched off (Figure 1.10). To sample the full range of k_x (k_x = −0.5 to 0.5 cycles/pixel) for the current value of k_y, a prephaser gradient pulse followed by a frequency-encoding gradient pulse are applied in the x-direction and the signal is sampled. This process is repeated for all of the required values of k_y (k_y = −0.5 to 0.5 cycles/pixel), so that the signal is sampled for all required pairs (k_x, k_y) comprising the 2D spatial frequency spectrum of the object. The process is called phase encoding because the phase of the transverse magnetization at a given position y is proportional to y after the field gradient G_{PE} has been applied. After the complete 2D spatial frequency spectrum (**k**-space) is sampled, the 2D inverse Fourier transform is used to reconstruct the image (Figure 1.11).

Alternative approaches for spatially localizing the signal

We have described the basic method of slice-selective excitation and the commonly used Fourier-based methods of frequency and phase encoding. While they are widely

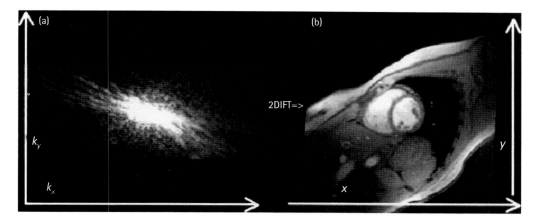

Figure 1.11

Two-dimensional (2D) image reconstruction by 2D Fourier transform. After sampling the 2D spatial frequency spectrum of an object over the 2D k-space by means of frequency encoding and phase encoding (a), 2D Fourier transformation of the sampled signal (raw data) is used to reconstruct the MR image (b). In this example, a short-axis image of the heart was acquired.

used, many refinements of these methods as well as different approaches have also been developed and applied with great success. For example, volume-selective, rather than slice-selective, RF pulses have been used for 'pencil beam' excitation to measure aortic pulse wave velocities.[3] Also, non-rectilinear sampling of **k**-space using radial or spiral trajectories has been used for real-time cine MRI and high-resolution MR coronary angiography.[4,5] Given the basic relationships between the spin-derived magnetization and RF and gradient pulses, a great variety of methods with different advantages and disadvantages have been developed for excitation and localization of the MRI signal.

Pulse sequences

Through the application of RF and gradient pulses to excite and spatially encode the MR signal, MR images can be acquired. The specific manner in which the pulses are played out is called the *pulse sequence*. By adjusting pulse sequence timing, RF pulse flip angles, gradient pulse areas, and numerous other parameters, many different types of images can be acquired. For the heart alone, an extensive array of specialized pulse sequences has been developed for imaging cardiac anatomy, left ventricular function, myocardial perfusion, coronary arteries, and other structures and functions. In this section, we describe a few of the basic sequences used for cardiac MRI.

Gradient-echo imaging

The two most basic MRI pulse sequences are the *gradient-echo* and *spin-echo* sequences. A timing diagram for a simple gradient-echo pulse sequence is shown in Figure 1.12, where the *x*-axis corresponds to time and the *y*-axis shows pulse amplitudes for the RF channel, slice-select (SS), frequency-encoding (FE), and phase-encoding (PE) gradients, and an analog-to-digital converter (ADC) for data sampling. To sample data for all of **k**-space, the module of pulses shown must be repeated N_{2D} times, where N_{2D} is the number of phase-encoding lines needed to reconstruct a 2D image. In successive repetitions, the amplitude of the phase-encoding gradient is changed to sample different lines of **k**-space. The time to repeat the pulses is called the repetition time, TR. The time from the center of the RF pulse to the echo peak is called the echo time, TE.

Within each repetition, the RF pulse and slice-select gradient perform slice-selective excitation, creating transverse magnetization in the chosen slice. The G_{PE} gradient pulse is played out to spatially encode the transverse magnetization in the phase-encoding direction. On the G_{FE} gradient channel, the prephaser pulse and frequency-encoding pulse are played out to spatially encode the magnetization in the orthogonal frequency-encoding direction. The prephaser gradient pulse causes initial phase incoherence of the transverse magnetization, and the frequency-encoding gradient subsequently rephases the transverse magnetization, which causes the gradient echo to peak at the echo time TE. The signal is sampled during application of the frequency-encoding gradient pulse. The signal is referred to as a gradient echo because gradient pulses are used to rephase the signal or echo at the center of the frequency-encoding gradient.

Short-TR gradient-echo imaging has played an important role in cardiac MRI for the past 10 years, since it has been the foundation for breath-hold cine MR imaging.[6] With the advent of steady-state free precession (SSFP) cine MRI, which has shorter scan times and improved

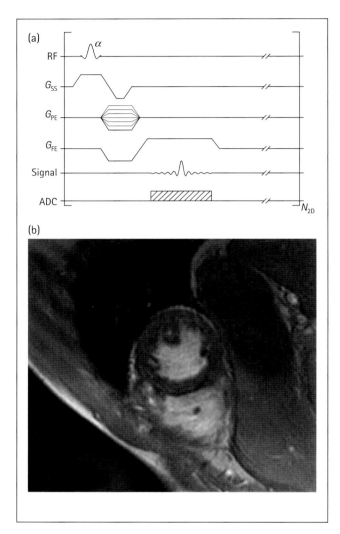

(a)

(b)

Figure 1.12
Timing diagram for a gradient-echo pulse sequence (a). Time is on the x-axis. An RF pulse with flip angle α and a gradient pulse G_{SS}, are used for slice-selective excitation. The frequency-encoding and phase-encoding gradients are used for spatial localization of the signal. The signal is dephased and rephased by the G_{FE} gradient pulses so that the echo peaks when phase coherence is achieved at the echo time TE. An analog-to-digital converter (ADC) is used to sample the signal. The sequence is repeated N_{2D} times, with different phase-encoding values, to sample all of the 2D k-space data. An example of a short-axis gradient-echo image of the heart is shown in (b).

image contrast, gradient-echo cine is no longer as widely used as it once was.[7] Nonetheless, it is still used often and its properties should be reviewed.

Short-TR gradient-echo cine MRI displays proton-density-weighted image contrast and is sensitive to inflow effects. As shown in Figure 1.12b, myocardium appears gray and, due to inflow of spins that have not been previously excited, the signal from blood has high intensity. Also, gradient-echo cine imaging can be sensitive to signal

loss due to inhomogeneity of the static magnetic field.[8] In the heart, inhomogeneity of the static magnetic field typically occurs in the vicinity of the posterior wall due to the interaction of the applied magnetic field with multiple tissues such as the heart, lung, and liver that have different magnetic susceptibilities. This extrinsic field inhomogeneity acts like a local gradient pulse, causing incoherence of transverse magnetization phase, shortening of $T2^*$, and signal loss artifacts. The amount of spin dephasing increases linearly with TE; thus, it is important to minimize TE in gradient-echo imaging to avoid these artifacts.[8]

Spin-echo imaging

The fundamental difference between gradient-echo and spin-echo imaging is that a spin-echo pulse sequence employs a refocusing RF pulse to eliminate signal loss due to static magnetic field inhomogeneity (Figure 1.13). The refocusing RF pulse, which is also commonly referred to as a 180° pulse, is placed at the time t = TE/2. During the time from the center of the slice-selective excitation RF pulse to TE/2, transverse magnetization accumulates phase due to static magnetic field inhomogeneity. The refocusing RF pulse flips the transverse magnetization about the M_y axis so that during the subsequent period of

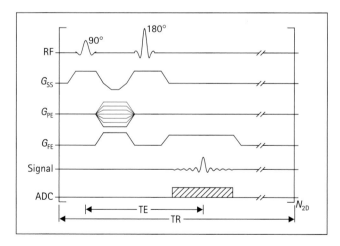

Figure 1.13
Timing diagram for a spin-echo pulse sequence. Time is on the x-axis. A 90° RF pulse and a simultaneously applied gradient pulse G_{SS} are used for slice-selective excitation. A second slice-selective RF pulse with a 180° flip angle is used to refocus transverse magnetization that lost phase coherence due to inhomogeneity of the static B_0 magnetic field. Frequency-encoding and phase-encoding gradients are used for spatial localization of the signal. The echo peaks and phase coherence occur at the echo time TE. The sequence is repeated N_{2D} times, with different phase-encoding values, to sample all of the 2D k-space data. The time to repeat the sequence is TR.

duration TE/2, phase accumulation due to static magnetic field inhomogeneity cancels the phase accumulation accrued during the initial period TE/2. The echo that refocuses at the time TE is referred to as a spin echo, and is significantly less sensitive than a gradient echo to signal loss from static field inhomogeneity.

Because spin-echo imaging is insensitive to field inhomogeneity, TE (and TR) can be widely adjusted to vary image contrast. Specifically, T1 weighting occurs when TR is short relative to T1 and TE is short relative to T2. T2 weighting occurs when TR is long and TE is long. Proton-density weighting is achieved when TR is long and TE is short. T2-weighted and proton-density-weighted images are typically acquired during a single acquisition, where spin echoes are acquired at both short and long TE.

While spin-echo pulse sequences generally have high signal-to-noise ratio (SNR) and are insensitive to field inhomogeneity, due to the use of extra RF and gradient pulses, spin-echo imaging is generally significantly slower than gradient-echo imaging. In cardiac MRI, a variant of the basic spin-echo sequence, the so-called black-blood fast spin-echo pulse sequence, currently plays an important role in imaging cardiac anatomy.[9] Diagrams demonstrating this technique are shown in Figures 1.14 and 1.15. Using R-wave detection of the ECG signal, a double inversion recovery pulse module is played out at end diastole. The first excitation pulse in this module is not slice-selective, and inverts the M_z component of the magnetization throughout the sensitive volume of the RF coil (i.e. essentially the whole body). Next, the second RF pulse, which is slice-selective, restores the initial value of M_z only for the imaging slice. During systole, two events occur that make blood in the image appear black. First, blood that was in the imaging slice flows out, and blood that was out of the imaging slice with inverted magnetization flows in. Second, T1 relaxation of the inverted magnetization occurs, so that the M_z of the blood in the imaging slice during mid diastole is nulled. Next, at mid diastole, a fast spin-echo sequence (Figure 1.15) is used to acquire image data. Here, a 90° slice-selective excitation pulse creates transverse magnetization $\mathbf{M}_{xy}$ from M_z. Then, a train of 180° slice-selective refocusing pulses creates a train of spin echoes. Each spin echo has a different phase-encoding value, so that multiple lines of **k**-space, typically 16–32 lines, are acquired per heart beat. Using a TR of 2 RR intervals, a complete image can be acquired during a 16-heartbeat breath-hold scan. An example demonstrating high-resolution imaging of cardiac anatomy from a breath-hold black-blood fast spin-echo acquisition is shown in Figure 1.14b.

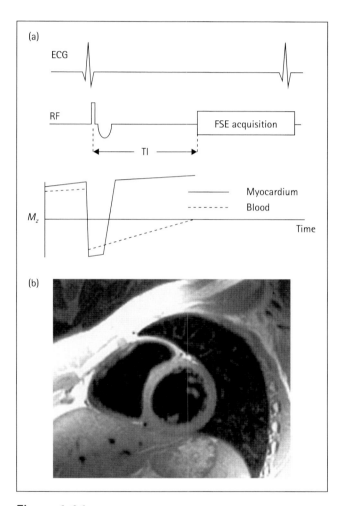

Figure 1.14
Schematic diagram for black-blood fast spin-echo imaging (a). Following an ECG trigger, a double inversion recovery (IR) RF pulse set is played out. The first IR pulse is nonselective, and inverts M_z throughout the body. The second IR pulse is slice-selective, and restores the initial M_z in the imaging slice but leaves M_z outside the imaging slice inverted. As the cardiac cycle proceeds to mid diastole, blood from outside the imaging slice enters the imaging slice. Also, the M_z of this blood relaxes to a null point. In mid diastole, after the inversion time TI, a fast spin-echo (FSE) sequence is used to image the heart. Blood appears black in the image because M_z is nulled when the RF excitation pulse of the FSE sequence is applied. An example of a short-axis black-blood fast spin echo is shown in (b).

Steady-state free precession (SSFP) imaging

Conventional gradient-echo imaging uses RF excitation pulses to create transverse magnetization from longitudinal magnetization, then samples the signal generated by precessing transverse magnetization while a gradient echo is formed. After data sampling, a gradient pulse is applied to cause phase incoherence of the transverse magnetization before the sequence is repeated. Use of such a gradi-

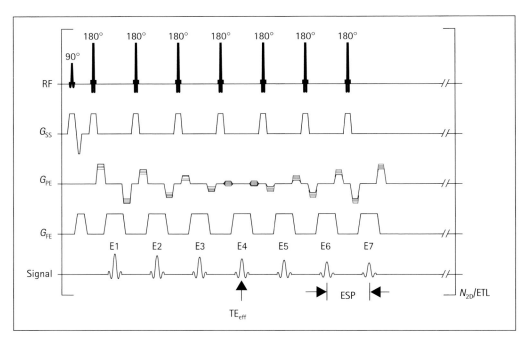

Figure 1.15
Timing diagram for a fast spin-echo pulse sequence. A 90° RF pulse and a simultaneously applied gradient pulse G_{SS} are used for slice-selective excitation. A series of 180° refocusing pulses with slice-select gradient pulses are used to refocus a train of spin echoes. Each echo has a unique phase-encoding value. The number of echoes per repetition, in this case 7, is called the echo train length (ETL). The time between successive echoes is called the echo spacing (ESP). The effective echo time TE_{eff} is the time from the center of the 90° RF excitation pulse to the echo with the minimum amount of phase encoding.

ent (in conjunction with proper adjustment of the phase of the RF pulses) is commonly called 'spoiling' the transverse magnetization.[10] Using this approach, the image signal and contrast in conventional gradient-echo imaging are essentially determined by the longitudinal magnetization. However, with the advent of state-of-the-art gradient hardware capable of fast slew rates and high gradient strengths, a technique that recycles, rather than spoils, the transverse magnetization can be used to achieve higher SNR and improved image contrast in the heart. This technique is usually called steady-state free precession (SSFP) imaging, but is also referred to as fast imaging with steady precession (FISP).[7]

To recycle transverse magnetization from sequence repetition to repetition without incurring image artifacts, the amount of phase accrued by the transverse magnetization during the time TR must be small. In practice, this is achieved by balancing the gradient pulses during each pulse sequence repetition to zero the gradient-induced phase accumulation and by using TR values of around 4 ms or less to minimize phase accumulation due to static magnetic field inhomogeneity (Figure 1.16). Under these conditions, and by applying higher RF pulse flip angles and RF phase cycling, cine images with a rather unique T2/T1-weighted image contrast are produced (Figure 1.16b). An additional property of balanced SSFP imaging is that these sequences are inherently insensitive to in-plane flow. Blood appears very bright in SSFP images because T2/T1 is large and because blood inflow occurs. Myocardium appears relatively dark on SSFP because T2/T1 is small. These signal properties combined with the short TR values lead to images with high blood–myocardium contrast in short acquisition times.

Segmented **k**-space imaging

Because the time to acquire most MR images is greater than a fraction of the cardiac cycle, image blurring due to cardiac motion is typically avoided by employing ECG gating and a technique called **k**-*space segmentation*. Specifically, R-wave detection of the ECG is used to define the cardiac cycle, and different segments of the image raw data (**k**-space data) are acquired in successive heartbeats. Blurring due to myocardial motion is avoided by acquiring the different segments at the same cardiac phase within successive heartbeats. Additional image artifacts due to respiratory motion are typically eliminated by acquiring data during suspended respiration. Accordingly, many cardiac MRI pulse sequences are designed to acquire ECG-gated images within a 10–20 s breathhold duration.

The segmented **k**-space method is used in many cardiac MRI pulse sequences, including black-blood fast spin-

(a)

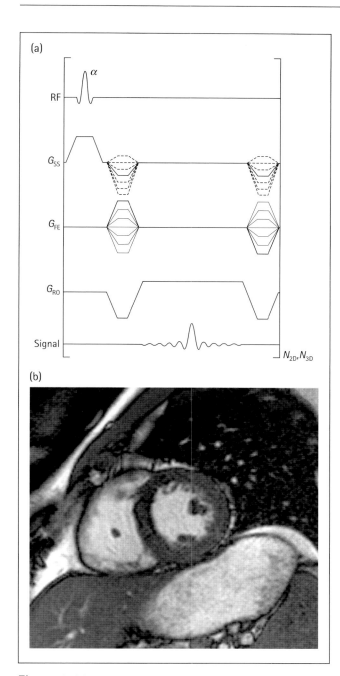

(b)

Figure 1.16
Timing diagram for steady-state free precession (SSFP) imaging (a). With the gradient systems available in state-of-the-art MRI scanners, TR times of less than 4–5 ms can be achieved for SSFP sequences. Using these TRs and balanced gradient waveforms, the amount of phase accumulated by the transverse magnetization during the time TR can be minimized, and this magnetization can therefore be recycled rather than spoiled, leading to higher signal-to-noise ratio and image contrast, and shorter scan times. Either 2D or 3D images can be acquired. An example of a 2D short-axis SSFP image of the heart is shown in (b).

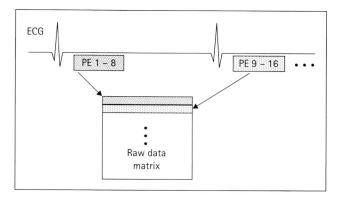

Figure 1.17
Segmented k-space acquisition. In an ECG-gated scan, data acquisition for a single image may be segmented across multiple heartbeats. This is typically done so that all k-space data for an image is temporally localized to a specific part of the cardiac cycle. In successive heartbeats of the acquisition, different segments of the k-space data are acquired. The total number of heartbeats per acquisition is the number of k-space lines per image divided by the number of lines per segment.

echo, gradient-echo cine, and SSFP cine. A diagram illustrating an example of k-space segmentation is shown in Figure 1.17, where the number of phase-encoding lines acquired per image per heartbeat is 8. If the total number of phase-encoding lines required per image is 128, then 16 heartbeats would be needed to acquire data for a complete image. If the TR for each sequence repetition was 5 ms, the nominal temporal resolution of each image would be 40 ms (8 ×5 ms). Synchronization of the pulse sequence to the ECG signal is used to determine the cardiac phase.

Signal-to-noise ratio, spatial resolution, and temporal resolution

In addition to detecting the MRI signal, receiver coils also pick up noise. The noise, which is of thermal origin, comes from fluctuating magnetic fields resulting from Brownian motion of electrons in the body and in the coil itself. The signal-to-noise ratio (SNR) is one of the fundamental measures of image quality. Images of a phantom illustrating relatively low and high SNR are shown in Figure 1.18. In this section, we review the factors that affect SNR in MR images, including spatial resolution and image acquisition time. In addition, we discuss the competing tradeoffs between SNR, image acquisition time, spatial resolution, and temporal resolution that are commonly encountered in cardiac MRI.

Factors that affect the SNR can be divided into those that affect signal and those that affect noise. Because the

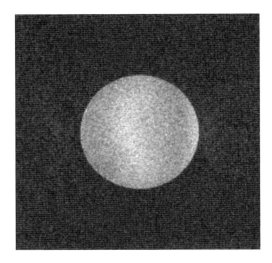 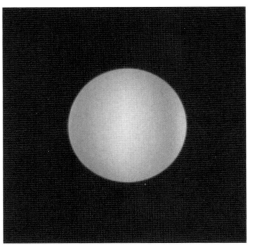

Figure 1.18
Signal-to-noise ratio (SNR). The SNR is one of the fundamental measures of image quality. Example images of a water-filled phantom with relatively low and high SNR are shown in (a) and (b), respectively. The images were acquired using 1 (a) and 32 (b) signal averages.

signal amplitude is directly proportional to the number of hydrogen atoms present, it is proportional to the image voxel size (determined by slice thickness and in-plane resolution). Additionally, the signal level is determined in a more complex way by other pulse sequence parameters such as timing (i.e. TE, TR, etc.) that affect the signal level at the readout time. The signal is also proportional to the number of averages, i.e. the number of times that each line of raw data is acquired. Factors that affect the noise include the number of averages and the time spent sampling each line of raw data. Specifically, the noise is inversely proportional to the square root of the number of signal averages and the data sampling time. The following equation summarizes the basic relationship between SNR and imaging parameters that can be readily adjusted:

$$SNR \propto \Delta x \Delta y \Delta z \sqrt{averages \times data\ sampling\ time}\ f(TE, TR, TI, etc.)$$

This equation has several important implications that can be illustrated by an example. Consider a case where we wish to improve the spatial resolution by a factor of 2, say by halving the slice thickness. The above equation indicates that this 2-fold increase in spatial resolution leads to a decrease in SNR by a factor of 2. To counter the SNR loss, the imaging time could be increased by performing more signal averaging. Since the relationship between SNR and signal averaging goes as the square root, the number of averages would need to increase by a factor of 4 in this example to exactly counter the signal loss. The increased number of averages could be achieved by increasing the total scan time. Alternatively, in a segmented **k**-space scan, the total scan time could be held constant and the temporal resolution of an image could be decreased by a factor of 4. This example and the SNR equation, more generally, describe the very practical tradeoffs that are commonly made between spatial resolution, SNR, scan time, and temporal resolution.

Other factors, such as the main field strength of the magnet, B_0, and the use of surface coils, also have a significant impact on the SNR. The signal is proportional to the square of B_0 and the noise is linearly proportional to B_0, so that the SNR is linearly proportional to B_0. Currently, the great majority of cardiac MRI is performed at a field strength of 1.5 T. However, considerable interest has recently been growing in cardiac MRI at 3 T. Also, it is important to use surface coil arrays to increase SNR in cardiac MRI. Most manufacturers supply 4- to 8-channel surface coil arrays, which typically lead to a 3- to 6-fold increase in SNR compared with receiving signal using the body coil of the MRI scanner.[11]

Summary of MRI terms introduced

MRI, NMR, spin, magnetic moment, gyroscope, Larmor precession frequency, applied magnetic field $\mathbf{B}_0$, spin $\frac{1}{2}$, low-energy parallel state, high-energy antiparallel state, radiofrequency RF, RF pulse $\mathbf{B}_1(t)$, Gd-DTPA, net magnetization M_z, equilibrium magnetization M_0, transverse magnetization $\mathbf{M}_{xy}$, 90° pulse, 180° pulse, T1, T2, T2*, longitudinal axis, transverse plane, magnetization transfer, chemical shift, chemical shift artifact, magnetic field gradient, frequency encoding, phase encoding, spatial frequency, Fourier transform.

Acknowledgement

The authors gratefully acknowledge the contribution of pulse sequence timing diagram figures by John P Mugler III, PhD and other figures by Jaime Mata, MS.

References

1. Wolff SD, Balaban RS. Magnetization transfer contrast (MTC) and tissue water proton relaxation in vivo. Magn Reson Med 1989; 10:135–44.

2. Simonetti OP, Kim RJ, Fieno DS, et al. An improved MR imaging technique for the visualization of myocardial infarction. Radiology 2001; 218:215–23.

3. Hardy CJ, Bolster BD Jr, McVeigh ER, et al. Pencil excitation with interleaved fourier velocity encoding: NMR measurement of aortic distensibility. Magn Reson Med 1996; 35:814–19.

4. Kerr AB, Pauly JM, Hu BS, et al. Real-time interactive MRI on a conventional scanner. Magn Reson Med 1997; 38:355–67 [Erratum 1998; 40:952–5].

5. Meyer CH, Hu BS, Nishimura DG, Macovski A. Fast spiral coronary artery imaging. Magn Reson Med 1992; 28:202–13.

6. Atkinson DJ, Edelman RR. Cineangiography of the heart in a single breath hold with a segmented turboFLASH sequence. Radiology 1991; 178:357–60.

7. Carr JC, Simonetti O, Bundy J, et al. Cine MR angiography of the heart with segmented true fast imaging with steady-state precession. Radiology 2001; 219:828–34.

8. Reeder SB, Faranesh AZ, Boxerman JL, McVeigh ER. In vivo measurement of T2* and field inhomogeneity maps in the human heart at 1.5 T. Magn Reson Med 1998; 39:988–98.

9. Simonetti OP, Finn JP, White RD, et al. 'Black blood' T2-weighted inversion-recovery MR imaging of the heart. Radiology 1996; 199:49–57.

10. Zur Y, Wood ML, Neuringer LJ. Spoiling of transverse magnetization in steady-state sequences. Magn Reson Med 1991; 21:251–63.

11. Bottomley PA, Lugo Olivieri CH, Giaquinto R. What is the optimum phased array coil design for cardiac and torso magnetic resonance? Magn Reson Med 1997; 37:591–9.

2

MR contrast agent basics

Robert M Weisskoff, Peter Caravan

Introduction

Approximately 25–30% of all magnetic resonance imaging (MRI) scans today use some kind of non-specific gadolinium (Gd)-based contrast agent, typically in order to make diseased tissues, primarily masses, appear brighter than the surrounding tissue. Cardiovascular applications, including angiography and functional imaging such as perfusion and myocardial viability, while growing quickly, still make up only a small fraction (< 10%) of those studies. In this chapter, we describe the general underlying chemistry and biophysics of contrast agents in clinical cardiovascular imaging. Since other chapters in the book focus on the specific applications of these agent for vascular and cardiac imaging, we focus here on the underlying mechanisms of action of these compounds, as well as some of the subtleties of how these agents behave in vivo.

While there are many kinds of external compounds that have been used to change signal properties in magnetic resonance, including hyperpolarized gases,[1,2] electron paramagnetic contrast agents,[3,4] potential pH-indicating agents,[5,6] magnetization-transfer-affecting agents,[7,8] and 'activatable' agents that change their MR properties based on the presence of enzymes,[9,10] we will focus primarily on agents that are injected into the body and use chelated metals to change the water relaxation properties. (Chapter 3 details the use of these and other technologies for molecular imaging with MRI.) The chelated, small-molecule Gd-based agents form the vast majority of 'MR contrast agents' clinically in use today and in the foreseeable future, and thus will form the bulk of the content of this chapter.

This chapter is organized in two broad sections. In the first, we summarize the general terminology used to describe contrast agents, and give an overview of MR contrast agents that are currently in routine clinical practice or being pursued commercially. The goal of this first section is to provide a working vocabulary about contrast agents for those working in cardiovascular MRI (CMR).

In the second section, we go into greater depth about both the chemistry and the biophysics of these agents, and about the physical and biological factors that affect their behavior in vivo. The goal of this second section is to give a broader summary of the current understanding of the underlying mechanisms, and point to some of the more recent literature in this area.

MR contrast agents: introduction

In this section, we outline the general terminology used to describe and characterize contrast agents in MRI. We characterize how the agents change the fundamental contrast on MR images by changing T1 and T2. Using this vocabulary, we then give a broad summary of the agents used in current clinical practice, as well as a number of agents that are under development in both commercial and academic settings.

Introduction to MRI biophysics

In this section, we describe the general vocabulary of contrast agents. This section assumes that the reader has a basic understanding of MRI vocabulary (see Chapter 1). Contrast agents shorten T1 and T2. While there are many mechanisms by which this occurs, and considerable chemistry, physical chemistry, and biophysics that can be applied to understand or predict these mechanisms, in many cases the effect of these mechanisms can be reduced to a single constant, called 'relaxivity'. The effect and definition of relaxivity is illustrated in Figure 2.1.

In Figure 2.1a, the effect of a typical contrast agent is shown on two hypothetical tissues, one with a T1 of 1200 ms (approximately that of heart muscle at 1.5 T),

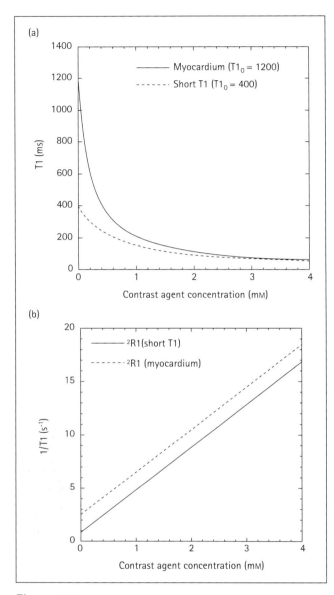

Figure 2.1
Change in (a) longitudinal relaxation time (T1) and (b) longitudinal relaxation rate (1/T1) for typical myocardial tissue (solid line, T1 = 1200 ms at 1.5 T and 37°C) and short T1 tissue (dashed line, T1 = 400 ms).

increase the rate of relaxation proportional to the amount of contrast agent:

$$\frac{1}{T1} = \frac{1}{T1_0} + r_1 C, \qquad (1)$$

where T1 is the observed T1 with contrast agent in the tissue, $T1_0$ is the T1 prior to addition of the contrast agent, C is the concentration of contrast agent, and r_1 is the molar longitudinal relaxivity (often just called the relaxivity). The conventional units of r_1 are $s^{-1}\,\mathrm{mM}^{-1}$. Thus the slope of 1/T1 as a function of contrast agent concentration (Figure 2.1b) reveals the relaxivity, in this case $4\,s^{-1}\,\mathrm{mM}^{-1}$. Figure 2.1b shows that the effect on relaxation rate is independent of the initial T1 of the tissue. That is, in terms of relaxation rate, the contrast agent has the same effect regardless of initial T1.

Transverse, or T2, relaxivity is defined in an analogous way:

$$\frac{1}{T2} = \frac{1}{T2_0} + r_2 C. \qquad (2)$$

For all medically used contrast agents, $r_2 > r_1$. As will be discussed in the section below on relaxation theory, r_1 and r_2 both depend on magnetic field strength and, temperature, and, with several exotic contrast agents, can be made to depend on pH, oxygenation, or even the presence of enzymes.

Effect on pulse sequence: Can there be too much of a good thing?

As will be discussed in greater detail in the section below on relaxation biophysics, contrast agent behavior in vivo is seldom as simple as the pure linear effect relaxation rate shown in Figure 2.1. However, even in the simple case of pure linear relaxation, the effect of the contrast agent on MR image is generally nonlinear. There are two sources of these nonlinearities in traditional spin-echo sequences: (a) T1 saturation and (b) T2 signal loss. Once the contrast agent forces T1 below about TR/2, increasing the contrast agent concentration will have little effect on increasing the available longitudinal magnetization because the tissue will have nearly fully recovered the magnetization before the next RF pulse. Furthermore, because contrast agents affect both T1 and T2 relaxation, at high enough concentration the contrast agent will reduce T2 to the order of TE, and thus increasing the contrast agent concentration will actually decrease MR image intensity.

These two effects are demonstrated for myocardial tissue in Figure 2.2 for both T1- and T2-weighted

and one with T1 = 400 ms. At low concentrations of contrast agent (left side of the graph), it appears that the contrast agent has a larger effect on the tissue with the longer T1. At higher concentrations of contrast agent (right side of Figure 2.1a), both tissues approach approximately the same T1. The simple way to quantify this effect is to consider the rate of relaxation, 1/T1. In the simplest cases, which characterize most cases found in medical imaging, the effect of the contrast agent is to

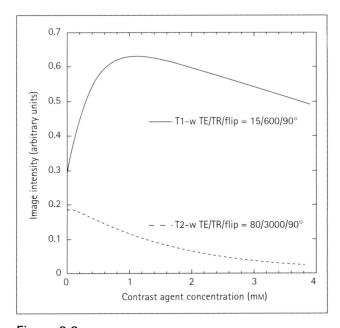

Figure 2.2
Effect of contrast agent on myocardial image intensity on T1-weighted and T2-weighted spin-echo scans. T1 weighting (TR = 600 ms) assumes a patient with a 100 BPM heart rate, and shows a linear increase in signal only for contrast agent concentration less than 0.5 mM. T2-weighted images (TR = 3 s) show only T2 signal loss effects due to contrast agent with no T1 enhancement, due to the long echo time of the T2-weighted sequence.

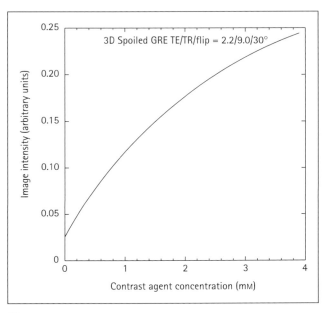

Figure 2.3
Effect of contrast agent on myocardial image intensity using a typical short-TR fast spoiled gradient-echo sequence. Because of the very short TE and short TR, monotonically increased image intensity is typical across the entire range on contrast agent concentrations typically found in clinical scans. (Compare Figure 2.2.)

sequences (myocardium was used for the solid curves in Figure 2.1). For the T1-weighted sequence (T1-w), TE/TR = 15/600 was used. In Figure 2.2, signal intensity begins to level out at a contrast agent concentration between 0.5 and 1.0 mM; on Figure 2.1a, this indeed is the range where the T1 of the myocardium has dropped to around 300 ms, or TR/2. At concentrations above 1 mM, the T1 effect is saturated, and the only *imaging* effect of the contrast agent is to make T2 shorter, and thus cause signal loss even on this T1-weighted sequence. Signal is lost because even a T1-weighted sequence has a finite TE, and thus T2 effects can creep in when T2 is short enough.

The signal intensity plateau on the T2-weighted scan (TE/TR = 80/3000: 'T2-w' in Figure 2.2) occurs at much lower contrast agent concentration, and, due to the long TR, the only real effect of the contrast agent is to reduce (rather than increase) signal intensity on this T2-weighted scan. However, this negative contrast can also be medically useful, and certain contrast agents (notably the iron oxide particles) create negative contrast exactly by providing enhanced T2 relaxation, and thus darker images on T2-weighted scans.

Although they are used somewhat less frequently in cardiac imaging, fast T1-weighted gradient-echo

sequences and especially 3D sequences typically have more linear image intensity enhancement as a function of contrast agent concentration. For example, the effect of contrast agent on the myocardium in a typical fast 3D spoiled gradient-echo sequence, TE/TR/flip = 2.2/9.0/30°, is graphed in Figure 2.3. Although image intensity grows more slowly than linearly at high concentration, at least it continues to grow even at high concentration.

Contrast agent zoology
Commercial contrast agents and those in development

Contrast agents evolved with the field of MRI, stemming from Lauturbur's use of manganese chloride in dogs in 1978.[11] Clinical trials for Gd-DTPA (gadopenetate, Magnevist) began in 1983,[12] shortly after the introduction of clinical MRI, and culminated in 1988 with Gd-DTPA becoming the first approved MRI contrast agent. As of March 2003, ten contrast agents have been approved for human use (Table 2.1). In addition, there are several oral contrast agents for gastrointestinal imaging that will not be discussed here.[13,14] The first generation of commercial contrast agents were the extracellular fluid agents (ECF

Table 2.1 Approved (March 2003) MR contrast agents: relaxivity, osmolality and viscosity (relevant references shown as superscripts)

Generic name	Product name	Chemical abbreviation	r_1, 0.5 T, 37°C (s^{-1} mM^{-1})	r_2, 0.5 T, 37°C (s^{-1} mM^{-1})	Osmolality[a] (osmol/kg)	Viscosity[a] (cP)
Gadopenetate	Magnevist	Gd-DTPA	3.8[91]		1.96[92]	2.9[92]
Gadoterate	Dotarem	Gd-DOTA	3.6[93]	4.8[93]	1.35[94] (4.02)[94]	2.0[94] (11.3)[94]
Gadodiamide	Omniscan	Gd-DTPA-BMA	3.9[94]		0.79[92] (1.90)[94]	1.4[92] (3.9)[94]
Gadoteridol	ProHance	Gd-HPDO3A	3.7[94]		0.63[94] (1.91)[94]	1.3[94] (3.9)[94]
Gadobutrol	Gadovist	Gd-DO3A-butrol	3.6[91]		0.57[91] (1.39)[92]	1.4[91] (3.7)[92]
Gadoversetamide	OptiMARK	Gd-DTPA-BMEA	4.7[95]		1.11[96]	2.0[96]
Gadobenate	MultiHance	Gd-BOPTA	4.4[97]	5.6[97]	1.97[98]	5.3[98]
Mangafodipir	Teslascan	Mn-DPDP	1.9[99]	2.2[99]	0.29[100]	0.7[100]
Ferumoxide	Feridex IV Endorem	AMI-25	24[57]	107[57]	0.2[101]	0.34[101]
Furucarbotran	Resovist	SHU555a	20[102]	190[102]	0.33[103]	1.0[103]

[a] All concentrations 0.5 M except for those in parentheses (1 M), Mn-DPDP (0.01 M), and AMI-25 (0.2 M).

agents),[15] followed by compounds designed for liver imaging.[16,17] Currently, there are several blood pool agents – that is, agents with longer distribution phase that remain in the blood for longer periods than the ECF agents – in clinical trials. At the preclinical stage, there are numerous exciting advancements in 'molecular imaging' agents:[18–20] compounds that detect pH change,[21,22] enzymatic activity,[23,24] and specific biomolecules (such as fibrin[25]) or receptors (such as $\alpha_v\beta_3$[26]). The majority of contrast agents used are Gd-based. Other metals are capable of providing contrast, and iron and manganese have been used in commercially approved agents. For the remainder of this chapter, we will focus only on those agents that are approved or in commercial trials.

Extracellular agents

The approved ECF agents are shown in Figure 2.4. These compounds exhibit three similar features: they all contain Gd, they all contain an 8-coordinate ligand binding to Gd, and they all contain a single water molecule coordination site to Gd. The multidentate ligand is required for safety.[27] It provides high thermodynamic stability and kinetic inertness with respect to metal loss, and enables the contrast agent to be excreted intact. This is important since these contrast agents are much less toxic than their sub-

stituents – that is, than either the chelating ligand or the Gd ion. For example, the DTPA ligand and gadolinium chloride both have LD_{50} of 0.5 mmol/kg in rats, while the Gd-DTPA complex has a safety margin nearly a factor of 20 higher, with LD_{50} of 8 mmol/kg.[15] (LD_{50} is the dose that has a roughly 50% chance to cause death.) As will be described in much greater detail in the section below on relaxation theory, the Gd ion and coordinated water molecule are essential to providing contrast. The high magnetic moment of Gd along with its relatively slow electronic relaxation rate make it an excellent relaxer of water protons. The proximity of the coordinated water molecule leads to efficient relaxation. The coordinated water molecule is in rapid chemical exchange (10^6 exchanges per second) with solvating water molecules.[28] This rapid exchange leads to a catalytic effect whereby the Gd complex effectively shortens the relaxation times of the bulk solution.

As outlined in Table 2.1, the extracellular agents have very similar properties. They are all very hydrophilic complexes with similar relaxivities and excellent safety profiles, and can be formulated at high concentrations. Because of the close similarity in their pharmacological behavior, MRI medical usage often just refers to these compounds as 'gadolinium'. An injection of any of these agents (with rare exceptions[29]) yields the same diagnostic information.

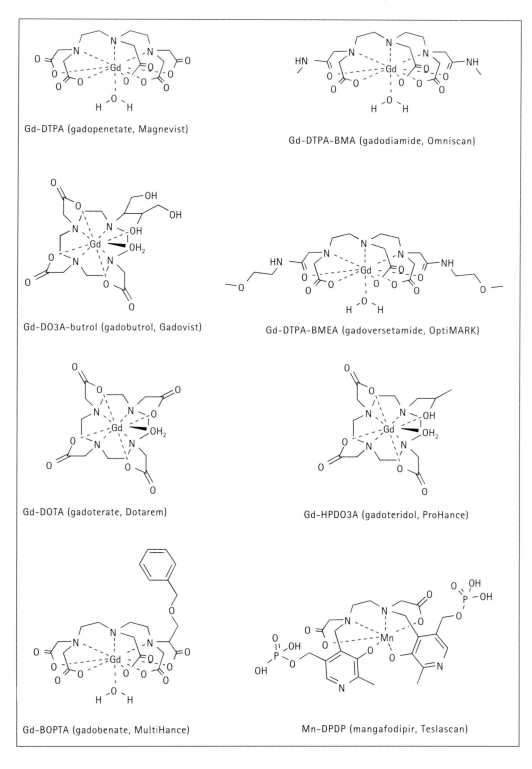

Figure 2.4
Structures of approved Gd- and Mn-based contrast agents.

Gd-DTPA (gadopenetate, Magnevist)

Gd-DTPA-BMA (gadodiamide, Omniscan)

Gd-DO3A-butrol (gadobutrol, Gadovist)

Gd-DTPA-BMEA (gadoversetamide, OptiMARK)

Gd-DOTA (gadoterate, Dotarem)

Gd-HPDO3A (gadoteridol, ProHance)

Gd-BOPTA (gadobenate, MultiHance)

Mn-DPDP (mangafodipir, Teslascan)

There are some differences among the physical properties. The diamide complexes have considerably lower thermodynamic stability (log $K \sim 17$ versus > 21 for other Gd complexes),[30,31] although this does not seem to affect their safety profile relative to the other agents. The nonionic (neutral) compounds (gadodiamide, gadoteridol, gadoversetamide, and gadobutrol) were designed to minimize the osmolality of the formulation. This was prompted by the distinct reduction in toxicity and side-effects brought on by the development of nonionic X-ray contrast media. However, for MRI, the injection volumes are much smaller than for X-ray, and thus the overall increase in osmolality after injection of an MR contrast agent is insignificant. One benefit of the nonionic compounds is the ability to formulate them at high concentration (1 M)[32] without drastically increasing the osmolality or viscosity (Table 2.1). These high-concentration formulations may be useful in fast dynamic studies such as brain perfusion and dynamic magnetic resonance angiography (MRA).

Liver agents

The ECF agents, like X-ray contrast agents, are cleared almost exclusively renally by glomerular filtration. It was recognized early on that altering the excretion pathway could allow liver imaging. Liver agents include the Gd-based compounds Gd-BOPTA (gadobenate, Multihance)[33,34] and Gd-EOB-DTPA (Eovist) (Figure 2.5),[35] the manganese complex Mn-DPDP (mangafodipir, Teslascan),[36] and the iron particle formulations AMI-25 (FeridexI.V., Endorem),[37] AMI-227 (Combidex, Sinarem),[38] and SHU555a (Resovist).[35] All of these compounds are available clinically, either in Europe and/or the USA, with the exception of Sinerem and Gd-EOB-DTPA, which are in an advanced stage of development. The different metal types have different mechanisms of action. The Gd compounds are taken up by hepatocytes[39] and cleared intact via the hepatobiliary system. The Gd complexes provide positive contrast (T1-weighted) of the hepatobiliary system. Mn-DPDP undergoes partial dissociation in vivo.[40] It is believed that endogenous zinc replaces the manganese ion. The free manganese is absorbed by the pancreas and hepatocytes in the liver and enables T1-weighted imaging of these organs. The iron oxide particles are taken up by the reticuloendothelial system and accumulate in the Kupffer cells in the liver.[38] As a result, even though these iron oxide agents generally create 'dark' signal, they create positive contrast for liver tumors, by leaving undiminished the signal from tumors that have a paucity of Kupffer cells. These iron agents are so-called superparamagnetic iron oxides (SPIO). These particles have a much greater effect on T2 and T2* than on T1 (Table 2.1). The SPIO agents are used with T2- or T2*-weighted sequences.

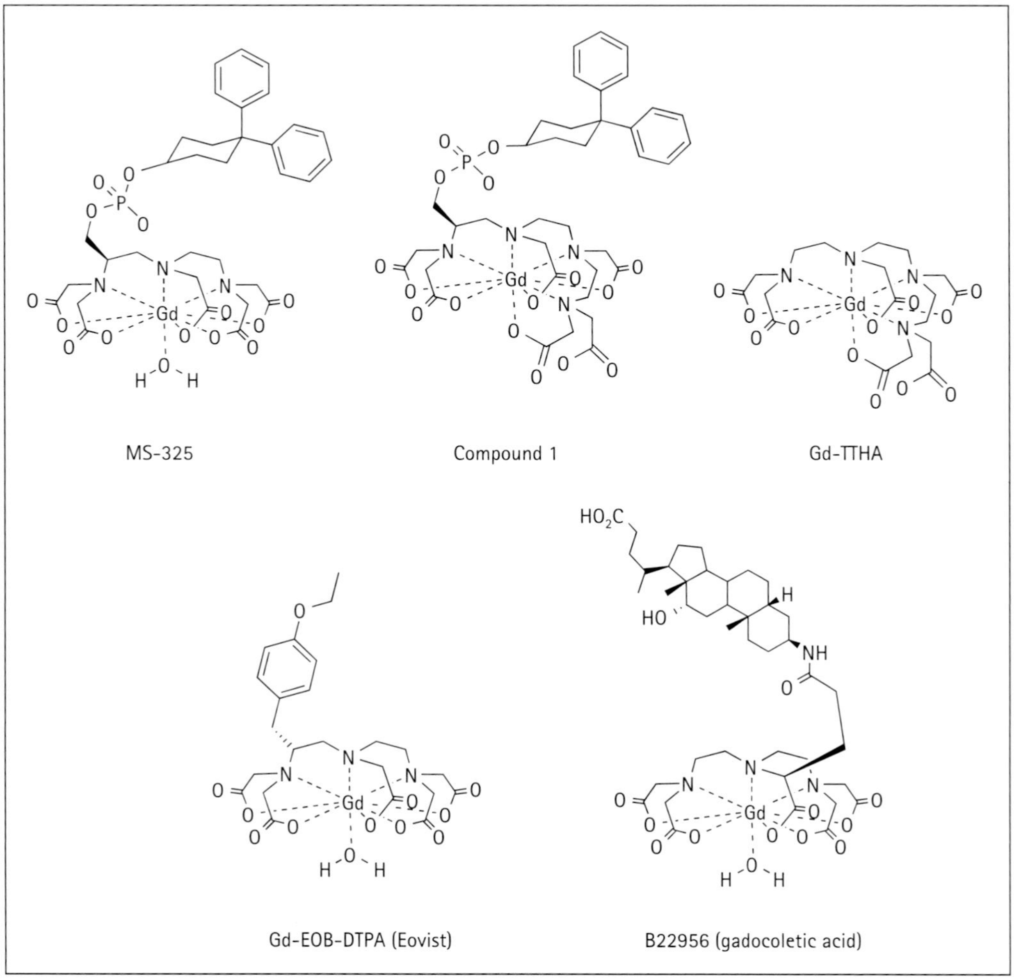

Figure 2.5
Structures of other molecular Gd agents.

MS-325

Compound 1

Gd-TTHA

Gd-EOB-DTPA (Eovist)

B22956 (gadocoletic acid)

Blood pool agents

Since most contrast agents are administered intra-venously, they are all potentially capable of imaging the blood vessels, and indeed the ECF agents described above are used routinely, if off-label, for angiography (see Chapter 15). The major drawback of the ECF agents for MRA is their pharmacokinetics. ECF agents rapidly leak out of the vascular space into all the interstitial spaces of the body. Angiography with ECF agents is thus typically limited to dynamic arterial studies. There has been considerable effort toward designing specific blood pool agents that would be tailored for vascular imaging. The ideal blood pool agent should remain in the vascular compartment and not leak out into the extracellular space. It should be capable of being given as a bolus such that a dynamic arterial image can be obtained. At the same time, it should have sufficient relaxivity and blood half-life that it is possible to obtain high-resolution steady-state images. As of March 2003, there are no approved blood pool agents. However, there are several in various stages of clinical development. Three approaches have been taken to design blood pool agents: protein binding, increased size, and ultrasmall iron oxide particles. These are discussed below.

MS-325[41] and B22956[42,43] are Gd-based compounds (Figure 2.5) that bind reversibly to serum albumin. Albumin is the most abundant protein in plasma, and its concentration is sufficiently high (600–700 μM) to bind enough contrast agent to have significant effects on blood T1. Reversible albumin binding serves four purposes: (1) the albumin slows the leakage of the contrast agent out of the intravascular space; (2) the reversible binding still allows a path for excretion – the unbound fraction can be filtered through the kidneys or taken up by hepatocytes; (3) the bound fraction is 'hidden' from the liver and kidneys, leading to an extended plasma half-life; and (4) the relaxivity of the contrast agent is increased 4- to 10-fold upon binding to albumin (see below). (Gd-BOPTA and Gd-EOB-DTPA have weak affinity for albumin

(~10% bound), which leads to a modest relaxivity increase relative to the ECF agents.)

The binding and relaxivity features of the Gd-based blood pool agents are listed in Table 2.2. Since binding affinity is moderate to weak for these compounds, the fraction bound to albumin will depend on the concentrations of albumin and the contrast agent. Immediately following injection, when the concentration of the contrast agent is high relative to albumin, there will be a greater free fraction. As the concentration of the contrast agent begins to stabilize (at ~0.5 mM), the fraction bound will become constant. The observed relaxivity will depend on the fraction bound; unlike ECF agents, T1 change in plasma is not linearly related to contrast agent concentration. Among the albumin-binding agents, MS-325 has a somewhat lower albumin affinity than B22956, although the majority of both are bound under steady-state conditions. The relaxivity of albumin-bound MS-325 is higher than that of B22956. MS-325 is cleared mainly renally excreted, while B22956 has significant biliary clearance as well as renal excretion.

Early work on blood pool compounds involved Gd covalently linked to macromolecules such as polylysine, dextran, or modified bovine serum albumin.[27] The large size of these compounds severely restricted diffusion out of the vascular space and led to very good vascular imaging properties. One major drawback was the very slow clearance of these agents in preclinical studies, as well as potential immunological response. This approach was modified by the synthesis of compounds that were large enough to be kept in the vascular compartment, but small enough to still be eliminated by glomerular filtration in the kidneys. Gadomer-17 (Figure 2.6) is an example of this type of blood pool agent.[44,45] Gadomer-17 is a large dendrimer (acting with the hydrodynamic properties of a ~17 kDa dendrimer) that contains 24 Gd complexes covalently linked. The dendritic (branching) approach to synthesis results in a compound that is approximately globular. The per-Gd relaxivity of Gadomer-17 is much

Table 2.2 Albumin binding and observed relaxivities (20 MHz) of MS-325, B22956, Gd-BOPTA, Gadomer-17, and P792 at 37°C (relevant references shown as subscripts)

	MS-325[a]	B22956[b]	Gd-BOPTA	Gadomer-17[c]	P792[d]
Agent type	Strong protein-binding	Strong protein-binding	Weak protein-binding	Increased size	Increased size
r_1 buffer (mM^{-1} s^{-1})	6.6[104]	6.5[43]	4.4[97]		39[105]
r_1 plasma (mM^{-1} s^{-1})	50[104]	27[43]	9.7[106]	18.7[107]	44.5[105]
% bound plasma	91[104]	95[43]			

[a] Data at 0.1 mM. [b] Data at 0.5 mM. [c] Relaxivity per Gd. [d] 4% HSA.

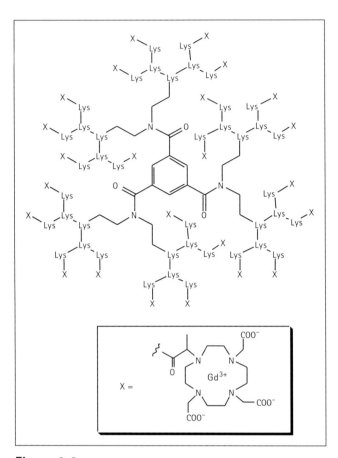

Figure 2.6
Structure of Gadomer-17.

higher than that of its monomeric units because of the slow tumbling of the molecule (see below). Using multiple Gd chelates to increase the size also increases the molecular relaxivity (24 Gd × 18.7 = molecular relaxivity of 450 s^{-1} mM^{-1}), which in turn means that lower doses can be given. Gadomer-17 is a neutral hydrophilic compound that has little affinity for plasma proteins. It appears to be excreted renally.

Another blood pool agent in clinical trials is P792 from Guerbet (Figure 2.7).[46,47] P792 can be viewed as a modified Gd-DOTA, where each acetate arm contains a large hydrophilic group. Increasing the molecular weight also increases the relaxivity, which (like the bound albumin or Gadomer-17) means that lower doses of Gd – compared with ECF agents – can be given to obtain comparable contrast. P792 has little affinity for plasma proteins and has predominantly renal clearance.

It should be noted that none of the Gd-based vascular agents described above is a 'true' blood pool compound. Although far superior to the ECF agents in terms of extravasation and relaxivity, there is still some fraction of the compound that leaks out into the extracellular space.

Iron oxide particles, on the other hand, are true blood pool agents.

The SPIO particles used for liver imaging are large enough to be recognized by the reticuloendothelial system (RES) and rapidly removed from the bloodstream. It was found that the smallest size fraction of these particles, the so-called ultrasmall iron oxide particles (USPIO), evaded the RES and could be used to image the blood pool.[14] Although smaller, these particles are still too large to passively leak out of the vascular space and make very good blood pool agents. Making ultrasmall particles not only changes the biodistribution of the compound, but also changes the relaxation phenomena. SPIO have a much greater effect on T2 than T1 (large r_2/r_1) and are used as T2 or T2* agents. USPIO have very good T1 relaxation properties (smaller r_2/r_1) and can be used for bright blood imaging (T1-weighted). The iron oxide particles are not excreted; the iron is eventually resorbed into the body. The iron particles in clinical trials are summarized in Table 2.3.

Many other mechanisms of action for contrast agents are being explored that lie beyond the scope of this chapter. Several for molecular-based imaging are described in greater detail in Chapter 27.

MR contrast agents: details

Relaxation theory

The first generation of contrast agents, the ECF agents, have very similar properties – so much so that 'gadolinium' is often used in casual reference to describe the use of any ECF agent in clinical practice. But not all gadolinium is the same. Figure 2.8 shows the field dependence of relaxivity for five contrast agents in 4.5% HSA solution. The ECF agents have superimposable relaxivities, but the newer contrast agents Gd-BOPTA and MS-325 have higher relaxivities and different field dependences. This section will attempt to make clear why contrast agents can differ in relaxivity and why relaxivity indeed depends on magnetic field and temperature.

Unlike nuclear agents or X-ray contrast agents, MRI contrast agents are imaged indirectly, by their effect on water relaxation rates, as described schematically in Equations (1) and (2) above. Since water is present at a very high concentration (55 000 mM) and the contrast agent is typically at much lower concentration (0.1–1 mM), the contrast agent must act catalytically to relax the water protons in order for there to be a measurable effect. Relaxivity, r_1 and r_2, thus describes this catalytic efficiency. In this section, we describe the molecular factors that determine relaxivity.[27,48] For discrete ions such

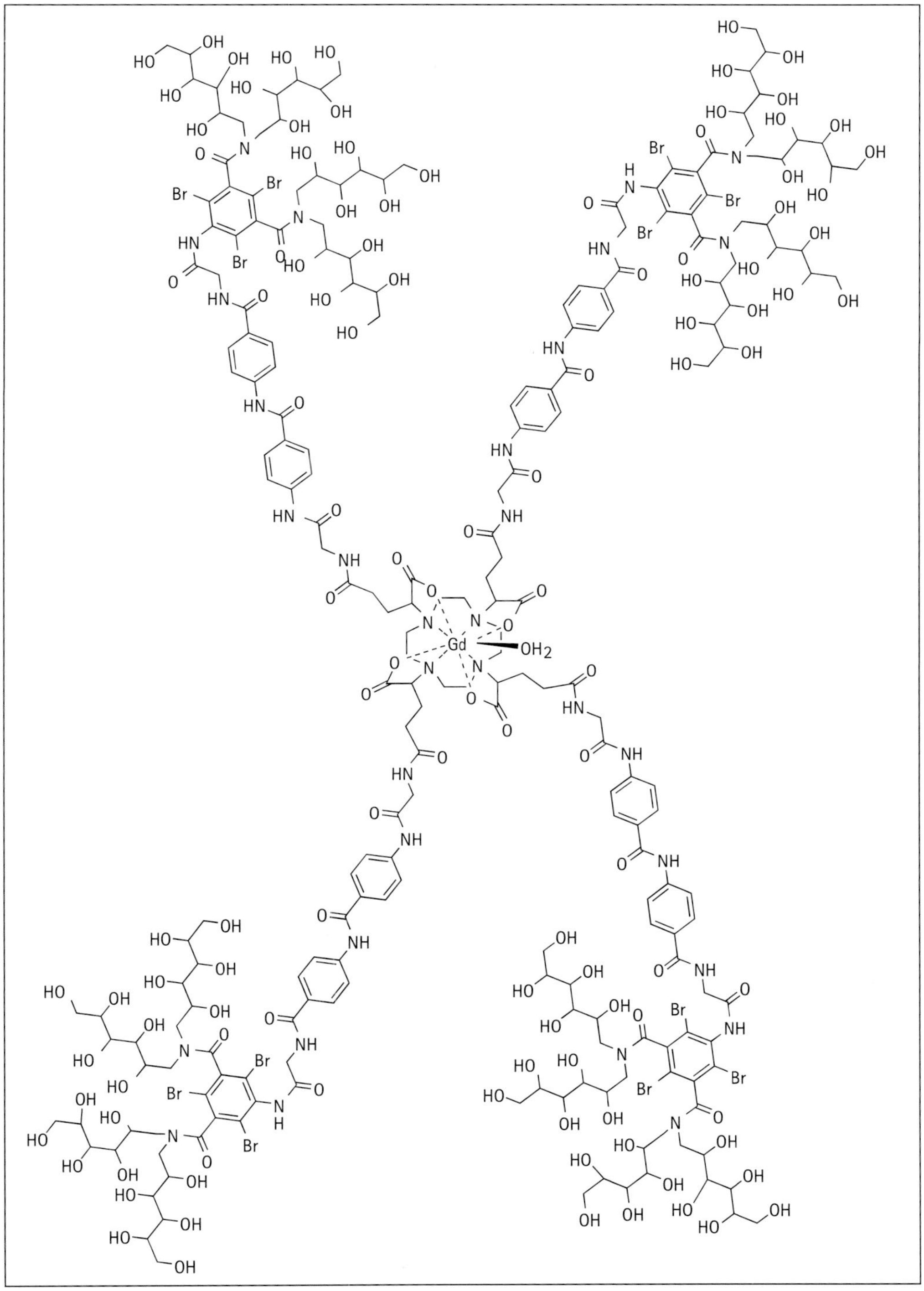

Figure 2.7
Structure of P792.

as Gd(III) and Mn(II), the factors influencing relaxivity are the same; for the iron oxide particles the relaxation mechanism is different and will be treated separately.

Relaxivity is often factored into inner- and outer-sphere. Inner-sphere relaxivity refers to the relaxation enhancement due to the exchangeable water(s) in the inner sphere. Outer-sphere relaxivity is that resulting from waters in the second and outer coordination spheres. This separation is often used because the inner-sphere component is easier to understand from a theoretical framework and because the inner-sphere component can often represent the majority of the overall relaxivity.

$$r_1 = \frac{\Delta(1/T_1)}{[\text{Gd}]} = r_1^{\text{IS}} + r_1^{\text{OS}} \qquad (3)$$

Table 2.3 Iron particle contrast agents: Relaxivities at 20 MHz (37°C) (relevant references shown as superscripts)

Generic name	Product name	Chemical abbreviation	Particle	r_1 $(s^{-1}\,mM^{-1})$	r_2 $(s^{-1}\,mM^{-1})$
Ferumoxide	Feridex IV, Endorem	AMI-25	SPIO	24[57]	107[57]
Furucarbotran	Resovist	SHU555a	SPIO	20[102]	190[102]
Ferumoxtran	Sinerem	AMI-227	USPIO	23[57]	51[57]
	Clariscan	NC100150	USPIO	25[108]	41[108]
		VSOP-C63	USPIO	30[109]	39[109]

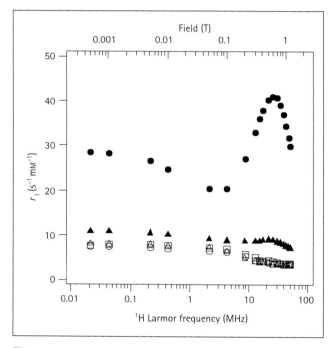

Figure 2.8
Relaxivities r_1 of 0.2 mM contrast agents in 4.5% HSA solution at 35°C, plotted as functions of magnetic field strength: open squares, Gd-DTPA (Magnevist); open circles, Gd-DTPA-BMA (Omniscan); open triangles, Gd-HPDO3A (ProHance); filled triangles, Gd-BOPTA (MultiHance); filled circles, MS-325.

The molecular factors influencing inner-sphere relaxivity are shown in Figure 2.9, which shows a water molecule coordinated to a metal ion M with a spin S. The water H atoms have spin I ($I = \frac{1}{2}$; for H), and the bound water is in equilibrium with the bulk water. To describe the dynamics of water binding and exchange, the average time that the bound water stays coordinated to metal ion is called the residency time τ_m; the residency time is the reciprocal of the water exchange rate, $k_{ex} = 1/\tau_m$. The distance through space between the ion and the proton is denoted by r (not to be confused with the relaxivities r_1 and r_2!). Also important in understanding relaxation are the electronic relaxation time of the metal ion, T_{1e} (sometimes referred to as τ_S), and the rotational correlation time τ_R. The relaxation mechanism is dipolar.

The contrast agent relaxes the water by acting as a local fluctuating magnet. The dipolar relaxation mechanism increases with the square of the magnetic moment μ_{eff}, which is proportional to its spin state, $\mu_{eff} \propto S(S + 1)$. Thus ions with large spin numbers such as Gd^{3+} ($S = \frac{7}{2}$) and Mn^{2+} ($S = \frac{5}{2}$), all other things being equal, produce larger relaxivity effects than ions with low spin numbers, such as Cu^{2+} ($S = \frac{1}{2}$). The size of the magnetic interaction falls off dramatically the farther away the water gets from the metal. This interaction falls off like the sixth power of the distance between the ion and the proton nucleus, and thus relaxation is proportional to $1/r^6$. The gadolinium ion is larger than the manganese ion, so r_{Gd-H} (~3.1 Å) < r_{Mn-H} (~2.9 Å). However, the Gd ion has a larger spin than manganese, which compensates for the longer ion–H distance; that is, $S(S + 1)/r^6$ is larger for Gd^{3+} than for Mn^{2+}.

In order for relaxation to be efficient, the local magnetic field (caused by the contrast agent) should be fluctuating at frequencies close to the proton Larmor frequency. The closer the fluctuating field is to the Larmor frequency, the more efficient will be the energy transfer and relaxation. There are three sources of the fluctuating field: electronic relaxation, rotational diffusion, and chemical exchange. Electronic relaxation is a fast process ($1/T_{1e}$ ranges from 10^5 to 10^{13} s^{-1}). As electrons within the ion traverse electronic states, a fluctuating field is set up. If electronic relaxation is too fast, then there will be little energy transfer to the proton. This has been likened to the incredibly rapid flapping wings of a hummingbird that have almost no effect on a nearby leaf.[27] As an example, the terbium and dysprosium ions Tb^{3+} and Dy^{3+}, which both have magnetic moments even greater than that of Gd^{3+}, are poor relaxation agents because they have too fast electronic relaxation rates. Ions such as Gd^{3+} and Mn^{2+} have symmetric electronic configurations (half-filled f and d shells, respectively), and these tend to have slower electronic relaxation rates.

Rotational diffusion is another source of fluctuation. As the contrast agent tumbles in solution, this too creates a fluctuating field. For spherical compounds, the

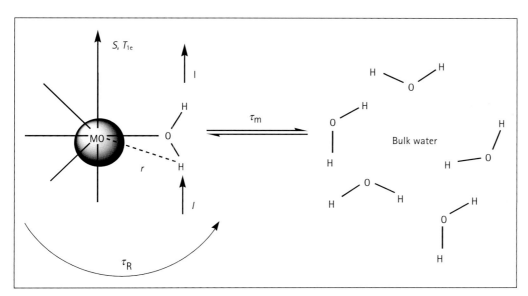

Figure 2.9
Molecular factors affecting relaxation.

rotational rate will increase as the size of the molecule is increased.

Finally, water exchange may also define the fluctuating field. If the water exchange rate is very fast, then this motion of the water drawing close and moving away from the ion will define the fluctuation. The rate of fluctuation is defined by a correlation time τ_c. The fastest rate will determine the correlation time:

$$\frac{1}{\tau_c} = \frac{1}{T_{1e}} + \frac{1}{\tau_R} + \frac{1}{\tau_m}. \quad (4)$$

In addition to its impact on the correlation time, water exchange plays another role in determining relaxivity. Until now, the discussion has involved describing the factors affect the relaxation of the water bound to the metal ion. However, once the coordinated water is relaxed, it must exchange with the bulk in order for the contrast agent to 'catalyze' the relaxation in many other water molecules in order to significantly affect bulk water relaxation. When the rate of water exchange is too slow, ultimately this will limit the contrast agent's relaxivity.

Finally, it is intuitive that if there are more water molecules directly coordinated to the ion, q, the relaxivity should increase proportionally. That is, while all of the agents described in Table 2.1 have only one water molecule coordinated by the ion, it is possible, both in theory and in practice, to have multiple coordination sites available for water.

Combining all of these factors together, inner-sphere relaxivity at a given field strength is described by the following equations:

$$r_1^{IS} = \frac{q/[H_2O]}{T_{1m} + \tau_m}, \quad (5)$$

$$\frac{1}{T_{1m}} = \frac{2}{15}\left(\frac{\mu_0}{4\pi}\right)^2 \hbar^2 \gamma_I^2 \gamma_S^2 \frac{S(S+1)}{r^6}\left[\frac{7\tau_c}{1+\omega_S^2\tau_c^2} + \frac{3\tau_c}{1+\omega_I^2\tau_c^2}\right], \quad (6)$$

where T_{1m} is the relaxation time of the inner-sphere water protons, γ_I and γ_S are the magnetogyric ratios of the proton and electron, respectively, μ_0 is the permeability of the vacuum, and $\hbar$ is Planck's constant divided by 2π. The field dependence in the square brackets in Equation (6) is given by ω_S and ω_I, the electron and proton Larmor frequencies in rad s^{-1}, respectively (the Larmor frequency is related to the external field by $\omega_{S,I} = \gamma_{S,I} B_0$).

The data in Figure 2.8, which show relaxivity as a function of external field strength, are referred to as nuclear magnetic relaxation dispersion (NMRD) profiles. Equations (5) and (6) go a long way to explaining the different NMRD profiles. Dispersion refers to how the relaxation rates disperse as a function of field, and this is a consequence of the Lorentzian functions in the square brackets in Equation (6). As the field (or frequency) is increased, at some point $\omega^2\tau_c^2 > 1$, and when this condition is met, the relaxivity will begin to decrease. Recall that the magnetogyric ratio of an electron is 658 times that of a proton, so the term with ω_S will disperse at lower frequencies than the term with ω_I. For the ECF agents in Figure 2.8, the NMRD shape is sigmoidal. By about 0.2 T (i.e. at all clinical imaging field strengths) the relaxivity is dropping as $\omega_S^2\tau_c^2$ becomes greater than 1. If the measurements were to continue to increasingly higher field strengths, then eventually the $3\tau_c/(1 + \omega_I^2\tau_c^2)$ term would disperse.

One way to increase relaxivity is to increase the correlation time τ_c. This increases the relaxation rate of the bound water ($1/T_{1m}$) and causes the denominator in Equation (5) to become smaller. This was the approach taken with protein-bound molecules (like MS-325, B22956, and, to a lesser extent, Gd-BOPTA) and larger molecular constructs like Gadomer-17 and P792. MS-325 binds to serum albumin and the bound complex thus has a much larger rotational correlation time. This binding increases τ_c and increases the relaxivity. A similar effect is seen for Gd-BOPTA, but since only about 10% of the Gd-BOPTA is bound to HSA, the NMRD curve is a roughly weighted average of the strongly protein-bound dispersion curve and the ECF dispersion curve.

Note, however, that the shape of the MS-325 profile is no longer sigmoidal. This effect arises because electronic relaxation also depends on field strength for gadolinium and manganese ions. At very low field strengths, the electronic relaxation time is constant, but as the field strength increases, the electronic relaxation time T_{1e} gets longer. So at low fields, the correlation time is dominated by electronic relaxation ($\tau_c \sim T_{1e}$), but as the field strength increases, T_{1e} is no longer the shortest correlation time. At higher fields, electronic relaxation is slower than rotation, and thus at high fields $\tau_c \sim \tau_R$. Thus, to understand the MS-325 NMRD profile, it must be considered in four parts. At low fields, the relaxivity does not change with field. At very low fields, the electronic relaxation rate is constant and $\omega_S^2 \tau_c^2 << 1$. As the field strength increases, $\omega_S^2 \tau_c^2 > 1$, and the relaxivity starts to decrease. T_{1e} increases as the field strength increases, so although the term $7\tau_c/(1 + \omega_S^2 \tau_c^2)$ in Equation (6) is approaching zero, the term $\dfrac{3\tau_c}{(1 + \omega_I^2)}$ is increasing and the relaxivity starts increasing at about 0.1 T. At ~1 T, $\omega_I^2 \tau_c^2 > 1$, and relaxivity starts to decline with field.

The field dependence of the transverse relaxivity r_2 is described by the following equations:

$$r_2^{IS} = \frac{q/[H_2O]}{\tau_m}\left[\frac{T_{2m}^{-2} + T_{2m}^{-1}\tau_m^{-1} + \Delta\omega_m^2}{\left(T_{2m}^{-1} + \tau_m^{-1}\right)^2 + \Delta\omega_m^2} \right], \quad (7)$$

$$\frac{1}{T_{2m}} = \frac{2}{15}\left(\frac{\mu_0}{4\pi}\right)^2 h^2\gamma_I^2\gamma_S^2\frac{S(S+1)}{r^6}\left[4\tau_c + \frac{13\tau_c}{1+\omega_S^2\tau_c^2} + \frac{3\tau_c}{1+\omega_I^2\tau_c^2}\right], (8)$$

For transverse relaxation, relaxivity also depends on the chemical shift $\Delta\omega_m$. However, for Gd and Mn complexes, the shift term is negligible and Equation (7) reduces to a dipolar transverse relaxation rate, $1/T_{2m}$:

$$r_2^{IS} = \frac{q/[H_2O]}{T_{1m} + \tau_m}. \quad (9)$$

This is a 'nondispersive' term; that is, a term that does not vanish at highest field strengths. This nondispersive term

has important consequences. For ECF agents where the correlation time is short, the term $\dfrac{3\tau_c}{(1+\omega_I^2\tau_c^2)}$ does not disperse at imaging field strengths and $1/T_{2m} = \dfrac{7}{6}\left(1/T_{1m}\right)$.

This translates directly into relaxivity for ECF agents, where r_2 is 15–20% higher than r_1 at any given frequency. For slowly tumbling complexes (e.g. blood pool agents), the term $\dfrac{3\tau_c}{(1+\omega_I^2\tau_c^2)}$ will begin to disperse at higher field strengths. For r_1, the relaxivity starts to drop at higher fields, but for r_2 the non-dispersive term means that transverse relaxivity stays constant (and there are other mechanisms that actually make it increase with increasing field strength). For slowly tumbling compounds, the ratio r_2/r_1 will thus increase at higher field strengths.

Data from MS-325 show this clearly (Figure 2.10). In the absence of albumin (triangles in Figure 2.10), MS-325 tumbles rapidly at 37°C with $\tau_R \sim 0.1$ ns. The r_1 and r_2 NMRD curves show that r_2 is 15–20% larger than r_1 and that over this magnetic field range (0.1–1.5 T) the relaxivities are relatively constant. In the presence of albumin, however, rotational diffusion is dramatically slowed, $\tau_R \sim 10$ ns. In this case, r_1 and r_2 rise as the correlation time increases with increasing field strength. At ~1 T, $\omega_I^2 \tau_c^2 > 1$

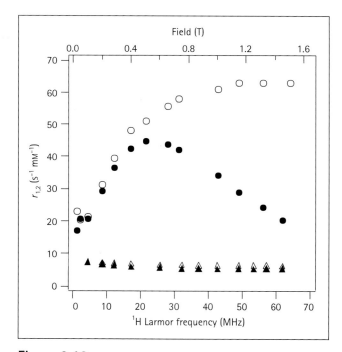

Figure 2.10
Longitudinal (r_1, filled symbols) and transverse (r_2, open symbols) relaxivities of MS-325 (0.1 mM) in the absence (triangles) or presence (circles) of 22.5% HSA at 37°C, as functions of field strength.

and r_1 starts to decline with increasing field strength. But because of the nondisperive $4\tau_c$ term in Equation (8), r_2 does not decrease with increasing field strength.

The above discussion might lead the unwary reader to conclude that r_1 goes to zero (i.e. no T1 relaxivity) at high enough fields. However, that is not the case, since the discussion up to this point has focused only on the inner-sphere term in the relaxivity, Equation (3). However, it is not only the water in the inner-sphere that provides relaxivity, but also the water molecules directly solvating the contrast agent (second-sphere water) and water diffusing nearby (outer-sphere water). These are usually grouped together as 'outer-sphere' relaxivity. The distinction between the two is one of timescales; water in the second sphere may have finite residency times longer than the translational diffusion constant of water, which defines true outer-sphere water. For water in the second sphere, relaxivity will depend on the same parameters that define inner-sphere relaxivity (second-sphere parameters will be denoted with a prime, e.g. q' = number of second-sphere waters). The differences are that there will be a larger number of second-sphere waters ($q' > q$) but the metal–hydrogen distance will be greater. The correlation time that defines second-sphere relaxivity will often be the residency time of the second-sphere water, unlike for inner-sphere relaxivity, where rotation often dominates. Outer-sphere relaxivity depends on the distance of closest approach of the water to the contrast agent and the diffusion constant of water.

The contribution of r_1^{OS} can be significant. For the ECF agents at medical imaging field strengths, about half the relaxivity stems from second- and outer-sphere waters. For ECF agents, the rotational correlation time is quite short, on the order of 50 ps at 37°C. This is similar to the lifetime of waters in the second-coordination sphere and not much longer than the diffusional correlation time. Although the distance from the ion to the second-sphere water protons is greater (recall the relevant magnetic field effects fall off like r^{-6}), there are more waters in the second-sphere than in the inner-sphere.

This effect is illustrated in Figure 2.11, where the NMRD profiles of Gd-DTPA (Figure 2.4), Gd-TTHA, MS-325 and compound (1) (Figure 2.5) are shown, recorded at 25°C and in PBS. Gd-TTHA is an analog of Gd-DTPA but with an additional carboxylate group to bind Gd, and is therefore $q = 0$. MS-325 is an analog of Gd-DTPA, but will have a longer rotational correlation time because it is larger (larger compounds tumble slower). Compound 1 is an analog of Gd-TTHA and MS-325 that was designed to contain no inner-sphere water. Figure 2.11 shows that the 'outer-sphere' (Gd-TTHA) contribution to relaxivity for Gd-DTPA is substantial; about half the relaxivity of Gd-DTPA is due to the outer-sphere water and about half stems from the inner-sphere

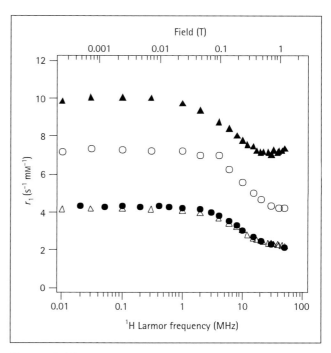

Figure 2.11
Longitudinal relaxivities r_1 of Gd-DTPA (open circles), Gd-TTHA (filled circles), MS-325 (filled triangles), and compound 1 (open triangles) in PBS at 25°C, as functions of field strength.

water. When the large lipophilic phosphodiester group is added to create MS-325 or compound 1, this has the primary effect of increasing the rotational correlation time. Increasing the rotational correlation time should increase the inner-sphere relaxivity, since this correlation time is the shortest for the inner-sphere water. But increasing the rotational correlation time should have little effect on the outer-sphere relaxivity, because the shortest correlation time here is the residency time of the second-sphere waters and the diffusion constant of water; changing the size of the molecule should not impact these parameters. Thus, in Figure 2.11, the relaxivity of MS-325 is increased relative to Gd-DTPA, but the relaxivity of compound 1 is the same as that of Gd-TTHA. The increase in MS-325 relaxivity in PBS is solely due to the inner-sphere water.

Outer-sphere relaxivity can be changed and increased. This is a function of second-sphere hydration. If the lifetime of the second-sphere water is long enough, then increases in the rotational correlation time will also have a positive effect on relaxivity. This has been shown for a $q = 0$ Gd complex bound to albumin, where the relaxivity was 23 s^{-1} mM^{-1} at 25°C.[49]

As improvements in contrast agent design continue to be made, τ_m, the inner-sphere water residency time, has become an increasingly important parameter of interest. For ECF agents, the water exchange rate is sufficiently fast that it does not affect relaxivity at 37°C. In terms of Equation (5), $T_{1m} \gg \tau_m$ in the denominator. When compounds tumble slowly, T_{1m} is decreased, and now the magnitude of τ_m may be important. It was originally thought that water exchange at Gd was exceedingly fast, ~10^9 s^{-1}. This is true for the simple aqua ion of Gd, but Merbach and co-workers[28,50–52] showed that for other Gd complexes, the water exchange rate varies and in general is slower than that of the aqua ion. For instance, at 37°C, the exchange rate at Gd-DTPA is ~10^7 s^{-1}, and that of Gd-DTPA-BMA is ~10^6 s^{-1}. There are other compounds where this rate can be as slow as 10^4 s^{-1} (i.e. a water residency time of 100 μs). The importance of this effect is that, no matter how much improvement is made in shortening T_{1m}, if the water does not exchange rapidly, then the compound will not produce significant relaxation. This is readily seen in the effect of temperature on relaxivity. Cooling the solution will make all processes slower. Lower temperatures will increase the rotational time and decrease T_{1m}. But lower temperatures will also increase the residency time τ_m. Equation (5) predicts that there will be an optimum temperature for relaxivity with a given contrast agent. To illustrate this, Figure 2.12 shows histograms of MS-325 relaxivity in the presence and absence of HSA as a function of temperature. In the absence of protein, cooling the sample increases r_1 because T_{1m} is much greater than τ_m; the benefit gained from shortening T_{1m} is greater than any offset by increasing τ_m. In the presence of protein, the opposite is true. Because MS-325 is bound to albumin, rotation is slow and T_{1m} is already

much shorter. Now the residency time of the inner-sphere water is limiting relaxivity (i.e. $\tau_m > T_{1m}$).

In order to create high-relaxivity compounds, different approaches have been tried. MS-325 and B22956 are small molecules that rely on albumin binding to slow rotation and increase relaxivity. P792 is designed to tumble more slowly by virtue of its size, and this leads to increased relaxivity. Gadomer-17 has higher relaxivity because of reduced tumbling and because there are multiple Gd centers per molecule. Studies done on multimeric Gd complexes suggest that the relaxivity gains per Gd center are additive.[45]

Other notable efforts have been to prepare contrast agents with more than one inner-sphere water ($q > 1$). This approach works well in pure water, but problems appear to occur in biological matrices. By increasing the number of waters, the number of donor atoms from the chelating ligand must be reduced. In most instances, the stability of the compound is affected and it may decompose in vivo and lose its Gd (or Mn). A second problem is that there are numerous endogenous ligands that have affinity for Gd (or Mn). An anion such as phosphate or citrate may bind to the Gd and displace the inner-sphere waters, greatly reducing the relaxivity of the complex. Notable exceptions to these two problems have been found in some compounds from Raymond and co-workers.[53]

Although increasing the molecular weight will increase the rotational correlation time for spherical molecules, this is more complicated for other shapes. For instance, there are several reports of Gd-DTPA linked to polylysine. Although these are high-molecular-weight polymers (50–250 kDa), the relaxivities per Gd are quite modest (10–13 s^{-1} mM^{-1}).[54] These linear polymers tumble very slowly end-over-end, but there are very fast motions along the chains. It is the fast motions that limit relaxivity. More spherical molecules such as dendrimers thus tend to have higher relaxivities. Noncovalent assemblies such as micelles and liposomes have been reported as well. Relaxivities of liposomal systems have been improved by adding excipients to increase the rigidity of the liposome, which serves to limit fast internal motions.[55,56]

A second factor to consider is the water exchange rate. If this is too slow, it may offset gains made from slowing down rotation. Gd-DTPA-BMA is known to have a relatively slow water exchange rate, and it has been shown that the amide functionality often confers slow water exchange properties. This is somewhat unfortunate, since DTPA bis(anhydride) is a very useful commercially available synthon that has been widely used to prepare novel contrast agents. The reaction of DTPA bis(anhydride) with a primary or secondary amine produces either a DTPA amide or a DTPA bis(amide). The Gd complexes of these have slower water exchange rates than Gd-DTPA.[27,48]

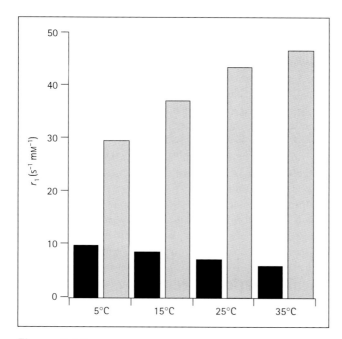

Figure 2.12
Longitudinal relaxivities r_1 of MS-325 in PBS (black bars) or human plasma (gray bars) as functions of temperature.

The iron oxide-based contrast agents have to be treated differently. These are not discrete molecules but crystals of iron oxide (Fe_3O_4) surrounded by a coating (often dextran). For Gd and Mn contrast agents with multiple ions, the relaxivity is additive for the number of ions in the compound; the spins of one Gd ion do not interact with the spins of another ion. For certain materials such as ferrites (iron oxides), the individual spins of each Fe build up cooperatively via quantum mechanical interactions to give the crystal a very large total spin, and thus the relaxivity will be a function of the number of spins. Such materials is called superparamagnetic, to describe their ferromagnetic-like properties, although superparamagnetic materials do not show any of the hysteresis of ferromagnetic materials.

The iron oxide particles consist of a core of one or more magnetic crystals of Fe_3O_4 embedded in a coating. Because these are materials rather than discrete molecules, there is a distribution of sizes. Ultrasmall particles of iron oxide (USPIO) have a single crystal core and a submicron diameter (e.g. ferumoxtran (Sinarem or AMI-227) has a crystal diameter of 4.3–4.9 nm and a global particle diameter of ~50 nm).[57] Small particles of iron oxide (SPIO) have cores containing more than one crystal of Fe_3O_4 and are larger than USPIOs but still submicron (e.g. ferumoxide (Enodrem or AMI-227) has a crystal diameter of 4.3–4.8 nm and a global particle diameter of ~200 nm).[57] USPIO and SPIO are small enough to form a stable suspension, and can be administered intravenously. The differences in their pharmacokinetic behavior have been described above. There are also large particles that are used for oral applications (e.g. Abdoscan, 50 nm crystals making up a 3 μm particle).[14]

There are no inner-sphere water molecules in iron particles, and relaxation of water arises from the water molecules diffusing near the particle. However, the mechanism of outer-sphere relaxation is different than described above. One feature is that the crystals have a net magnetization, and as the external field is increased, this magnetization is increased (this is true as well for Gd, but the effect is much smaller). The modulation of this net magnetization can cause proton relaxation (so-called Curie spin relaxation). Theories describing the field dependence of iron oxide relaxivity have been reported.[14]

There are some generalities about relaxivity in these particles. For the USPIOs, the longitudinal relaxivity r_1 can be quite high, and these can function as effective T1 agents. The ratio r_2/r_1 for USPIOs is significantly larger than for Gd complexes and r_2 increases with increasing magnetic field. When there is aggregation of crystals, which is the case in SPIOs, longitudinal relaxivity tends to decrease (r_1 drops) and transverse relaxivity increase (r_2 increases). Thus, both for the particles themselves and for aggregates of particles, the ratio r_2/r_1 typically increases as with the size of the particles or aggregates increases,

although the T2-relaxivity as a function of particle size can be quite complicated (see, e.g. references 58 and 59). The effect of aggregation of crystals is that the aggregate itself can be considered a large magnetized sphere whose magnetic moment increases with increasing field strength. This gives rise to susceptibility effects, and the SPIOs can act as T2* relaxation agents. This has important consequences when considering the effects of contrast agent compartmentalization on imaging (see below).

Weissleder and co-workers have developed chemistry for making modified iron oxides, the so-called crosslinked iron oxides (CLIO). This has enabled the production of a number of targeted molecular imaging agents.[60–64]

Relaxation biophysics

As is apparent from the previous section, a number of chemical factors influence the effectiveness with which Gd, Mn, or Fe can catalyze the relaxation of water, and that even in the pristine environment of the test tube, the exact relaxivity of any compound is difficult (and, in truth, currently impossible) to predict a priori. This situation is only compounded in vivo by the wide variety of environments that biological protons and the contrast agents are found. The complexities of biological relaxivity in NMR were recognized in the 1950s and 1960s,[65–68] culminating in the use of a chemical exchange model for characterizing biological compartment exchange by Hazelwood et al.[69] Transverse (T2) relaxation in vivo is made even more complex by the various outer-sphere effects that are not at all well modeled by Equation (8). The additional outer-sphere effects are potentially so large, and so poorly predicted by earlier models, that these effects are often characterized independently as 'susceptibility contrast' mechanisms, and both Monte Carlo modeling (see, e.g. reference 70) and more recently exact analytical approaches[71] have been used to predict or explain these effects.

A detailed explanation of all of the effects of these contrast agents is well beyond the scope of this chapter, and a review[72] is available for the reader interested in a more detailed survey of the field. The remainder of this section includes brief mention of the issues and how they relate to CMR applications.

Local variation in relaxivity, water exchange and T1

The simple relaxivity equation (Equation 1) is not necessarily that simple in a biological setting, and even describing the effects on an MR pulse sequence with a single 'relaxivity' can be misleading. The value of the relaxivity (i.e. the proportionality constant between 1/T1 and concentration) can be affected in vivo, and there is also the more complicated effect of local compartmentalization of the contrast agent and the ability of all of tissue water to experience the inner-sphere effects of the agent. In this section, we briefly touch on the issue of whether biology can affect relaxation per se, and then discuss in somewhat more depth the effects of compartmentalization and water exchange on the magnitude of MR signal changes due to the presence of the contrast agent. The actual relaxivity within a compartment might be affected by the biological mileau. For some compounds, with strong or weak albumin binding (e.g. MS-325, B22956, and Gd-BOPTA), local variations in the albumin concentration will affect the amount of contrast agent bound to albumin and thus affect the overall relaxivity. For example, in the plasma space, albumin concentration is typically high (0.6–0.7 mM) compared with the extracellular space in the normal heart (0.2–0.3 mM), and some spaces (e.g. cerebrospinal fluid, CSF) have almost no albumin. As shown in Figure 2.10, for example, at 1.5 T, MS-325 charges its relaxivity from 20 s^{-1} mM^{-1} to 6 s^{-1} mM^{-1} depending on whether it is in the plasma or in CSF. Even for the conventional ECF Gd-based agents in extreme settings, the actual relaxivity could vary. For example, Stanisz and Henkelman[73] showed that in extremely turgid media, which might characterize some biological compartments, the relaxivity of Gd-DTPA can be affected when the macromolecular concentration is high enough. However, no study to date using quantitative methods to compare both the relaxivity and the concentration of contrast agent in specific biological compartments has found a relaxivity in vivo that differs from its temperature-matched in vitro value.[74] Since local binding of ECF agents would also enhance relaxivity by slowing down tumbling (as it does with MS-325 and B22956 locally binding to albumin), investigators have also postulated that binding in specific disease states might occur in vivo even for the nonspecific ECF agents. So far, however, no reproducible evidence of in vivo binding that affects relaxivity has been shown for any of the extracellular agents.

Of much greater impact is the effect of biological compartmentalization of a T1 agent. Except for pathological situations, most contrast agents in use today are excluded from intact cells. That is, with the exception of opsinization of iron oxide particles[75] and the uptake of Mn into cells,[76] most chelates are designed to keep the heavy metal out of cells. Thus, the normal situation in most cardiovascular settings is that contrast agent will be locally concentrated in extracellular spaces. As a result, the simple relaxivity equations do not necessarily hold.

To get some sense of the magnitude of the issue, consider a 1 mM solution of any Gd-based ECF contrast agent. In a simple test tube, it takes an average of about 3 μs for water to diffuse between Gd ions,[72] and thus in the time of a typical imaging TE or TR (for T2 or T1, respectively), a given water molecule may interacts with thousands or millions of Gd ions, and all water molecules will interact with approximately the same number of Gd ions. Now if that same 1 mM solution is compartmentalized solely within the cardiac microvasculature – as it might be in the first pass in a perfusion study – it takes between 2–20 s for most of the water in the tissue (90% of it is extravascular) to physically diffuse into the microvasculature. Thus, most of the water in the tissue does not have the opportunity to be relaxed by the Gd in the typical TR of an imaging acquisition. As a net result, the actual signal enhancement is typically less than that predicted by using Equation (1) with the assumption that the contrast agent is uniformly distributed throughout the tissue.

As a useful simplification of the biologically complex process of water diffusion through a biological compartment, and water exchange through the semipermeable membranes that separate compartments, the concept of 'water exchange' and exchange time τ between compartments is frequently used.[69] When the contrast agent is compartmentalized, or in the more general case that contrast agent concentration is different between two or more compartments because of delivery kinetics (such as first-pass perfusion and myocardial viability imaging paradigms), the water exchange rate and the size of the compartments will determine the effect of the contrast agent on the MR signal.

While the algebra is straightforward, even in the simplest case of two compartments with a single exchange constant, the general formula describing the effect of water relaxation is too algebraically complex to be included here. However, the limiting behavior in two cases can help describe the situations where this exchange strongly affects contrast and when it can, for all intents and purposes, be ignored.

In the first case, water moves so fast between the biological compartments that the net effect is as if the contrast agent were uniformly spread throughout the whole tissue. This regime, called 'fast exchange', occurs whenever the exchange rate 1/τ between the compartments is much faster than the difference in relaxation rates between the compartments.[77] For example, in the blood itself, the red cell, due both to high water permeability across the red cell membrane and to the very small size of the red cell, has a relatively short exchange time, on the order of 5–10 ms.[78] As a result, even though the intact red cell membrane prevents most MR contrast agents from entering the cell, as long as the plasma T1 is longer than 20 ms (which it is even in the first pass of most contrast agents), the two compartments of the blood (plasma plus red cells) will remain in fast exchange, and thus the blood will behave for MRI purposes as if the contrast agent were spread uniformly through the blood. In this case, in general, the effective relaxation rate will be the weighted average of the relaxation in the two compartments. That is, if for compartment i the volume fraction is f_i, the initial T1 is $T1_i$ and the concentration of agent is C_i (which could be zero), then the whole tissue together will behave like

$$\frac{1}{T1} = f_1\left(\frac{1}{T1_1} + r_1 C_1\right) + f_2\left(\frac{1}{T1_2} + r_2 C_2\right). \quad (10)$$

In the second case, water moves much more slowly between the compartments. This case, called 'slow exchange', occurs whenever the water exchange rate is much slower than the difference in relaxation rates between the compartments. In this case, a single relaxation time, and thus a single relaxivity, are meaningless, because the two microscopic compartments will relax with their own relaxation times.

An example of these two limiting cases of slow and fast exchange as a function of contrast agent concentration is shown in Figure 2.13. This graph assumes that a typical Gd-based ECF agent with a relaxivity of 4 s^{-1} mM^{-1} is in the extracellular space (20%) and excluded from the intracellular space (80%). The graph shows the effect on signal intensity with a typical, T1-weighted sequence that might be used for perfusion imaging (TR = 800 ms) or a myocardial viability study. (The concentration range shown on this curve is met easily during a 0.1 mmol/kg injection of an ECF agent on the first pass.) Thus, water

mobility can have a dramatic effect on signal intensity on cardiac MRI scans.

As noted by several researchers,[79,80] the choice of MRI pulse sequence can dramatically affect the dependence of contrast enhancement on the exact details of water mobility. For example, gradient-echo sequences with short TR and high flip angle show much reduced sensitivity to exchange. This effect is demonstrated in Figure 2.14, for a TE/TR/flip = 2/10/30° spoiled gradient-echo sequence under the same biological parameters as Figure 2.13. As is typical in MRI, we don't get something for nothing. Comparing Figure 2.14 with Figure 2.13, we find that the reduced difference between slow and fast exchange has come at the expense of signal (the y-axis). For some applications, detecting the smallest amount of contrast difference is paramount; for other applications, notably quantitative ones, insensitivity to exchange leads to more accurate assessment even when the lower signal-to-noise ratio is take into account.

Very few biological compartments show true slow exchange, except at extremely high concentration of contrast agent. However, the intermediate case, when exchange is neither slow nor fast ('intermediate exchange'), occurs very commonly. In the intermediate case, the relaxation behavior will also appear biexponential, though both the apparent compartment size and the effective T1 of the two compartments will vary from their biological size and T1.

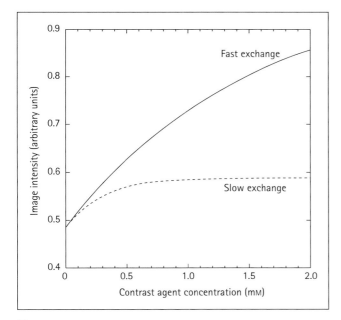

Figure 2.13
Impact of extremes of water exchange on MR signal for a typical ECF agent in the myocardium. Fast exchange (solid line) shows much larger signal increases than slow exchange (dashed line). It is assumed that the agent is restricted to the extracellular space (20% by volume), r_1 = 4 s^{-1}mM^{-1}, and the spin-echo sequence TR = 800 ms.

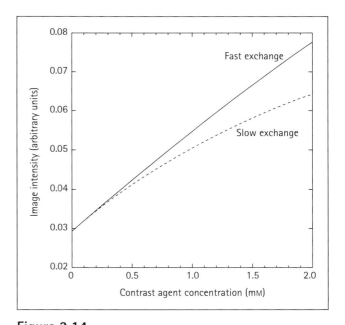

Figure 2.14
Impact of extremes of water exchange on MR signal is reduced by using fast gradient-echo sequences. Fast exchange (solid line) shows only slight signal increases than slow exchange (dashed line). It is assumed that the agent is restricted to the extracellular space (20% by volume), r_1 = 4 s^{-1} mM^{-1}, and the fast gradient-echo sequence TR/flip = 10/30°.

Most nonpathological biological tissues without a contrast agent present, ignoring the effects of blood flow,[81] are in fast exchange between the compartments, and thus appear to have primarily monoexponential decay in longitudinal relaxation. As contrast agent is added to one or more compartments, the exchange, regime moves from fast exchange to intermediate exchange, and, in occasional cases, even into slow exchange. Note that because 'fast' or 'slow' exchange depends on the T1s of the compartments, the same biological compartments can be in fast or slow exchange depending on the concentration of contrast agent. Note that the modeling of this shape does allow for the estimation of water exchange times in vivo (see, e.g. reference 82).

Of course, even characterizing the simplest piece of human tissue as having only one or two compartments is clearly an oversimplification, and careful, high-precision measurements of tissues has demonstrated much more than biexponential behavior, allowing the creation of a whole spectrum of relaxation times within any real tissue. Nevertheless, models that incorporate two compartments have been very useful for explaining (or optimizing imaging parameters to avoid the need to explain) the effects of biological water mobility on contrast-enhanced scans.

While the exact relationship between contrast agent concentration and signal change thus depends strongly on the biological compartmentalization of the water and the contrast agent, as well the pulse sequence used for imaging, the clinical significance of these effects also depends strongly on the application. For qualitative applications, especially for those that depend on simple questions ('Is the septum significantly brighter than the rest of the heart?' for myocardial viability, or 'Does the septum remain completely dark during the first pass of a contrast agent?' in a so-called first-pass perfusion study), the quantitative details of the amount of enhancement for a given amount of contrast agent are relatively minor. However, for more quantitative questions ('What degree of enhancement always correlates to dead myocardium?' or 'What is the perfusion in ml/100 g/min?'), the details of relaxation, and especially the changes in relaxation biophysics that may occur in abnormal physiology, may become important.

Susceptibility induced changes in apparent T2

The second broad type of effect that arise from biological compartmentalization is susceptibility contrast. For these effects, the contrast agent causes microscopic field inhomogeneity on a biological scale of tens of nanometers to micrometers rather than on the chemical scale of angstroms to nanometers. There are two effects that have been used in cardiovascular MRI studies. In the first, proton diffusion through these inhomogeneities (often called 'mesoscopic' inhomogeneities[71] since the scale of the inhomogeneities is of the same order as the scale of the water's Brownian motion), causes the protons to dephase from one another due the different magnetic fields that they experience during their random walks. In the second, even in the absence of water diffusion, the field inhomogeneity causes intravoxel dephasing and thus signal loss on gradient-echo images due to the different microscopic magnetic fields within the voxel.

The complexity of estimating the size of these two effects is exacerbated by the wide range of potential biological compartments in which the water and the contrast agent may reside. While the strengths of the perturbing magnetic fields are directly proportional to the agent's concentration, usually expressed through the agent's molar susceptibility constant χ, the actual magnitude and even direction of the magnetic field shifts depend strongly on the size and the shape of the biological compartment in which the contrast agent resides,[83] and the size of the susceptibility contrast effect depends on how the water diffuses through the tissue. In vivo, predicting these effects and quantifying their results remains an active area of research.

Given the inherent difficulty in quantifying these effects, it may seem surprising that the susceptibility effect would be useful in clinical MRI. However, because the susceptibility T2 effect does not require water to pass into the hydration sphere of the contrast agent, large effects can be observed even when the contrast agent is compartmentalized in a very small tissue compartment. For example, first-pass brain perfusion imaging (so-called PWI[84]) relies on the susceptibility effect due to the compartmentalization of currently approved extracelluar Gd-based agents. The small blood volume in the brain (4% in gray matter, 2% in white matter) and the relatively limited water exchange between the extravascular and intravascular spaces in the brain ultimately limit the size of signal changes due to any T1-based contrast agent at acceptable doses. The susceptibility-based T2 and T2* effects, however, can be much larger – as much as a 50% signal drop in normal gray matter at the same dose – due to the 'action at a distance' effect possible with the outer-sphere effect. Thus, especially in cases of slow exchange and small compartments available for the contrast agent, susceptibility contrast may be the medically relevent contrast mechanism of choice. At present, these larger effects, however, are accompanied by potentially larger uncertainty in the absolute quantitation, especially when there is underlying pathology. Nevertheless, as with the potential limits on quantitation in myocardial perfusion and viability imaging, the appeal of routine qualitative imaging using these effects has been demonstrated consistently over the past decade.

Safety

The safety of MR, contrast agents, which of themselves offer no direct therapeutic benefit, is always a question of appropriate medical concern. The Gd-based chelates are among the safest injectible compounds in current medical use, and certainly have a reputation for being safer, especially in terms of reduced nephrotoxicity, than their X-ray contrast agent counterparts. (There is limited use of Gd chelates as X-ray contrast agents reported in the literature because of this.[85]) Nevertheless, both the heavy-metal (Gd)[86] and the chelate have potential toxic effects, and have demonstrated acute toxicity in animal studies at high enough doses. A further review of the various animal studies is given by Lauffer.[87]

The safety record of the four longest approved Gd-based agents (Gd-DTPA, Gd-DTPA-BMA, Gd-HPDO3A, and Gd-DOTA) have been reviewed by Runge.[88] He found that the four agents had approximately the same overall adverse event rates, with nausea (1–2%) and hives (1%) leading the list. Nearly all adverse events with these agents are transient, mild, and self-limiting. Nevertheless, there are reports of serious adverse reactions, including life-threatening anaphylactoid reactions and death, with these agents. The best estimate puts the rate of these events at between 1 in 200 000 and 1 in 400 000 patients.[89] While also very safe, the safety record for Fe-based and Mn-based[90] agents is growing, but (due in part to their much smaller market share), is currently less well documented. The Gd-based ECF contrast agents have been studied and most are approved for pediatric use in pediatric patients above 2 years, although there are differences in their approval wording. The package inserts for these agents should always be consulted for the latest safety information.

Summary

A large number of contrast agents have been approved for MRI in the past 15 years, and a significant number of new agents, including blood pool and tissue-specific agents, that are potentially relevant for CMR are currently in development. The MRI behavior of these agents, which often is summarized by a single effectiveness parameter, r_1, is actually quite complex, in terms of both the underlying chemistry and the biophysics in vivo. While many elements of that complexity remain active areas of research – both for understanding existing agents and for creating new agents and new uses for those agents – the relative safety and ease of use of these agents has brought them into routine use in many medical applications of MRI. As CMR expands clinically, no doubt the use of MR contrast agents will expand as well.

References

1. Salerno M, Altes TA, Mugler JP, et al. Hyperpolarized noble gas MR imaging of the lung: potential clinical applications. Eur J Radiol 2001; 40:33–44.

2. Mugler JP, Driehuys B, Brookeman JR, et al. MR imaging and spectroscopy using hyperpolarized ^{129}Xe gas: preliminary human results. J Magn Reson Med 1997; 37:809–15.

3. Ardenkjaer Larsen JH, Laursen I, Leunbach I, et al. EPR and DNP properties of certain novel single electron contrast agents intended for oximetric imaging. J Magn Reson 1998; 133:1–12.

4. Krishna MC, English S, Yamada K, et al. Overhauser enhanced magnetic resonance imaging for tumor oximetry: coregistration of tumor anatomy and tissue oxygen concentration. Proc Natl Acad Sci USA 2002; 99:2216–21.

5. Løkling KE, Fossheim SL, Skurtveit R, et al. pH-sensitive paramagnetic liposomes as MRI contrast agents: in vitro feasibility studies. Magn Reson Imaging 2001; 19:731–8.

6. Raghunand N, Zhang S, Sherry AD, et al. In vivo magnetic resonance imaging of tissue pH using a novel pH-sensitive contrast agent, GdDOTA-4AmP. Acad Radiol 2002; Suppl 2:S481–3.

7. Aime S, Barge A, Delli Castelli D, et al. Paramagnetic lanthanide(III) complexes as pH-sensitive chemical exchange saturation transfer (CEST) contrast agents for MRI applications. Magn Reson Med 2002; 47:639–48.

8. Ward KM, Aletras AH, Balaban RS. A new class of contrast agents for MRI based on proton chemical exchange dependent saturation transfer (CEST). J Magn Reson 2000; 143:79–87.

9. Louie AY, Hüber MM, Ahrens ET, et al. In vivo visualization of gene expression using magnetic resonance imaging. Nat Biotechnol 2000; 18:321–5.

10. Perez JM, Josephson L, O'Loughlin T, et al. Magnetic relaxation switches capable of sensing molecular interactions. Nat Biotechnol 2002; 20:816–20.

11. Lauterbur PC, Dias MHM, Rudin AM. Augmentation of tissue water proton spin-lattice relaxation rates by in vivo addition of paramagnetic ions. In: Frontiers in Biological Energetics (Papers from International Symposium). New York: Academic Press, 1978, p752.

12. Carr DH, Brown J, Bydder GM, et al. Intravenous chelated gadolinium as a contrast agent in NMR imaging of cerebral tumors. Lancet 1984; i:484–6.

13. Schwert DD, Davies JA, Richardson N. Non-gadolinium-based MRI contrast agents. Top Curr Chem 2002; 221(Contrast Agents I):165–99.

14. Muller RN, Roch A, Colet J-M, et al. Particulate magnetic contrast agents. In: Chemistry of Contrast Agents in Medical Magnetic Resonance Imaging Bognor Regis, UK: John Wiley and Sons 2001: 417–35.

15. Gries H. Extracellular MRI contrast agents based on gadolinium. Top Curr Chem 2002; 221(Contrast Agents I):1–24.

16. Low RN. Contrast agents for MR imaging of the liver. J Magn Reson Imaging 1997; 7:56–67.

17. Mahfouz A-E, Hamm B, Taupitz M. Contrast agents for MR imaging of the liver: a clinical overview. Eur Radiol 1997; 7:507–13.

18. Weissleder R, Mahmood U. Molecular imaging. Radiology 2001; 219:316–33.

19. Lowe MP. MRI contrast agents: the next generation. Aust J Chem 2002; 55:551–6.

20. Aime S, Cabella C, Colombatto S, et al. Insights into the use of paramagnetic Gd(III) complexes in MR-molecular imaging investigations. J Magn Reson Imaging 2002; 16:394–406.

21. Aime S, Crich SG, Botta M, et al. A macromolecular Gd(III) complex as pH-responsive relaxometric probe for MRI applications. Chem Commun 1999; 16:1577–8.

22. Lowe MP, Parker D, Reany O, et al. pH-dependent modulation of relaxivity and luminescence in macrocyclic gadolinium and europium complexes based on reversible intramolecular sulfonamide ligation. J Am Chem Soc 2001; 123:7601–9.

23. Louie AY, Huber MM, Ahrens ET, et al. In vivo visualization of gene expression using magnetic resonance imaging. Nat Biotechnol 2000; 18:321–5.

24. Nivorozhkin AL, Kolodziej AF, Caravan P, et al. Enzyme-activated Gd^{3+} magnetic resonance imaging contrast agents with a prominent receptor-induced magnetization enhancement. Angew Chem Int Ed 2001; 40:2903–6.

25. Flacke S, Fischer S, Scott MJ, et al. Novel MRI contrast agent for molecular imaging of fibrin: implications for detecting vulnerable plaques. Circulation 2001; 104:1280–5.

26. Sipkins DA, Cheresh DA, Kazemi MR, et al. Detection of tumor angiogenesis in vivo by $\alpha_v\beta_3$-targeted magnetic resonance imaging. Nat Med 1998; 4:623–6.

27. Caravan P, Ellison JJ, McMurry TJ, et al. Gadolinium(III) chelates as MRI contrast agents: structure, dynamics, and applications. Chem Rev 1999; 99:2293–352.

28. Powell DH, Ni Dhubhghaill OM, Pubanz D, et al. High-pressure NMR kinetics. Part 74. Structural and dynamic parameters obtained from ^{17}O NMR, EPR, and NMRD studies of monomeric and dimeric Gd^{3+} complexes of interest in magnetic resonance imaging: an integrated and theoretically self-consistent approach. J Am Chem Soc 1996; 118:9333–46.

29. Bashir A, Gray ML, Boutin RD, et al. Glycosaminoglycan in articular cartilage: in vivo assessment with delayed Gd(DTPA)(2−)-enhanced MR imaging. Radiology 1997; 205:551–8.

30. Kumar K, Tweedle MF. Ligand basicity and rigidity control formation of macrocyclic polyamino carboxylate complexes of gadolinium(III). Inorg Chem 1993; 32:4193–9.

31. White DH, DeLearie LA, Moore DA, et al. The thermodynamics of complexation of lanthanide(III) DTPA-bisamide complexes and their implication for stability and solution structure. Invest Radiol 1991; 26(Suppl 1):S226–8.

32. Tombach B, Heindel W. Value of 1.0-M gadolinium chelates: review of preclinical and clinical data on gadobutrol. Eur Radiol 2002; 12:1550–6.

33. Kirchin MA, Pirovano GP, and Spinazzi A. Gadobenate dimeglumine (Gd-BOPTA). Invest Radiol 1998; 33:798–809.

34. Davies BE, Kirchin MA, Bensel K, et al. Pharmacokinetics and safety of gadobenate dimeglumine (multihance) in subjects with impaired liver function. Invest Radiol 2002; 37:299–308.

35. Mintorovitch J, Shamsi K. Eovist injection and Resovist Injection: two new liver-specific contrast agents for MRI. Oncology (Huntingt) 2000; 14(6 Suppl 3):37–40.

36. Jung G, Heindel W, Krahe T, et al. Influence of the hepatobiliary contrast agent mangafodipir trisodium (Mn-DPDP) on the imaging properties of abdominal organs. Magn Reson Imaging 1998; 16:925–31.

37. Clement O, Siauve N, Cuenod CA, et al. Liver imaging with feru-moxides (Feridex): fundamentals, controversies, and practical aspects. Top Magn Reson Imaging 1998; 9:167–82.

38. Wang YX, Hussain SM, Krestin GP. Superparamagnetic iron oxide contrast agents: physicochemical characteristics and applications in MR imaging. Eur Radiol 2001; 11:2319–31.

39. Pascolo L, Cupelli F, Anelli PL, et al. Molecular mechanisms for the hepatic uptake of magnetic resonance imaging contrast agents. Biochem Biophys Res Commun 1999; 257:746–52.

40. Schmidt PP, Toft KG, Skotland T, et al. Stability and transmetalation of the magnetic resonance contrast agent MnDPDP measured by EPR. J Biol Inorg Chem 2002; 7:241–8.

41. Lauffer RB, Parmelee DJ, Dunham SU, et al. MS-325: albumin-targeted contrast agent for MR angiography. Radiology 1998; 207:529–38.

42. La Noce A, Stoelben S, Scheffler K, et al. B22956/1, a new intravascular contrast agent for MRI: first administration to humans – preliminary results. Acad Radiol 2002; 9(Suppl 2):S404–6.

43. Cavagna FM, Lorusso V, Anelli PL, et al. Preclinical profile and clinical potential of gadocoletic acid trisodium salt (B22956/1), a new intravascular contrast medium for MRI. Acad Radiol 2002; 9(Suppl 2):S491–4.

44. Dong Q, Hurst DR, Weinmann HJ, et al. Magnetic resonance angiography with gadomer-17. An animal study original investigation. Invest Radiol 1998; 33:699–708.

45. Nicolle GM, Toth E, Schmitt-Willich H, et al. The impact of rigidity and water exchange on the relaxivity of a dendritic MRI contrast agent. Chemistry 2002; 8:1040–8.

46. Port M, Corot C, Raynal I, et al. Physicochemical and biological evaluation of P792, a rapid-clearance blood-pool agent for magnetic resonance imaging. Invest Radiol 2001; 36:445–54.

47. Gaillard S, Kubiak C, Stolz C, et al. Safety and pharmacokinetics of p792, a new blood-pool agent: results of clinical testing in non-patient volunteers. Invest Radiol 2002; 37:161–6.

48. Toth E, Helm L, Merbach AE. Relaxivity of gadolinium(III) complexes: theory and mechanism. In: Chemistry of Contrast Agents in Medical Magnetic Resonance Imaging. 2001: 45–119.

49. Caravan P, Greenfield MT, Li X, et al. The Gd^{3+} complex of a fatty acid analogue of DOTP binds to multiple albumin sites with variable water relaxivities. Inorg Chem 2001; 40:6580–7.

50. Micskei K, Helm L, Brucher E, et al. Oxygen-17 NMR study of water exchange on gadolinium polyaminopolyacetates $[Gd(DTPA)(H_2O)]^{2-}$ and $[Gd(DOTA)(H_2O)]^-$ related to NMR imaging. Inorg Chem 1993; 32:3844–50.

51. Micskei K, Powell DH, Helm L, et al. Water exchange on gadolinium (aqua)(propylenediamine tetraacetate) complexes $[Gd(H_2O)_8]^{3+}$ and $[Gd(PDTA)(H_2O)_2]^-$ in aqueous solution: a variable-pressure, -temperature and -magnetic field oxygen-17 NMR study. Magn Reson Chem 1993; 31:1011–20.

52. Southwood-Jones RV, Earl WL, Newman KE, et al. Oxygen-17 NMR and EPR studies of water exchange from the first coordination sphere of gadolinium(III) aquoion and gadolinium(III) propylenediaminetetraacetate. J Chem Phys 1980; 73:5909–18.

53. Cohen SM, Xu J, Radkov E, et al. Syntheses and relaxation properties of mixed gadolinium hydroxypyridinonate MRI contrast agents. Inorg Chem 2000; 39:5747–56.

54. Spanoghe M, Lanens D, Dommisse R, et al. Proton relaxation enhancement by means of serum albumin and poly-L-lysine labeled with DTPA–gadolinium(3+): relaxivities as a function of molecular weight and conjugation efficiency. Magn Reson Imaging 1992; 10:913–17.

55. Glogard C, Stensrud G, Hovland R, et al. Liposomes as carriers of amphiphilic gadolinium chelates: the effect of membrane composition on incorporation efficacy and in vitro relaxivity. Int J Pharm 2002; 233:131–40.

56. Glogard C, Stensrud G, Klaveness J. Novel high relaxivity colloidal particles based on the specific phase organisation of amphiphilic gadolinium chelates with cholesterol. Int J Pharm 2003; 253:39–48.

57. Jung CW, Jacobs P. Physical and chemical properties of superparamagnetic iron oxide MR contrast agents: ferumoxides, ferumoxtran, ferumoxsil. Magn Reson Imaging 1995; 13:661–74.

58. Weisskoff RM, Zuo CS, Boxerman JL, et al. Microscopic susceptibility variation and transverse relaxation: theory and experiment. Magn Reson Med 1994; 31:601–610.

59. Hardy P, Henkelman RM. On the transverse relaxation rate enhancement induced by diffusion of spins through inhomogeneous fields. Magn Reson Med 1991; 17:348–56.

60. Wunderbaldinger P, Josephson L, Weissleder R. Crosslinked iron oxides (CLIO): a new platform for the development of targeted MR contrast agents. Acad Radiol 2002; 9(Suppl 2):S304–6.

61. Schellenberger EA, Hogemann D, Josephson L, et al. Annexin V-CLIO: a nanoparticle for detecting apoptosis by MRI. Acad Radiol 2002; 9(Suppl 2):S310–11.

62. Kang HW, Josephson L, Petrovsky A, et al. Magnetic resonance imaging of inducible E-selectin expression in human endothelial cell culture. Bioconjug Chem 2002; 13:122–7.

63. Josephson L, Kircher MF, Mahmood U, et al. Near-infrared fluorescent nanoparticles as combined MR/optical imaging probes. Bioconjug Chem 2002; 13:554–60.

64. Ichikawa T, Hogemann D, Saeki Y, et al. MRI of transgene expression: correlation to therapeutic gene expression. Neoplasia 2002; 4:523–30.

65. Zimmerman JR, Brittin WE. Nuclear magnetic resonance studies in multiple phase systems: lifetime of a water molecule in an adsorbing phase on silica gel. J Phys Chem 1957; 61:1328–33.

66. McConnell HM, Reaction rates by nuclear magnetic resonance. J Chem Phys 1958; 28:430.

67. Woessner DE, Zimmerman JR. Nuclear transfer and anisotropic motional spin phenomena: Relaxation time temperature dependence studies of water adsorbed on silica gel. IV. J Phys Chem 1963; 35:1590–1600.

68. Leigh JS. Relaxation times in systems with chemical exchange: some exact solutions. J Magn Reson 1971; 4:308–11.

69. Hazlewood C, Chang D, Nichols B, et al. Nuclear magnetic resonance transverse relaxation times of water protons in skeletal muscle. Biophys J 1974; 14:583–605.

70. Boxerman JL, Hamberg LM, Rosen BR, et al. MR contrast due to intravascular magnetic susceptibility perturbations. Magn Reson Med 1995; 34:555–66.

71. Sukstanskii AL, Yablonskiy DA. Theory of FID NMR signal dephasing induced by mesoscopic magnetic field inhomogeneities in biological systems. J Magn Reson 2001; 151:107–17.

72. Donahue K, Weisskoff RM, Burstein D. Water diffusion and exchange as they influence contrast enhancement. J Magn Reson Imag 1997; 7:102–10.

73. Stanisz GJ, Henkelman RM. Gd-DTPA relaxivity depends on macromolecular content. Magn Reson Med 2000; 44:665–7.

74. Donahue KM, Burstein D, Manning WJ, et al. Studies of Gd-DTPA relaxivity and proton exchange rates in tissue. Magn Reson Med 1994; 32:66–76.

75. Moore A, Weissleder R, Bogdanov A. Uptake of dextran-coated monocrystalline iron oxides in tumor cells and macrophages. J Magn Reson Imaging 1997; 7:1140–5.

76. Bremerich J, Saeed M, Arheden H, et al. Normal and infarcted myocardium: differentiation with cellular uptake of manganese at MR imaging in a rat model. Radiology 2000; 216:524–30.

77. McLaughlin AC, Leigh JS. Relaxation times in systems with chemical exchange. J Magn Reson 1973; 9:296–304.

78. Wright GA, Hu BS, Macovski A. Estimating oxygen saturation of blood in vivo with MR imaging at 1.5 T. J Magn Reson Imaging 1991; 1:275–83.

79. Donahue KM, Weisskoff RM, Chesler DA, et al. Improving MR quantification of regional blood volume with intravascular T1 contrast agents: accuracy, precision and water exchange. Magn Reson Med 1996; 36:858–67.

80. Kim YR, Rebro KJ, Schmainda KM. Water exchange and inflow affect the accuracy of T1-GRE blood volume measurements: implications for the evaluation of tumor angiogenesis. Magn Reson Med 2002; 47:1110–20.

81. Detre J, Leigh J, Williams D, et al. Perfusion Imaging. Magn Reson Med 1992; 23:37–45.

82. Landis CS, Li X, Telang FW, et al. Equilibrium transcytolemmal water-exchange kinetics in skeletal muscle in vivo. Magn Reson Med 1999; 42:467–78.

83. Chu SC, Xu Y, Balschi JA, et al. Bulk magnetic susceptibility shifts in NMR studies of compartmentalized samples: use of paramagnetic reagents. Magn Reson Med 1990; 13:239–62.

84. Rosen BR, Belliveau JW, Vevea JM, et al. Perfusion imaging with NMR contrast agents. Magn Reson Med 1990; 14:249–65.

85. Peña CS, Kaufman JA, Geller SC, et al. Gadopentetate dimeglumine: a possible alternative contrast agent for CT angiography of the aorta. J Comput Assist Tomogr 1999; 23:23–4.

86. Luckey TD, Venugopal B. Metal Toxicity in Mammals, Vol 1. New York: Plenum, 1977.

87. Lauffer R. MRI contrast agents: basic principles. In: Clinical Magnetic Resonance Imaging (Edelman R, Hesselink J, Zlatkin MB, eds). Philadelphia: WB Saunders, 1996.

88. Runge VM. Safety of Approved MR Contrast Media for Intravenous Injection. J Magn Reson Imaging 2000; 12:205–13.

89. Carr JJ. Magnetic resonance contrast agents for neuroimaging: safety issues. Neuroimaging Clin North Am 1994; 4:43–54.

90. Federle M, Chezmar J, Rubin DL, et al. Efficacy and safety of mangafodipir trisodium (MnDPDP) injection for hepatic MRI in adults: results of the US Multicenter phase III clinical trials. Efficacy of early imaging. J Magn Reson Imaging 2000; 12:689–701.

91. Vogler H, Platzek J, Schuhmann-Giampieri G, et al. Pre-clinical evaluation of gadobutrol: a new, neutral, extracellular contrast agent for magnetic resonance imaging. Eur J Radiol 1995; 21:1–10.

92. Tweedle MF, Hagan JJ, Kumar K, et al. Reaction of gadolinium chelates with endogenously available ions. Magn Reson Imaging 1991; 9:409–15.

93. Aime S, Anelli PL, Botta M, et al. Synthesis, characterization, and 1/T1 NMRD profiles of gadolinium(III) complexes of monoamide derivatives of DOTA-like ligands. X-ray structure of the 10-[2-[2-hydroxy-1-(hydroxymethyl)ethyl]amino]-1-[(phenylmethoxy)-methyl]-2-oxoethyl]-1,4,7,10-tetraazacyclododecane-1,4,7-triacetic acid–gadolinium(III) complex. Inorg Chem 1992; 31:2422–8.

94. Tweedle MF. Physicochemical properties of gadoteridol and other magnetic resonance contrast agents. Invest Radiol 1992; 27(Suppl 1):2–6.

95. Periasamy M, White D, DeLearie L, et al. The synthesis and screening of nonionic gadolinium(III) DTPA–bisamide complexes as magnetic resonance imaging contrast agents. Invest Radiol 1991; 26(Suppl 1):S217–20.

96. OptiMARK Package Insert. St Louis, MO: Mallinckrodt, Inc.

97. Uggeri F, Aime S, Anelli PL, et al. Novel contrast agents for magnetic resonance imaging. Synthesis and characterization of the ligand BOPTA and its Ln(III) complexes (Ln = Gd, La, Lu). X-ray structure of disodium (TPS-9-145337286-C-S)-[4-carboxy-5,8,11-tris(carboxymethyl)-1-phenyl-2-oxa-5,8,11-triazatridecan-13-oato(5−)]gadolinate(2−) in a mixture with its enantiomer. Inorg Chem 1995; 34:633–42.

98. Multihance Package Insert. Konstanz: Bracco-Byk Gulden.

99. Tirkkonen B, Aukrust A, Couture E, et al. Physicochemical characterisation of mangafodipir trisodium. Acta Radiol 1997; 38(4 Pt 2):780–9.

100. Teslascan Package Insert. Princeton: Amersham Health.

101. FeridexIV Package Insert. Wayne NJ: Berlex.

102. Bremer C, Allkemper T, Baermig J, et al. RES-specific imaging of the liver and spleen with iron oxide particles designed for blood pool MR-angiography. J Magn Reson Imaging 1999; 10:461–7.

103. Resovist Package Insert. Berlin: Schering Diagnostics.

104. Lauffer RB, Parmelee DJ, Dunham SU, et al. MS-325: albumin-targeted contrast agent for MR angiography. Radiology 1998; 207:529–38.

105. Port M, Corot C, Raynal I, et al. Physicochemical and biological evaluation of P792, a rapid-clearance blood-pool agent for magnetic resonance imaging. Invest Radiol 2001; 36:445–54.

106. de Haën C, Gozzini L. Soluble-type hepatobiliary contrast agents for MR imaging. J Magn Reson Imaging 1993; 3:1993.

107. Clarke SE, Weinmann HJ, Dai E, et al. Comparison of two blood pool contrast agents for 0.5-T MR angiography: experimental study in rabbits. Radiology 2000; 214:787–94.

108. Kellar KE, Fujii DK, Gunther WH, et al. NC100150 Injection, a preparation of optimized iron oxide nanoparticles for positive-contrast MR angiography. J Magn Reson Imaging 2000; 11:488–94.

109. Taupitz M, Schnorr J, Abramjuk C, et al. New generation of monomer-stabilized very small superparamagnetic iron oxide particles (VSOP) as contrast medium for MR angiography: preclinical results in rats and rabbits. J Magn Reson Imaging 2000; 12:905–11.

3

Cardiac magnetic resonance spectroscopy

Stefan Neubauer

Introduction

Cardiac magnetic resonance imaging (MRI) has in recent years been developed with great success. However, this technique uses the ^{1}H nucleus in water (H_2O) and fat (CH_2 and CH_3 groups) molecules as its only signal source. ^{1}H-MRI of the heart is an excellent method for obtaining anatomical and functional information, but offers little biochemical insight into the state of cardiac tissue. In contrast, cardiac magnetic resonance spectroscopy (MRS) allows the study of many other nuclei with a nuclear spin, i.e. with an uneven number of protons, neutrons, or both. Importantly, MRS is the only available method for the noninvasive study of cardiac metabolism without the need for the application of external radioactive tracers, as are required for example for positron emission tomography (PET). Table 3.1 summarizes information on nuclei of interest for the metabolic study of cardiac tissue by MRS: these include ^{1}H (protons from metabolites other than water and fat), ^{13}C, ^{23}Na, and ^{31}P (which is the most widely studied nucleus). Noninvasive imaging of cardiac metabolism is a long-standing cardiologists' dream, and, theoretically, many clinical questions can be answered with cardiac MRS. The main reason why MRS has not yet fulfilled its promise in clinical cardiology is related to its two fundamental physical limitations: the nuclei studied with MRS have a much lower MR sensitivity than ^{1}H and are present in concentrations that are several orders of magnitude lower than those of ^{1}H nuclei of water and fat (Table 3.1). The direct consequence of this is that, while MR spectra can be obtained from the human heart, the temporal and spatial resolution of MRS is many times lower than that of MRI, and therefore high-resolution metabolic imaging by MRS has not yet found its way into mainstream cardiology.

MRS has been a standard method in experimental cardiology ever since the first ^{31}P-MR spectrum from an isolated heart was obtained by Radda's group in 1977,[1] and since then MRS has been used for the study of many aspects of cardiac metabolism. Other pioneering groups in this field were those of Ingwall[2] and Jacobus.[3] A large body of literature exists on experimental applications of MRS to the heart, and the overwhelming majority of publications on cardiac MRS report on experimental animal work. An introduction to the experimental applications of MRS is important even for a clinical textbook, so that the principles of MRS can be explained in well-defined experimental settings. This then allows us to extrapolate them to clinical applications that might become feasible in the future, if the technical challenges presently limiting the clinical utility of MRS are overcome. While this chapter should enable the reader to understand the principles of MRS and its clinical potential, comprehensive reviews on MRS are available for those interested in greater detail.[4–7]

Table 3.1 Properties of nuclei relevant to cardiac MRS			
Nucleus	Natural abundance (%)	Relative MR sensitivity (%)	Myocardial tissue concentrations
^{1}H	99.98	100	H_2O 110 M; up to ~ 90 mM (CH_3–^{1}H of creatine)
^{13}C	1.1	1.6	Labelled compounds, several mM
^{23}Na	100	9.3	10 mM (intracellular); 140 mM (extracellular)
^{31}P	100	6.6	Up to ~18 mM (PCr)

Physics of MRS

The most extensively studied nucleus in cardiac MRS is
[31]P, while the most widely used animal model is the isolated buffer-perfused rodent heart. The basic principles of
MRS (for a textbook on the general physical principles of
Magnetic Resonance Spectroscopy, see reference 8) will
therefore be derived from ^{31}P-MRS in the isolated heart
model; these principles apply to MRS of all nuclei. MRS is
performed using an MR spectrometer, which consists of a
high-field vertical or horizontal superconducting magnet
(currently up to 18 T) with a bore size ranging between
~5 cm and ~1 m. The magnet bore holds the nucleus-
specific probe head with the radiofrequency (RF) coils,
which are used for MR excitation and signal reception.
The magnet is interfaced with a control computer, a magnetic field gradient system, and an RF transmitter and
receiver. The first step in an MRS experiment is to
homogenize the magnetic field with shim gradients (hence
the term 'shimming'), since MRS requires much higher
magnetic field homogeneity than MRI. An RF impulse is
then sent into the RF coils for spin excitation. The resulting MR signal, the free induction decay (FID), is then
recorded by a computer. The FID describes the relation
between time and signal intensity, and typically shows an
exponential signal decrease over time. After signal acquisition, the FID is subjected to a mathematical manipulation
termed 'Fourier transformation', which results in an MR
spectrum, relating resonance frequency and signal intensity. As mentioned, the main limitation of MRS is its low
sensitivity, and thus many FIDs have to be signal-averaged
to obtain MR spectra with a sufficient 'signal-to-noise
ratio' (SNR, defined as signal amplitude divided by the
standard deviation of background noise). The required
number of acquisitions ('iterations') depends on various
factors, predominantly the metabolite concentration in
the sample, the 'filling factor' (the mass of the observed
object relative to the coil size), the natural abundance of
the nuclear isotope under study, its relative MR sensitivity
(Table 3.1), the pulse angle, and the pulse repetition time
(TR). Typically, for a perfused rat heart experiment at
7–12 T, 100–200 FIDs are acquired and signal-averaged.
In MRS, it is important to account for the effects of partial
saturation when selecting pulse angles and TR: a full MR
signal from a given nucleus can only be obtained when the
nucleus is excited from a fully relaxed spin state, i.e. when
a time of at least $5 \times T1$ has passed since the previous
excitation (for example, T1 of phosphocreatine at 7 T is
~3 s, requiring a TR of 15 s; at 1.5 T, T1 ~4.4 s, requiring
a TR of 22 s); 'fully relaxed' spectra can therefore only be
obtained with long TRs, leading to prohibitively long
acquisition times. Since the initial part of the FID contains
most of the information on the signal, the use of shorter
TRs yields spectra with higher SNR for a given acquisition
time, but in these spectra, part of the signal is lost due to

saturation effects ('partially saturated spectra'). Since the
T1s of ^{31}P metabolites such as phosphocreatine and ATP
are significantly different (T1 of phosphocreatine is ~2–3
times that of ATP), the extent of saturation also varies for
different ^{31}P resonances. Thus, when quantifying partially
saturated spectra, 'saturation factors' need to be used for
correction. These factors are determined for each metabolite by comparing fully relaxed and saturated spectra. In
practice, TRs and pulse angles for CMS are chosen to yield
acceptable measurement times at a ~20–50% degree of
saturation. Larger degrees of saturation (i.e. very short
TRs) make the quantification of spectra unreliable.

A typical ^{31}P-MR spectrum from an isolated, beating rat
heart, obtained in 5 min at 7 T with a TR of 1.93 s and a
pulse angle of 45°, is shown in Figure 3.1. A ^{31}P-MR spectrum shows six resonances, corresponding to the three [31]P
atoms of ATP (the resonance at the right shoulder of the
α-P ATP peak represents the P atom of NAD[+]), phosphocreatine, inorganic phosphate and monophosphate esters
(mostly AMP and glycolytic intermediates). Although
there are many more ^{31}P-containing metabolites present
in the heart, the reason why only this limited number of
[31]P resonances is visible is that ^{31}P nuclei need to be
present above a certain concentration threshold
(~0.6 mM) as well as free in solution. In contrast, immobi-
lized metabolites (e.g. plasma membrane phosphates) give

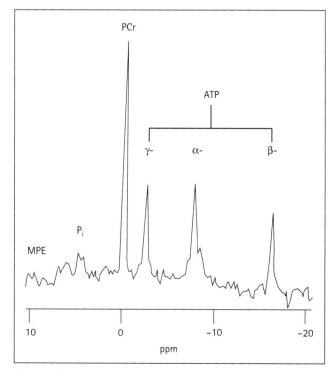

Figure 3.1
^{31}P-MR spectrum of an isolated, buffer-perfused rat heart
obtained within 5 min at 7 T. PCr, phosphocreatine; P_i, inorganic
phosphate; MPE, monophosphate esters.

no quantifiable MR signal due to very short T2 values; such metabolites only contribute to the broad 'baseline hump' of ^{31}P spectra. In MR spectroscopy, 'chemical shift' describes the phenomenon in which different metabolites resonate at distinct frequencies, allowing their discrimination from each other. Chemical shift is quantified relative to the B_0 field in parts per million (ppm). The physical reason for this phenomenon is that different positions in the molecule are subject to subtle differences in local magnetic field strength, spreading the resonance frequencies of ^{31}P metabolites over a range of ~30 ppm. After correction for saturation, quantification of experimental ^{31}P spectra is straightforward: The area under each resonance is proportional to the amount of each ^{31}P nucleus in the sample, and metabolite resonances are therefore quantified by integrating peak areas. This is typically achieved by using Lorentzian line curve-fitting algorithms. Relative metabolite levels are calculated directly (such as the phosphocreatine/ATP ratio), but absolute metabolite concentrations are generally evaluated by comparing the tissue ^{31}P-resonance areas with those of an external ^{31}P reference standard. The most widely used standard is phenylphosphonate, which generates an additional peak in the spectrum not overlapping with any of the naturally abundant ^{31}P resonances.[2,9,10] A fundamental advantage over destructive methods such as traditional biochemical methods, where the tissue has to be frozen and extracted, is that the MRS measurement is noninvasive. This allows for the sequential acquisition of spectra, and the dynamic response of energy metabolites to ischemia, hypoxia, or inotropic stimulation can be followed in one experiment, so that, in contrast to wet chemical analysis, each heart can serve as its own control, and the number of required experiments is drastically reduced.

Experimental animal studies

^{31}P-MRS studies

^{31}P-MRS is suitable for the repeated study of cardiac high-energy phosphate metabolism, to noninvasively monitor the energetic state of the heart (see above for metabolites visible in a ^{31}P spectrum). ATP is the only substrate for all energy-consuming reactions in the cell. Phosphocreatine, the other major high-energy phosphate compound, acts as an energy reservoir and has at least two additional roles: First, it serves as an energy transport molecule in the 'creatine kinase (CK)/phosphocreatine energy shuttle'[11,12] (Figure 3.2). The high-energy phosphate bond is transferred from ATP to creatine at the site of ATP production (i.e. the mitochondria), yielding phosphocreatine and ADP. This reaction is catalyzed by the mitochondrial creatine kinase isoenzyme (CK$_{Mito}$). Phosphocreatine, which is a smaller molecule than ATP, then diffuses through the cytoplasm to the site of ATP utilization, the myofibrils, where the back-reaction occurs, ATP is reformed and is used for contraction. This reaction is catalyzed by the myofibrillar-bound MM-creatine kinase isoenzyme (CK-MM). Free creatine then diffuses back to the mitochondria. This 'energy shuttle' is required because the low free cytosolic ADP concentration (40–80 μM) does not provide the necessary capacity for back-diffusion to the mitochondria,[11,13] while free creatine is present at concentrations that are at least two orders of magnitude greater. The second crucial cellular function of phosphocreatine and CK is to maintain free cytosolic ADP at low concentration. Free ADP cannot be measured directly, but is calculated from the CK equilibrium assumption:

$$[ADP] = \frac{[ATP] \times [creatine]}{[PCr] \times [H^+] \times K_{eq}},$$

where [...] denotes concentration, PCr is phosphocreatine, [H$^+$] is the intracellular hydrogen ion concentration, and K_{eq} is the equilibrium constant of the CK reaction.

A low free cytosolic ADP concentration is required for normal cardiac function, because ADP determines the free-energy change of ATP hydrolysis (ΔG, in kJ mol^{-1}), a measure of the amount of energy released from ATP hydrolysis:

$$\Delta G = \Delta G_o + RT \ln \frac{[ADP] \times [P_i]}{[ATP]},$$

where ΔG_o is the standard free-energy change at 37°C, R is the universal gas constant, T is the temperature in Kelvin, and P$_i$ is inorganic phosphate.

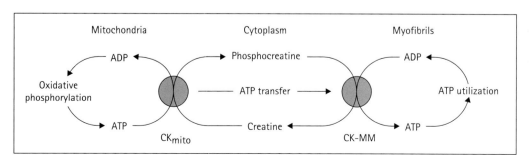

Figure 3.2
The creatine kinase-phosphocreatine energy shuttle. For details, see text.

In the normal heart, ΔG is ~ -58 kJ mol^{-1}. Many intracellular enzymes such as SR-Ca^{2+}-ATPase will not function properly below a threshold value for ΔG of about -52 kJ mol^{-1}.

When ATP is hydrolyzed, inorganic phosphate is formed: ATP $\rightleftharpoons$ ADP + P$_i$. Inorganic phosphate increases when ATP utilization exceeds ATP production, for example during ischemia. ^{31}P-CMS also allows the quantification of intracellular pH (pH$_i$), from the chemical shift difference between phosphocreatine and inorganic phosphate, which is pH-sensitive.

^{31}P-MRS has been widely used for the study of cardiac energy metabolism under various experimental conditions. In isolated perfused heart, the effects of perfusion with various metabolic substrates have been studied: for example, phosphocreatine concentrations are higher for pyruvate and/or fatty acid substrates and for perfusion with blood (phosphocreatine/ATP ratio $\sim$1.5–2.0) than when glucose is the only substrate (phosphocreatine/ATP ratio $\sim$1.3).[2] A much debated subject is the effect of changes in cardiac workload on cardiac energetics. While moderate changes in workload do not alter energetics,[14] substantial increases do, and, under these conditions, phosphocreatine levels decline.[15,16] ATP content remains constant with varying workload, due to the CK equilibrium favoring ATP synthesis over phosphocreatine synthesis by a factor of $\sim$100. Thus, for any stress situation, including ischemia, ATP will only decrease when phosphocreatine levels are substantially depleted, and this is why the phosphocreatine/ATP ratio is a sensitive indicator of the energetic state of the heart. ^{31}P-MRS has been widely used to study the changes of myocardial energy metabolism in ischemia and reperfusion (e.g. Clarke et al[17]). A related injury model is hypoxia/reoxygenation; hypoxia differs from ischemia in that only oxygen supply is stopped while perfusion and substrate supply are maintained. Figure 3.3 shows an example of the changes in cardiac energy metabolism during control, hypoxia, and reoxygenation: after 30 min of hypoxia, ATP resonances are reduced by $\sim$50%, phosphocreatine by $\sim$80%, and inorganic phosphate and monophosphate esters have increased. During reoxygenation, inorganic phosphate shows full, phosphocreatine partial, and ATP no recovery. We showed that, when hearts are pretreated with a Ca^{2+} antagonist, changes in energetics are attenuated: verapamil protected hearts from the effects of hypoxic injury.[18] An important study by Clarke et al[17] demonstrated that changes of energetics after the onset of ischemia occur extremely rapidly: the decrease of phosphocreatine and the increase of inorganic phosphate were amongst the very earliest metabolic responses in myocardial ischemia, changing only seconds after its onset, while ATP and pH$_i$ are much slower to decrease, i.e. only after several minutes. In this study, a temporal resolution of 12 s was achieved by summing spectra from several experiments. This study demonstrates that, if we were successful in detecting the changes in energetics in human myocardium with high temporal and spatial resolution, we could directly image parameters that detect myocardial ischemia within seconds after its onset. No other diagnostic approach currently achieves this.

A unique aspect of ^{31}P-MRS is the measurement of the rate and velocity of chemical reactions in vivo, using the

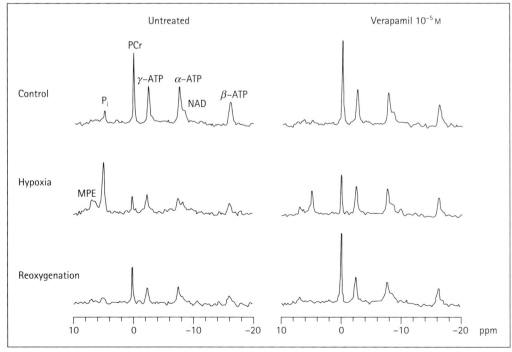

Figure 3.3
^{31}P-MR spectra from an untreated perfused rat heart and a heart treated with verapamil during control, at the end of 30 min of hypoxia, and at the end of 30 min of reperfusion. NAD, nicotine adenine dinucleotide. For details, see text. (Reproduced from Neubauer S, Ingwall JS. J Mol Cell Cardiol 1989; 21:1163–78,[18] with permission from Academic Press Limited.)

magnetization (saturation) transfer method (see, e.g. reference 19). In heart, the CK and ATP synthesis reactions can be quantified. It was shown, for example, that CK reaction velocity, a measure of ATP transfer from mitochondria to myofibrils, correlates with cardiac workload.[15] During recovery after ischemia, CK reaction velocity is closely correlated with recovery of mechanical function.[20] It is important to apply this method to the human heart,[21] which has yet to be done in patients with heart disease.

Experimental ^{31}P-MRS studies have substantially contributed to our understanding of the role of energetics in heart failure. Various heart failure models have been examined, such as the spontaneously hypertensive rat,[22] the Syrian cardiomyopathic hamster,[23,24] furazolidone-induced cardiomyopathy in the turkey,[25] and, as the clinically most relevant model, chronic coronary artery ligation in the rat[19] and pig.[26] Uniformly, and independently of the etiology of heart failure, the failing myocardium shows a characteristic energetic phenotype: reduced phosphocreatine, unchanged or moderately (by <30%) reduced ATP, unchanged or increased inorganic phosphate, and substantially reduced CK reaction velocity (parameters measured with ^{31}P-MRS). Furthermore, total creatine content and total and mitochondrial CK activities are decreased and fetal BB- and MB-CK isoenzymes increase (parameters measured with other biochemical techniques). These changes are likely to contribute to the impairment of contractile reserve in failing myocardium, most likely due to the failure to maintain appropriate ΔG values during inotropic stimulation.[27] Horn et al[28] have provided strong evidence for a causal role of cardiac energetics in chronically infarcted rat hearts. Rats were treated with a creatine analogue, β-guanidinopropionate, following myocardial infarction (MI) for 2 months. This led to an 85% depletion of phosphocreatine content as measured by ^{31}P-MRS. Under these conditions, failing rat hearts were unable to maintain normal ATP homeostasis, and ATP levels declined; this was not observed for nonfailing hearts. Remarkably, when rats were pretreated with β-guanidinopropionate and phosphocreatine was depleted before MI was induced, the 24-hour mortality rate of left anterior descending (LAD) coronary artery ligation was 100%, as compared with a standard mortality in this model of 40%. These results show that failing hearts with severely depleted phosphocreatine levels cannot maintain normal ATP homeostasis and that high phosphocreatine levels are required to survive the stress of an acute MI, demonstrating the importance of the CK/phosphocreatine system under acute and chronic cardiac stress conditions. Results of these experimental ^{31}P-MRS investigations have led scientists to study the failing human myocardium by ^{31}P-MRS (see below).

Most experimental ^{31}P-MRS studies were performed without spatial localization or with the crude localization achieved with surface coils. However, spectroscopic imaging in one[29] or three[30] dimensions has also been reported, allowing the noninvasive measurement of regional heterogeneity of cardiac energy metabolism (Figure 3.4). In large animals such as the dog and pig, Zhang and co-workers[31,32] were able to obtain ^{31}P spectra from five distinct voxels spanning the left ventricular wall, thereby examining transmural heterogeneity of energy metabolism. These studies suggest that during cardiac stress, energetic changes are more pronounced in the subendocardium than in the subepicardium.

Other MRS-detectable nuclei (^{1}H, ^{13}C, [23]Na)

[1]H shows the highest MR sensitivity of all MR-detectable nuclei, as well as high natural abundance (Table 3.1). In principle, many metabolites can be detected by ^{1}H-MRS, since ^{1}H is contained in a large number of metabolites, the most relevant of which are creatine, lactate, carnitine, taurine and CH_3 and CH_2 resonances of lipids.[33–35] Particularly promising is the noninvasive measurement of total creatine,[36,37] which, in conjunction with ^{31}P-MRS should allow the noninvasive determination of the ultimately relevant energetic parameters, namely free ADP and ΔG of ATP hydrolysis. Furthermore, tissue oxygenation can be probed noninvasively by ^{1}H-MRS, using the oxymyoglobin and deoxymyoglobin resonances.[38] However, ^{1}H-MRS is technically demanding, and pulse sequences suppressing the strong ^{1}H signal from water are required. The complex ^{1}H spectra show overlapping resonances, many of which still have to be characterized. However, because of the high sensitivity of signal detection, of all MRS-detectable nuclei, ^{1}H-MRS may in the long term have the greatest potential for clinical application.

The ^{13}C nucleus has a low natural abundance (~1%). Thus, for a ^{13}C-MRS experiment, the heart has to be supplied with ^{13}C-labelled compounds such as [1-^{13}C]glucose. Typically, these are added to perfusion media or infused into a coronary artery during a defined study protocol. Substrate utilization by the heart[39,40] is then investigated, or the activities of key enzymes or entire metabolic pathways are quantified (e.g. citric acid cycle flux, pyruvate dehydrogenase flux, and β-oxidation of fatty acids[41–44]). ^{13}C-MRS studies have allowed the study of intermediary metabolism in animal models of heart disease. However, clinical applications have yet to be reported for the heart, because of the following methodological limitations: (1) the MR sensitivity of the ^{13}C nucleus is too low to allow for spatially resolved detection in a reasonable measuring time; (2) the required high concentrations of exogenous ^{13}C-labelled precursors are unphysiological;

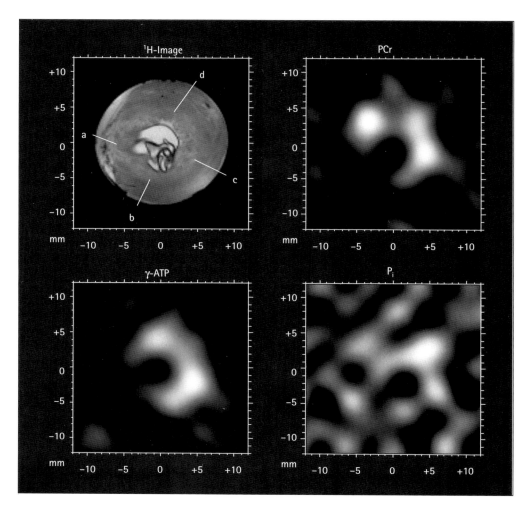

Figure 3.4
Central slices of a 3D ^{31}P chemical shift imaging experiment in an isolated, chronically infarcted rat heart (12 T, nominal voxel size 54 μl). On the ^{1}H image (upper left), the infarcted area in the anterior wall ('a') appears just barely brighter than the unaffected myocardium. In ^{31}P images, however, the infarcted area can be identified due to the complete absence of phosphocreatine (PCr; upper right) and of γ-ATP (lower left). Inorganic phosphate (P_i) cannot be detected due to its low concentration (lower right). (Reproduced from Von Kienlin M et al. Magn Reson Med 1998; 39:731–41,[30] with permission from John Wiley & Sons, New York.)

and (3) for in vivo studies, it is necessary to infuse the ^{13}C-labelled compounds directly into a coronary artery.

^{23}Na-MRS is the only noninvasive method that can evaluate changes in intra- and extracellular Na^+ during cardiac injury.[45,46] Maintenance of the sarcolemmal Na^+ concentration gradient (~140 mM extracellular versus ~10 mM intracellular) is a requirement for normal cardiac function. During membrane depolarization, Na^+ enters the cardiomyocyte through the 'fast' Na^+ channel; Na^+ is removed from the cell by high-capacity Na^+/K^+-ATPase. Additionally, Na^+ is transported via $Na^+–Ca^{2+}$ and $Na^+–H^+$ exchange mechanisms. A ^{23}Na spectrum from the heart shows only one peak representing the total Na^+ signal. For intra- and extracellular Na^+ pools to be discriminated, paramagnetic shift reagents, such as $[DyTTHA]^{3-}$ or $[TmDOTP]^{5-}$, have to be added to the perfusate. These high-molecular-weight chelate complexes are distributed in the extracellular compartments but do not enter the intracellular space. Na^+ in the close vicinity of shift reagents undergoes a downfield chemical shift of its resonance frequency (Figure 3.5). This method has been used experimentally to examine the mechanisms of

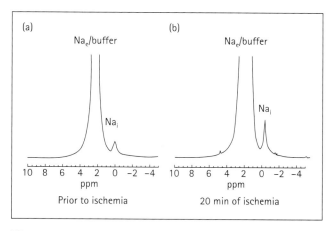

Figure 3.5
^{23}Na-MR spectra from an isolated rat heart: (a) during perfusion with buffer containing shift reagent and (b) in the same heart after 20 min of ischemia. The unshifted Na peak at 0 ppm represents the intracellular Na pool (Na_i). The shifted peak at 2.5 ppm arises predominantly from Na in the buffer (in the surrounding bath) and from Na in the extracellular myocardial space (Na_e). (Reproduced from Weidensteiner C et al. Magn Reson Med 2002; 48:89–96,[54] with permission from John Wiley & Sons, New York.)

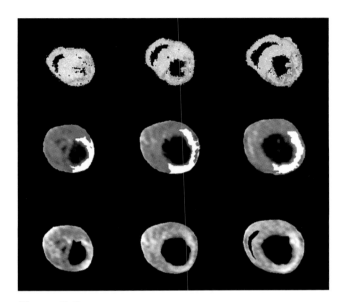

Figure 3.6
Bottom row: Three adjacent slices of a 3D ^{23}Na-MRI dataset in an isolated rat heart 4 weeks post myocardial infarction after segmentation. Middle row: The region with signal elevation of double standard deviation over mean in the ^{23}Na image is delineated in white, and is chosen for infarct size measurement. Top row: corresponding histological slices with stained infarcted area. The area of increased ^{23}Na signal intensity closely matches the histological scar area ($r = 0.91$; $p < 0.0001$). (Reproduced from Horn M et al. Magn Reson Med 2001; 45:756–64,[52] with permission from John Wiley & Sons, New York.)

intracellular Na^+ accumulation in ischemia–reperfusion injury[47,48] or the mechanisms of ventricular fibrillation, which is preceded by accumulation of intracellular Na^+.[49] It would be highly desirable to develop ^{23}Na-MR shift reagents for clinical use, but these are currently not yet available. Experimental MR imaging of total ^{23}Na (which does not require the use of shift reagents) was first reported by DeLayre et al.[50] In acute ischemia, the total myocardial ^{23}Na-MRI signal increases due to the breakdown of ion homeostasis (see above) and the formation of both intra- and extracellular edema (see e.g. reference 51). Furthermore, we have shown that the total Na signal remains significantly elevated during chronic scar formation in the rat post-MI model[52] because of the expansion of the extracellular space in scar (Figure 3.6), and the area of elevated ^{23}Na signal correlated closely with histologically determined infarct size. In contrast, ^{23}Na content is not elevated in akinetic but stunned or hibernating myocardium.[52] These experiments form the basis for our hypothesis that ^{23}Na-MRI may allow detection of myocardial viability without the use of external contrast agents (such as are required for 'late enhancement' Gd-DTPA viability imaging[53]). Due to the relatively high sensitivity of ^{23}Na and its short T1, allowing for rapid TRs, total

^{23}Na-MRI appears feasible in humans (see below). We recently also reported, for the first time, on ^{23}Na-MR chemical shift imaging of intracellular Na (Na_i) in perfused hearts, using a ^{23}Na-MR shift reagent.[54] In hearts with an acute occlusion of the LAD coronary artery, we demonstrated a local Na_i signal increase in the anterior wall in the range of 60–110% compared with remote, normoxic tissue.

Experimental MRS studies in genetically manipulated mice

In recent years, interest in experimental MRS has been steadily growing, largely due to the advent of genetically manipulated mice. Transgenic technology is providing new strains of mice in which key metabolic regulators are either deleted (knockout) or overexpressed, and these new models are likely to offer new insight into the mechanisms regulating cardiac metabolism in the normal and failing heart. MRS is an ideal technique to study the metabolic consequences of genetic alterations in the perfused heart model (see, e.g. references 55 and 56), and techniques for MRS in mice in vivo are also being developed by a number of groups around the world. This will be illustrated by several recent important examples.

Combined assessment of cardiac metabolism and function in anaesthetized mice in vivo has been reported, maintaining close to physiological heart rates of ~600 bpm,[57] and using spatially localized ^{31}P-MRS with 1D chemical shift imaging to obtain cardiac ^{31}P-MR spectra at 4.7 T. The phosphocreatine/ATP ratio was found to be 2.0 ± 0.2, a value similar to that reported for human heart. The MR-determined ejection fraction was $65 \pm 7\%$. Thus, cardiac function and metabolism can now be measured simultaneously in mice in vivo at physiological heart rates. This approach should find widespread use for the study of new genetically manipulated mouse models with altered cardiac metabolism. The finding of similar phosphocreatine/ATP ratios for human and mouse suggests that the mouse is an appropriate model for studies of cardiac energetics.

Mice with knockout of CK genes ('single' M-CK or 'double' M- and mitochondrial CK knockout) provide new insight into the role of CK in heart.[58,59] Isolated perfused hearts from mice with double-CK knockout (residual CK activity 3% of control) show unchanged isovolumic function, a ~30% reduction in phosphocreatine levels, and a 99% reduction in CK flux, i.e. of high-energy phosphate bond shuttling between ATP and phosphocreatine. Thus, these hearts have almost no functional CK shuttle, with the CK shuttle rate being 9% of that of ATP production rate by mitochondria. Compared with wild-type controls, these mice show greater increases in free ADP levels under metabolic stress[60] and cannot improve their free-energy change of ATP hydrolysis when perfused with an optimal substrate (pyruvate). While this study nicely demonstrates the metabolic consequences of CK knockout, this model, like many other gene knockout models, is characterized by major ultrastructural changes, including increased mitochondrial mass and shortening of intracellular diffusion distances.[61] Thus, in the CK knockout model, the structural adaptations occurring in response to CK knockout are revealing more about the true function of CK in heart than phenotype measurements of cardiac function or metabolism.

The GLUT4 protein is the predominantly insulin-sensitive sarcolemmal glucose transporter, responsible for a substantial portion of overall glucose uptake by the heart. Mice with knockout of GLUT4 have been shown to develop severe left ventricular hypertrophy and a 30% loss of systolic function. ^{31}P-MRS studies of these mice in vivo[62] have shown a ~60% increase in the cardiac phosphocreatine/ATP ratio, and, as ATP levels were unchanged, a ~60% increase in phosphocreatine and total creatine levels (Figure 3.7). This is a remarkable finding in that this is the only condition described so far where phosphocreatine or total creatine levels are increased to supernormal values, and this has occurred in the setting of

left ventricular hypertrophy, where, typically, phosphocreatine levels are decreased. The molecular mechanisms behind this unusual finding of increased phosphocreatine and creatine content require further study.

^{1}H-MRS is also beginning to make contributions to noninvasive phenotyping of the metabolic consequences of genetic manipulation: the myoglobin knockout mouse was demonstrated to show complete absence of the ^{1}H-MRS signals for myoglobin.[63] It is predicted that in the coming years the number of research centres using a combination of MRI and MRS methods to noninvasively phenotype genetically manipulated mice will grow rapidly.

Clinical studies

Methods for clinical cardiac MRS

Almost all previous human cardiac MR spectroscopy studies have interrogated the ^{31}P nucleus. Clinical cardiac spectroscopy faces major technical challenges, and this is the main reason for the slow progress with the method. To be clinically practical, the total examination time (for both imaging and spectroscopy) should not be more than 1 hour, and thus time for signal acquisition is limited. The heart is a rapidly moving organ, currently requiring gating to the heartbeat, and, when resolution is further improved, ultimately to respiration as well.[64] Clinical MR systems operate at 1.5 T (more recently also 3 T), i.e. at a considerably lower field than the equivalent animal systems. The cardiac muscle lies behind the chest wall skeletal muscle, which by itself creates a strong ^{31}P signal that requires suppression. This necessitates the use of localization techniques. Localization methods proposed for the MRS study of the human heart include DRESS (depth-resolved surface coil spectroscopy), rotating frame, 1D-CSI (chemical shift imaging), ISIS (image-selected in vivo spectroscopy), and 3D-CSI (Figure 3.8). A full review of these methods is available elsewhere.[65] Most of the methodological contributions to human cardiac MRS have been pioneered by Bottomley et al.[66–68] Although less comfortable for the patient, most MRS studies have been performed in a prone position rather than supine: this reduces motion artifacts as well as the distance from the heart to the surface coil, thus improving sensitivity. For most spectroscopic techniques, a stack of ^{1}H scout images is first obtained, which is used to select the spectroscopic volume(s). The low sensitivity of ^{31}P-MRS has required large voxel sizes, typically ~30 ml. A typical ^{31}P-MR spectrum of a healthy volunteer is shown in Figure 3.9. Compared with the rat heart spectrum, the SNR is lower, and two additional resonances are detected: 2,3-diphosphoglycerate (2,3-DPG), due to the presence of blood (erythrocytes) in the interrogated voxel, and phosphodi-

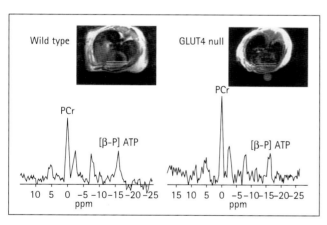

Figure 3.7
Image-guided, spatially localized ^{31}P MRS of an intact mouse. Representative axial [1]H-MR images (above) and ^{31}P-MR spectra (below) acquired in the same examination without repositioning the animals are presented from a wild-type (left) and a GLUT4 knockout (right) mouse. ^{31}P-MR spectra from the cardiac regions (slice thickness 1 mm) annotated on the ^{1}H spin-echo, axial MR images indicate the relative myocardial content of phosphocreatine (PCr) and ATP under these noninvasive, lightly sedated conditions. Note that the heart is larger and the myocardial phosphocreatine/ATP ratio is higher in the GLUT4 knockout than in the wild-type animal. (Reproduced from Weiss RG et al. FASEB J 2002; 16:613–15,[62] with permission from the Federation of American Societies for Experimental Biology, Bethesda, MD.)

esters (PDE), a signal due to membrane as well as serum phospholipids. The 2,3-diphosphoglycerate resonances overlap with the inorganic phosphate peak, which therefore cannot be detected in blood-contaminated human ^{31}P-MR spectra, and thus intracellular pH also cannot be determined; intracellular inorganic phosphate and pH will ultimately be detectable in human myocardium when spatial resolution is sufficient to avoid significant blood contamination of ^{31}P spectra. Relative quantification of human ^{31}P spectra is immediately straightforward, and the phosphocreatine/ATP and phosphodiester/ATP peak area ratios are calculated. Phosphocreatine/ATP is considered an index of the energetic state of the heart (see the section above on experimental animal studies). The meaning of the phosphodiester/ATP ratio remains poorly understood, and this ratio may not change with cardiac disease. Human ^{31}P resonances require correction for the effects of partial saturation according to the principles described for experimental MRS. At 1.5 T, the phosphocreatine T1 is $\sim 4.4 \pm 0.5$ s, and that of ATP is $\sim 2.4 \pm 0.4$ s.[65] Experimental studies suggest that [31]P T1 values remain constant in the presence of cardiac disease,[19,20] but this remains to be studied in detail. [31]P spectra also require correction for the amount of blood contamination: blood contributes signal to the ATP, 2,3-diphosphoglycerate, and phosphodiester resonances of a cardiac ^{31}P spectrum. As human blood spectra show an ATP/2,3-diphosphoglycerate area ratio of ~ 0.11 and a phosphodiester/ 2,3-diphosphoglycerate area ratio of ~ 0.19, for blood correction, the ATP resonance area of cardiac spectra is reduced by 11% of the 2,3-diphosphoglycerate resonance area, and the phosphodiester resonance area is reduced by 19% of the 2,3-diphosphoglycerate resonance area.[69] [31]P metabolite ratios in blood also change in the presence of disease,[70] which should be taken into account when blood-correcting spectra. Blood correction will hopefully no longer be required when voxel sizes are further reduced to allow acquisition of uncontaminated spectra. For area integration of resonances in human ^{31}P spectra, a time-domain or frequency-domain Lorentzian line-fitting algorithm is applied.

Absolute quantification of phosphocreatine and ATP is technically demanding, but is clearly a necessity in the long term, as the phosphocreatine/ATP ratio cannot detect simultaneous decreases in both phosphocreatine and ATP, which occur, for example, in the failing[71] or in the infarcted non-viable[72] myocardium. In principle, absolute ^{31}P metabolite levels can be quantified by obtaining simultaneous signal from a ^{31}P standard as well as estimates of myocardial mass based on MRI.[67] An alternative approach[68] uses simultaneous acquisition of a ^{1}H spectrum, which is used to calibrate the ^{31}P signal to the tissue water proton content. Von Kienlin and colleagues[73] have developed an advanced technique, SLOOP (spectral localization with optimum pointspread function), that

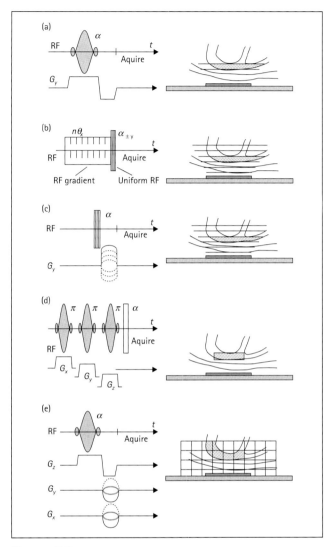

Figure 3.8
Basic pulse sequences for localized cardiac MRS with surface coils. (a) DRESS (Depth-resolved surface coil spectroscopy): a single section parallel to the plane of the surface coil is selected by applying an MR imaging gradient G in the presence of a modulated radiofrequency (RF) excitation pulse of flip angle α. (b) The 'rotating frame' MR method uses the gradient inherent in a surface coil to simultaneously spatially encode spectra from multiple sections parallel to the surface coil by means of the application of a θ flip angle pulse, which is stepped in subsequent applications of the sequence. (c) 1D-CSI (one-dimensional chemical shift imaging) similarly encodes multiple sections but uses an MR imaging gradient whose amplitude is stepped. (d) ISIS (image-selected in vivo spectroscopy) localizes to a single volume with selective inversion pulses applied with G_x, G_y and G_z MR imaging gradients; all eight combinations of the three pulses must be applied and the resultant signals added and subtracted. (e) A section-selective 3D-CSI (three-dimensional chemical shift imaging) sequence employs MR imaging section selection in one dimension and phase encoding in two dimensions. (Reproduced from Bottomley P. Radiology 1994; 191:593–612,[65] with permission from the Radiological Society of North America.)

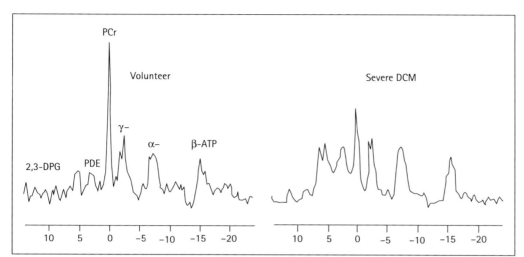

Figure 3.9
^{31}P-MR spectra from the human heart of a volunteer and of a patient with dilated cardiomyopathy (DCM). The reduction of the phosphocreatine (PCr) resonance in the patient is apparent. (Reproduced from Neubauer S et al. Eur Heart J 1995; 16(Suppl O):115–18,[106] with permission from WB Saunders Company Ltd.)

achieves both better compartment matching by allowing curved regions of interest that are better suiting the shape of the heart, and absolute quantification with high accuracy. This method requires the use of a ^{31}P reference standard, flip angle calibration, precise B_1 field mapping and determination of myocardial mass in the interrogated voxel. This technique is now being put to use in clinical studies of heart disease (see below).

In the long term, it will also be important to combine ^{31}P- and ^{1}H-MRS in human cardiac spectroscopy for measurement of the ultimately energetically relevant parameters free ADP and ΔG of ATP hydrolysis, as described in canine myocardium.[36] Another highly relevant energetic parameter that has so far escaped measurement in human myocardium is the rate and extent of ATP transfer from the site of ATP production (the mitochondria) to the site of ATP utilization (the myofibrils). As described above, in isolated perfused hearts, this can be quantified using the saturation transfer method. This measurement has previously been impractical in humans, since direct implementation of the experimental method would lead to measurement times of several hours. Bottomley et al[74] have developed the FAST (four-angle saturation transfer) method, which allows measurement of creatine kinase flux in ~30 min. This employs acquisition of four spectra under partially saturated conditions. In two acquisitions, one of the exchanging species is saturated. The other two employ a control saturation. Each pair of saturations is applied with two different flip angles, and the equilibrium magnetization, relaxation times, and reaction rates are calculated from these measurements. CK reaction rates were found to be 0.29 ± 0.06 s^{-1} in healthy volunteers. It will be important to apply this method in clinical studies.

Due to its distance from the ^{31}P surface coil, it has previously been impossible to interrogate the posterior wall of the human heart. However, Pohmann and von Kienlin[75] have implemented acquisition-weighted ^{31}P chemical shift imaging in volunteers at 2 T. Acquisition weighting significantly reduced the signal contamination between adjacent voxels, and it was possible to obtain human heart ATP and phosphocreatine images with 16 ml spatial resolution within 30 min (Figure 3.10). Furthermore, for the first time, ^{31}P spectra from the posterior wall could be obtained. If implemented at higher field (3 or 4 T) in the future, this method might make higher-resolution cardiac ^{31}P metabolic imaging a reality.

A major technical development effort is required to make clinical cardiac MRS more practical and relevant. This will include advances in coil and sequence design, and implementation of MRS at higher field strengths.[76,77] A major effort will also be required to develop generally accepted technical standards for the acquisition and processing of human cardiac MRS, so that measurements from different centers can be compared directly.

Normal human myocardium

In normal human heart, the phosphocreatine/ATP ratio is ~1.8,[65] although, due to the different methods being used, the range of 'normal' phosphocreatine/ATP ratios reported in the literature is considerable, ranging from about 1.1 to 2.4. This underscores the need for developing generally accepted methodological standards. Using SLOOP (see above) for absolute concentration measurements, we have reported that phosphocreatine levels in normal human myocardium are 9.0 ± 1.2 and ATP levels 5.3 ± 1.2 mmol/kg wet weight. These numbers agree with measurements in animal hearts in vivo.[18,71] There is some debate as to whether high-energy phosphate levels decrease with advancing age,[78] but larger systematic studies on this issue are still outstanding.

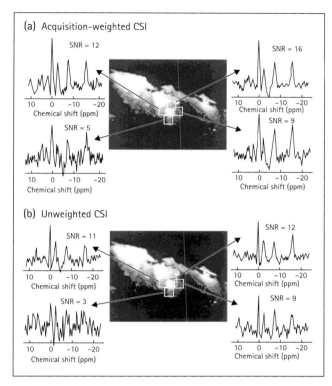

Figure 3.10
Results of (a) acquisition-weighted and (b) unweighted ^{31}P chemical shift imaging (CSI) experiments on a healthy volunteer. For both experiments, four spectra from the same voxel positions are shown. The nominal voxel size was $2.5 \times 2.5 \times 4.0$ cm^3, and each experiment consisted of 2048 scans synchronized to the heartbeat. SNR, signal-to-noise ratio. The spectra obtained with acquisition weighting show a considerably higher phosphocreatine/ATP ratio and a higher SNR for the phosphocreatine and ATP signals. Also, high-resolution spectra from the posterior wall can be obtained. (Reproduced from Pohmann R, von Kienlin M. Magn Reson Med 2001; 45:817–26,[75] with permission from John Wiley & Sons, New York.)

Ischemic heart disease

This is potentially the largest field for clinical application of ^{31}P-MRS, mainly with regard to two aspects: detection of exercise induced ischemia and assessment of myocardial viability.

Detection of exercise-induced ischemia

A decrease in phosphocreatine and an increase in inorganic phosphate are amongst the very earliest metabolic responses in myocardial ischemia (see above), changing within seconds after reduction of oxygen supply. Thus, if we were able to detect these metabolites in human myocardium with high temporal and spatial resolution, we would come close to the 'ideal' diagnostic tool for detecting exercise-induced regional ischemia (i.e. highly sensitive, no intravenous agents, no radiation). Such a 'biochemical stress test' would allow the detection of the regional biochemical consequences of myocardial ischemia at rest and during exercise and recovery. While high-resolution metabolic imaging for this approach is not yet feasible, in selected patients with large anterior wall territories, which become ischemic on exercise, the principal feasibility has been demonstrated: Weiss et al[79] (Figure 3.11) showed that in patients with high-grade LAD stenosis, phosphocreatine/ATP ratios were normal at rest; phosphocreatine/ATP decreased during hand grip exercise (a 30–35% increase in cardiac work) from 1.5 ± 0.3 to 0.9 ± 0.2, and returned towards normal during recovery from exercise. After revascularization (percutaneous transluminal coronary angioplasty (PTCA) or bypass operation), phosphocreatine/ATP ratios no longer changed with exercise. These findings were reproduced by Yabe et al,[80] who also demonstrated that a decrease in phosphocreatine/ATP ratios could only be detected in patients with reversible defects on thallium scintigraphy (presumably viable myocardium) but not in

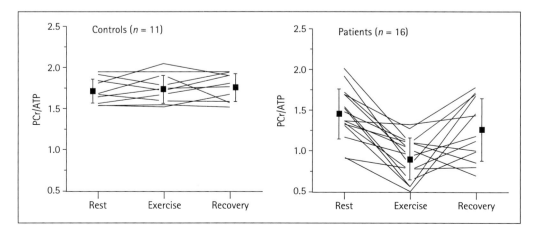

Figure 3.11
Phosphocreatine (PCr)/ATP ratios at rest and during handgrip exercise and recovery in controls and in patients with stenosis of the left anterior descending coronary artery. PCr/ATP decreased in patients but not in healthy volunteers. (Reproduced from Weiss RG et al. N Engl J Med 1990; 323:1593–600.[79] © 1990 Massachusetts Medical Society)

those with fixed thallium defects (presumably scar), where phosphocreatine/ATP was already reduced at rest.[72] If high spatial (1–5 ml) and temporal (stress duration <15 min) resolution for this approach could be achieved, then there is no doubt that this method would find its way into routine cardiology. A ^{31}P-MRS stress test would, for example, allow the noninvasive study of the efficiency of revascularization procedures or of various anti-anginal therapies. To speculate, a 'phosphocreatine threshold' may emerge as a clinically relevant parameter, representing the level of exercise achievable without a decrease in myocardial phosphocreatine concentrations, allowing objective fine-tuning of anti-anginal therapy. Another important clinical application of ^{31}P-MRS stress testing has been reported by Pohost's group:[81] the pathophysiologic mechanisms of exercise-induced chest pain in women with normal coronary arteries remain debated, but microvascular dysfunction and subsequent tissue ischemia in the absence of macroscopic coronary stenoses has been postulated as a likely cause. In 7 of 35 women with chest pain and normal coronary arteries, the phosphocreatine/ATP ratio decreased by 29% ± 5% during handgrip exercise (Figure 3.12). These findings, for the first time, provide direct evidence of exercise-induced myocardial ischemia in a subgroup of women with chest

pain and normal coronary arteries. ^{31}P-MRS stress testing may facilitate the development and monitoring of treatment for this ubiquitous condition.

Assessment of myocardial viability

The second area for potential clinical application of ^{31}P-MRS in ischemic heart disease is the assessment of myocardial viability. Akinetic (i.e. noncontracting) myocardium, supplied by a stenotic coronary artery, may be non-viable (scarred), in which case revascularization by PTCA or bypass grafting cannot improve contractility and is probably of little or no clinical benefit. Alternatively, akinetic myocardium may be viable (i.e. biochemically and morphologically largely intact), in which case it is either stunned or hibernating. Hibernating myocardium has downregulated contractility to reduce energy needs, thereby adjusting the balance between oxygen supply and demand.[82] Stunned myocardium is transiently and reversibly dysfunctional in spite of reperfusion after a reversible ischemic insult. Both biochemical[19] and ^{31}P-MRS[29,83] measurements in animal models have shown that myocardial scar tissue contains negligible amounts of ATP (<1% of normal levels), while in stunned and hibernat-

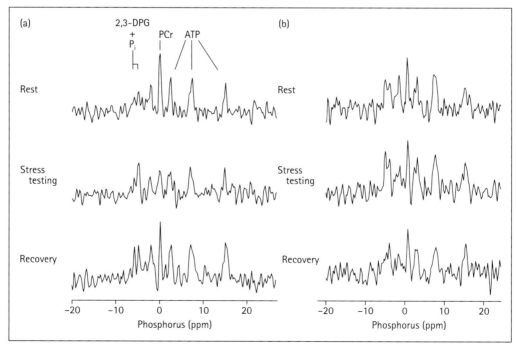

Figure 3.12

Results of ^{31}P-MRS in two women with chest pain and coronary artery stenosis of 20% or less. The woman whose results are shown in (a) had a significant decrease (27%) in the phosphocreatine/ATP ratio during stress testing, whereas the woman whose results are shown in (b) did not (a decrease of 1%). The peaks of phosphocreatine (PCr), ATP, and inorganic phosphate (P$_i$) plus 2,3-diphosphoglycerate (2,3-DPG) are identified in (a). In (b), there is little change in the phosphocreatine/ATP ratio from period to period. (Reproduced from Buchthal S et al. N Engl J Med 2000; 342:829–35.[81] © 2000 Massachusetts Medical Society)

ing[84] myocardium, ATP levels remain close to normal. Therefore, a noninvasive method that allows measurement of myocardial ATP levels with high spatial (1–5 ml) and acceptable temporal (<30 min) resolution should be ideal for evaluation of myocardial viability. Only three clinical studies have previously addressed this issue: Kalil-Filho et al[85] studied 29 patients with anterior infarction 4 and 39 days after MI. All patients showed akinetic anterior myocardium, which had recovered function at the time of the second examination. Phosphocreatine/ATP ratios were normal in stunned myocardium (1.51 ± 0.17 versus 1.61 ± 0.18 in volunteers), and did not change during the recovery of contractile function (1.51 ± 0.17 versus 1.53 ± 0.17). These observations were confirmed by Beer et al,[86] who also showed that in patients with nonviable infarcts, failing to recover regional contractile function after 6 months, ^{31}P-spectra showed complete absence of a phosphocreatine resonance. While these initial observations are interesting, loss of myocardial tissue (such as following a nonviable infarct leading to necrosis and scar formation) leads primarily to reductions in both phosphocreatine and ATP; thus, fundamentally, the extent of viable tissue loss cannot be detected using the phosphocreatine/ATP ratio. This requires measurement of absolute concentrations of high-energy phosphates. Only one clinical study on viability has previously attempted this: Yabe et al[72] showed that absolute myocardial ATP content was significantly reduced in patients with fixed thallium defects (nonviable myocardium) but was unchanged in patients with reversible defects (viable myocardium). While these initial results are promising, technical advances are required to achieve the necessary resolution to make ^{31}P-MRS evaluation of viability clinically practical. Viability assessment by ^{31}P-MRS only requires obtaining spectra at rest, and thus a high-resolution approach should be more easily achievable than for a biochemical stress test for detection of exercise-induced ischemia at rest and stress, where acquisition times are more limited.

A promising new technique for viability detection is measurement of the total creatine content by localized ^{1}H-MRS.[36,87] Scar tissue shows an almost complete loss of total creatine. Due to the higher MR sensitivity of ^{1}H and because the concentration of creatine CH_3 protons is ~10-fold higher than the ^{31}P concentrations of ATP, the resolution of ^{1}H-MRS is superior to that of ^{31}P-MRS, currently at ~1 ml. On the other hand, several methodological problems associated with ^{1}H-MRS (see above) remain to be solved until the method can clinically be more widely applied.

As described above for experimental animal studies, [23]Na-MRI may allow the detection of myocardial viability without the use of external contrast agents, since the myocardial [23]Na signal is elevated in both acute necrosis and chronic scar. Due to the 100% natural abundance, the relatively high MR sensitivity (9.3% of ^{1}H) and tissue concentration (~140 mM extracellular, ~10 mM intracellular) of [23]Na, and its short T1 (~30 ms at 1.5 T), allowing for short TR, next to ^{1}H, [23]Na offers the highest MRI resolution of all MR-detectable nuclei. [23]Na-MRI of total Na content has been established in humans with a resolution of up to 392 µl,[88,89] using an ECG-triggered 3D spoiled gradient-echo sequence (FLASH), with an acquisition time of ~1 hour (Figure 3.13). We have applied this method to study patients 8 days (subacute) and over 6 months (chronic) after acute MI, and have obtained the first in vivo [23]Na-MR images of infarcted human myocardium.[90] All patients after subacute infarction and

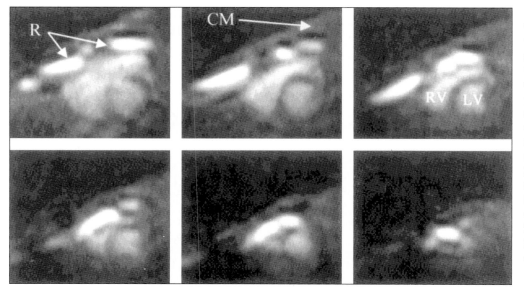

Figure 3.13

[23]Na-MRI of the human heart: six consecutive short-axis, ECG-gated FLASH images of a healthy male volunteer, showing the chest muscle (CM), ribs (R), right and left atrium, and the complete right (RV) and left (LV) ventricles. The in-plane resolution was 3.5 mm × 7.0 mm and the acquisition time 49 min. (Reproduced from Pabst T et al. Magn Reson Med 2001; 45:164–6,[89] with permission from John Wiley & Sons, New York.)

12 of 15 patients with chronic infarction had an area of elevated ^{23}Na signal intensity that correlated significantly with wall motion abnormalities. In a follow-up study, we are currently investigating whether an increased Na content accurately predicts myocardial viability, i.e. recovery of contractile function after 6 months. Further improvement of the spatial resolution of ^{23}Na-MRI (which currently requires minimum voxel volumes that are two orders of magnitude larger than those of ^{1}H-MRI late enhancement techniques) by the use of faster gradients, improved coils and higher field strength, as well as mapping of absolute Na content, are important requirements if ^{23}Na-MRI is to become a mainstream clinical viability assessment technique.

Thus, in principle, ^{31}P-MRS, ^{1}H-MRS and ^{23}Na-MRI/MRS provide an armamentarium of diagnostic tests that might in the future become an ideal approach for viability assessment. Unlike currently used techniques, such as dobutamine echocardiography, thallium scintigraphy, and positron emission tomography, the MRS approach has fundamental advantages: it is radiation-free, does not require the application of intravenous agents, and does not require stressing the heart, but instead provides intrinsic contrast for distinction between viable and nonviable myocardium. Furthermore, we believe that the mechanisms of contrast are fully understood – which cannot be said, for example, for the Gd-DTPA late enhancement technique. However, substantially higher resolution will first have to be achieved (see below) before systematic clinical studies comparing MRS with traditional methods of viability assessment can be undertaken.

Valvular heart disease

Experimental studies suggest alterations in myocardial energy metabolism for advanced left ventricular hypertrophy.[31,91] Accordingly, studying patients with left ventricular hypertrophy due to aortic stenosis or incompetence, Conway et al[92] demonstrated reduced phosphocreatine/ATP ratios (1.10 ± 0.32 versus 1.50 ± 0.20 in volunteers; mean $\pm$ SD) only when clinical signs of heart failure were present, while phosphocreatine/ATP ratios remained unchanged (1.56 ± 0.15) for clinically asymptomatic stages. Similarly, in patients with aortic valve disease, we showed a reduction of phosphocreatine/ATP ratios only for New York Heart Association (NYHA) classes III and IV but not for NYHA classes I and II.[93] For the same degree of heart failure, energy metabolism appeared to be affected more in aortic stenosis (pressure overload) than in aortic incompetence. In aortic stenosis, reductions in phosphocreatine/ATP ratios correlated with left ventricular end-diastolic pressures and also with end-diastolic wall stress.[93] Using the recently developed

SLOOP technique for absolute quantification (see above), we have reported unchanged absolute ATP concentrations and a 28% decrease in phosphocreatine concentrations in patients with aortic stenosis.[94] It is also possible to use ^{31}P-MRS to follow the time course of recovery of cardiac energetics during regression of hypertrophy following surgical valve replacement.[95] Patients with aortic valve stenosis were studied before and 40 weeks after surgery. During this time, the phosphocreatine/ATP ratio increased from 1.28 ± 0.17 to 1.47 ± 0.14 (control subjects 1.43 ± 0.14). Thus, cardiac energy metabolism normalized completely 9 months after valve replacement. It is conceivable that ^{31}P-MRS may in the future provide clinical information aiding the optimum timing for valve replacement. This question will have to be answered by a long-term prospective clinical study on this subject involving large numbers of patients.

Hypertension and 'athlete's heart'

Only three studies have examined patients with left ventricular hypertrophy due to chronic hypertension. Lamb et al[96] demonstrated reduced phosphocreatine/ATP ratios in patients with hypertension both at rest and during dobutamine-stress testing. Furthermore, phosphocreatine/ATP ratios correlated inversely with indices of diastolic function (E deceleration peak). In contrast, two other studies showed no significant changes in cardiac energetics in hypertension.[78,94] It is likely that differences in patient characteristics, such as severity and duration of hypertension, are responsible for this discrepancy, since experimental data clearly suggest that cardiac energetics are impaired in long-standing hypertension.[97] In advanced hypertensive heart disease, ^{31}P-MRS should allow the energetic correlates of hypertrophy regression during various forms of antihypertensive therapy to be followed.

Interestingly, 'physiological' hypertrophy in the athlete's heart differs from hypertrophy due to pathological causes in that the myocardial phosphocreatine/ATP ratio remains normal at rest and during stress;[98,99] experimental work in rats subjected to exercise training had predicted this finding.[100] The molecular mechanisms underlying these differences in energy metabolism between physiological and pathological myocardial hypertrophy are an important area for future research.

Heart failure

Experimental studies (see above) have universally shown reduced phosphocreatine, total creatine, and CK reaction velocity in chronically failing myocardium (see e.g. references 19 and 24). Initial clinical ^{31}P-MRS studies, however, which did not grade patients for the severity of heart failure and included mild stages, failed to detect significant reductions in phosphocreatine/ATP ratios.[101–104] Hardy et al[105] first demonstrated that the myocardial phosphocreatine/ATP ratio is significantly reduced (from 1.80 ± 0.06 to 1.46 ± 0.07) in symptomatic patients with heart failure of ischemic or nonischemic origin. We reported that the decrease of phosphocreatine/ATP ratios in dilated cardiomyopathy correlated with the clinical severity of heart failure according to NYHA class[69] and also with left ventricular ejection fraction.[106] Thus, phosphocreatine/ATP ratios decrease for the more symptomatic stages of heart failure (see also Figure 3.9) but remain normal initially. However, in heart failure, both phosphocreatine and ATP levels decrease in parallel,[71] and this cannot be detected by measurement of phosphocreatine/ATP ratios. Using the SLOOP technique for absolute quantification (see above), we have studied patients with heart failure due to dilated cardiomyopathy (ejection fraction 18%), and found that absolute phosphocreatine levels were reduced by 51% and ATP levels by 35%, while the phosphocreatine/ATP ratio decreased by 25% only.[94] Furthermore, we observed significant correlations between left ventricular volumes/ejection fraction and energetics, with the highest correlations being observed for phosphocreatine and the weakest for the phosphocreatine/ATP ratio. Thus, we demonstrated for the first time using noninvasive ^{31}P-MRS that ATP levels are significantly reduced in heart failure, and that the true extent of changes in energy metabolism in heart failure is underestimated when phosphocreatine/ATP ratios are measured rather than absolute concentrations. Therefore, measurement of absolute concentrations of high-energy phosphates should become the standard approach for human ^{31}P-MRS studies in heart failure as well as for other cardiac pathologies.

The energy-deprivation hypothesis in heart failure has recently gained fresh support, since an analysis of heart failure trials from the past decade shows that any treatment that is energy-costly (e.g. β-receptor mimetic and phosphodiesterase inhibitor drugs), while increasing cardiac output in the short term, has ultimately increased mortality, while any treatment that is energy-sparing (e.g. beta-blockers, angiotensin-converting enzyme (ACE) inhibitors, and angiotensin II receptor blockers), has improved survival in long-term studies. For clinical heart failure trials, it would thus be highly attractive to monitor the early energetic response of the myocardium to new classes of agents for the treatment of heart failure, and it is conceivable that the phosphocreatine/ATP ratio or absolute concentrations of phosphocreatine and ATP may be powerful surrogate parameters for mortality in heart failure trials. This hypothesis will be tested in the coming years. Our initial observation was that in 6 patients with

dilated cardiomyopathy treated with standard medical therapy including ACE inhibitors, digitalis, diuretics, and, in 4 patients, β-blockers, clinical recompensation occurred over 3 months. Over this time, the phosphocreatine/ATP ratio of the patients improved significantly from 1.51 ± 0.32 to 2.15 ± 0.27.[69] Apart from this early anecdotal evidence, no systematic study has been published so far using ^{31}P-MRS to monitor cardiac energetics during heart failure treatment. However, the first treatment trial using ^{31}P-MRS to monitor cardiac energetics has been reported in Friedreich's ataxia. This primarily neurological disease often leads to cardiomyopathy, due to deficiency of the mitochondrial protein frataxin, leading to deficient mitochondrial respiration and increased free-radical damage. Lodi et al[107] reported on patients with Friedreich's ataxia, who were treated with antioxidants (coenzyme Q and vitamin E) for 6 months. During this time, the myocardial phosphocreatine/ATP ratio increased from 1.34 ± 0.59 to 2.02 ± 0.43, demonstrating that cardiac energy metabolism was markedly improved by antioxidative treatment. Analogous heart failure trials are urgently awaited.

In line with the concept that energy-sparing forms of therapy improve prognosis in heart failure is our observation that phosphocreatine/ATP ratios hold prognostic information on the survival of patients with heart failure that extends beyond the prognostic relevance of clinical and hemodynamic variables. We showed that in dilated cardiomyopathy, the myocardial phosphocreatine/ATP ratio was a better predictor of long-term survival than left ventricular ejection fraction or NYHA class[108] (Figure 3.14).

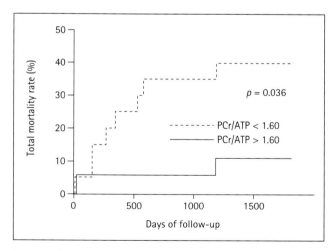

Figure 3.14
Kaplan–Meier life table analysis for total mortality of dilated cardiomyopathy patients divided into two groups split by the myocardial phosphocreatine (PCr)/ATP ratio (< 1.60 versus > 1.60). Patients with an initially low PCr/ATP ratio showed increased mortality over the study period of, on average, 2.5 years. (Reproduced from Neubauer S et al. Circulation 1997; 96:2190–6,[108] with permission from the American Heart Association.)

Thus, ^{31}P-MRS may become a tool for prognosis evaluation in heart failure. It is possible that determination of CK reaction velocity in heart failure will provide an even more relevant energetic index, but presently this parameter has been measured in volunteers only,[74] and studies in heart failure are eagerly awaited.

Cardiac transplantation

Experimental reports showed that ^{31}P-MRS can detect cardiac transplant rejection in animal models.[109,110] Thus, the hope had been that MRS might allow noninvasive diagnosis and monitoring of the degree of transplant rejection, reducing the need for repetitive biopsies. However, while phosphocreatine/ATP ratios were reduced in human transplanted hearts with histological evidence of rejection, there was no correlation with biopsy histology scores.[111] Phosphocreatine/ATP ratios also decrease during the first few weeks after transplantation as a result of transient perioperative myocardial ischemia,[112] slowly recovering thereafter. Thus, phosphocreatine/ATP ratios obtained at rest cannot predict transplant rejection. However, measurement of absolute concentrations of ATP and phosphocreatine may be more promising: myocyte mass is reduced by active rejection, and thus, while the phosphocreatine/ATP ratio may be unaltered, absolute ATP and phosphocreatine levels may be reduced. The transplanted heart also develops transplant vasculopathy, and Evanochko et al[113] hypothesized that ^{31}P-MRS stress measurements would therefore be a more sensitive indicator. They studied transplanted patients with rest and stress ^{31}P-MRS. Of 25 patients, 10 showed a substantial decrease in the phosphocreatine/ATP ratio of 26% ± 4% during exercise. Results of studies correlating absolute concentration measurements and stress testing with biopsy scores are eagerly awaited, since a reliable noninvasive test for accurate prediction of the degree of transplant rejection would be clinically highly relevant.

Genetic heart disease

One of the most promising areas for clinical cardiac ^{31}P-MRS is the noninvasive phenotyping of cardiomyopathies due to specific gene defects. While much work needs to be done, it is conceivable that specific gene defects may eventually be identifiable by a specific metabolic profile, as detected noninvasively by MRS. Most work in this area has so far concentrated on hypertrophic cardiomyopathy (HCM). HCM is, in most cases, due to well-characterized genetic mutations associated with substantial increases in left ventricular wall thickness and structural disarray of myofibrils.[114] Experimental studies of a transgenic mouse model of HCM suggest an alteration of cardiac energetics.[115] Similarly, human studies in HCM[79,103,104,116–118] have shown reduced phosphocreatine/ATP ratios in myocardial tissue affected by hypertrophy. The largest group of HCM patients has so far been reported by Jung et al,[119] who demonstrated that young, asymptomatic patients with HCM show a significantly reduced phosphocreatine/ATP ratio, indicating that energetic imbalance occurs at an early stage of the disease process. In follow-up work, they reported that HCM patients with a familial history of the disease, i.e. with an inherited genetic defect, showed a more pronounced derangement of energetics (phosphocreatine/ATP ratio 1.81 ± 0.28) than those patients without a family history (phosphocreatine/ATP ratio 2.10 ± 0.39).[120] In the future, large patient cohorts with HCM and identified specific gene defects will have to be studied to test the hypothesis that metabolic phenotyping using ^{31}P-MRS can noninvasively predict the specific genetic mutation present in individual HCM patients. As a technical point, future studies in HCM patients should also include absolute quantification of regional ATP and phosphocreatine content, since regional myocyte loss in HCM may not be detectable by measurement of metabolite ratios. Combined ^{31}P- and ^{1}H-MRS studies should enable us to determine whether reduced phosphocreatine content in HCM is due to relative myocardial ischemia (normal total creatine) or loss of total creatine, a phenomenon characteristic of other forms of hypertrophy.[4]

Another interesting recent study in this area has reported on patients with Becker muscular dystrophy, (BMD) an X-chromosome linked disease associated with the absence or altered expression of dystrophin in cardiac and skeletal muscle, as well as on female carriers of the disease.[121] BMD may lead to the development of cardiomyopathy and heart failure. Both patients (phosphocreatine/ATP ratio 1.55 ± 0.33) as well as apparently healthy female carriers (1.37 ± 0.25) showed significantly lower phosphocreatine/ATP ratios than control subjects (2.44 ± 0.33), although all of the carriers and most of the patients had well-preserved left ventricular function (Figure 3.15). This suggests that in the heart, energetic imbalance occurs early in the disease process and may contribute to the development of contractile dysfunction in BMD.

Conclusions and future perspective

MRS spectroscopy is a unique noninvasive method, allowing multiple insights into cardiac metabolism in normal

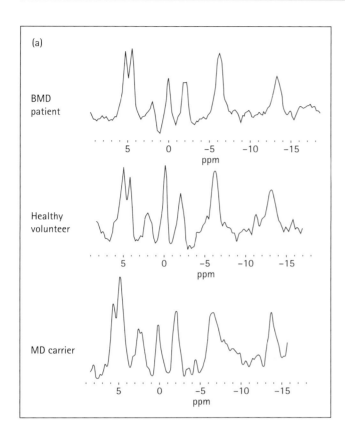

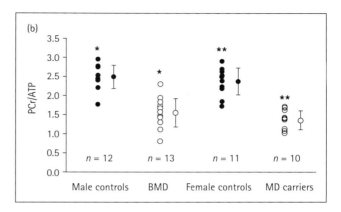

Figure 3.15
(a) Examples of spectra from a patient with Becker muscular dystrophy (BMD), a female carrier of muscular dystrophy (MD), and a healthy volunteer. (b) Phosphocreatine/ATP ratio for patients with BMD and carriers of muscular dystrophy (MD) as compared with control subjects. $*p < 0.05$; $**p < 0.0001$. (Reproduced from Crilley J et al. J Am Coll Cardiol 2000; 36:1953–8,[121] with permission from Elsevier Science Inc, New York.)

and diseased heart. As outlined in this chapter, on theoretical grounds, MRS provides a wealth of information that should be directly clinically relevant for patient management. The question then remains why cardiac MRS has not yet found its way into routine clinical practice – and, in fact, whether it ever will in the future or whether it will remain a research tool for academic centres with special interest. The main obstacle to the routine implementation of cardiac MRS has been and still is its technical complexity and limited resolution. Thus, a major technological effort is required to improve spatial resolution for ^{31}P studies from currently ~25 to ~1 ml voxel sizes. Furthermore, the temporal resolution has to be improved from 20–30 min to 3–5 min of acquisition time. Also, high-SNR spectra need to be acquired so that measurement variability is reduced to <5%, and standardized acquisition and quantification protocols will have to be developed and agreed upon. This would then provide clinicians with measurements that are universally accepted and that they can trust and base their clinical decisions on.

This author believes that, with a major dedicated technological development effort focused on coil design, on sequence design, and in particular on high-field magnets, these goals should be achievable in coming years, so that high-resolution metabolic imaging may become part of standard diagnostic pathways in patients with ischemic heart disease, heart failure, valve disease, and genetic cardiomyopathy.

Acknowledgements

The author would like to thank the following colleagues (listed in alphabetical order) for their contributions over many years of collaboration on MRS: Meinrad Beer, Kieran Clarke, Georg Ertl, Jane Francis, Axel Haase, Dietbert Hahn, Michael Horn, Kai Hu, Joanne S Ingwall, Markus von Kienlin, Kurt Kochsiek, Christine Lorenz, Saul Myerson, Thomas Pabst, Steffen Petersen, Matthew Robson, Stefan Roell, Jörn Sandstede, Rolf Sauter, Michaela Scheuermann-Freestone, Juergen Schneider, Matthias Spindler, Rong Tian, Hugh Watkins, and Frank Wiesmann.

References

1. Garlick PB, Radda GK, Seeley PJ. Phosphorus NMR studies on perfused heart. Biochem Biophys Res Commun 1977; 74:1256–62.

2. Ingwall JS. Phosphorus nuclear magnetic resonance spectroscopy of cardiac and skeletal muscles. Am J Physiol 1982; 242:H729–44.

3. Jacobus WE, Taylor GJT, Hollis DP, Nunnally RL. Phosphorus nuclear magnetic resonance of perfused working rat hearts. Nature. 1977; 265:756–8.

4. Neubauer S. High-energy phosphate metabolism in normal, hypertrophied and failing human myocardium. Heart Failure Rev 1999; 4:269–80.

5. Pohost GM, Meduri A, Razmi RM, et al. Cardiac MR spectroscopy in the new millennium. Rays 2001; 26:93–107.

6. Beyerbacht HP, Vliegen HW, Lamb HJ, et al. Phosphorus magnetic resonance spectroscopy of the human heart: current status and clinical implications. Eur Heart J 1996; 17:1158–66.

7. Weiss RG, Kalil-Filho R, Bottomley PA. Clinical cardiac magnetic resonance spectroscopy. In: Cardiovascular Magnetic Resonance (Manning WJ, Pennell DJ, eds). Philadelphia: Churchill Livingstone, 2001:437–46.

8. Gadian DG. NMR and its Applications to Living Systems, 2nd edn. New York: Oxford University Press, 1995.

9. Neubauer S, Ertl G, Krahe T, et al. [Experimental and clinical possibilities of MR spectroscopy of the heart]. Z Kardiol 1991; 80:25–36.

10. Clarke K, Stewart LC, Neubauer S, et al. Extracellular volume and transsarcolemmal proton movement during ischemia and reperfusion: a ^{31}P NMR spectroscopic study of the isovolumic rat heart. NMR Biomed 1993; 6:278–86.

11. Wallimann T, Wyss M, Brdiczka D et al. Intracellular compartmentation, structure and function of creatine kinase isoenzymes in tissues with high and fluctuating energy demands: the 'phosphocreatine circuit' for cellular energy homeostasis. Biophys J 1992; 281:21–40.

12. Ingwall JS, Kramer MF, Fifer MA, et al. The creatine kinase system in normal and diseased human myocardium. N Engl J Med 1985; 313:1050–4.

13. Jacobus WE. Respiratory control and the integration of heart high-energy phosphate metabolism by mitochondrial creatine kinase. Annu Rev Physiol 1985; 47:707–25.

14. Balaban RS, Kantor HL, Katz LA, Briggs RW. Relation between work and phosphate metabolite in the in vivo paced mammalian heart. Science 1986; 232:1121–3.

15. Bittl JA, Ingwall JS. Reaction rates of creatine kinase and ATP synthesis in the isolated rat heart. A ^{31}P NMR magnetization transfer study. J Biol Chem 1985; 260:3512–17.

16. Zhang J, Duncker DJ, Xu Y, et al. Transmural bioenergetic responses of normal myocardium to high workstates. Am J Physiol. 1995; 268:H1891–905.

17. Clarke K, O'Connor AJ, Willis RJ. Temporal relation between energy metabolism and myocardial function during ischemia and reperfusion. Am J Physiol 1987; 253:H412–21.

18. Neubauer S, Ingwall JS. Verapamil attenuates ATP depletion during hypoxia: ^{31}P NMR studies of the isolated rat heart. J Mol Cell Cardiol 1989; 21:1163–78.

19. Neubauer S, Horn M, Naumann A, et al. Impairment of energy metabolism in intact residual myocardium of rat hearts with chronic myocardial infarction. J Clin Invest 1995; 95:1092–100.

20. Neubauer S, Hamman BL, Perry SB, et al. Velocity of the creatine kinase reaction decreases in postischemic myocardium: a ^{31}P-NMR magnetization transfer study of the isolated ferret heart. Circ Res 1988; 63:1–15.

21. Bottomley PA, Hardy CJ. Mapping creatine kinase reaction rates in human brain and heart with 4 tesla saturation transfer ^{31}P NMR. J Magn Reson 1992; 99:443–8.

22. Bittl JA, Ingwall JS. Intracellular high-energy phosphate transfer in normal and hypertrophied myocardium. Circulation 1987; 75:I96–101.

23. Buser PT, Camacho SA, Wu ST, et al. The effect of dobutamine on myocardial performance and high-energy phosphate metabolism at different stages of heart failure in cardiomyopathic hamsters: a ^{31}P MRS study. Am Heart J 1989; 118:86–91.

24. Nascimben L, Friedrich J, Liao R, et al. Enalapril treatment increases cardiac performance and energy reserve via the creatine kinase reaction in myocardium of Syrian myopathic hamsters with advanced heart failure. Circulation 1995; 91:1824–33.

25. Liao R, Nascimben L, Friedrich J, et al. Decreased energy reserve in an animal model of dilated cardiomyopathy. Relationship to contractile performance. Circ Res 1996; 78:893–902.

26. Zhang J, Wilke N, Wang Y, et al. Functional and bioenergetic consequences of postinfarction left ventricular remodeling in a new porcine model. MRI and ^{31}P-MRS study. Circulation 1996; 94:1089–100.

27. Ingwall JS. Is cardiac failure a consequence of decreased energy reserve? Circulation 1993; 87(Suppl VII):58–62.

28. Horn M, Remkes H, Stromer H, et al. Chronic phosphocreatine depletion by the creatine analogue β-guanidinopropionate is associated with increased mortality and loss of ATP in rats after myocardial infarction. Circulation 2001; 104:1844–9.

29. Friedrich J, Apstein CS, Ingwall JS. ^{31}P nuclear magnetic resonance spectroscopic imaging of regions of remodeled myocardium in the infarcted rat heart. Circulation 1995; 92:3527–38.

30. Von Kienlin M, Rösch C, Le Fur Y, et al. Three-dimensional ^{31}P magnetic resonance spectroscopic imaging of regional high-energy phosphate metabolism in injured rat heart. Magn Reson Med. 1998; 39:731–41.

31. Zhang J, Merkle H, Hendrich K, et al. Bioenergetic abnormalities associated with severe left ventricular hypertrophy. J Clin Invest 1993; 92:993–1003.

32. Liu J, Wang C, Murakami Y, et al. Mitochondrial ATPase and high-energy phosphates in failing hearts. Am J Physiol Heart Circ Physiol 2001; 281:H1319–26.

33. Ugurbil K, Petein M, Madian R, et al. High resolution proton NMR studies of perfused rat hearts. FEBS Lett 1984; 167:73–8.

34. Balschi JA, Hetherington HP, Bradley EL Jr, Pohost GM. Water-suppressed one-dimensional ^{1}H NMR chemical shift imaging of the heart before and after regional ischemia. NMR Biomed 1995; 8:79–86.

35. Balschi JA, Hai JO, Wolkowicz PE, et al. ^{1}H NMR measurement of triacylglycerol accumulation in the post-ischemic canine heart after transient increase of plasma lipids. J Mol Cell Cardiol 1997; 29:471–80.

36. Bottomley PA, Weiss RG. Noninvasive localized MR quantification of creatine kinase metabolites in normal and infarcted canine myocardium. Radiology 2001; 219:411–18.

37. Schneider J, Fekete E, Weisser A, Neubauer S, von Kienlin M. Reduced ^{1}H-NMR visibility of creatine in isolated rat hearts. Magn Reson Med 2000; 43:497–502.

38. Kreutzer U, Mekhamer Y, Chung Y, Jue T. Oxygen supply and oxidative phosphorylation limitation in rat myocardium in situ. Am J Physiol Heart Circ Physiol 2001; 280:H2030–7.

39. Solomon MA, Jeffrey FM, Storey CJ, et al. Substrate selection early after reperfusion of ischemic regions in the working rabbit heart. Magn Reson Med. 1996; 35:820–6.

40. Malloy CR, Jones JG, Jeffrey FM, et al. Contribution of various substrates to total citric acid cycle flux and anaplerosis as determined by ^{13}C isotopomer analysis and O_2 consumption in the heart. Magma 1996; 4:35–46.

41. Lewandowski ED. Cardiac carbon 13 magnetic resonance spectroscopy: On the horizon or over the rainbow? J Nucl Cardiol 2002; 9:419–28.

42. Lewandowski ED, Kudej RK, White LT, et al. Mitochondrial preference for short chain fatty acid oxidation during coronary artery constriction. Circulation 2002; 105:367–72.

43. Burgess SC, Babcock EE, Jeffrey FM, et al. NMR indirect detection of glutamate to measure citric acid cycle flux in the isolated perfused mouse heart. FEBS Lett 2001; 505:163–7.

44. Weiss RG. ^{13}C-NMR for the study of intermediary metabolism. Magma 1998; 6:132.

45. Springer CS Jr, Pike MM, Balschi JA, et al. Use of shift reagents for nuclear magnetic resonance studies of the kinetics of ion transfer in cells and perfused hearts. Circulation 1985; 72:IV89–93.

46. Kohler SJ, Perry SB, Stewart LC, et al. Analysis of ^{23}Na NMR spectra from isolated perfused hearts. Magn Reson Med 1991; 18:15–27.

47. Van Emous JG, Vleggeert-Lankamp CL, Nederhoff MG, et al. Postischemic $Na^+–K^+$-ATPase reactivation is delayed in the absence of glycolytic ATP in isolated rat hearts. Am J Physiol Heart Circ Physiol 2001; 280:H2189–95.

48. Clarke K, Cross HR, Keon CA, et al. Cation MR spectroscopy (^7Li, ^{23}Na, ^{39}K and ^{87}Rb). Magma 1998; 6:105–6.

49. Neubauer S, Newell JB, Ingwall JS. Metabolic consequences and predictability of ventricular fibrillation in hypoxia. A ^{31}P- and ^{23}Na-nuclear magnetic resonance study of the isolated rat heart. Circulation 1992; 86:302–10.

50. DeLayre JL, Ingwall JS, Malloy C, Fossel ET. Gated sodium-23 nuclear magnetic resonance images of an isolated perfused working rat heart. Science 1981; 212:935–6.

51. Kim RJ, Lima JAC, Chen EL, et al. Fast ^{23}Na magnetic resonance imaging of acute reperfused myocardial infarction. Potential to assess myocardial viability. Circulation 1997; 95:1877–85.

52. Horn M, Weidensteiner C, Scheffer H, et al. Detection of myocardial viability based on measurement of sodium content: A ^{23}Na-NMR study. Magn Reson Med 2001; 45:756–64.

53. Kim RJ, Wu E, Rafael A, et al. The use of contrast-enhanced magnetic resonance imaging to identify reversible myocardial dysfunction. N Engl J Med 2000; 343:1445–53.

54. Weidensteiner C, Horn M, Fekete E, et al. Imaging of intracellular sodium with shift reagent aided ^{23}Na CSI in isolated rat hearts. Magn Reson Med 2002; 48:89–96.

55. Spindler M, Saupe KW, Christe ME, et al. Diastolic dysfunction and altered energetics in the αMHC403/+ mouse model of familial hypertrophic cardiomyopathy. J Clin Invest 1998; 101:1775–83.

56. Cross HR, Lu L, Steenbergen C, et al. Overexpression of the cardiac Na^+/Ca^{2+} exchanger increases susceptibility to ischemia/reperfusion injury in male, but not female, transgenic mice. Circ Res 1998; 83:1215–23.

57. Chacko VP, Aresta F, Chacko SM, Weiss RG. MRI/MRS assessment of in vivo murine cardiac metabolism, morphology, and function at physiological heart rates. Am J Physiol Heart Circ Physiol. 2000; 279:H2218–24.

58. Saupe KW, Spindler M, Hopkins JC, et al. Kinetic, thermodynamic, and developmental consequences of deleting creatine kinase isoenzymes from the heart. Reaction kinetics of the creatine kinase isoenzymes in the intact heart. J Biol Chem 2000; 275:19 742–6.

59. Van Dorsten FA, Nederhoff MG, Nicolay K, Van Echteld CJ. ^{31}P NMR studies of creatine kinase flux in M-creatine kinase-deficient mouse heart. Am J Physiol 1998; 275:H1191–9.

60. Saupe KW, Spindler M, Tian R, Ingwall JS. Impaired cardiac energetics in mice lacking muscle-specific isoenzymes of creatine kinase. Circ Res 1998:898–907.

61. Kaasik A, Veksler V, Boehm E, et al. Energetic crosstalk between organelles: architectural integration of energy production and utilization. Circ Res 2001; 89:153–9.

62. Weiss RG, Chatham JC, Georgakopolous D, et al. An increase in the myocardial PCr/ATP ratio in GLUT4 null mice. FASEB J 2002; 16:613–15.

63. Merx MW, Flogel U, Stumpe T, et al. Myoglobin facilitates oxygen diffusion. FASEB J 2001; 15:1077–9.

64. Kozerke S, Schar M, Lamb HJ, Boesiger P. Volume tracking cardiac ^{31}P spectroscopy. Magn Reson Med 2002; 48:380–4.

65. Bottomley PA. MR spectroscopy of the human heart: the status and the challenges. Radiology 1994; 191:593–612.

66. Bottomley PA. Noninvasive study of high-energy phosphate metabolism in human heart by depth-resolved ^{31}P NMR spectroscopy. Science 1985; 229:769–72.

67. Bottomley PA, Hardy CJ, Roemer PB. Phosphate metabolite imaging and concentration measurements in human heart by nuclear magnetic resonance. Magn Reson Med 1990; 14:425–34.

68. Bottomley PA, Atalar E, Weiss RG. Human cardiac high-energy phosphate metabolite concentrations by 1D-resolved NMR spectroscopy. Magn Reson Med 1996; 35:664–70.

69. Neubauer S, Krahe T, Schindler R, et al. ^{31}P magnetic resonance spectroscopy in dilated cardiomyopathy and coronary artery disease. Altered cardiac high-energy phosphate metabolism in heart failure. Circulation 1992; 86:1810–18

70. Horn M, Neubauer S, Bomhard M, et al. ^{31}P-NMR spectroscopy of human blood and serum: results from volunteers and patients with congestive heart failure, diabetes mellitus and hyperlipidemia. Magma 1993; 1:55–60.

71. Shen W, Asai K, Uechi M, et al. Progressive loss of myocardial ATP due to a loss of total purines during the development of heart failure in dogs: a compensatory role for the parallel loss of creatine. Circulation 1999; 100:2113–18.

72. Yabe T, Mitsunami K, Inubushi T, Kinoshita M. Quantitative measurements of cardiac phosphorus metabolites in coronary artery disease by ^{31}P magnetic resonance spectroscopy. Circulation 1995; 92:15–23.

73. Meininger M, Landschutz W, Beer M, et al. Concentrations of human cardiac phosphorus metabolites determined by SLOOP ^{31}P NMR spectroscopy. Magn Reson Med 1999; 41:657–63.

74. Bottomley PA, Ouwerkerk R, Lee RF, Weiss RG. Four-angle saturation transfer (FAST) method for measuring creatine kinase reaction rates in vivo. Magn Reson Med 2002; 47:850–63.

75. Pohmann R, von Kienlin M. Accurate phosphorus metabolite images of the human heart by 3D acquisition-weighted CSI. Magn Reson Med 2001; 45:817–26.

76. Lee RF, Giaquinto R, Constantinides C, et al. A broadband phased-array system for direct phosphorus and sodium metabolic MRI on a clinical scanner. Magn Reson Med 2000; 43:269–77.

77. Hetherington HP, Luney DJ, Vaughan JT, et al. 3D ^{31}P spectroscopic imaging of the human heart at 4.1 T. Magn Reson Med 1995; 33:427–31.

78. Okada M, Mitsunami K, Inubushi T, Kinoshita M. Influence of aging or left ventricular hypertrophy on the human heart: contents of phosphorus metabolites measured by ^{31}P MRS. Magn Reson Med 1998; 39:772–82.

79. Weiss RG, Bottomley PA, Hardy CJ, Gerstenblith G. Regional myocardial metabolism of high-energy phosphates during isometric exercise in patients with coronary artery disease. N Engl J Med 1990; 323:1593–600.

80. Yabe T, Mitsunami K, Okada M, et al. Detection of myocardial ischemia by ^{31}P magnetic resonance spectroscopy during handgrip exercise. Circulation 1994; 89:1709–16.

81. Buchthal SD, den Hollander JA, Merz CN, et al. Abnormal myocardial phosphorus-31 nuclear magnetic resonance spectroscopy in women with chest pain but normal coronary angiograms. N Engl J Med 2000; 342:829–35.

82. Vanoverschelde JLJ, Wijns W, Borgers M, et al. Chronic myocardial hibernation in humans. Circulation 1997; 95:1961–71.

83. von Kienlin M, Rosch C, Le Fur Y, et al. Three-dimensional ^{31}P magnetic resonance spectroscopic imaging of regional high-energy phosphate metabolism in injured rat heart. Magn Reson Med 1998; 39:731–41.

84. Flameng W, Vanhaecke J, Van Belle H, et al. Relation between coronary artery stenosis and myocardial purine metabolism, histology and regional function in humans. J Am Coll Cardiol 1987; 9:1235–42.

85. Kalil-Filho R, de Albuquerque CP, Weiss RG, et al. Normal high-energy phosphate ratios in stunned human myocardium. J Am Coll Cardiol 1997; 30:1228–32.

86. Beer M, Sandstede J, Landschutz W, et al. Altered energy metabolism after myocardial infarction assessed by ^{31}P-MR-spectroscopy in humans. Eur Radiol 2000; 10:1323–8.

87. Bottomley P, Lee SYH, Weiss RG. Proton MR spectroscopy of creatine in myocardial infarction. In: Proceedings of ISMRM 4th Scientific Meeting, New York, 1996:426.

88. Parrish TB, Fieno DS, Fitzgerald SW, Judd RM. Theoretical basis for sodium and potassium MRI of the human heart at 1.5 T. Magn Reson Med 1997; 38:653–61.

89. Pabst T, Sandstede J, Beer M, et al. Optimization of ECG-triggered 3D ^{23}Na MRI of the human heart. Magn Reson Med 2001; 45:164–6.

90. Sandstede JJ, Pabst T, Beer M, et al. Assessment of myocardial infarction in humans with ^{23}Na MR imaging: comparison with cine MR imaging and delayed contrast enhancement. Radiology 2001; 221:222–8.

91. Wexler LF, Lorell BH, Momomura S, et al. Enhanced sensitivity to hypoxia-induced diastolic dysfunction in pressure-overload left ventricular hypertrophy in the rat: role of high-energy phosphate depletion. Circ Res 1988; 62:766–75.

92. Conway MA, Allis J, Ouwerkerk R, et al. Detection of low phosphocreatine to ATP ratio in failing hypertrophied human myocardium by ^{31}P magnetic resonance spectroscopy. Lancet 1991; 338:973–6.

93. Neubauer S, Horn M, Pabst T, et al. Cardiac high-energy phosphate metabolism in patients with aortic valve disease assessed by ^{31}P-magnetic resonance spectroscopy. J Invest Med 1997; 45:453–62.

94. Beer M, Sandstede J, Landschütz W, et al. Absolute concentrations of myocardial high-energy phosphate metabolites in normal, hypertrophied and failing human myocardium, measured non-invasively with ^{31}P-SLOOP-magnetic resonance spectroscopy. J Am Coll Cardiol 2002; 40:1267–74.

95. Beyerbacht HP, Lamb HJ, van Der Laarse A, et al. Aortic valve replacement in patients with aortic valve stenosis improves myocardial metabolism and diastolic function. Radiology 2001; 219:637–43.

96. Lamb HJ, Beyerbacht HP, van der Laarse A, et al. Diastolic dysfunction in hypertensive heart disease is associated with altered myocardial metabolism. Circulation 1999; 99:2261–7.

97. Perings SM, Schulze K, Decking U, et al. Age-related decline of PCr/ATP-ratio in progressively hypertrophied hearts of spontaneously hypertensive rats. Heart Vessels 2000; 15:197–202.

98. Pluim BM, Chin JC, De Roos A, et al. Cardiac anatomy, function and metabolism in elite cyclists assessed by magnetic resonance imaging and spectroscopy. Eur Heart J 1996; 17:1271–8.

99. Pluim BM, Lamb HJ, Kayser HW, et al. Functional and metabolic evaluation of the athlete's heart by magnetic resonance imaging and dobutamine stress magnetic resonance spectroscopy. Circulation 1998; 97:666–72.

100. Spencer RG, Buttrick PM, Ingwall JS. Function and bioenergetics in isolated perfused trained rat hearts. Am J Physiol 1997; 272:H409–17.

101. Schaefer S, Gober JR, Schwartz GG, et al. In vivo phosphorus-31 spectroscopic imaging in patients with global myocardial disease. Am J Cardiol 1990; 65:1154–61.

102. Auffermann W, Chew WM, Wolfe CL, et al. Normal and diffusely abnormal myocardium in humans: functional and metabolic characterization with P-31 MR spectroscopy and cine MR imaging. Radiology 1991; 179:253–9.

103. de Roos A, Doornbos J, Luyten PR, et al. Cardiac metabolism in patients with dilated and hypertrophic cardiomyopathy: assessment with proton-decoupled P-31 MR spectroscopy. J Magn Reson Imaging 1992; 2:711–19.

104. Masuda Y, Tateno Y, Ikehira H, et al. High-energy phosphate metabolism of the myocardium in normal subjects and patients with various cardiomyopathies – the study using ECG gated MR spectroscopy with a localization technique. Jpn Circ J 1992; 56:620–6.

105. Hardy CJ, Weiss RG, Bottomley PA, Gerstenblith G. Altered myocardial high-energy phosphate metabolites in patients with dilated cardiomyopathy. Am Heart J 1991; 122:795–801.

106. Neubauer S, Horn M, Pabst T, et al. Contributions of ^{31}P-magnetic resonance spectroscopy to the understanding of dilated heart muscle disease. Eur Heart J 1995; 16(Suppl O):115–18.

107. Lodi R, Hart PE, Rajagopalan B, et al. Antioxidant treatment improves in vivo cardiac and skeletal muscle bioenergetics in patients with Friedreich's ataxia. Ann Neurol 2001; 49:590–6.

108. Neubauer S, Horn M, Cramer M, et al. Myocardial phosphocreatine-to-ATP ratio is a predictor of mortality in patients with dilated cardiomyopathy. Circulation 1997; 96:2190–6.

109. Haug CE, Shapiro JI, Chan L, Weil RD. P-31 nuclear magnetic resonance spectroscopic evaluation of heterotopic cardiac allograft rejection in the rat. Transplantation 1987; 44:175–8.

110. Fraser CD Jr, Chacko VP, Jacobus WE, et al. Early phosphorus 31 nuclear magnetic resonance bioenergetic changes potentially predict rejection in heterotopic cardiac allografts. J Heart Transplant 1990; 9:197–204.

111. Bottomley PA, Weiss RG, Hardy CJ, Baumgartner WA. Myocardial high-energy phosphate metabolism and allograft rejection in patients with heart transplants. Radiology 1991; 181:67–75.

112. van Dobbenburgh JO, de Jonge N, Klopping C, et al. Altered myocardial energy metabolism in heart transplant patients: consequence of rejection or a postischemic phenomenon? In: Proceedings of SMRM. New York: Society of Magnetic Resonance in Medicine, 1993:1093.

113. Evanochko WT, Buchthal SD, den Hollander JA, et al. Cardiac transplant patients response to the ^{31}P MRS stress test. J Heart Lung Transplant 2002; 21:522–9.

114. Spirito P, Seidman CE, McKenna WJ, Maron BJ. The management of hypertrophic cardiomyopathy. N Engl J Med 1997; 336:775–85.

115. Spindler M, Saupe KW, Christe ME, et al. A murine model of familial hypertrophic cardiomyopathy shows a markedly impaired response to inotropic stimulation. Circulation 1996; 94(8 Suppl I):I-433 (abst).

116. Rajagopalan B, Blackledge MJ, McKenna WJ, et al. Measurement of phosphocreatine to ATP ratio in normal and diseased human heart by ^{31}P magnetic resonance spectroscopy using the rotating frame-depth selection technique. Ann NY Acad Sci 1987; 508:321–32.

117. Sakuma H, Takeda K, Tagami T, et al. ^{31}P MR spectroscopy in hypertrophic cardiomyopathy: comparison with Tl-201 myocardial perfusion imaging. Am Heart J 1993; 125:1323–8.

118. Sieverding L, Jung WI, Breuer J, et al. Proton-decoupled myocardial ^{31}P NMR spectroscopy reveals decreased PCr/Pi in patients with severe hypertrophic cardiomyopathy. Am J Cardiol 1997; 80(3A):34A–40A.

119. Jung WI, Sieverding L, Breuer J, et al. ^{31}P NMR spectroscopy detects metabolic abnormalities in asymptomatic patients with hypertrophic cardiomyopathy. Circulation 1998; 97:2536–42.

120. Jung WI, Hoess T, Bunse M, et al. Differences in cardiac energetics between patients with familial and nonfamilial hypertrophic cardiomyopathy. Circulation 2000; 101:E121.

121. Crilley JG, Boehm EA, Rajagopalan B, et al. Magnetic resonance spectroscopy evidence of abnormal cardiac energetics in Xp21 muscular dystrophy. J Am Coll Cardiol 2000; 36:1953–8.

4

Quantitative image analysis

Nael F Osman

Introduction

Cardiac magnetic resonance (CMR) provides excellent image quality of the heart that surpasses that of echocardiography and provides a potential tool for more accurate diagnosis. The advantages of CMR, however, are not limited to better image quality – it can also provide unique ways to quantify many useful diagnostic indicators. Such an ability to quantify is significant for improving the diagnosis of cardiac disease and its consequent treatment. Automatic quantification improves the objectiveness of the diagnosis or screening process and makes it less observer-dependent, therefore reducing inter- and intra-observer variability.

CMR is rich in the number of methods for quantifying some indicators: these methods can be classified into *direct* methods – performed in the imaging stage – or *indirect* methods – requiring extra processing on the acquired images. Direct quantification is that which is performed by the imaging technique with little postprocessing necessary to produce the targeted measurements. For example, phase contrast (PC)[1,2] is a well-known direct technique where a pulse sequence encodes the motion of the protons into the phase of the acquired image. The acquired images then show the motion of protons at each pixel, and the motion measurements appear in the image itself. However, it is often hard to find a direct method that will directly encode certain indicator in the acquired images. When this is the case, it is possible to obtain intermediate images that reveal the desired features, but relatively sophisticated techniques are then necessary for quantification. For example, the size of the heart can be assessed by an experienced physician with CMR images. However, producing a number would require some image processing. Direct quantification is not the subject of this chapter, which will present some of the methods for analyzing CMR images and producing useful measurements.

Quantification is extremely useful in the clinical environment, provided the methods used to extract the measurements satisfy several criteria. These criteria, in general, are:

1. *Automation*: this is an important feature that makes the measurements independent of the observer. In general, it is hard to measure the degree of automation, but the fewer steps that are required from the observer, the more automated is the technique. It should be borne in mind that the degree of automation is an important determinant of the objectiveness of the quantification technique. This contrasts with the usual misunderstanding that quantification *alone* makes a technique objective. In fact, if quantification is dependent on a human observer to produce the measurements, these measurements would inherent qualitative assessment from the human factor.

2. *Speed*: the algorithm should be able to produce measurements in a relatively short time relative to the imaging time. Algorithms that require several hours for image analysis would be useless for clinical applications, where large numbers of subjects are imaged. Even for research applications, where time is not as big a factor as in clinical applications, a long time for analysis could limit the number of subject in a studied population.

3. *Reproducibility*: this feature relates to intra-observer variability. While reproducibility is related to automation, they are not equivalent. A fully automated process is definitely reproducible. A semi-automated technique, however, might or might not be reproducible, depending on the sensitivity of measurements to the user.

4. *Accuracy*: this is perhaps the most important feature, because none of the others would be important were the technique inherently erroneous. Determining the accuracy of a technique is done by comparing with a gold standard, or using phantom experiments and simulations.

Quantification techniques have been developed to analyze different types of CMR. For example, it is possible to quantify perfusion of the blood from first-pass contrast images, global function from cine images, or regional contractility from MR tagging. We will therefore focus our attention on describing methods for measuring the mechanical function of the heart – both global and regional function. The main function of the heart, of course, is to pump the blood that circulates in the body. This is achieved by the contraction of the wall muscle during systole. It is important, therefore, to be able to measure the efficiency of the heart by measuring global function. At the same time, measuring the regional contractility of the muscle is important in the assessment of specific diseases, such as coronary heart disease (CHD).

Global function

The CMR scanner is capable of imaging a selected volume that includes the heart at in any orientation. This is accomplished usually by acquiring multiple slices that cover a specific volume, which provides a 3D view of the anatomy, or by acquiring a 3D volume.[3,4] The acquisition of the volume that covers the heart enables measurement of global quantities, such as ventricular mass, ventricular volume, and ejection fraction. These global measurements are obtained by marking the region of the heart muscle in the CMR images by segmenting the image based on anatomy. Many computer algorithms have been developed to automatically segment CMR images of the heart and the vascular system,[4] and even some commercial packages are available and are used routinely to analyze the images.

Segmentation

To produce some of the global measurements of the heart, such as the mass of the ventricle, or the volume in the left ventricle (LV) at different instants of the cardiac cycle, it is important to separate the heart from other anatomical structures. This is accomplished in 2D images of the heart by attempting to identify the location of points on contours at the boundaries of the heart muscle, i.e. the epicardium and endocardium.[3–6] This identification is the most difficult part of the process, and is usually done using active contours, which are typically initialized close to the boundaries. Then, a computer algorithm deforms the contours, based on the intensity of the images, to converge at the edge of the heart.

Segmentation is a straightforward step, but because of its reliance on the intensity of the image, it is very sensitive

to noise and intensity variations due to blood flow and coil sensitivities. The segmentation of the LV is more prone to fail at the endocardium due to the papillary muscles and the heterogeneity of the blood intensity. Better imaging using *steady-state free precession (SSFP)*[7–10] enhances the contrast between the tissue and blood and reduces the error in identifying the endocardium. Identification of the epicardium is better suited for segmentation because of the delineation of the myocardium from the cavity of the lungs. The points of insertion for the right ventricle (RV) and the inferior side of the LV (away from the lungs) are more problematic.

Recently, commercial software called MASS (Medis, Inc., The Netherlands) has been introduced for segmentation. The tool uses more sophisticated steps (as described in Figures 4.1 and 4.2) for carrying out the segmentation in a robust and user-friendly way. Since the segmentation is not completely reliable, the tool provides simple ways to correct for errors in segmentations.

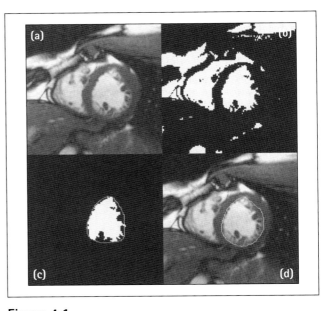

Figure 4.1
Example of contour detection steps for endocardial contour detection using the MASS software package.[5] (a) Result of automated LV center detection. The LV center detection is based on the Hough transform and is carried out using information from all available slices such that the position and orientation of the long axis of the LV is obtained. (b) An optimal threshold for the image is detected automatically. (c) The thresholded region closest to the detected center point is used to generate an initial estimation of the endocardial boundary. This contour is generated as a smooth convex hull around the thresholded region. The generated contour serves as a model for the next contour detection step. (d) The final edge detection step is based on graph searching techniques. During this step, the contour is constrained to lie in close proximity to the model contour. Large irregularities of the contour are avoided by penalty costs for sidestepping the contour. (Courtesy of RJ van der Geest.)

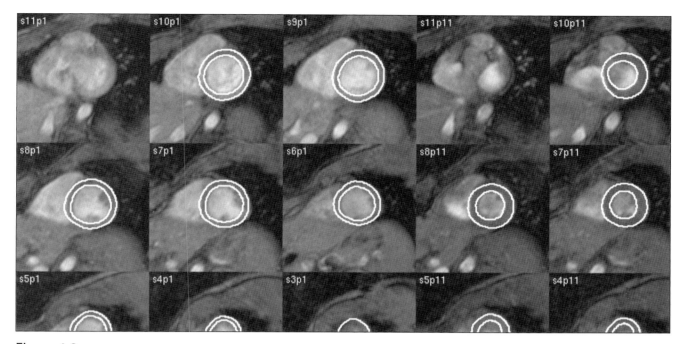

Figure 4.2
In this example, a 'time-series AAM' contour detection method was used to perform simultaneous detection of LV endocardial and epicardial contours in CMR images of a full cardiac cycle.[11] This illustration shows an example of results obtained by this method for multiple slices in an end-diastolic and end-systolic image. By integrating temporal information in the contour detection method, the segmentation result is guaranteed to describe a time-continuous cardiac motion pattern. Using this method, artifacts in individual images hardly influence the contour detection result. Further research is being carried out to extend AAM contour detection for 3D time series. (Courtesy of RJ van der Geest.)

Upon segmenting the heart at a specific cardiac phase, the contours are used as initialization for the contours in the subsequent cardiac phases and neighboring slices as well. These contours define the geometry of the LV wall muscle during the cardiac cycle.

Global measurements

Based on the identification of the heart contours, global measurements are straightforward. From the contours of the endocardium, the volume of the LV cavity is measured using Simpson's rule at different cardiac phases. The volumes of the cavity at end-systole and end-diastole (ESV and EDV) are determined based on the largest and smallest volumes. By measuring the percentage change in volume at end-systole relative to end-diastole, the ejection fraction (EF) of the heart is then measured. Mathematically, $EF = 100 \times (EDV - ESV)/EDV$ %. However, the entire blood ejection volume can be determined from the sequence, which is useful for demonstrating important periods in the cardiac cycle, such as systole, isovolumetric relaxation time, early diastole, and late diastole.

Regional function

In contrast to global function, which provides a collective assessment of the function of the heart, regional measurements provide assessments of specific regions of the heart, which is useful for diagnosis of CHD and might be an accurate predictor of future cardiac events. It is conceivable that symptoms of cardiac disease could occur regionally before being detected by global measurements.

Perhaps there is no other modality equal to CMR in its ability to image regional motion inside the wall muscle. With CMR, we can measure rapid motion, such as the flow of the blood using *phase contrast (PC)*, which is sometimes called *velocity encoding*. Relatively slower motion, such as that of the myocardium, can be imaged using *MR tagging*.[12–15] Other techniques, such as *stimulated echo (STE)*[16,17] and *displacement encoding with stimulated echo (DENSE)*[18–20] can give higher resolution for regional strain – but at the expense of longer imaging times. DENSE might be able to produce measurements directly without the need for complicated postprocessing, similar to phase contrast.

The main issue in regional measurement is the resolution of the image. Higher resolution of regional function can cost longer imaging and postprocessing time. Since the current abilities of MRI exceed the existing methods for assessing regional function, it is not clear what is the sufficient resolution and its impact on health care.

Regional function from cine images

Based on the segmentation of cine images as described previously, it is possible to measure one of the important regional function parameters, namely wall thickening. Wall thickening is simply the change in the thickness of the LV wall during the cardiac cycle, which is the distance between the endocardium and epicardium. By identifying the contours of the epicardium and the endocardium, computation of the distance becomes straightforward. However, some issues must be considered. The images of the heart represent a short-axis (or long-axis) slice of the heart. Since the image plane is, in fact, fixed relative to heart motion, the measured wall thickening would not represent the actual thickening of the wall. The perceived wall thickening is caused by through-motion of the heart since different regions of the wall will appear on the image plane during the cardiac cycle. This can cause in some cases a faked impression of wall thickening. An accurate measure of wall thickening in a region should also track the motion of that region. Unfortunately, tracking the motion from cine images is very difficult and very time-consuming. This can be done using another technology, namely MR tagging.

MR tagging

Cine images of the heart can reveal the motion of the wall and changes in the thickness during systole. However, as well as being unable to track the motion of tissue, the cine images cannot be used to measure directly the details of motion inside the wall muscle or the rotation and torsion of the ventricle. To be able to measure these details directly requires the use of some anatomical landmarks, such as the papillary muscle or the insertion of the RV at the LV, or the implantation of markers. The former would complicate the quantification, since automatic identification of the anatomy requires human intervention. Adding physical markers is a better choice, since it allows control of the shape and distribution of the marker for easier automatic identification. On the other hand, insertion of physical markers is an invasive procedure and impractical for clinical applications. Moreover, the physical markers could influence the motion of the heart, and hence distort the measurements.

MR tagging was introduced by Zerhouni et al[15] in 1988 and Axel and Dougherty[13,14] in 1989. This technique places *nonphysical* markers noninvasively inside the tissue by manipulating the magnetization of the tissue using special encoding pulses. These markers, called *tags*, appear in the acquired images as dark lines. The tags are generated by

modulating the magnetization of the heart that lasts for a fraction of a second. The tags therefore appear on the acquired images and accompany the motion of the myocardium during the cardiac cycle. This ability to place markers in the tissue is *unique* to CMR. The advantages of MR tagging are enormous: it is noninvasive and temporary, and can be easily designed in different shapes. Because it is possible to design MR tags of regular shapes, they can be used for automatic quantification of strain. Therefore, MR tags not only show the motion of the myocardium, but also can be designed in such a way that automatic analysis of motion is possible.

Tagging generation and images

The most common form of tagging is accomplished through the use of a special sequence called *spatial modulation of magnetization (SPAMM)*. This sequence modulates the magnetization at different locations in order to produce an image of the heart that is modulated by a specific regular pattern. The basic components of a SPAMM sequence are a collection of RF pulses separated by gradient pulses and followed by crushers. As a result, a collection of parallel tag lines appears. These lines are orthogonal to the direction of the gradients; for example, a gradient in the horizontal direction generates vertical tags. In addition, the separation of the tag lines is dependent on the gradient pulses: the stronger the gradients, the closer the tag lines. However, the sharpness of the tag lines depends on the number of RF pulses. The broadest tag lines are generated by using two RF pulses and one gradient, which is called 1–1 SPAMM. In this case, the actual shape of the tag intensity is sinusoidal. Because of its dull intensity pattern, this sequence is not often used – except in the case of *complementary SPAMM (CSPAMM)*.[21–24]

The SPAMM pulse sequence, as explained previously, generates one set of tag lines. Typically, the sequence is applied twice with two different sets of magnetic gradients, orthogonal to each other. This results in the generation of two sets of lines crossing each other and appearing as a regular *grid*.

Since the initial interest in analyzing the heart was during systole, MR tags were designed to analyze this period. The tagging pulse sequence is usually obtained after the QRS complex in the ECG, indicating end-diastole. This results in marking the tissue when the LV is completely filled with blood and ready to contract. The tagging sequence is then followed by pulse sequences to acquire a cine image of the heart during systole. The time during a single heartbeat is usually insufficient, and both tagging and imaging sequences must be repeated several times until all images are reconstructed. This usually requires up to 12 heartbeats in many cases. During this time, the chest cannot move in order to guarantee the repetitiveness of the heartbeats. This is guaranteed by asking the subject to hold his/her breath

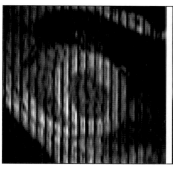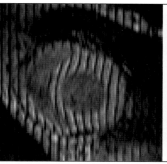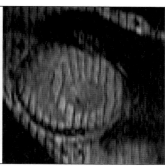

Figure 4.3
An example of tagged CMR images during the cardiac cycle. Typically, the tag lines are not visible throughout the whole cardiac cycle. This can be seen in the fading of the lines by the end of early diastole.

during that time; however, this can fail if arrhythmias occur. This image acquisition over several heartbeats is called *segmented* imaging.

Figure 4.3 shows tagged images acquired during systole. As can be seen, the tag lines bend, revealing the motion of the myocardium.

Analysis of tagged images using HARP

A number of tools have been developed that are capable of measuring regional function, but many are too slow to be used in a clinical setting. Recently, a new method called

harmonic phase (HARP) imaging has been developed that shortens the analysis time to a fraction of a minute.[25–29]

Basic concepts

HARP analysis is based on filtering the images in such a way that complex images are generated. A complex image is an image that can be split into two components: magnitude and phase. With HARP, it was proved[25] that the phase images have a direct relation to the motion and deformation of the tags, and thus to the motion of the myocardium. The filtering of the tagged images, however, can be problematic. Figure 4.4 shows a tagged CMR image in (a) and a corresponding image, called the Fourier image, in (b). The

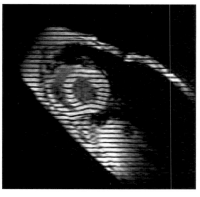

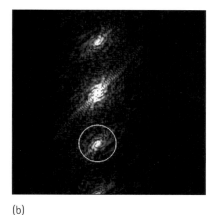

Figure 4.4
A tagged CMR image (a) and its Fourier image (b), which shows harmonic peaks. By filtering the circled peak in (b), the resulting image is a complex image that can be split into a magnitude image (c) and harmonic phase (HARP) image (d). Notice the bending of the dark bands of the HARP image similar to the original tagged image.

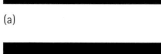

(a)   (b)

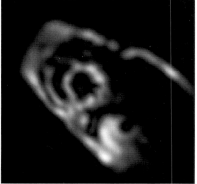

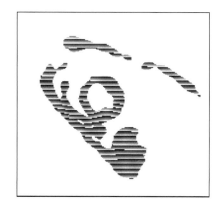

(c)   (d)

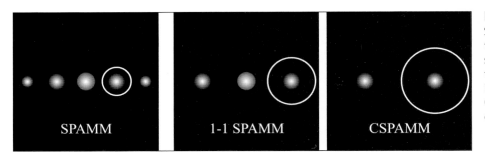

Figure 4.5
Spectral peak formation for different tag patterns. As can be seen, the selected pattern affects the design of the filter to extract the harmonic images. The largest filter occurs with CSPAMM because of the elimination of the central peak.

Fourier image shows multiple bright spots, which are call *harmonic peaks*. These harmonic peaks are related to the existence of tag lines. In the HARP technique, one of these harmonic peaks is selected by using a filter that suppresses the other peaks. As a result, a complex image is generated, from which a phase image is obtained.

The shape of the filter is a key element in the HARP method. The filter is centered at the first harmonic peak, whose location is related to the tag separation – and thus known a priori. The size of the filter is selected to avoid overlapping with other peaks. In routine practice, the diameter of the circular filter is the same as the distance from the origin (as shown in Figure 4.5a). This is not, however, an optimal situation for measuring motion. In general, the larger the filter, the better the resolution of the resulting complex image. This can be achieved by eliminating the other peaks by modifying the tagging process. Using a 1–1 SPAMM sequence, all the other harmonic peaks are removed except for the first-harmonic peak and the peak at the origin (Figure 4.5b). In case of CSPAMM, the peak at the origin is also removed by subtracting two tagged MR images with different tag pattern, and the filter can be designed larger with higher resolution of motion (Figure 4.5c). Kuijer et al[30] showed that HARP with CSPAMM improves the accuracy and resolution of motion measurements using HARP.

Motion tracking

The phase images of HARP are also useful for tracking motion. The basic concept here is that the phase of any point in the tissue does not change over time, and it is possible then to track the motion of a point simply by determining the position in the images at different cardiac phases that satisfy this condition. This concept can be easily implemented and is capable of tracking the motion of any point in a fraction of a second. Figure 4.6 shows a tagged heart and the trajectories of motion of different points during the cardiac cycle.

Mesh tracking

It is possible to track multiple points that segment the heart using the HARP tracking method. A mesh that segments the LV into a number of segments can be built at one timeframe – preferably close to end-systole. Each of the points that constitute the mesh is tracked through the other timeframes. The mesh, therefore, seems to deform with the motion of the heart. The changes in the geometry of the mesh can then be measured. Figure 4.7 shows a mesh constructed at a given timeframe and the resulting deformations.

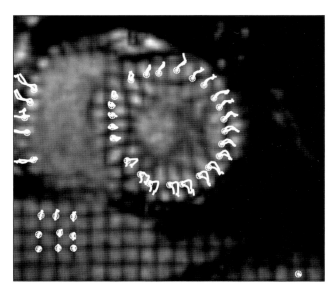

Figure 4.6
The motion of points can be tracked using HARP at different timeframes in a fraction of a second. The curves show the trajectories of motion for a number of selected points (circles). Each trajectory can be tracked in a fraction of a second. Notice the motion of the lateral side of the LV toward the septum during systole.

Regional measurements

Because of the ability to track the myocardium from tagged CMR images, the number of measurements that can be obtained is substantial. These measurements include the *strain* and the *strain rate*. Strain is usually defined as the change in the length of an object per unit length. For example, if a fiber of 5 mm length decreases to 4 mm, i.e. a loss of 1 mm, the resulting strain is −20%, with the negative sign indicating a reduction in length. The strain measurement, however, describes one-dimen-

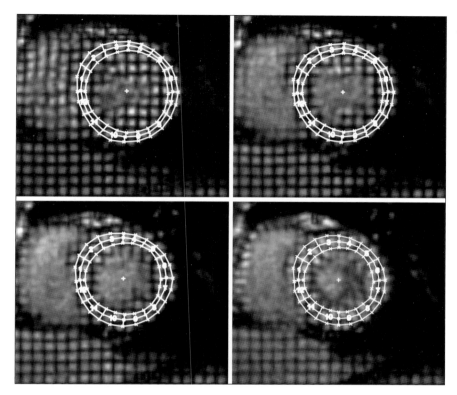

Figure 4.7
The tracked points of a mesh deform the mesh in accordance with the motion of the LV during the cardiac cycle.

sional objects of a given length. For the heart and the wall muscle, there are no obvious elongated fibers, and the strains in specific directions must be computed.

Significant local strains include circumferential shortening, radial thickening, and longitudinal compression. Figure 4.8 shows the geometric meaning of these strains. Another set of strain measurements is that of principal strain values. These strains are the maximum changes in length regardless of direction. It is typical for the directions of these strains to differ from the principal directions of the heart (circumferential, radial, and longitudinal directions). This difference is small in normal hearts, but not in dysfunctional hearts.

The HARP method can measure the local strain of tissue by measuring the frequency of the tag lines.

Figure 4.9 gives an example of this. Assume that a piece of tissue resembles a fiber with a tagging pattern, as shown. Note that the number of tags per unit length is called the *frequency* of the tag pattern. If this piece of tissue contracts (as does the myocardial tissue during systole), the tag lines become closer to each other and the tag frequency increases in proportion to that contraction. Similarly, the stretching of this tissue has the opposite effect: the frequency decreases in proportion to the stretching. Hence, by measuring the change in tag frequency, we can measure local strain.

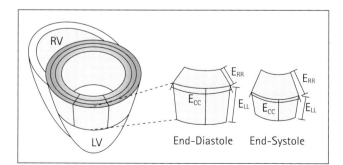

Figure 4.8
An illustration showing the direction of the strains in the myocardium.

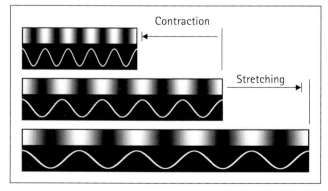

Figure 4.9
An illustration showing the relation between local strain and tag frequency. The contraction of a tagged fiber in the middle would increase the tagging frequency (density of tag lines) as shown in the top fiber. Stretching, on the other hand, causes a reduction in local frequency (bottom).

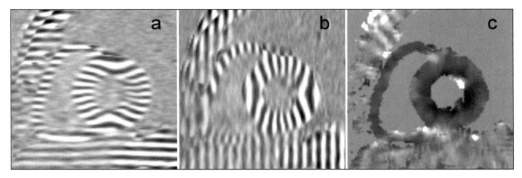

Figure 4.10

CSPAMM images with horizontal (a) and vertical (b) sinusoidal tagging patterns. The images were obtained with steady-state free precession (SSFP) imaging combined with myocardial tagging. Using HARP, the circumferential strain (E_{CC}) map (c) was calculated from these CSPAMM images. The gray background corresponds to $E_{CC} = 0$ (no strain). Dark regions correspond to negative strain (shortening). Note the clear transmural gradient in the circumferential strain. (Courtesy of J Zwanenburg and JPA Kuijer.)

Because CMR typically acquires 2D images of the heart, 2D motion can be observed on the cine image of a slice. This motion also has strain values; however, these computations are confined to a 2D plane, and do not represent the actual 3D motion of the heart. Nevertheless, because of its simplicity, this has been the preferred method of analysis. Figure 4.10 shows two tagged MR images with orthogonal tag directions (a and b). From the two images, a map showing the circumferential shortening was computed from changes in the tag frequency (c).

The measured strain can be represented numerically by plotting the changes in local strain during the cardiac cycle. By tracking the motion of different regions of the heart using a mesh, the regional strains are measured on the trajectory of motion. The resulting plots, as shown in Figure 4.11, are curves representing the evolution of strain with time at different segments.

Another mechanical characteristic that can be determined from tracking the motion of the heart is the twist of the base relative to the apex of the heart, called *torsion*.

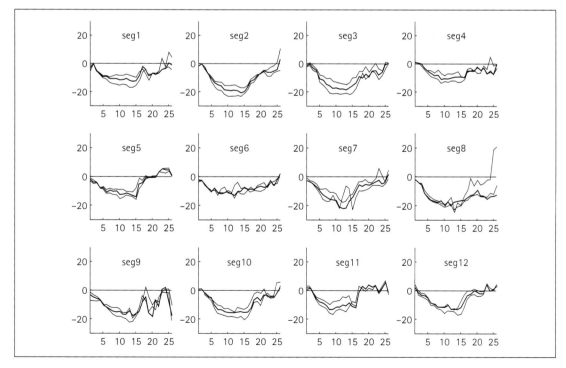

Figure 4.11

The temporal evolution of strain during the cardiac cycle is determined at different segments by using a tracked mesh to follow the deformation of the heart. The bold line shows the strain at midwall, while the other lines represent the endocardial and epicardial strains. Notice the transmural difference in strain.

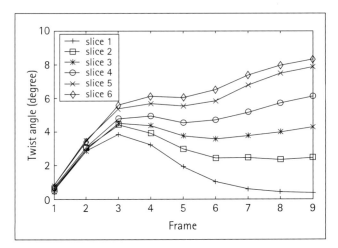

Figure 4.12
The typical cardiac twist at different mid-ventricular slices, where slice 1 is the most basal. The difference in twist between the slices is the ventricular torsion.

Due to the direction of the myocardial fibers, the heart shows a torsion that increases during systole to reach a maximum. This torsion is followed by rapid untwisting during the isovolumetric relaxation period and during diastole. Figure 4.12 shows the rotation of different slices around the middle of the LV. The variation rotation between the slices, which causes the torsion of the LV, can be seen. It has been shown that measuring LV torsion can be useful for detecting aortic stenosis.[24]

Software tools for tagging analysis

HARP methods have been implemented in a user-friendly software package that enables easy analysis of tagged CMR images. This software was developed for research needs and is currently being implemented for commercial applications (Diagnosoft Inc, Palo Alto, CA, USA). The key element of this new software package is fast automated analysis. The total analysis of a study is decreased in the commercial version so that the analysis of an entire study requires less than 10 minutes. The main time-consuming steps are image importing and building the mesh. Tracking and strain analysis are accomplished in seconds. Figure 4.13 shows a screen shot of the program.

Measuring global function from tagging

Global measurements are commonly used in clinical practice because they are easy to obtain, and local function can be estimated intuitively from global function, while the estimation of global from local function is difficult. Up to now, estimates of regional function have relied on tedious and time-consuming analysis; however, with the advent of fast techniques for analyzing regional function, it should be possible even to use regional function to estimate global function.

Tracking of the mesh using HARP can be used to measure global function. The tracked subendocardium can be used to mark the ventricular cavity, and the volume can be measured from multislices using Simpson's rule. It is then possible to determine the EDV and ESV, as well as the EF.[31] The advantage of this approach is that it eliminates the need for untagged images – thus reducing imaging time – and it is more automatic since segmentation is required in only one timeframe, which can be selected to be optimal for automatic segmentation.

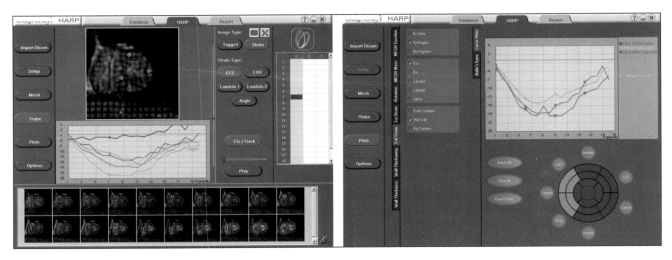

Figure 4.13
Screen shots of the HARP tool for the analysis of tagged images in a single slice. The resulting measurements can be presented at different segments and in different formats, as seen in the right window.

Future directions

Quantitative imaging

A reduction in imaging time and analysis, partially by incorporating measurements into the imaging sequence, serves a great benefit by shortening the total quantification time. Direct quantitative imaging is perhaps the ultimate goal for the efficient measurement of different regional parameters.

The ability of CMR to produce measurements directly with no postprocessing is not new. Phase contrast has an intensity that is proportional to velocity in the image. No sophisticated computations are required as with MR tagging. The new technique called *displacement encoding using stimulated echo (DENSE)*[18–20] is another example of direct imaging, with phase images directly related to the displacement of the cardiac tissue. It is even possible to image contractility directly without measuring displacement. For example, *strain-encoded (SENC)*[32,33] imaging can reveal the local distribution of strain directly in acquired CMR images with no lengthy postprocessing. SENC images, in this case, do not reveal motion or velocity, but rather the contractility of the muscle.

Composite images

The number of measurements that can be produced by CMR is rich, but, at the same time, long imaging times are required to obtain these and other CMR images separately. For CMR to be more cost-effective, imaging sessions must be completed rapidly and efficiently. Thus, it would be of benefit to combine two different imaging modalities; for example, contrast images used in perfusion or viability imaging, and tagging images measuring motion. Other combinations are also possible.

Using composite images will be challenging for quantification, since this entails more sophisticated image processing in order to acquire the same amount of information as obtained from the two (or more) imaging methods separately. This requires decoupling of the features of the different methods. For example, when combining tagging with contrast, it is important to differentiate whether the lack of intensity in a region is caused by the contrast agent or the MR tags. Perhaps other combinations would be more efficient.

Conclusions

In conclusion, many techniques have been developed for analyzing CMR images. Characterized by compelling image quality or unique imaging features, the output of the techniques is progressively becoming more reliable. CMR is considered to be the gold standard for determining and measuring regional function, and it is getting ever closer to clinical applications due to the introduction of fast analysis tools.

Acknowledgements

The author would like to thank Li Pan, Joost Kuijer, and Robert van der Geest for providing some of the figures and insights. I would also like to thank Mary McAllister for her great help in preparing this chapter.

References

1. Pelc LR, Sayre J, Yun K, et al. Evaluation of myocardial motion tracking with cine-phase contrast magnetic resonance imaging. Invest Radiol 1994; 29:1038–42.

2. Pelc NJ, Drangova M, Pelc LR, et al. Tracking of cyclic motion with phase-contrast cine MR velocity data. J Magn Reson Imaging 1995; 5:339–45.

3. van der Geest RJ, Reiber JH. Quantification in cardiac MRI. J Magn Reson Imaging 1999; 10:602–8.

4. van der Geest RJ, de Roos A, van der Wall EE, Reiber JH. Quantitative analysis of cardiovascular MR images. Int J Card Imaging 1997; 13:247–58.

5. van der Geest RJ, Buller VG, Jansen E, et al. Comparison between manual and semiautomated analysis of left ventricular volume parameters from short-axis MR images. J Comput Assist Tomogr 1997; 21:756–65.

6. Mitchell SC, Lelieveldt BP, van der Geest RJ, et al. Multistage hybrid active appearance model matching: segmentation of left and right ventricles in cardiac MR images. IEEE Trans Med Imaging 2001; 20:415–23.

7. Alfakih K, Thiele H, Plein S, et al. Comparison of right ventricular volume measurement between segmented *k*-space gradient-echo and steady-state free precession magnetic resonance imaging. J Magn Reson Imaging 2002; 16:253–8.

8. Peters DC, Ennis DB, McVeigh ER. High-resolution MRI of cardiac function with projection reconstruction and steady-state free precession. Magn Reson Med 2002; 48:82–8.

9. Herzka DA, Kellman P, Aletras AH, et al. Multishot EPI-SSFP in the heart. Magn Reson Med 2002; 47:655–64.

10. Thiele H, Nagel E, Paetsch I, et al. Functional cardiac MR imaging with steady-state free precession (SSFP) significantly improves endocardial border delineation without contrast agents. J Magn Reson Imaging 2001; 14:362–7.

11. Lelieveldt B, Mitchell S, Bosch J, et al. Time-continuous segmentation of cardiac image sequences using active appearance motion models. In: Information Processing in Medical Imaging IPMI-2001 (Insana M, Leahy R, eds). Berlin: Springer-Verlag, 2001: 446–52.

12. Axel L. Noninvasive measurement of cardiac strain with MRI. Adv Exp Med Biol 1997; 430:249–56.

13. Axel L, Dougherty L. MR imaging of motion with spatial modulation of magnetization. Radiology 1989; 171:841–5.

14. Axel L, Dougherty L. Heart wall motion: improved method of spatial modulation of magnetization for MR imaging. Radiology 1989; 172:349–50.

15. Zerhouni E, Parish D, Rogers W, et al. Human heart: tagging with MR imaging – a method for noninvasive assessment of myocardial motion. Radiology 1988; 169:59–63.

16. Frahm J, Hanicke W, Bruhn H, et al. High-speed STEAM MRI of the human heart. Magn Reson Med 1991; 22:133–42.

17. Fischer SE, Stuber M, Scheidegger MB, Boesiger P. Limitations of stimulated echo acquisition mode (STEAM) techniques in cardiac applications. Magn Reson Med 1995; 34:80–91.

18. Aletras AH, Balaban RS, Wen H. High-resolution strain analysis of the human heart with fast-DENSE. J Magn Reson 1999; 140:41–57.

19. Aletras AH, Ding S, Balaban RS, Wen H. DENSE: displacement encoding with stimulated echoes in cardiac functional MRI. J Magn Reson 1999; 137:247–52.

20. Aletras AH, Wen H. Mixed echo train acquisition displacement encoding with stimulated echoes: an optimized DENSE method for in vivo functional imaging of the human heart. Magn Reson Med 2001; 46:523–34.

21. Fischer SE, McKinnon GC, Scheidegger MB, et al. True myocardial motion tracking. Magn Reson Med 1994; 31:401–13.

22. Stuber M, Spiegel MA, Fischer SE, et al. Single breath-hold slice-following CSPAMM myocardial tagging. Magma 1999; 9:85–91.

23. Stuber M, Nagel E, Fischer SE, et al. Quantification of the local heartwall motion by magnetic resonance myocardial tagging. Comput Med Imaging Graph 1998; 22:217–28.

24. Stuber M, Scheidegger MB, Fischer SE, et al. Alterations in the local myocardial motion pattern in patients suffering from pressure overload due to aortic stenosis. Circulation 1999; 100:361–8.

25. Osman NF, Kerwin WS, McVeigh ER, Prince JL. Cardiac motion tracking using CINE harmonic phase (HARP) magnetic resonance imaging. Magn Reson Med 1999; 42:1048–60.

26. Osman NF, McVeigh ER, Prince JL. Imaging heart motion using harmonic phase MRI. IEEE Trans Med Imaging 2000; 19:186–202.

27. Osman NF, Prince JL. Visualizing myocardial function using HARP MRI. Phys Med Biol 2000; 45:1665–82.

28. Garot J, Bluemke DA, Osman NF, et al. Fast determination of regional myocardial strain fields from tagged cardiac images using harmonic phase MRI. Circulation 2000; 101:981–8.

29. Garot J, Bluemke DA, Osman NF, et al. Transmural contractile reserve after reperfused myocardial infarction in dogs. J Am Coll Cardiol 2000; 36:2339–46.

30. Kuijer JP, Jansen E, Marcus JT, et al. Improved harmonic phase myocardial strain maps. Magn Reson Med 2001; 46:993–9.

31. Dornier C, Ivancevic MK, Lecoq G, et al. Assessment of the left ventricle ejection fraction by MRI tagging: comparisons with cine MRI and coronary angiography. In: Proceedings of International Society of Magnetic Resonance in Medicine ISMRM, Honolulu, HI, 2002.

32. Osman NF, Sampath S, Atalar E, Prince JL. Imaging longitudinal cardiac strain on short-axis images using strain-encoded MRI. Magn Reson Med 2001; 46:324–34.

33. Osman NF, Sampath S, Derbyshier JA, et al. Real-time SENC for the detection of regional dysfunction during dobutamine stress test. In: Proceedings of Society of Cardiovascular MRI (SCMR) Fifth Annual Scientific Sessions, Orlando, FL, 2002.

5

Real-time CMR and parallel imaging

Daniel K Sodickson

Introduction

The challenges and the benefits of rapid magnetic resonance imaging (MRI) are nowhere more apparent than in the field of cardiac imaging. Cardiac motion, respiratory motion, and blood flow all constrain the viable window of data acquisition in cardiac MRI (CMR). Accurate characterization of the patterns of motion and flow may require still greater speed and temporal resolution. Fortunately, technological and methodological improvements have to a great extent kept pace with this demand for speed, allowing accelerations of data acquisition by several orders of magnitude over the decades since the introduction of MRI. Meanwhile, cardiac and respiratory gating techniques, as well as other methods of motion correction, have allowed many forms of cardiac imaging to proceed on longer timescales. Nevertheless, the ongoing development of ungated real-time cardiac imaging applications has continued to push the leading edge of imaging speed, and to put MR hardware and software to the test.

This chapter will outline some of the principal methods now in use for rapid and real-time CMR. The emphasis will rest upon basic principles and current trends, rather than upon rigorous completeness. Rapid CMR is an area of vigorous ongoing research, and many valiant and potentially valuable techniques will of necessity be overlooked, or will receive only brief mention here. In fact, the very number and variety of existing rapid imaging approaches presents an opportunity that will constitute a theme of this chapter: the opportunity for synergy, for combinations of disparate approaches with distinct underlying mechanisms to yield ever greater imaging speed.

We will begin with a survey of three basic categories of real-time imaging techniques used for CMR: rapid Cartesian data trajectories, non-Cartesian trajectories, and parallel imaging. For each of these categories, we will outline the fundamental modes of data acquisition and image reconstruction, and will discuss particular issues that may attend practical implementations. We will also sketch briefly some of the broader repertoire of fast imaging approaches that may play a role in real-time cardiac imaging, and will discuss enabling technologies for real-time imaging systems. Finally, we will attempt to survey some of the range of existing applications of real-time CMR.

Techniques

Rapid Cartesian trajectories

Signal data acquired on a regular grid have for some time been the standard for bread-and-butter applications of MRI. As described elsewhere in this book, such data may be obtained using well-defined discrete gradient steps, and the resulting k-space pattern may be described by simple integer indices in a Cartesian axis system. As a result, image reconstruction can be comparatively simple and efficient, sometimes involving no more than a fast Fourier transform. The leftmost panel of Figure 5.1a shows an example of a simple Cartesian data set, acquired with regularly stepped phase-encoding gradients and constant-length readout gradients.

One of the earliest Cartesian acquisition techniques to be used for real-time imaging was the echo planar imaging (EPI) technique.[1] In EPI, multiple gradient echoes are read out after a single spin excitation, with each readout occurring in the opposite direction to the last, resulting in a rapid back-and-forth raster pattern of data acquisition (Figure 5.1b, left). All the data in a pure EPI acquisition are accumulated in a single shot. There is no need to wait for spin relaxation prior to acquisition of each line of data, resulting in a high intrinsic speed. This high speed allowed early real-time cardiac imaging in animals and humans.[2,3] However, as is the case with most rapid imaging approaches, the high speed of EPI comes at a price. Since magnetization from the same excitation remains in the transverse plane for the duration of the sequence, phase

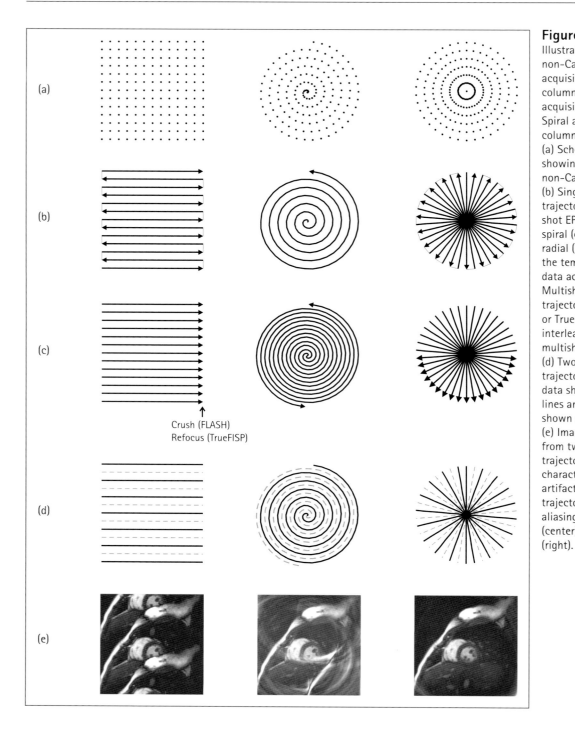

Figure 5.1

Illustration of Cartesian and non-Cartesian data acquisition strategies. Left column: Cartesian acquisition. Center column: Spiral acquisition. Right column: Radial acquisition. (a) Schematic data matrices, showing basic Cartesian and non-Cartesian patterns. (b) Single-shot acquisition trajectories: Cartesian single-shot EPI (left); single-shot spiral (center); single-shot radial (right). Arrows indicate the temporal direction of data acquisition. (c) Multishot acquisition trajectories: Cartesian FLASH or TrueFISP (left); two-interleave spiral (center); multishot radial (right). (d) Twofold undersampled trajectories, with acquired data shown as solid black lines and omitted data shown as dashed gray lines. (e) Images reconstructed from twofold undersampled trajectories, showing characteristic undersampling artifacts for each class of trajectory: coherent linear aliasing (left); spiral aliasing (center); radial streaking (right).

errors can accumulate over the entire sequence, and the advantages of a short acquisition window in single-shot EPI are partially offset by its comparative sensitivity to a variety of artifacts relating to susceptibility, motion, and flow. The alternating direction of EPI readouts also can produce artifacts unless careful calibration is performed. These effects, combined with the common practice of sampling in the presence of time-varying gradients in order to maximize speed, can require more complex image reconstruction algorithms than are generally called for with many other Cartesian trajectories.

A different approach to rapid Cartesian imaging is represented in the FLASH[4,5] family of sequences, which were also introduced and used for fluoroscopic acquisitions[6,7] relatively early in the development of fast imaging approaches. In FLASH and similar sequences (Figure 5.1c, left), short excitation pulses are each followed by a single readout. The small flip angle of pulses, in combination with spoiler gradients to crush any residual transverse magnetization at the end of the readout, allow rapid repetition (short TR) and a brisk imaging speed. As a result of the need for multiple radiofrequency (RF) pulses, imaging times can be inherently longer for these sequences than for EPI. However, since less time is available for accumulation of phase errors following any given excitation, FLASH sequences have a desirable robustness. Other tradeoffs include a comparatively low signal-to-noise ratio (SNR) for very low flip angles and high speeds, and a comparatively low inherent T2 contrast, which may nevertheless be enhanced in a preparation phase prior to readout of the data.

Hybrid approaches intermediate between the EPI and the FLASH approaches were subsequently proposed and used with success for real-time cardiac imaging. In segmented or interleaved EPI sequences,[8,9] each excitation pulse is followed by multiple readouts in the style of EPI, but a more modest number of readouts per excitation is used, and the full signal data set is acquired in multiple shots in the style of FLASH acquisitions. This approach combines some of the speed and SNR advantages of EPI with the robustness of FLASH-like sequences.

In recent times, steady-state free precession (SSFP) or TrueFISP[10,11] sequences have become popular for real-time imaging. (Alternate names are used by various manufacturers, including FIESTA and Balanced FFE.) Interestingly, this family of sequences are not inherently the fastest of available techniques; however, the availability of high-performance fast gradient systems has allowed the SSFP sequences to be used effectively for real-time imaging. SSFP sequences refocus all the magnetization at the end of each readout, rather than spoiling it with crusher gradients (Figure 5.1c, left). As a result of this refocusing, higher flip angles may be used than are typical in FLASH sequences. Refocusing can also come at a cost: for excessively long TE, tissue that has moved or undergone other irreversible modulation since the time of excitation cannot be completely refocused, and stereotypic artifacts result. Fast gradients allow reduced TE, greatly enhancing sequence performance. One of the most attractive features of SSFP sequences for cardiac imaging is the high intrinsic contrast they provide between blood and myocardium, which results from a combination of T1 and T2 effects. An increasing number of cardiac cine imaging studies have recently been reported using TrueFISP,[12,13] and these have been followed by real-time implementations.[14,15]

Figure 5.2a and b show examples of real-time cardiac images obtained using Cartesian segmented EPI and TrueFISP sequences.

Non-Cartesian trajectories

Non-Cartesian acquisitions (Figure 5.1, center and right-hand columns) take a modified path through data space as compared with the regular Cartesian path (Figure 5.1, left-hand column). As a result, non-Cartesian acquisitions generally have properties quite distinct from those of Cartesian acquisitions, and many of these properties have been shown to be advantageous for real-time applications.

Spiral trajectories[16,17] have been used extensively for real-time imaging. A sample spiral trajectory is shown in the central panel of Figure 5.1a. The lack of sharp transitions in the oscillating gradient patterns required to generate a spiral allows efficient use even of gradients with limited switching rates, and high switching rates may be employed for still greater speed. For real-time implementations, data are typically acquired continuously during the long spiral readout (Figure 5.1b, center), which again promotes speed, but which also, as in the case of EPI, allows phase errors to accumulate. Also as for EPI, multi-shot spiral acquisitions, with interleaved spiral trajectories following separate RF pulses (Figure 5.1c, center), may be used to control these errors. The appearance of artifacts in spiral acquisitions may differ from the Cartesian case, due to the altered order and weighting of points in k-space. Rather than resulting in localized distortions or signal loss, for example, effects such as off-resonance shifts may result in blurring in images obtained from spiral acquisitions. A typical spiral trajectory begins in the center

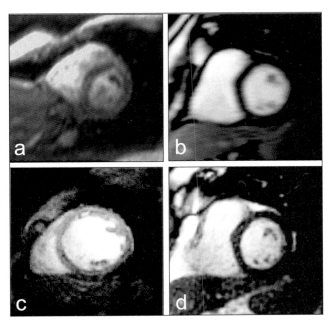

Figure 5.2

Examples of real-time short-axis cardiac images obtained using (a) Cartesian segmented EPI, (b) Cartesian TrueFISP, (c) spiral, and (d) radial TrueFISP pulse sequences. ((a) adapted from Bornstedt et al. Magn Res Imaging 2001; 14:300–5 with permission of John Wiley & Sons, Inc.,[85] Figure 3. (c) adapted from Kaji et al J Am Coll Cardiol 2001; 38:527–33.,[90] Figure 1. (b,d) courtesy of Orlando Simonetti. Radiology 2001; 221:827–36.[27])

of k-space, and works its way symmetrically outward, but reverse-spiral trajectories with different relaxation weighting have also been explored.[18,19] Spiral trajectories require specialized image reconstruction procedures, since the irregular sampling precludes the use of a simple fast Fourier transform. Various reconstruction procedures have been proposed. Regridding algorithms[20,21] that map the data to a Cartesian grid are most frequently used.

A variant of another non-Cartesian sampling pattern – the radial trajectory – was used to generate the very first MR images.[22,23] Radial trajectories were subsequently reintroduced and further explored for their comparative insensitivity to motion.[24] Sample radial acquisition trajectories are shown in the right column of Figure 5.1. Such trajectories may be implemented with a single radial readout per RF pulse (Figure 5.1c, right), or in multiple-readout or even single-shot mode (Figure 5.1b, right). As is the case for spiral trajectories, radial image reconstructions are more complex than for the Cartesian case, typically involving either regridding procedures or projection-reconstruction algorithms analogous to those used in X-ray computed tomography (CT).

The motion insensitivity of radial trajectories results in part from their intrinsic oversampling of the center of k-space, which is traversed by each angular readout or 'projection'. This redundancy also represents an underlying inefficiency in data acquisition – the number of acquired data points needed in principle to generate an image of a given matrix size is generally larger than for Cartesian acquisitions. Nevertheless, radial trajectories have had a recent resurgence for real-time imaging applications, in part because of their undersampling behavior.[25]

When Cartesian acquisitions are undersampled, i.e. when intermediate lines of k-space data are omitted as shown in Figure 5.1d (left), such that the spacing of lines exceeds the Nyquist limit, the resulting images show well-defined aliasing artifacts (Figure 5.1e, left). This aliasing results from the inability of the Fourier transform operation to separate certain regularly spaced points in the image plane based only on the undersampled spatial frequency data. As is shown in Figure 5.1e, the regular pattern of Cartesian undersampling results in coherent overlap of spatially separated image regions, which can obscure important structures. The appearance of undersampling artifacts is notably different in many non-Cartesian trajectories, however. For example, the lack of a regular Cartesian grid structure to the acquired and the omitted data in undersampled spiral (Figure 5.1d, center) and radial (Figure 5.1d, right) trajectories results in a spreading of aliasing artifact among multiple spatial positions, producing the characteristic spiral or radial streaking artifacts shown in Figure 5.1e.

For undersampled radial trajectories in particular, it has been recognized that significant degrees of undersampling may be tolerated without obscuring important cardiac or vascular anatomy, and without compromising effective spatial resolution.[25,26] (The undersampled radial image at the right in Figure 5.1e, for example, is clearly preferable to the aliased Cartesian and spiral images at the left and center.) As a result, smaller data sets may be acquired, restoring the speed and efficiency of radial trajectories and, in recent times, enabling real-time cardiac imaging. Undersampled radial (or 'undersampled projection reconstruction') techniques have been combined with real-time TrueFISP sequences to yield high contrast between blood and myocardium.[27–29] Further accelerations have been achieved using combinations of radial undersampling with multi-echo readouts.[29]

Figure 5.2c and d show examples of real-time cardiac images obtained using a spiral imaging sequence and a radial TrueFISP sequence, respectively. The radial TrueFISP image was obtained with a number of radial projections equal to the number of Cartesian phase-encoding lines in the Cartesian TrueFISP image of Figure 5.2b, resulting in an increased spatial resolution (2.3 mm × 2.3 mm versus 2.3 mm × 6 mm) at the same temporal resolution (55 ms/frame). Figure 5.3 shows another comparison of Cartesian and radial TrueFISP (or balanced FFE) sequences. Motion of the myocardium during systole results in severe ghosting artifacts in the Cartesian systolic image (Figure 5.3c), whereas the corresponding radial systolic image (Figure 5.3d) displays more minor and clinically acceptable radial streaking artifacts.[28]

Parallel imaging

The concept of undersampling leads naturally to the topic of parallel imaging. It is clear from the example of undersampled projection reconstruction that the acquisition of smaller data sets reduces acquisition time. This is actually a result of the fact that, regardless of the particular k-space trajectory taken, MR data acquisition traditionally occurs in a sequential order, point by point or line by line. In Cartesian trajectories, each line of data requires separate application of a switched field gradient and in some cases an RF pulse. Even in single-shot spiral trajectories without sharp gradient transitions, data are acquired sequentially at different evolution times during the extended readout. As a consequence of this sequential strategy, traditional MR acquisition speed has been limited by the maximum switching rates of gradients and pulses. Physical limits are set by the performance of the gradient and RF amplifiers, while potentially more stringent physiologic constraints result from the need to avoid neuromuscular stimulation or excessive deposition of RF power in tissue.

Parallel imaging seeks to circumvent these constraints on speed by acquiring some portion of the data *simultaneously*, rather than in a traditional sequential order.

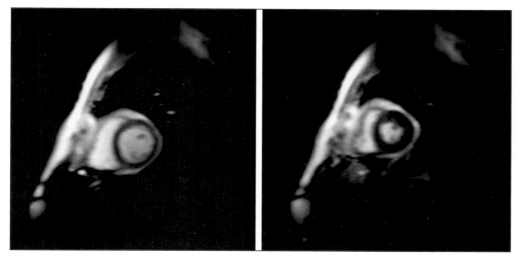

Figure 5.7
Real-time Cartesian TrueFISP cardiac images, accelerated by a factor of 1.5 to 15 frames/s using a self-calibrating generalized parallel imaging technique.[51] A flexible four-element array contoured to the chest wall was used for this study, and substantial motion of the chest wall and the diaphragm occurred over the course of the respiratory cycle, as can be appreciated from the two distinct timeframes shown. Use of self-calibration allowed accurate accelerated images to be obtained at all timeframes, despite motion of the coil array, which would confound a fixed calibration.

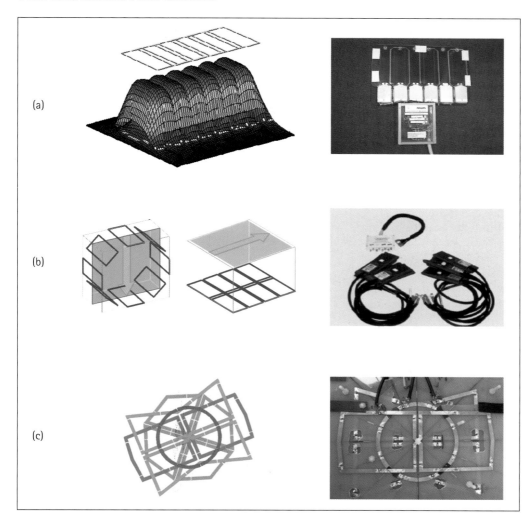

(a)

(b)

(c)

Figure 5.8
Selected parallel imaging coil array designs. (a) A prototype linear six-element array for cardiac imaging (Philips Medical Systems, Best, Netherlands[54]). A schematic of the conductor arrangement and simulated coil sensitivities are shown to the left of a photograph of the array. (b) An eight-element array with independently positionable elements (Nova Medical, Inc., Wakefield, MA, photograph courtesy of Patrick Ledden). Two possible array configurations – an encircling configuration and a two-dimensional stacked arrangement – are shown alongside a picture of the array. (c) A prototype four-element array with concentric crossed elements,[57] departing from the traditional loop design. The conductor pattern template and a photograph are shown.

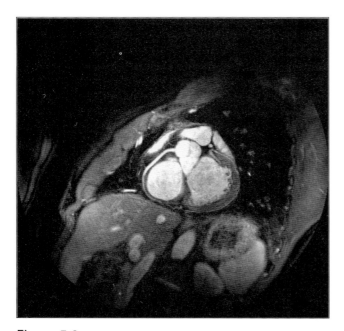

Figure 5.9
Maximum-intensity projection of a twofold accelerated three-dimensional data set showing the right coronary artery in a healthy adult subject, obtained using a generalized self-calibrating spiral parallel imaging technique, PARS (parallel imaging with augmented radius in k-space).[62,63] A navigator-gated and corrected, ECG-triggered three-dimensional spiral pulse sequence[109] was used to acquire MR signal data at a rate of one interleaf per R–R interval, and a total of 40 spiral interleafs were acquired. Although this particular implementation used cardiac triggering and respiratory gating, self-calibrating non-Cartesian parallel imaging techniques hold great promise for real-time cardiac imaging. (MIP image provided by Ernest Yeh and Matthias Stuber.)

Other means of using temporal information from dynamic image sets have also been proposed. Techniques such as UNFOLD[67] and SLAM[68] introduce temporal modulations into the acquired k-space data in order to remove aliasing artifacts in individually under-sampled frames. In fact, UNFOLD has been used to reduce residual streaking artifacts in real-time cardiac imaging techniques using undersampled projection reconstruction.[29] Similar principles have been used to increase acceleration or remove residual aliasing artifacts in parallel imaging.[69,70]

Partial Fourier approaches use the conjugate symmetry of k-space data to reconstruct images with full k-space coverage from asymmetrically sampled data, allowing as much as twofold accelerations of data acquisition. Partial Fourier techniques have been used for cardiac fluoroscopy.[71,72]

Alternatively, one may depart from Fourier encoding entirely. Selective RF pulses have been used to produce non-Fourier modulations of magnetization that represent objects more compactly than is possible with traditional Fourier coefficients. As a result, fewer encoding steps are required for a given image resolution, and imaging time may be reduced. Examples include wavelet encoding[73,74] and SVD encoding,[75] which have been used for dynamic adaptive imaging.

Given the range of techniques that are available in principle for accelerated data acquisition, the choice of a particular recipe for real-time cardiac imaging can be a dauntingly flexible one. If a sequence with desirable contrast properties does not have sufficient speed for a desired frame rate at a target spatial resolution, one may always consider adding an ancillary acceleration technique, so long as that technique does not exhaust the baseline reserves of image SNR. In practice, the choice of real-time tools may often be dictated by available hardware and software resources.

Enabling technologies

The ongoing development of strong, rapidly switched gradient systems has been a cornerstone for progress in real-time imaging. Given the canonical tradeoff between SNR and imaging speed, coils and coil arrays designed for high SNR in target cardiac image planes also play a crucial role. As discussed earlier, the advent of parallel imaging has placed new demands on coil design. The maximum acceleration and SNR that may be achieved in a parallel imaging study scales with the number of independent coil arrays available for imaging. Partly as a consequence of this, the number of commercially available receivers has been growing in recent years, from a heretofore typical number of four to a more luxurious eight on several current systems, with higher numbers being discussed.

Particularly as the number of independent receiver channels grows, the configuration of the data pipeline becomes increasingly important, since large quantities and high rates of incoming data must be accommodated. Furthermore, many real-time imaging applications call for real-time visualization. Integrated hardware and software for rapid image reconstruction and display has played an enabling role in making potentially complex image reconstructions practical with low latency from acquisition to display.[76,77]

In short, routine real-time applications require an integrated real-time imaging system. Various custom systems have been constructed at particular research centers over the years.[78–81] By now, many manufacturers have incorporated real-time components and capabilities into their commercial systems.

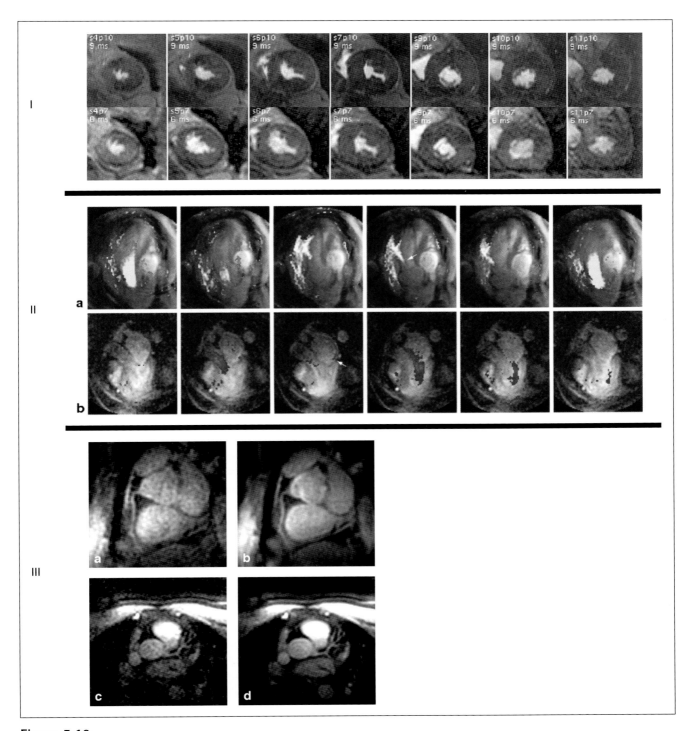

Figure 5.10

A sampling of real-time cardiac imaging applications. (I) Left ventricular (LV) function assessment.[87] Short-axis images acquired with conventional Cartesian cine gradient echo (top) and real-time segmented EPI (bottom) acquisitions are shown, including diastolic frames of all slices covering the LV in a patient with LV hypertrophy. (II) Real-time color flow.[96] Image sequences from three-chamber views of (a) a patient with aortic insufficiency and (b) a patient with mitral regurgitation are shown. These consecutive frames are acquired in 180 ms each, which is the true frame rate. A sliding window reconstruction and display operates at 18 frames/s. In series (a), aortic regurgitation is observed throughout diastole (frames 3–5). In series (b), mitral regurgitation is observed during diastole (frames 2–3). (III) Coronary MR angiography without ECG gating or breathholding.[100] Images were obtained using interleaved spiral (a,b) and interleaved echo-planar (c,d) pulse sequences, without (a,c) and with (b,d) adaptive averaging. ((I) reproduced from Plein et al. Magn Res Imaging 2001; 14:23–30,[87] Figure 2. (II) reproduced from Nayak et al. Magn Res Med 2000; 43:251–8,[96] Figure 9. (III) reproduced from Hardy et al,[100] Figure 4 with permission from John Wiley & Sons, Inc.)

Applications

One of the most popular uses of real-time CMR has been in the area of left-ventricular function assessment. Numerous recent studies[14,15,81–91] have used real-time techniques to characterize ventricular volume, ejection fraction, mass, and wall motion, both at rest and under physiologic or pharmacologic stress. Good correlation has been demonstrated with CMR cine studies, whose breath-holding and ECG gating requirements may be dispensed with in real-time studies. Good correlation with and complementarity to echocardiography has also been demonstrated. In a further emulation and supplementation of echocardiographic capabilities, flow-encoded MR sequences have been implemented in real time.[92–97]

Interventional and intravascular applications[98] place a high demand on image acquisition speed, and these applications have for some time served as a motivating force for real-time technique and system development. Interventional approaches are the subject of other chapters in this volume.

Real-time imaging has also begun to play an enabling role for MR coronary angiography. Low-resolution real-time scanning may be used in an interactive mode for rapid identification of target image planes, which are then subjected to slower high-resolution scanning.[99] Alternatively, information from real-time coronary artery scans may be coregistered and averaged to yield improved SNR or spatial resolution.[100] As the speed of real-time imaging techniques increases, direct high-resolution real-time coronary MR scans are beginning to become feasible.[101]

Interactive scan planning, with the user steering through a volume in real time to identify target anatomy, represents one example of the type of supporting role that real-time techniques can play once they are effectively integrated into an imaging system. Another example is evident in the routine use of navigators,[102–105] which generally employ some form of rapid selective excitation and one-dimensional readout to track the motion of a tissue interface. Information about the motion of the interface may then be incorporated in real time for the correction of slice positions or the registration of data. Rapid 'pencil beam' excitations may also be used for direct real-time visualization of interface motion, analogous to M-mode echocardiography.[79,106] Knowledge obtained from real-time studies may also aid in the effective placement of navigators in practical imaging examinations.[107]

Figure 5.10 shows a sampling of examples of real-time cardiac imaging applications (offered with the caveat that representative still-frame images tend not to do justice to dynamic series, which are best viewed in real time). So far, we have discussed these applications in relative isolation. However, integration of many structural and functional studies into a single examination will also require high speed and efficiency.[108] It stands to reason, then, that integrated real-time imaging capabilities will form an important part of that Holy Grail of CMR: the comprehensive cardiac exam.

In summary, after two decades of development in the techniques and technologies of rapid MRI, a rich arsenal of tools for real-time imaging exists, and many of those tools are becoming increasingly available to clinical users of MR systems. As CMR moves further into the clinical mainstream, real-time imaging capabilities can be expected to continue to provide access to the benefits of CMR at short timescales.

Acknowledgements

The following colleagues are acknowledged for kindly providing figure materials: A Bornstedt, O Simonetti, S Kaji, B Hu, T Schaeffter, C McKenzie, P Ledden, M Ohliger, E Yeh, M Stuber, S Plein, K Nayak, B Hu, and C Hardy.

References

1. Mansfield P. Multiplanar image formation using NMR spin echoes. J Phys C 1977; 10:L55.

2. Doyle M, Rzedzian R, Mansfield P, Coupland RE. Dynamic NMR cardiac imaging in a piglet. Br J Radiol 1983; 56:925–30.

3. Chapman B, Turner R, Ordidge RJ, et al. Real-time movie imaging from a single cardiac cycle by NMR. Magn Reson Med 1987; 5:246–54.

4. Haase A, Frahm J, Matthaei K. FLASH imaging: rapid NMR imaging using low flip angles. J Magn Reson 1986; 67:258–66.

5. Matthaei D, Haase A, Henrich D, Duhmke E. Cardiac and vascular imaging with an MR snapshot technique. Radiology 1990; 177:527–32.

6. Riederer SJ, Tasciyan T, Farzaneh F, et al. MR fluoroscopy: technical feasibility. Magn Reson Med 1988; 8:1–15.

7. Wright RC, Riederer SJ, Farzaneh F, et al. Real-time MR fluoroscopic data acquisition and image reconstruction. Magn Reson Med 1989; 12:407–15.

8. McKinnon GC. Ultrafast interleaved gradient-echo-planar imaging on a standard scanner. Magn Reson Med 1993; 30:609–16.

9. Davis CP, McKinnon GC, Debatin JF, et al. Single-shot versus interleaved echo-planar MR imaging: application to visualization of cardiac valve leaflets. J Magn Reson Imaging 1995; 5:107–12.

10. Oppelt A, Graumann R, Barfuss H, et al. FISP: a new fast MRI sequence. Electromedica 1986; 54:15–18.

11. Duerk JL, Lewin JS, Wendt M, Petersilge C. Remember true FISP? A high SNR, near 1-second imaging method for T2-like contrast in interventional MRI at .2 T. J Magn Reson Imaging 1998; 8:203–8.

12. Barkhausen J, Ruehm SG, Goyen M, et al. MR evaluation of ventricular function: true fast imaging with steady-state precession versus fast low-angle shot cine MR imaging: feasibility study. Radiology 2001; 219:264–9.

13. Carr JC, Simonetti O, Bundy J, et al. Cine MR angiography of the heart with segmented true fast imaging with steady-state precession. Radiology 2001; 219:828–34.

14. Lee VS, Resnick D, Bundy JM, et al. Cardiac function: MR evaluation in one breath hold with real-time true fast imaging with steady-state precession. Radiology 2002; 222:835–42.

15. Barkhausen J, Goyen M, Ruhm SG, et al. Assessment of ventricular function with single breath-hold real-time steady-state free precession cine MR imaging. AJR 2002; 178:731–5.

16. Ahn BC, Kim JH, Cho ZH. High-speed spiral-scan echo planar NMR imaging. IEEE Trans Med Imaging 1986; 5:2–7.

17. Meyer CH, Hu BS, Nishimura DG, Macovski A. Fast spiral coronary artery imaging. Magn Reson Med 1992; 28:202–13.

18. Block W, Pauly J, Nishimura D. RARE spiral T2-weighted imaging. Magn Reson Med 1997; 37:582–90.

19. Bornert P, Aldefeld B, Eggers H. Reversed spiral MR imaging. Magn Reson Med 2000; 44:479–84.

20. O'Sullivan JD. A fast sinc function gridding algorithm for Fourier inversion in computer tomography. IEEE Trans Med Imaging 1985; 4:200–7.

21. Jackson JI, Meyer CH, Nishimura DG, Macovski A. Selection of a convolution function for Fourier inversion using gridding. IEEE Trans Med Imaging 1991; 10:473–8.

22. Lauterbur P. Image formation by induced local interactions: examples employing nuclear magnetic resonance. Nature 1973; 242:190–1.

23. Lauterbur P, Lai C-M. Zeugmatography by reconstruction from projections. IEEE Trans Nucl Sci 1980; 27:1227–31.

24. Glover GH, Pauly JM. Projection reconstruction techniques for reduction of motion effects in MRI. Magn Reson Med 1992; 28:275–89.

25. Peters DC, Korosec FR, Grist TM, et al. Undersampled projection reconstruction applied to MR angiography. Magn Reson Med 2000; 43:91–101.

26. Peters DC, Epstein FH, McVeigh ER. Myocardial wall tagging with undersampled projection reconstruction. Magn Reson Med 2001; 45:562–7.

27. Shankaranarayanan A, Simonetti OP, Laub G, et al. Segmented k-space and real-time cardiac cine MR imaging with radial trajectories. Radiology 2001; 221:827–36.

28. Schaeffter T, Weiss S, Eggers H, Rasche V. Projection reconstruction balanced fast field echo for interactive real-time cardiac imaging. Magn Reson Med 2001; 46:1238–41.

29. Larson AC, Simonetti OP. Real-time cardiac cine imaging with SPIDER: steady-state projection imaging with dynamic echo-train readout. Magn Reson Med 2001; 46:1059–66.

30. Roemer PB, Edelstein WA, Hayes CE, et al. The NMR phased array. Magn Reson Med 1990; 16:192–225.

31. Carlson JW. An algorithm for NMR imaging reconstruction based on multiple RF receiver coils. J Magn Reson 1987; 74:376–80.

32. Hutchinson M, Raff U. Fast MRI data acquisition using multiple detectors. Magn Reson Med 1988; 6:87–91.

33. Kelton JR, Magin RL, Wright SM. An algorithm for rapid image acquisition using multiple receiver coils. In: Proceedings of the 8th Annual Meeting of the Society for Magnetic Resonance in Medicine, Amsterdam, 1989: 1172.

34. Kwiat D, Einav S, Navon G. A decoupled coil detector array for fast image acquisition in magnetic resonance imaging. Med Phys 1991; 18:251–65.

35. Carlson JW, Minemura T. Imaging time reduction through multiple receiver coil data acquisition and image reconstruction. Magn Reson Med 1993; 29:681–7.

36. Sodickson DK, Manning WJ. Simultaneous acquisition of spatial harmonics (SMASH): fast imaging with radiofrequency coil arrays. Magn Reson Med 1997; 38:591–603.

37. Pruessmann KP, Weiger M, Scheidegger MB, Boesiger P. SENSE: sensitivity encoding for fast MRI. Magn Reson Med 1999; 42:952–62.

38. Weiger M, Pruessmann KP, Scheidegger MB, Boesiger P. Cardiac real-time acquisition using coil sensitivity encoding. In: Proceedings of 6th Scientific Meeting of the International Society for Magnetic Resonance in Medicine, Sydney, 1998: 803.

39. Weiger M, Pruessmann KP, Boesiger P. Cardiac real-time imaging using SENSE. SENSitivity Encoding scheme. Magn Reson Med 2000; 43:177–84.

40. Sodickson DK, Stuber M, Botnar RM, et al. SMASH real-time cardiac MR imaging at echocardiographic frame rates. In: Proceedings of 7th Scientific Meeting of the International Society for Magnetic Resonance in Medicine, Philadelphia, 1999: 387.

41. Jakob PM, Griswold MA, Edelman RR, et al. Accelerated cardiac imaging using the SMASH technique. J Cardiovasc Magn Reson 1999; 1:153–7.

42. Pruessmann KP, Weiger M, Boesiger P. Sensitivity encoded cardiac MRI. J Cardiovasc Magn Reson 2001; 3:1–9.

43. Sodickson DK, McKenzie CA, Li W, et al. Contrast-enhanced 3D MR angiography with simultaneous acquisition of spatial harmonics: a pilot study. Radiology 2000; 217:284–9.

44. Weiger M, Pruessmann KP, Kassner A, et al. Contrast-enhanced 3D MRA using SENSE. J Magn Reson Imaging 2000; 12:671–7.

45. Kyriakos WE, Panych LP, Kacher DF, et al. Sensitivity profiles from an array of coils for encoding and reconstruction in parallel (SPACE RIP). Magn Reson Med 2000; 44:301–8.

46. Sodickson DK, McKenzie CA. A generalized approach to parallel magnetic resonance imaging. Med Phys 2001; 28:1629–43.

47. Pruessmann KP, Weiger M, Bornert P, Boesiger P. Advances in sensitivity encoding with arbitrary k-space trajectories. Magn Reson Med 2001; 46:638–51.

48. Sodickson DK. Tailored SMASH image reconstructions for robust in vivo parallel MR imaging. Magn Reson Med 2000; 44:243–51.

49. Jakob PM, Griswold MA, Edelman RR, Sodickson DK. AUTO-SMASH: a self-calibrating technique for SMASH imaging. Magma 1998; 7:42–54.

50. Heidemann RM, Griswold MA, Haase A, Jakob PM. VD-AUTO-SMASH imaging. Magn Reson Med 2001; 45:1066–74.

51. McKenzie CA, Yeh EN, Ohliger MA, et al. Self-calibrating parallel imaging with automatic coil sensitivity extraction. Magn Reson Med 2002; 47:529–38.

52. Sodickson DK, Griswold MA, Jakob PM, et al. Signal-to-noise ratio and signal-to-noise efficiency in SMASH imaging. Magn Reson Med 1999; 41:1009–22.

53. Griswold MA, Jakob PM, Edelman RR, Sodickson DK. A multicoil array designed for cardiac SMASH imaging. Magma 2000; 10:105–13.

54. Creemers HMM, Sodickson DK. Design of new receive coils for fast cardiac imaging. J Cardiovasc Magn Reson 1999; 1:278–9 (abst).

55. Weiger M, Pruessmann KP, Leussler C, et al. Specific coil design for SENSE: a six-element cardiac array. Magn Reson Med 2001; 45:495–504.

56. Lee RF, Westgate CR, Weiss RG, et al. Planar strip array (PSA) for MRI. Magn Reson Med 2001; 45:673–83.

57. Ohliger MA, Greenman R, McKenzie CA, Sodickson DK. Concentric coil arrays for spatial encoding in parallel MRI. In: Proceedings of 9th Scientific Meeting of the International Society for Magnetic Resonance in Medicine, Glasgow, 2001: 21.

58. Willig J, Brown R, Eagan T, Shvartsman S. Perfectly sinusoidal SMASH field shapes from birdcage sectors. In: Proceedings of 9th Scientific Meeting of the International Society for Magnetic Resonance in Medicine, Glasgow, 2001: 696.

59. Ohliger M, Yeh E, McKenzie C, Sodickson D. Fundamental physical constraints on the performance of parallel magnetic resonance imaging. In: Proceedings of 10th Scientific Meeting of the International Society for Magnetic Resonance in Medicine, Honolulu, 2002: 2387.

60. Wiesinger F, Pruessmann K, Boesiger P. Inherent limitation of the reduction factor in parallel imaging as a function of field strength. In: Proceedings of 10th Scientific Meeting of the International Society for Magnetic Resonance in Medicine, Honolulu, 2002: 191.

61. Reykowski A, Schnell W, Wang J. Simulation of SNR limit for SENSE related reconstruction techniques. In: Proceedings of 10th Scientific Meeting of the International Society for Magnetic Resonance in Medicine, Honolulu, 2002: 2385.

62. Yeh E, McKenzie C, Lim D, et al. Parallel imaging with augmented radius in k-Space (PARS). In: Proceedings of 10th Scientific Meeting of the International Society for Magnetic Resonance in Medicine, Honolulu, 2002: 2399.

63. Yeh E, Stuber M, McKenzie C, et al. Self-calibrated spiral parallel imaging. In: Proceedings of 10th Scientific Meeting of the International Society for Magnetic Resonance in Medicine, Honolulu, 2002: 2390.

64. Rasche V, Holz D, Proksa R. MR fluoroscopy using projection reconstruction multi-gradient-echo (prMGE) MRI. Magn Reson Med 1999; 42:324–34.

65. Webb AG, Liang ZP, Magin RL, Lauterbur PC. Applications of reduced-encoding MR imaging with generalized-series reconstruction (RIGR). J Magn Reson Imaging 1993; 3:925–8.

66. Chandra S, Liang ZP, Webb A, et al. Application of reduced-encoding imaging with generalized-series reconstruction (RIGR) in dynamic MR imaging. J Magn Reson Imaging 1996; 6:783–97.

67. Madore B, Glover GH, Pelc NJ. Unaliasing by Fourier-encoding the overlaps using the temporal dimension (UNFOLD), applied to cardiac imaging and fMRI. Magn Reson Med 1999; 42:813–28.

68. Rehwald WG, Kim RJ, Simonetti OP, et al. Theory of high-speed MR imaging of the human heart with the selective line acquisition mode. Radiology 2001; 220:540–7.

69. Kellman P, Epstein FH, McVeigh ER. Adaptive sensitivity encoding incorporating temporal filtering (TSENSE). Magn Reson Med 2001; 45:846–52.

70. Madore B. Using UNFOLD to remove artifacts in parallel imaging and in partial-Fourier imaging. Magn Reson Med 2002; 48:493–501.

71. Debbins JP, Riederer SJ, Rossman PJ, et al. Cardiac magnetic resonance fluoroscopy. Magn Reson Med 1996; 36:588–95.

72. Kerr AB, Pauly JM, Nishimura DG. Partial k-space acquisition for real-time MR imaging. In: Proceedings of 6th Scientific Meeting of the International Society for Magnetic Resonance in Medicine, Sydney, 1998: 1945.

73. Panych LP, Jakab PD, Jolesz FA. Implementation of wavelet-encoded MR imaging. J Magn Reson Imaging 1993; 3:649–55.

74. Weaver JB, Xu Y, Healy DM, Driscoll JR. Wavelet-encoded MR imaging. Magn Reson Med 1992; 24:275–87.

75. Zientara GP, Panych LP, Jolesz FA. Dynamically adaptive MRI with encoding by singular value decomposition. Magn Reson Med 1994; 32:268–74.

76. Morgan PN, Iannuzzelli RJ, Epstein FH, Balaban RS. Real-time cardiac MRI using DSP's. IEEE Trans Med Imaging 1999; 18:649–53.

77. Eggers H, Proksa R. Multiprocessor system for real-time convolution interpolation reconstruction. In: Proceedings of 7th Scientific Meeting of the International Society for Magnetic Resonance in Medicine, Philadelphia, 1999: 95.

78. Holsinger AE, Wright RC, Riederer SJ, et al. Real-time interactive magnetic resonance imaging. Magn Reson Med 1990; 14:547–53.

79. Hardy CJ, Darrow RD, Nieters EJ, et al. Real-time acquisition, display, and interactive graphic control of NMR cardiac profiles and images. Magn Reson Med 1993; 29:667–73.

80. Kerr AB, Pauly JM, Hu BS, et al. Real-time interactive MRI on a conventional scanner. Magn Reson Med 1997; 38:355–67.

81. Yang PC, Kerr AB, Liu AC, et al. New real-time interactive cardiac magnetic resonance imaging system complements echocardiography. J Am Coll Cardiol 1998; 32:2049–56.

82. Weber OM, Eggers H, Spiegel MA, et al. Real-time interactive magnetic resonance imaging with multiple coils for the assessment of left ventricular function. J Magn Reson Imaging 1999; 10:826–32.

83. Setser RM, Fischer SE, Lorenz CH. Quantification of left ventricular function with magnetic resonance images acquired in real time. J Magn Reson Imaging 2000; 12:430–8.

84. Nagel E, Schneider U, Schalla S, et al. Magnetic resonance real-time imaging for the evaluation of left ventricular function. J Cardiovasc Magn Reson 2000; 2:7–14.

85. Bornstedt A, Nagel E, Schalla S, et al. Multi-slice dynamic imaging: complete functional cardiac MR examination within 15 seconds. J Magn Reson Imaging 2001; 14:300–5.

86. Nayak KS, Pauly JM, Nishimura DG, Hu BS. Rapid ventricular assessment using real-time interactive multislice MRI. Magn Reson Med 2001; 45:371–5.

87. Plein S, Smith WH, Ridgway JP, et al. Qualitative and quantitative analysis of regional left ventricular wall dynamics using real-time magnetic resonance imaging: comparison with conventional breath-hold gradient echo acquisition in volunteers and patients. J Magn Reson Imaging 2001; 14:23–30.

88. Plein S, Smith WH, Ridgway JP, et al. Measurements of left ventricular dimensions using real-time acquisition in cardiac magnetic resonance imaging: comparison with conventional gradient echo imaging. Magma 2001; 13:101–8.

89. Schalla S, Nagel E, Lehmkuhl H, et al. Comparison of magnetic resonance real-time imaging of left ventricular function with conventional magnetic resonance imaging and echocardiography. Am J Cardiol 2001; 87:95–9.

90. Kaji S, Yang PC, Kerr AB, et al. Rapid evaluation of left ventricular volume and mass without breath-holding using real-time interactive cardiac magnetic resonance imaging system. J Am Coll Cardiol 2001; 38:527–33.

91. Schalla S, Klein C, Paetsch I, et al. Real-time MR image acquisition during high-dose dobutamine hydrochloride stress for detecting left ventricular wall-motion abnormalities in patients with coronary arterial disease. Radiology 2002; 224:845–51.

92. Guilfoyle DN, Gibbs P, Ordidge RJ, Mansfield P. Real-time flow measurements using echo-planar imaging. Magn Reson Med 1991; 18:1–8.

93. Hu BS, Pauly JM, Nishimura DG. Localized real-time velocity spectra determination. Magn Reson Med 1993; 30:393–8.

94. Irarrazabal P, Hu BS, Pauly JM, Nishimura DG. Spatially resolved and localized real-time velocity distribution. Magn Reson Med 1993; 30:207–12.

95. Gatehouse PD, Firmin DN, Collins S, Longmore DB. Real time blood flow imaging by spiral scan phase velocity mapping. Magn Reson Med 1994; 31:504–12.

96. Nayak KS, Pauly JM, Kerr AB, et al. Real-time color flow MRI. Magn Reson Med 2000; 43:251–8.

97. Wetzel SG, Lee VS, Tan AG, et al. Real-time interactive duplex MR measurements: application in neurovascular imaging. AJR 2001; 177:703–7.

98. Lardo AC. Real-time magnetic resonance imaging: diagnostic and interventional applications. Pediatr Cardiol 2000; 21:80–98.

99. Hardy CJ, Darrow RD, Pauly JM, et al. Interactive coronary MRI. Magn Reson Med 1998; 40:105–11.

100. Hardy CJ, Saranathan M, Zhu Y, Darrow RD. Coronary angiography by real-time MRI with adaptive averaging. Magn Reson Med 2000; 44:940–6.

101. Nayak KS, Pauly JM, Yang PC, et al. Real-time interactive coronary MRA. Magn Reson Med 2001; 46:430–5.

102. Ehman RL, Felmlee JP. Adaptive technique for high-definition MR imaging of moving structures. Radiology 1989; 173:255–63.

103. Sachs TS, Meyer CH, Hu BS, et al. Real-time motion detection in spiral MRI using navigators. Magn Reson Med 1994; 32:639–45.

104. Wang Y, Rossman PJ, Grimm RC, et al. Navigator-echo-based real-time respiratory gating and triggering for reduction of respiration effects in three-dimensional coronary MR angiography. Radiology 1996; 198:55–60.

105. McConnell MV, Khasgiwala VC, Savord BJ, et al. Prospective adaptive navigator correction for breath-hold MR coronary angiography. Magn Reson Med 1997; 37:148–52.

106. Pearlman JD, Hardy CJ, Cline HE. Continual NMR cardiography without gating: M-mode MR imaging. Radiology 1990; 175:369–73.

107. Danias PG, Stuber M, Botnar RM, et al. Relationship between motion of coronary arteries and diaphragm during free breathing: lessons from real-time MR imaging. AJR 1999; 172:1061–5.

108. Plein S, Ridgway JP, Jones TR, et al. Coronary artery disease: assessment with a comprehensive MR imaging protocol – initial results. Radiology 2002; 225:300–7.

109. Bornert P, Stuber M, Botnar RM, et al. Direct comparison of 3D spiral vs. Cartesian gradient-echo coronary magnetic resonance angiography. Magn Reson Med 2001; 46:789–94.

6

Myocardial function and stress imaging

Eike Nagel

Introduction

Global left-ventricular (LV) function and size, as well as left-ventricular mass, are used to determine the diagnoses and the prognoses of patients with cardiovascular disease. An important example is the size of the left ventricle, since it has been shown that an enlargement of LV volume after myocardial infarction is related to an increased risk for LV remodeling and heart failure.[1] In addition, an accurate determination of LV mass helps to correctly classify patients with LV hypertrophy or cardiomyopathy.

In recent years, cardiac magnetic resonance (MR) imaging (CMR) has become the accepted reference standard for the assessment of global LV volumes and mass, since CMR methods are both accurate and highly reproducible.[2] With advances in high-resolution breathhold techniques for the visualization of myocardial motion, this application has gained widespread acceptance for the assessment of LV function and regional wall motion. These techniques can be used to detect, localize, and quantitate myocardial infarction, in combination with infarct imaging (see Chapter 6) hibernating myocardium can be assessed, and stress examinations allow the detection of ischemic myocardium.

This chapter will discuss indications for the assessment of LV function; it will describe different imaging sequences and strategies, such as free breathing, breath-holding and real-time imaging. Standardized procedures for anatomical planning of the basic views as well as the visual and quantitative assessment of the images will be supplied. Normal values for the assessment of LV function and mass are given and potential pitfalls discussed. The rationale of stress imaging, image interpretation, and caveats of dobutamine stress imaging will be discussed and related to the newest literature. Practical recommendations for patient setup and how to perform stress examinations are given. The chapter ends with topics currently under investigation, such as the combination of wall motion and perfusion.

Indications for the assessment of LV function

The imaging strategy has to be chosen according to the indication of the CMR study (Table 6.1). On one hand,

Table 6.1 Imaging strategies for different indications		
Indication	*Imaging strategy*	*Quantification*
Rapid evaluation of global LV function	Minimal data set: 3 short axes, 2 long axes	If visually normal: area–length ejection fraction
Determination of LV mass	Full coverage; slice gap (2–4 mm) possible	Full quantification
Accurate determination of LV function: follow-up studies valvular heart disease myocarditis myocardial infarction	Full coverage; slice gap (2–4 mm) possible	Full quantification
Detection of stress-induced wall motion abnormalities	Minimal data set: 3 short axes, 2 long axes	Visual (see comments in text on quantification of stress MR)

full coverage of the left ventricle with a series of short-axis slices is the most reproducible and accurate approach. On the other hand, data acquisition as well as postprocessing of such a large data set require considerable time. As an alternative, a minimal data set can be acquired that should at least cover the 17 segments suggested by the American Heart Association/American College of Cardiology (AHA/ACC)[3] (Figure 6.1), which can be achieved by acquiring a minimum of three short axes and one long-axis view. We recommend a minimal data set consisting of five views: three short axes, a four-chamber view, and a two-chamber view. Such a data set can be acquired in

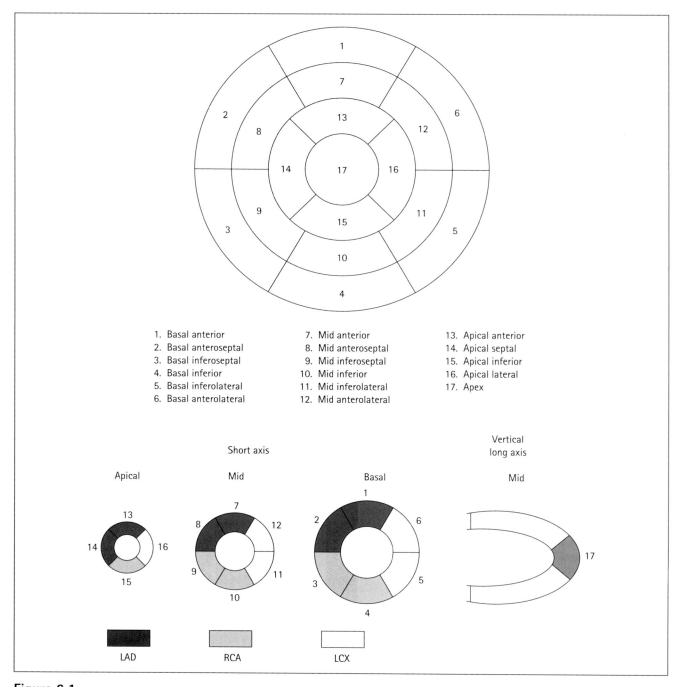

1. Basal anterior
2. Basal anteroseptal
3. Basal inferoseptal
4. Basal inferior
5. Basal inferolateral
6. Basal anterolateral

7. Mid anterior
8. Mid anteroseptal
9. Mid inferoseptal
10. Mid inferior
11. Mid inferolateral
12. Mid anterolateral

13. Apical anterior
14. Apical septal
15. Apical inferior
16. Apical lateral
17. Apex

Figure 6.1
Left-ventricular segmentation (according to AHA/ACC statements).[3] The anterior insertion point of the right ventricle is used as a starting point and determines the segment border between 1 and 2, 7 and 8, as well as 13 and 14. The segments are assigned to specific coronary arteries according to the graph.

five breathholds lasting ~10 s each, and thus the examination time is ~2–3 min. This approach is very robust, is easy to quantify, and covers most myocardial segments twice.

In many patients sent for a CMR study, the assessment of LV function is not the primary goal; however, a rapid determination of LV function should be performed whenever possible. In these patients, it is important to classify LV ejection fraction as normal, mildly, or severely depressed, and to detect regional wall motion abnormalities at rest. This can be done with a minimal data set covering all 17 segments. If no wall motion abnormalities are seen, area–length ejection fraction (see below) is usually adequate to generate a basic quantification. In contrast, patients sent for the determination of LV mass or for an accurate determination of LV function, such as those with valvular heart disease, myocarditis, or after myocardial infarction, require full coverage of the LV and quantification of all slices using Simpson's method (see below). For these indications, MRI is regarded as the reference standard due to its high accuracy and reproducibility, and thus care needs to be taken to achieve this accuracy and to be able to detect small changes over time. If the patient is sent for a stress examination, a minimal data set covering all 17 segments is adequate, since the data need to be acquired during each stress level. Image evaluation for stress CMR is usually visual.

Basics for the assessment of LV function

Hardware

For the assessment of LV function, the MR scanner should be a ≥1 T whole-body scanner. For stress examinations, preferably 1.5 T should be used. The gradients should have a strength of ≥30 mT/m and a speed of ≥75 mT/m/ms.

Even though cardiac examinations can be performed with the body coil integrated into the scanner, a much better signal-to-noise ratio (SNR) is achieved with specific cardiac phased array coils usually consisting of 4–6 elements placed around the thorax of the patient. We recommend the use of such a coil for all cardiac examinations.

An electrocardiogram (ECG) or vectorcardiogram[4] is required for all cardiovascular examinations, and is used for triggering/gating of the image acquisition and for monitoring of the patient.

For stress examinations, blood pressure monitoring devices are also required (see below).

Sequences

For the assessment of LV function sequences that fulfil the following requirements have to be applied:[5]

- strong contrast between blood and endocardium;
- good contrast between epicardium and surrounding structures (lung, liver, etc.);
- in-plane resolution ~2 mm × 2 mm or better;
- slice thickness ~8 mm or better;
- temporal resolution <50 ms.

In general, these requirements are fulfilled by all gradient-echo sequences, for example standard gradient-echo, segmented *k*-space (turbo) gradient-echo, echo-planar imaging (EPI), hybrid sequences (turbo gradient-echo echo-planar imaging), and steady-state free precession (SSFP) techniques. Images can be acquired during free breathing or during short breathholding. ECG triggering, retrospective ECG gating, or real-time imaging is needed to account for cardiac motion. From this variety of possibilities, most users currently choose a few standard strategies.

Turbo gradient-echo (TFE, FLASH) / segmented *k*-space gradient-echo

This sequence type has been the standard sequence until recently. Most data on normal values and most clinical studies have been performed with such sequences. Typically, a *k*-space segmentation of 12–16 is applied, and thus each image is acquired during 12–16 heartbeats. To minimize artifacts from breathing motion, breathholding is required during this period. A range of typical scan parameters is listed in Table 6.2. With such sequences, all of the requirements mentioned above can be fulfilled with minimal scan time; for example, five imaging planes can be covered well within 3 min. Thus, this sequence can also be used during stress examinations.

Steady-state free precession (BFFE, FIESTA, TrueFISP)

Today's state-of-the-art scanners are equipped with SSFP techniques. This sequence offers a better delineation of the endo- and epicardium within even shorter scan times when compared with turbo gradient-echo imaging. Typically, breath hold durations of 8–12 heartbeats are used. The sequence parameters are listed in Table 6.2. Whereas such sequences are used as the 'work horse' in most centers today, one should keep in mind potential differences in normal values in comparison with turbo gradient-echo techniques.

Table 6.2 Standard sequence parameters

	Turbo gradient-echo: multishot /segmented	Steady-state free precession (SSFP): multishot /segmented	Real time imaging (SSFP): single-shot
Motion suppression	Prospective / retrospective ECG, breathholding	Prospective / retrospective ECG, breathholding	None
Range of TE / TR / flip (ms / ms / °)	~3 / ~6 / 20–30	< 2 / < 4 / 50–60	< 2 / < 4 / 50–60
Approximate spatial resolution (mm^3)	$2 \times 2 \times 8$	$2 \times 2 \times 8$	$(3–4) \times (3–4) \times 10$
Approximate temporal resolution (ms)	< 50	< 40	~60 (35^a)
Approximate scan duration	10–15 s	12 s (6 s^a)	2–3 RR intervals

^{a} With the use of parallel imaging.

Real-time imaging

Most real-time techniques are faster versions of turbo gradient-echo or SSFP techniques. Real-time imaging[6,7] has been shown to achieve similar or superior image quality when compared with echocardiography.[7] It also permits an accurate determination of LV ejection fraction[8,9] and allows the detection of wall motion abnormalities during stress examinations.[10] However, this reduction in measurement time, which allows the acquisition of all data in real time (and thus without ECG triggering or breathholding), can only be achieved by reductions in spatial and temporal resolution. As a result, current real-time techniques do not yet fulfil the basic requirements set forth above, and therefore should not be used for routine scanning. Potential applications, however, are in those patients who are unable to hold their breath.

Comparison of different sequences

The major differences between turbo gradient-echo and SSFP techniques are the differences in generating contrast. Whereas for the former, the signal of the blood depends on the inflow of magnetized spins, in the latter, contrast is independent of flow. This has advantages especially in patients with low ejection fraction (slow flow) and for the assessment of long-axis views, since the blood flows parallel to the slice, rather than orthogonal to it. Thus, the use of SSFP techniques has considerably enhanced image quality especially in these patients and views (Figure 6.2).[11] In addition, the flow independence allows one to visualize slowly flowing blood (e.g. behind trabeculae and papillary muscles). As a consequence, wall thickness is usually measured to be thinner with steady-state tech-

niques in comparison with turbo gradient-echo. This needs to be kept in mind when using normal values derived from different sequences.

In a direct comparison of the contrast achieved between blood and endocardium for different echocardiographic and CMR techniques, it can be shown that, even with state-of-the-art echo techniques such as second-harmonic imaging and contrast-enhanced echocardiography, contrast is much lower with echo in comparison with CMR (Figure 6.3). Interestingly, this holds true for both long-axis and short-axis views with SSFP techniques, whereas long-axis views acquired with turbo gradient-echo techniques do not show superior contrast for the reasons given above.

Motion suppression

ECG

Since CMR data are acquired during several heartbeats (except for real-time imaging), data acquisition needs to be synchronized to the ECG. Usually, cardiac triggering is applied. With this technique, the R-wave is used to start data acquisition always at the same timepoint within the ECG. An alternative approach is a continuous data acquisition with retrospective distribution of the data to different parts of the cardiac cycle (retrospective gating).

Breathing motion

Breathholding is the preferred method for motion suppression for the assessment of LV function. Since the diaphragmatic position is more reproducible and stable in mid-expiration in comparison with inspiration, we use repetitive mid-expiratory positions at the German Heart

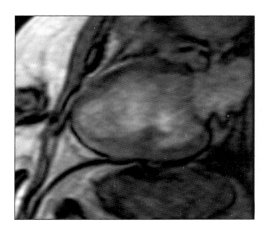
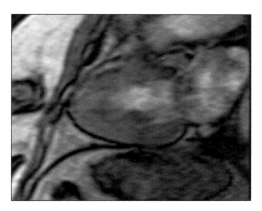
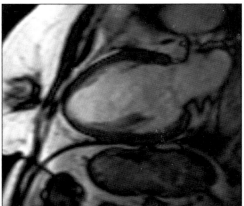
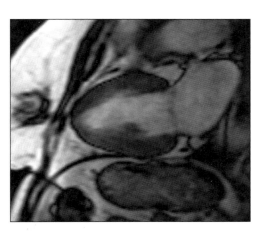

Figure 6.2
Comparison of turbo gradient-echo (top row) with steady-state free precession (SSFP) (bottom row). Note the superior contrast between the blood and the endocardium, and the epicardium versus surrounding structures, with SSFP. The mitral valve is delineated much more clearly with SSFP.

Institute in Berlin. However, despite the reduction of breathhold duration from ~20 to ~10–12 heartbeats, occasionally patients who are unable to hold their breath are encountered. In these cases, several data acquisitions (usually three or four) during free breathing are performed and signal averaging is used to obtain images. The acquisition duration is ~2 min per view. Thus, this approach cannot be used in combination with high-dose stress. Alternatively, navigators can be used to minimize artifacts from breathing motion.[12] Real-time imaging with its limitations of spatial and temporal resolution is also becoming a useful alternative to signal averaging or navigator approaches.

Planning
Definition of standard imaging planes

For cardiac examinations, the following standard imaging planes are usually chosen. Typically, these are double-angulated and follow the anatomy of the heart, rather than the body.

Short-axis view (SAX)

Short-axis views transect the LV perpendicular to its long axis (which is defined by the LV apex and the midpoint of the mitral valve) (Figure 6.4). (Some authors define the short axis as an axis parallel to the mitral value annulus.)

Four-chamber view (4-CH) / horizontal long-axis view (HLA)

A four-chamber view or horizontal long-axis view transects the LV through the apex and the midpoint of the mitral valve. It also covers the left atrium, right ventricle and right atrium at their maximal diameters (Figure 6.4).

Two-chamber view (2-CH) / vertical long-axis view (VLA)

A two-chamber view is a long-axis view perpendicular to the four-chamber view covering the anterior and inferior wall of the LV (Figure 6.4).

Standard procedure to acquire the basic imaging planes

See Figure 6.5 for the planning steps. We usually start with a transverse data set searching for a slice that contains part

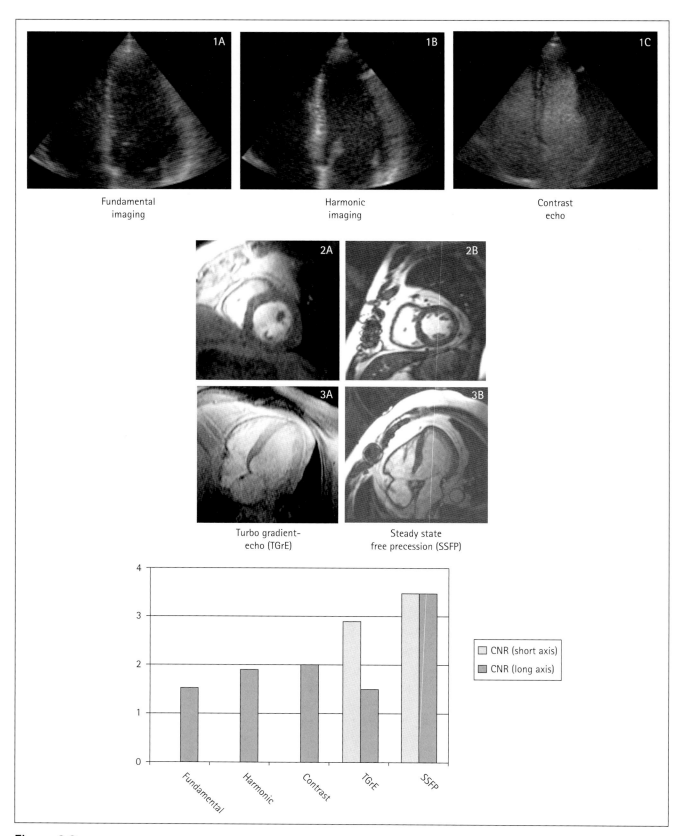

Figure 6.3
Contrast-to-noise ratio (CNR) for different echocardiographic and CMR techniques.

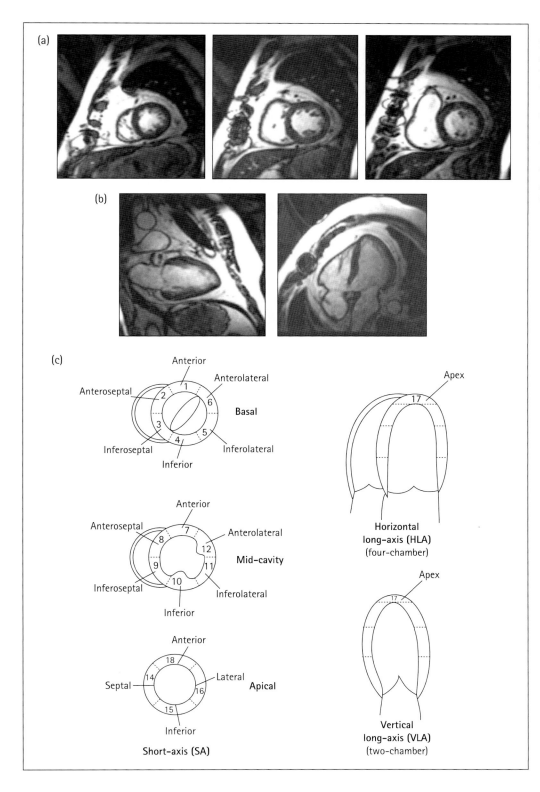

Figure 6.4

Standard views and segments. (a) Short-axis views (left to right: apex, equator, base). (b) Vertical long-axis view (two-chamber) (left) and horizontal long-axis view (four-chamber) (right). (c) Segmentation according to the American Heart Association/American College of Cardiology.[3]

of the mitral valve and a large proportion of the LV, most favorably the apex (in patients with a vertical heart axis, two different slices need to be chosen: one imaging the mitral value, one imaging the apex). In this slice, we define a single angulated ('pseudo-RAO') view cutting

through the LV apex and the midpoint of the mitral valve. This scan is already acquired in the same breathhold position as the diagnostic images to optimize planning for this diaphragmatic position. We also use multiphase imaging for this step of planning to plan the next steps on the

(a)

(b)

(c)

(d)

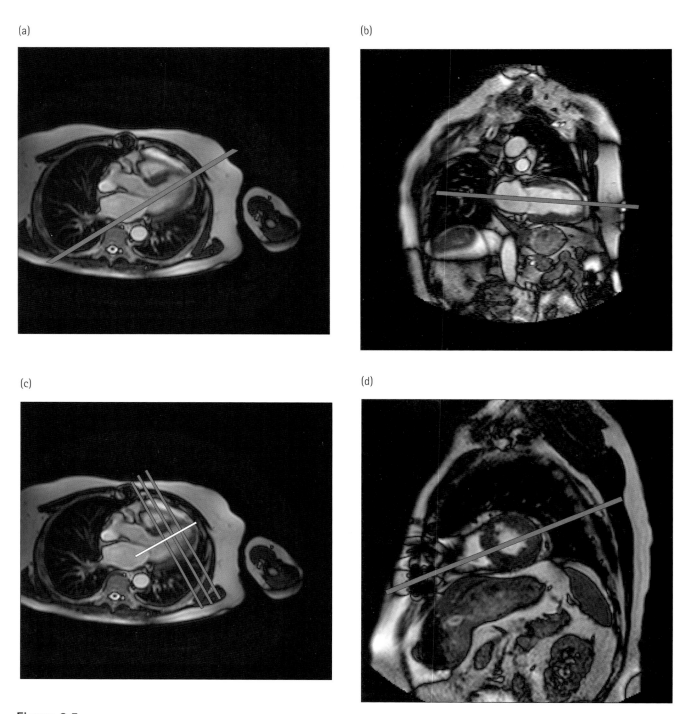

Figure 6.5

Planning steps. (a) On a transverse slice containing the mitral valve, a single angulated scan is planned through the apex and the midpoint of the mitral valve. (b) On the resulting 'pseudo-RAO', a second angulation is added again through the apex and the midpoint of the mitral valve. (c) The resulting double-angulated 'pseudo-4CH view' is used to define short-axis views that transverse a line connecting the apex and the midpoint of the mitral valve. (d) On the short-axis views, the four-chamber view is planned through the largest extension of the right ventricle and the midpoint of the LV.

Continued on next page

(e)

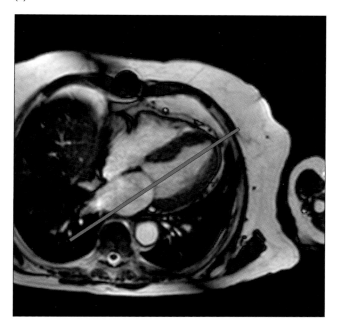

Figure 6.5 Continued
(e) The resulting horizontal long-axis view is used to define the vertical long-axis view.

end-systolic images (allowing to correct for the motion of the basal plane – see below). On the end-systolic image of this view, we plan a double-angulated view ('pseudo-4CH'), again cutting through the LV apex and the midpoint of the mitral valve. On this double-angulated view (end-systole), which usually contains parts of the right ventricle and the atria (thus 'pseudo-4CH'), we plan the short-axis views, which transect the LV perpendicular to its long axis. To achieve this, we draw a line from the apex to the midpoint of the mitral valve and plan the next views perpendicular to this line. This line is also used to determine the position of the short-axis planes relative to the long axis of the LV. If a complete coverage is to be achieved, the most basal plane should be just basal to the mitral valve in the end-diastolic frame. If only three short-axis views are to be acquired, we place the apical slice on 25% of the length between the apex and the valvular plane, and the basal slice on 75% of this distance. The third plane is placed in the middle of the two.

Alternatively to the method described above, real-time imaging can be used to achieve the basic imaging planes. Again angulations should be altered step by step and breathing position should be identical to the position required for high-resolution scanning.

Interpretation of LV function

For most indications, visual assessment is used. Whereas this is sufficient to classify ejection fraction as roughly normal, mildly, or severely depressed and to grade wall motion as normo-, hypo-, a-, or dyskinetic, one should keep in mind that always all segments need to be assessed and that an accurate assessment requires quantification. This can be achieved by using the area–length method, which is integrated into most scanners. This approach, however, should only be used to generate an approximation in patients without wall motion abnormalities. Accurate assessment of end-diastolic volume, end-systolic volume and LV mass require a three-dimensional analysis. Usually Simpson's rule is used, where epi- and endocardial contours are traced at end-diastole (defined as the first temporal frame directly after the R-wave of the ECG) and end-systole (defined as the temporal frame at which the image shows the smallest LV cavity area, usually ~300 ms after the R-wave). Papillary muscles are excluded from the LV volume and included with the LV mass. Special attention is required for the basal slice (see below). End-diastolic and end-systolic volumes (ESV and ESV) are calculated by summation of the volume of each slice (determined by area × (slice thickness + slice gap)) for all slices. Stroke volume (SV) is calculated as EDV − ESV, and ejection fraction (EF) as (SV/EDV) × 100%. Cardiac output is SV multiplied by heartrate. The LV end-diastolic mass is obtained from the volume of the LV muscle tissue including the interventricular septum multiplied by the specific myocardial weight ($1.05\ g/cm^3$). For right-ventricular volumes, the procedure is the same as for the LV. Right-ventricular mass, however, refers only to the mass of the free wall and excludes the septum. Usually indices for body weight or body surface area, rather than absolute values, are used. According to DuBois and DuBois,[13] body-surface area (BSA, in m^2) can be calculated as $[\text{weight (kg)}]^{0.425} \times [\text{height (cm)}]^{0.725} \times 0.007184.$

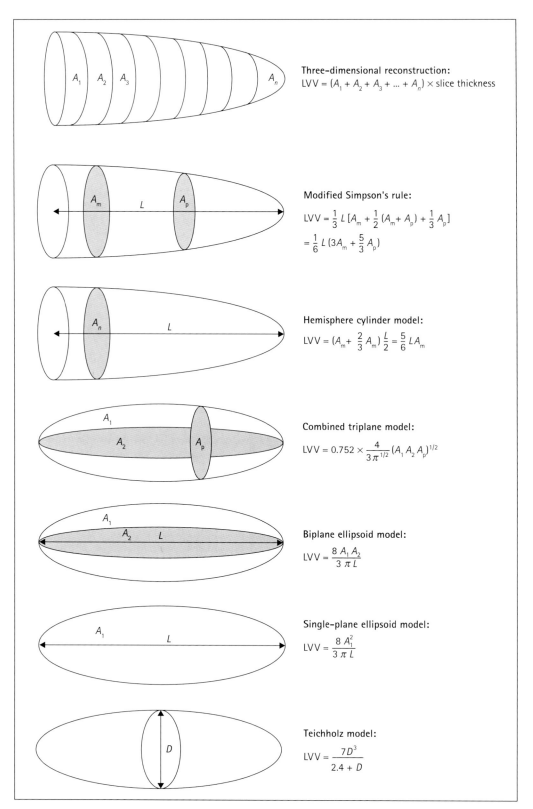

Figure 6.6
Potential models for quantification of LV volumes. (Reproduced from Thiele et al. J Cardiovasc Magn Reson 2002; 4:327–39[14] with permission from Marcel Dekker Inc.)

Alternatively, models can be used in combination with SSFP techniques[14] (but not turbo gradient-echo imaging, since contrast between blood and endocardium is insufficient for long axis views); however, these models need to take all three dimensions into account (Figure 6.6). Advantages are more rapid evaluation (and data acquisition), as well as the use of long-axis views, which account accurately for long-axis changes. Disadvantages in the use of models are that not all of the myocardium is analyzed and small changes in the angulations or breathhold position of long-axis views have a larger influence on the determination of wall thickness and area, in comparison with short-axis views.

Regional wall motion can best be assessed using the centerline method, in which wall thickness and thickening are calculated from the endo- and epicardial contours

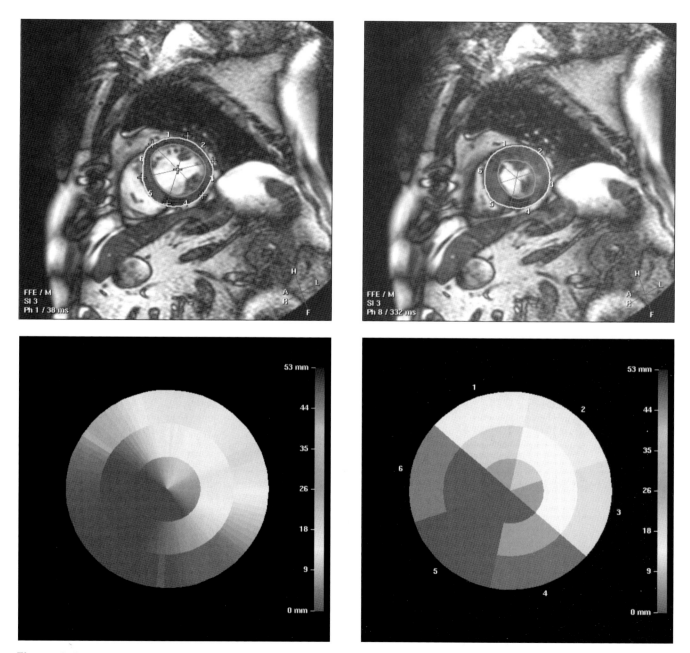

Figure 6.7
Patient with occlusion of the right coronary artery and inferoseptal myocardial infarction. Upper row: segmentation of the end-diastolic (left) and end-systolic (right) endo- and epicardial contours and placement of six equiangular segments starting from the anterior right-ventricular septal insertion. The papillary muscles are excluded from the wall. Bottom row: Bull's-eye plot for three short-axis views displaying the endocardial wall motion. Note the reduction of wall motion in the inferior and inferoseptal regions in all three slices.

for 100 equidistant segments for each view.[15] The result can be demonstrated using a bull's-eye plot. In such a plot, the outer segments present the most basal LV level (Figure 6.7). The further one moves towards the center of the plot, the more one looks at the apical level. Specific regions can then be assigned to specific coronary artery perfusion territories (see Figure 6.1).

Normal values of LV function

Normal values are dependent on age, gender, and body size.[16–18] Thus, reference values should be specified for age and gender and be normalized to body size (Tables 6.3–6.6).

Pitfalls and solutions
Basal slice

The largest potential source of error for an accurate determination of LV volumes is the decision whether or not to include the basal slice in the volumes.[19] In the normal heart, the basal slice moves considerably more toward the apex during systolic contraction.[20,21] Thus, more slices

Table 6.3 Normal ventricular values (mean ± 1 SD, with 95% confidence intervals in parentheses).

	All (n = 75)			*Males* (n = 47)			*Females* (n = 28)		
LVEDV(ml)	121	± 34	(55–187)	136	± 30	(77–195)	96	± 23	(52–141)
RVEDV(ml)	138	± 40	(59–217)	157	± 35	(88–227)	106	± 24	(58–154)
LVESV(ml)	40	± 14	(13–67)	45	± 14	(19–72)	32	± 9	(13–51)
RVESV(ml)	54	± 21	(12–96)	63	± 20	(23–103)	40	± 14	(12–68)
IVSM (g)	54	± 13	(28–80)	61	± 11	(40–82)	42	± 8	(26–58)
LVFWM (g)	104	± 27	(44–150)	117	± 22	(75–159)	82	± 19	(46–119)
LVTM (g)	158	± 39	(82–234)	178	± 31	(118–238)	125	± 26	(75–175)
RVFWM (g)	46	± 11	(25–67)	50	± 10	(30–70)	40	± 8	(24–55)
LVEF (%)	67	± 5	(57–78)	67	± 5	(56–78)	67	± 5	(56–78)
RVEF (%)	61	± 7	(47–76)	60	± 7	(47–74)	63	± 8	(47–80)
LVSV (ml)	82	± 23	(36–127)	92	± 21	(51–33)	65	± 16	(33–97)
RVSV (ml)	84	± 24	(37–1331)	95	± 22	(52–138)	66	± 16	(35–98)
LVTM/LVEDV (g/ml)	1.33	± 0.18	(0.98–1.68)	1.34	± 0.19	(0.96–1.71)	1.31	± 0.16	(0.99–1.63)
RVM/RVEDV (g/ml)	0.35	± 0.06	(0.23–0.47)	0.33	± 0.06	(0.21–0.44)	0.38	± 0.05	(0.28–0.48)
LVTM/RVM	3.46	± 0.66	(2.16–4.76)	3.64	± 0.72	(2.23–5.04)	3.17	± 0.43	(2.33–4.01)
CO (l/min)	5.2	± 1.4	(2.42–8.05)	5.8	± 3.0	(2.82–8.82)	4.3	± 0.9	(2.65–5.98)

LV, left-ventricular; RV, right-ventricular; EDV, end-diastolic volume; ESV, end-systolic volume; IVSM, interventricular septal mass; FWM, free wall mass; LVTM, LV total mass; EF, ejection fraction; SV, stroke volume; RVM, RV mass; CO, cardiac output (Reprinted from Lorenz et al. J Cardiovasc Magn Reson 1999; 1:7–21[16] with permission from Marcel Dekker Inc.)

Table 6.4 Normal ventricular values (mean ± 1 SD, with 95% confidence intervals in parentheses) normalized to body surface area (BSA).

	All (n = 75)			*Males* (n = 47)			*Females* (n = 28)		
LVEDV/BSA (ml/m²)	66	± 12	(44–89)	69	± 11	(47–92)	61	± 10	(41–81)
RVEDV/BSA (ml/m²)	75	± 13	(49–101)	80	± 13	(55–105)	67	± 10	(48–87)
LVTM/BSA (g/m²)	87	± 12	(64–109)	91	± 11	(70–113)	79	± 8	(63–95)
LVFWM/BSA (g/m²)	57	± 8	(40–73)	60	± 8	(44–76)	52	± 6	(40–64)
IVSM/BSA (g/m²)	30	± 4	(21–38)	31	± 4	(23–39)	27	± 4	(20–34)
RVFWM/BSA (g/m²)	26	± 5	(17–34)	26	± 5	(16–36)	25	± 4	(18–33)
LVSV/BSA (ml/m²)	45	± 8	(29–61)	47	± 8	(32–62)	41	± 8	(26–56)
RVSV/BSA (ml/m²)	46	± 8	(30–62)	48	± 8	(32–64)	42	± 8	(27–57)
CO/BSA (l/min/m²)	2.9	± 0.6	(1.74–4.03)	3.0	± 0.6	(1.74–4.20)	2.8	± 0.5	(1.75–3.80)

For abbreviations, see Table 6.3.
(Reprinted from Lorenz et al. J Cardiovasc Magn Reson 1999; 1:7–21[16] with permission from Marcel Dekker Inc.)

Table 6.11 Dobutamine termination criteria.

- Submaximal heart rate reached $[(220 - \text{age}) \times 0.85]$
- Blood pressure decrease > 20 mmHg systolic below baseline systolic blood pressure or decrease > 40 mmHg from a previous level
- Blood pressure increase > 240/120 mmHg
- Intractable symptoms
- New or worsening wall motion abnormalities in at least two adjacent LV segments (out of 17)
- Complex cardiac arrhythmias

(Reproduced from Nagel et al. J Cardiovasc Magn Reson 2001; 3:267–81[5] with permission from Marcel Dekker Inc.)

The monitoring of blood pressure, cardiac rhythm and patients' symptoms can be done either by placing standard equipment outside the scanner room connected to the patient with special extensions through a waveguide in the RF cage or by using special CMR-compatible equipment, which exists at many CMR sites. A defibrillator and all drugs for emergency treatment must be available at the CMR site. A specific problem for patient monitoring within the magnet is the difficulty in assessing changes of ST segments from the ECG (the magnetized blood flowing through the aorta exerts an electric current occurring at the same time as the ST segment). However, since wall motion abnormalities precede ST changes,[33,34] and such abnormalities can be readily detected with CMR, monitoring is effective without a diagnostic ECG. This requires an online assessment of wall motion during image reconstruction performed immediately after image acquisition. Several guidelines recommend an additional use of oximetry for monitoring purposes. In our experience, the value of this is only as an alternative rhythm control, which, however, is no longer required with the extremely reliable vector ECG[4] used in our institution.

Accuracy of stress testing
Viability

By using low-dose dobutamine, which stimulates wall thickening without inducing ischemia (10 µg/kg body

weight/min), Baer et al have shown good results for CMR for the detection of viable myocardium when compared with positron emission tomography (PET)[35] and transesophageal echocardiography (sensitivity 81% and specificity 100%) in a study of 43 patients.[36] The prediction of functional recovery 4–6 months after revascularization yielded a sensitivity of 89% and a specificity of 94% when an increase in systolic wall thickening of 2 mm or more was observed during stress CMR, which are essentially identical to the sensitivity and specificity of PET.[37] Similar results have been found by Sandstede et al.[38] in 25 patients.

Thus, low-dose dobutamine stress CMR is a valid tool for the detection of viable myocardium, and can compete with transesophageal echocardiography and PET; however, current data stem from single centers only, and multicenter studies in larger numbers of patients are required to fully evaluate this technique.

Newer approaches to determine viable myocardium (see Chapter 8) may replace dobutamine stress testing for this indication; however, integrated assessment of viability and ischemia in one stress test without the need for contrast agents is possible with dobutamine and remains of interest for some indications.

Stress-induced wall motion abnormalities for the diagnosis of ischemia

Echocardiographic detection of wall motion abnormalities during high-dose dobutamine stress, or during exercise, has been shown to be an accurate diagnostic tool for the screening of patients with suspected coronary artery disease. Sensitivities and specificities have been reported to lie within the ranges of 54–96% and 60–100%, respectively,[39] depending on the pretest likelihood of disease and the experience of the stress center. However, the value of stress echocardiography is limited by a rate of 10–15% for nondiagnostic results,[39] low specificities for the basal–lateral and basal–inferior segments of the LV,[40] and very low reproducibility of test results.[41]

Using CMR, good results (Table 6.12) have been found for the detection of wall motion abnormalities at

Table 6.12 Sensitivity and specificity of high-dose dobutamine stress CMR

Ref	Sensitivity (%)	Specificity (%)	n (vs angiography)	Dobutamine dose
42	91	—	25	20
43	85	—	26	20
49	91	80	39	20
45	86	86	172	40
47	83	83	41	40
58	87	86	45	40

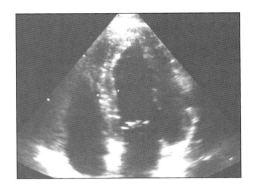
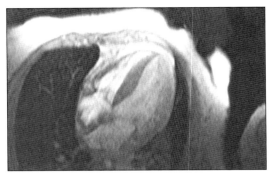
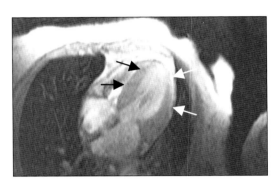

Figure 6.10
Dobutamine stress echocardiography versus dobutamine stress CMR. Top row: end-diastole. Bottom row: end-systole. Only high-dose stress images are shown. Note the wall motion abnormality seen with CMR (turbo gradient-echo technique; right), but missed with echocardiography (second-harmonic imaging; left). (Reproduced from Nagel et al. Circulation 1999; 99:763–70.[45])

intermediate doses of dobutamine (maximum 20 μg/kg body weight/min i.v.).[42–44] However, echocardiographic studies have shown that high-dose dobutamine and additional atropine are required to ensure high sensitivity. In a prospective study of 208 patients with suspected coronary artery disease, high-dose dobutamine/atropine (40 μg/kg body weight/min plus up to 1 mg atropine i.v.) stress was used, and echocardiography and CMR (Figure 6.10) were compared with angiography for the detection of significant coronary artery disease (>50% angiographic diameter stenosis).[45] In this study, significant improvements in sensitivity (86% versus 74%), specificity (86% versus 70%), and diagnostic accuracy (86% versus 73%) of CMR versus transthoracic echocardiography were found. These differences were most pronounced in patients who had moderate echocardiographic image quality.[46] The results were comparable when echocardiographic image quality was good or very good. In a different study by Hundley et al,[47] patients with nondiagnostic echocardiograpic image quality were assessed with a similar protocol, and 94% of them could be adequately examined with CMR yielding a sensitivity and specificity of 83% in those patients who also underwent angiographic assessment.

Since high-dose dobutamine stress CMR is highly accurate and can be performed in less than 30 min, it is increasingly replacing dobutamine stress echocardiography for the detection of coronary artery disease, in patients with nondiagnostic or suboptimal echocardiographic image quality.

Recommendations for CMR stress testing

Image acquisition

It is of special importance to explain to the patient not only the course of the examination but also the breathhold procedure. Written informed consent must be obtained in advance from all patients. A venous line (≥ 18-gauge) should be placed in the cubital vein, and blood pressure and heart rate should be monitored on the contralateral arm.

Viability (low-dose dobutamine)

As time for image acquisition is not limited by the stress regime, low-dose dobutamine (≤ 10 μg dobutamine/kg body weight/min) studies can be performed with standard gradient-echo or SSFP sequences, even though breathhold techniques should be used whenever possible. Five standard views should be acquired. Images are acquired at rest and during each stress level. The stress protocol is shown in Table 6.8; monitoring and contraindications are listed in Tables 6.9 and 6.10.

Wall motion abnormalities (high-dose dobutamine)

For high-dose dobutamine stress tests, breathhold cine imaging of the same views as recommended for low-dose dobutamine studies should be peformed. Imaging starts immediately after increasing the dobutamine dose. To achieve an adequate number of phases also during tachycardia, the temporal resolution needs to be ~25 frames/s (<40 ms). Studies published so far have used a spatial resolution of around 2×2 mm or better, with a slice thickness of 6–10 mm. Images are acquired and reviewed at rest and during each stress level. For the stress protocol and details concerning monitoring, contraindications and termination criteria refer to Tables 6.8–6.11.

Image interpretation

Viability

For viability studies, quantitative assessment is required. A minimal end-diastolic wall thickness of > 5 mm with resting thickening or resting akinesia with an improvement of systolic wall thickening of $\geqslant$ 2 mm during dobutamine stimulation are the diagnostic criteria for viable myocardium.[35–37]

Wall motion abnormalities for the diagnosis of ischemia

For image interpretation, multiple synchronized cine loop display is recommended, optimally allowing the display of all views at each dose level simultaneously. The ventricle is analyzed for 17 segments per stress level, which are visually or quantitatively evaluated according to the standards suggested by the American Society of Echocardiography.[48] Image quality is graded as good, acceptable, or bad, and the number of diagnostic segments is reported. Segmental wall motion is classified as normokinetic, hypokinetic, akinetic, or dyskinetic, and assigned 1–4 points. The sum of points is divided by the number of analyzed segments and yields a wall motion score. Normal contraction results in a wall motion score of 1; a higher score is indicative of wall motion abnormalities. During dobutamine stress with increasing doses, a lack of increase in wall motion or systolic wall thickening or a decrease in wall motion or thickening are both regarded as pathological findings (Figure 6.11).

Quantitative regional wall motion

A quantitative analysis of wall motion and systolic thickening is possible, and has shown good results in small studies.[49,50] Further improvements in diagnostic accuracy and reproducibility may be achieved with online or rapid offline analysis of myocardial tagging,[51] which allows quantification of regional three-dimensional myocardial motion.

Combination of different methods

In general, a combination of different imaging methods can be used within a CMR examination. Combined determination of wall motion and perfusion has been demonstrated in animals[52] and in small numbers of patients.[53,54] A comprehensive protocol including perfusion, wall motion, infarct imaging, and coronary artery imaging, has recently been presented.[55] However, preliminary data in larger patient populations have not shown any superiority of a combined approach in comparison with dobutamine stress or perfusion alone[56]

Training

For adequate image acquisition and interpretation, as well as patient care during stress, specific training is required. This includes the ability to perform the scan, to interpret the images immediately after acquisition during the scan, to stop the test if new wall motion abnormalities occur, and to perform cardiopulmonary resuscitation, as well as the ability to adequately react to other emergency situations that may occur during stress testing, such as severe angina pectoris, cardiac arrhythmias, or bronchoconstriction. There is an advantage for physicians or technicians who have trained in dobutamine stress echocardiography, since they fulfil all of the above requirements and have a trained eye for the detection of wall motion abnormalities. Current guidelines do not specifically address training for stress examinations.[5,57]

Conclusions and outlook

CMR of LV volume, mass, and function has become the reference standard. Today's standard ECG-triggered breathhold techniques (turbo gradient-echo and SSFP) can be used routinely to achieve high-resolution, high-contrast images reproducibly. Real-time techniques can be used in specific cases. Whereas rapid evaluations of ejection fraction and regional wall motion are possible from a minimal data set, accurate assessment requires full coverage and quantification of the LV. Dobutamine stress imaging can be safely and reliably used to detect ischemic myocardium in a broad range of patients, and is superior to echocardiography due to better image quality.

Future developments will integrate rapid (online) quantification of regional wall motion and faster stress protocols. It remains to be seen whether a combination of wall motion with perfusion has advantages over a single stress test alone and whether low-dose dobutamine stress

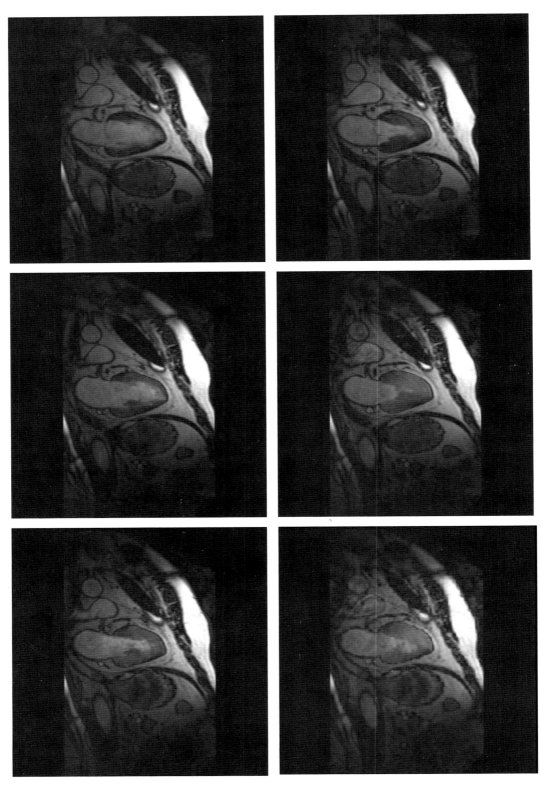

Figure 6.11
Dobutamine stress CMR: example of myocardial ischemia. All images were acquired with the turbo gradient-echo technique at 1.5 T. Left column: end-diastole. Right column: end-systole. Top row: rest. Middle row: intermediate dobutamine stress (20 µg/kg body weight/min). Bottom row: maximal stress. Note the wall motion abnormality apical inferior at maximum stress – also seen at rest, but not at intermediate stress. This was regarded as a biphasic response with hibernating myocardium and stress-induced ischemia.

remains a useful tool despite advances in delayed enhancement techniques.

References

1. White H, Norris R, Brown M, et al. Left ventricular end-systolic volume as the major determinant of survival after recovery from myocardial infarction. Circulation 1987; 76:44–51.

2. Bogaert JG, Bosmans HT, Rademakers FE, et al. Left ventricular quantification with breath-hold MR imaging: comparison with echocardiography. Magma 1995; 3:5–12.

3. Cerqueira MD, Weissman NJ, Dilsizian V, et al. Standardized myocardial segmentation and nomenclature for tomographic imaging of the heart: a statement for healthcare professionals from the Cardiac Imaging Committee of the Council on Clinical Cardiology of the American Heart Association. Circulation 2002; 105:539–42.

4. Fischer S, Wickline S, Lorenz C. Novel real-time R-wave detection algorithm based on the vectorcardiogram for accurate gated magnetic resonance acquisitions. Magn Reson Med 1999; 42:361–70.

5. Nagel E, Lorenz C, Baer F, et al. Stress cardiovascular magnetic resonance: consensus panel report. J Cardiovasc Magn Reson 2001; 3:267–81.

6. Lorenz CH, Fischer SE, Mens G, et al. Interactive cardiac scan planning on a standard clinical MR scanner. In: Proceedings of the International Society for Magnetic Resonance in Medicine, Sydney, 1998: 1958 (abst).

7. Yang PC, Kerr AB, Liu AC, et al. New real-time interactive cardiac magnetic resonance imaging system complements echocardiography. J Am Coll Cardiol 1998; 32:2049–56.

8. Scheidegger MB, Spiegel M, Stuber M, et al. Assessment of cardiac wall thickening and ejection fraction from real time cardiac MR images in patients with left ventricular dysfunction. In: Proceedings of the International Society for Magnetic Resonance in Medicine, Sydney, 1998: 554 (abst).

9. Nagel E, Schneider U, Schalla S, et al. Magnetic resonance real-time imaging for the evaluation of left ventricular function. J Cardiovasc Magn Reson 2000; 2:7–14.

10. Schalla S, Klein C, Paetsch I, et al. Real-time MR image acquisition during high-dose dobutamine hydrochloride stress for detecting left ventricular wall-motion abnormalities in patients with coronary arterial disease. Radiology 2002; 224:845–51.

11. Thiele H, Nagel E, Paetsch I, et al. Functional cardiac MR imaging with steady-state free precession (SSFP) significantly improves endocardial border delineation without contrast agents. J Magn Reson Imaging 2001; 14:362–7.

12. Bellenger NG, Gatehouse PD, Rajappan K, et al. Left ventricular quantification in heart failure by cardiovascular MR using prospective respiratory navigator gating: comparison with breath-hold acquisition. J Magn Reson Imaging 2000; 11:411–17.

13. Dubois D, Dubois E. A formula to estimate the approximate surface area if height and weight are known. Arch Intern Med 1916; 17:863–71.

14. Thiele H, Paetsch I, Schnackenburg B, et al. Improved accuracy of quantitative assessment of left ventricular volume and ejection frac-

15. Sheehan F, Stewart D, Dodge H. Variability in the measurement of regional left ventricular wall motion from contrast agent angiograms. Circulation 1983; 86:550–9.

16. Lorenz C, Walker E, Morgan V, et al. Normal human right and left ventricular mass, systolic function, and gender differences by cine magnetic resonance imaging. J Cardiovasc Magn Res 1999; 1:7–21.

17. Marcus J, de Waal L, Götte M, et al. MRI-derived left ventricular function parameters and mass in healthy young adults: relation with gender and body size. Int J Cardiac Imaging 1999; 15:411–19.

18. Sandstede J, Lipke C, Beer M, et al. Age- and gender-specific differences in left and right ventricular cardiac function and mass determined by cine magnetic resonance imaging. Eur Radiol 2000; 10:438–42.

19. Marcus J, Götte M, Dewaal L, et al. The influence of through-plane motion on left ventricular volumes measured by magnetic resonance imaging: implications for image acquisition and analysis. J Cardiovasc Magn Res 1999; 1:1–6.

20. Rogers WJ, Shapiro W, Weiss J, et al. Quantification of and correction for left ventricular systolic short-axis shortening by magnetic resonance tissue tagging and slice isolation. Circulation 1991; 84:721–31.

21. Stuber M, Nagel E, Fischer SE, et al. Systolic long axis contraction of the human myocardium. Proceedings of the Society of Magnetic Resonance 1995:1419 (abst).

22. Zerhouni EA. Myocardial tagging by magnetic resonance imaging. Coron Artery Dis 1993; 4:334–9.

23. Axel L, Dougherty L. Heart wall motion: Improved method of spatial modulation of magnetization for MR imaging. Radiology 1989; 172:349–50.

24. Buchalter MB, Weiss JL, Rogers WJ, et al. Noninvasive quantification of left ventricular rotational deformation in normal humans using magnetic resonance imaging myocardial tagging. Circulation 1990; 81:1236–44.

25. Rademakers FE, Buchalter MB, Rogers WJ, et al. Dissociation between left ventricular untwisting and filling. Accentuation by catecholamines. Circulation 1992; 85:1572–81.

26. Dong S, Hees P, Siu C, et al. MRI assessment of LV relaxation by untwisting of rate: a new isovolumic phase measure of tau. Am J Physiol 2001; 281:H2002–9.

27. Stuber M, Scheidegger MB, Fischer SE, et al. Alterations in the local myocardial motion pattern in patients suffering from pressure overload due to aortic stenosis. Circulation 1999; 100:361–8.

28. Dong SJ, MacGregor JH, Crawley AP, et al. Left ventricular wall thickness and regional systolic function in patients with hypertrophic cardiomyopathy. A three-dimensional tagged magnetic resonance imaging study. Circulation 1994; 90:1200–9.

29. Nagel E, Stuber M, Lakatos M, et al. Cardiac rotation and relaxation after anterolateral myocardial infarction. Coron Artery Dis 2000; 11:261–7.

30. Picano E, Mathias WJ, Pingitore A, et al. Safety and tolerability of dobutamine–atropine stress echocardiography: a prospective, multicentre study. Echo Dobutamine International Cooperative Study Group. Lancet 1994; 344:1190–2.

31. Mertes H, Sawada SG, Ryan T, et al. Symptoms, adverse effects, and complications associated with dobutamine stress echocardiography. Experience in 1118 patients. Circulation 1993; 88:15–19.

32. Wahl A, Gollesch A, Paetsch I, et al. Safety and feasibility of high-dose dobutamine–atropine stress MRI for diagnosis of myocardial ischemia: experience in 650 consecutive patients. Circulation 2002; abst.

33. Heyndrickx C, Baic H, Nelkins P, et al. Depression of regional blood flow and wall thickening after brief coronary occlusion. Am J Physiol 1978; 234:H653–60.

34. Picano E. Symptoms and Signs of Myocardial Ischemia. Berlin: Springer-Verlag, 1997.

35. Baer FM, Voth E, Schneider CA, et al. Comparison of low-dose dobutamine–gradient-echo magnetic resonance imaging and positron emission tomography with [^{18}F]fluorodeoxyglucose in patients with chronic coronary artery disease. A functional and morphological approach to the detection of residual myocardial viability. Circulation 1995; 91:1006–15.

36. Baer FM, Voth E, LaRosee K, et al. Comparison of dobutamine transesophageal echocardiography and dobutamine magnetic resonance imaging for detection of residual myocardial viability. Am J Cardiol 1996; 78:415–19.

37. Baer FM, Theissen P, Schneider CA, et al. Dobutamine magnetic resonance imaging predicts contractile recovery of chronically dysfunctional myocardium after successful revascularization. J Am Coll Cardiol 1998; 31:1040–8.

38. Sandstede JJ, Bertsch G, Beer M, et al. Detection of myocardial viability by low-dose dobutamine cine MR imaging. Magn Reson Imaging 1999; 17:1437–43.

39. Geleijnse ML, Fioretti PM, Roelandt JR. Methodology, feasibility, safety and diagnostic accuracy of dobutamine stress echocardiography. J Am Coll Cardiol 1997; 30:595–606.

40. Bach DS, Muller DW, Gros BJ, Armstrong WF. False positive dobutamine stress echocardiograms: characterization of clinical, echocardiographic and angiographic findings. J Am Coll Cardiol 1994; 24:928–33.

41. Hoffmann R, Lethen H, Marwick T, et al. Analysis of interinstitutional observer agreement in interpretation of dobutamine stress echocardiograms. J Am Coll Cardiol 1996; 27:330–6.

42. Pennell DJ, Underwood SR, Manzara CC, et al. Magnetic resonance imaging during dobutamine stress in coronary artery disease. Am J Cardiol 1992; 70:34–40.

43. Baer FM, Voth E, Theissen P, et al. Gradient-echo magnetic resonance imaging during incremental dobutamine infusion for the localization of coronary artery stenoses. Eur Heart J 1994; 15:218–25.

44. van Rugge FP, van der Wall EE, de Roos A, Bruschke AV. Dobutamine stress magnetic resonance imaging for detection of coronary artery disease. J Am Coll Cardiol 1993; 22:431–9.

45. Nagel E, Lehmkuhl HB, Bocksch W, et al. Noninvasive diagnosis of ischemia-induced wall motion abnormalities with the use of high-dose dobutamine stress MRI: comparison with dobutamine stress echocardiography. Circulation 1999; 99:763–70.

46. Nagel E, Lehmkuhl HB, Klein C, et al. [Influence of image quality on the diagnostic accuracy of dobutamine stress magnetic resonance imaging in comparison with dobutamine stress echocardiography for the noninvasive detection of myocardial ischemia]. Z Kardiol 1999; 88:622–30.

47. Hundley W, Hamilton C, Thomas M, et al. Utility of fast cine magnetic resonance imaging and display for the detection of myocardial ischemia in patients not well suited for second harmonic stress echocardiography. Circulation 1999; 100:1697–702.

48. Rina IL, Balody GJ, Hanson P, et al. Guidelines for clinical exercise testing laboratories. Circulation 1995; 91:912.

49. van Rugge FP, van der Wall EE, Spanjersberg SJ, et al. Magnetic resonance imaging during dobutamine stress for detection and localization of coronary artery disease. Quantitative wall motion analysis using a modification of the centerline method. Circulation 1994; 90:127–38.

50. van der Geest RJ, Buller VGM, Jansen E, et al. Comparison between manual and semiautomated analysis of left ventricular volume parameters from short-axis MR images. J Comput Assist Tomogr 1997; 21:756–65.

51. Power T, Kramer C, Shaffer A, et al. Breath-hold dobutamine magnetic resonance myocardial tagging: normal left ventricular response. Am J Cardiol 1997; 80:1203–7.

52. Kraitchman DL, Wilke N, Hexeberg E, et al. Myocardial perfusion and function in dogs with moderate coronary stenosis. Magn Reson Med 1996; 35:771–80.

53. Bremerich J, Buser P, Bongartz G, et al. Noninvasive stress testing of myocardial ischemia: comparison of MRI perfusion and wall motion analysis to ^{99m}TcMIMI SPECT, relation to coronary angiography. Eur Radiol 1997; 7:990–5.

54. Sensky PR, Jivan A, Hudson NM, et al. Coronary artery disease: combined stress MR imaging protocol–one-stop evaluation of myocardial perfusion and function. Radiology 2000; 215:608–14.

55. Plein S, Ridgway JP, Jones TR, et al. Coronary artery disease: assessment with a comprehensive MR imaging protocol – initial results. Radiology 2002; 225:300–7.

56. Wahl A, Roethemeyer S, Paetsch I, et al. Simultaneous assessment of wall motion and myocardial perfusion during high dose dobutamine stress MRI improves diagnostis of ischemia in patients with known coronary artery disease. J Cardiovasc Magn Reson 2002; 4:136–7 (abst).

57. Pohost G, Higgins C, Grist T, et al. Guidelines for credentialing in cardiovascular magnetic resonance (CMR). J Cardiovasc Magn Reson 2000; 2:233–4.

58. Schmidt M, Joachims M, Theissen P, et al. Comparison of dobutamine-stress magnetic resonance imaging and dipyridamole-TL-201-SPECT as alternative strategies for the detection of coronary artery disease in patients not suitable for echocardiography. Nuklearmedizin 2001; 40:198–206.

7

CMR of myocardial perfusion

Jürg Schwitter

Introduction

In coronary artery disease (CAD) clinical decisions regarding the need for angioplasty or bypass surgery are ideally based on both coronary stenosis anatomy and its hemodynamic significance.[1] In addition, the severity and extent of perfusion abnormalities relate to the patient's prognosis.[2–4] Therefore, diagnostic tests for the assessment of myocardial perfusion such as single-photon emission computed tomography (SPECT) play a key role in patient management. However, the method suffers from attenuation artifacts[5,6] and its spatial resolution is limited. Further, scintigraphic techniques expose patients to radiation, which becomes important if such techniques are to be used to screen patients for the presence of CAD. Conversely, magnetic resonance (MR) perfusion imaging, lacking this radiation burden, would allow for broader screening and, moreover, for monitoring of patients over time to yield information on the progression of the disease.

Physiological aspects

Physical exercise or pharmacological β-adrenergic stimulation increase myocardial oxygen demand and cause ischemia in cases where increased oxygen demand is not met by an increased blood supply. In this case, diastolic and later on systolic cardiac function deteriorates, and ultimately the patient may experience typical angina. Based on experimental studies in the mid-1980s, it was recognized that coronary stenoses with $\geq$ 50% diameter reduction limit maximal hyperemic flow, thus causing ischemia during situations of increased oxygen demand.[7] Therefore, $\geq$ 50% diameter stenoses are typically considered hemodynamically significant, and in general such stenoses are treated by interventions. Moreover, data from the pre-intervention era, i.e. from the Coronary Artery Surgery Study (CASS) registry and others indicate that

complications such as myocardial infarctions are more frequent in vessels with significant stenoses.[8–10] With respect to the prognostic significance of coronary stenoses, considerably larger data bases are available when using noninvasive methods for the assessment of the coronary circulation. In a meta-analysis comprising > 12 000 patients, the extent and severity of myocardial perfusion defects assessed during exercise or pharmacologically induced hyperemia were strong predictors of future cardiac events.[2] Accordingly, noninvasive imaging techniques such as SPECT/positron emission tomography (PET) imaging or MR perfusion imaging are aimed at assessing myocardial perfusion during hyperemia. In the case of abnormalities during vasodilation, further tests for viability assessment are added involving rest–redistribution/reinjection studies for SPECT, [^{18}F]-fluorodeoxyglucose uptake studies for PET, or delayed enhancement studies for cardiac MR imaging (CMR).[11]

Growing evidence indicates that at a preclinical stage of CAD, maximum vasodilator capacity, i.e. coronary flow reserve (CFR), is impaired in patients with cardiovascular risk factors but anatomically normal coronary arteries (< 50% diameter stenoses).[12] Since evaluation of CFR, defined as hyperemic flow divided by resting flow, necessitates quantification of myocardial blood flow, PET is typically used for assessment of CFR. The concept of CFR can also be pursued by CMR, given the possibility to quantitatively measure blood flow or at least to obtain estimates of flow that linearly correlate with flow over a large range (encompassing resting and hyperemic condition). Since CFR is limited in the presence of a significant coronary stenosis ($\geq$ 50% diameter reduction without relevant collateral flow), CFR also yields reliable diagnostic information.[13,14] Interestingly, several studies using PET demonstrated that hyperemic flow data correlated strongly with percentage area stenosis on coronary angiography and correlations were as high as those observed for CFR data.[15–18] In agreement with these observations, hyperemic MR perfusion data prooved highly accurate in the detection of CAD.[19]

The high spatial resolution of MR perfusion imaging allows one to differentiate contrast medium (CM) wash-in in subendocardial and subepicardial layers,[20] which may help to better understand coronary pathophysiology, for example in syndrome X.[21] Finally, the superiority of subendocardial hyperemic data over transmural hyperemic data for the detection of CAD has been reported.[19]

Technical aspects

For the detection of perfusion abnormalities, most experience is with the so-called CM first-pass approaches. With these techniques, a bolus of CM is injected into a peripheral or central vein and its effect on myocardial signal is monitored with fast MR pulse sequences. The most commonly used CM are the extravascular gadolinium-based chelates, and accordingly they are combined with heavily T1-weighted pulse sequences. As alternatives to these CM first-pass approaches, blood oxygen level-dependent (BOLD) techniques,[22,23] spin labeling techniques,[24–27] and magnetization transfer techniques[28] are also under investigation to assess myocardial perfusion. A schematic of the various pulse sequences for perfusion assessment is given in Table 7.1.

Common to all CM first-pass techniques either under development or in clinical routine are the requirements

to: (1) provide high spatial resolution to become sensitive for small subendocardial perfusion deficits; (2) provide adequate cardiac coverage to allow for assessment of the extent of perfusion deficits; (3) feature high CM sensitivity to generate optimum contrast between normally and abnormally perfused myocardium during CM passage. Finally, acquisition of perfusion data should occur every 1–2 heartbeats to allow for calculation of various parameters of perfusion (see below). To fulfil these requirements, speed of data acquisition and time-efficient magnetization preparation are of paramount importance, since passage of CM during hyperemic conditions only lasts 5–10 s. Cardiac motion during this time period is typically eliminated by ECG triggering, while breathing motion is minimized by a breathhold maneuver. Such control of motion preserves the high spatial resolution of the MR perfusion data on the order of 1–3 mm × 1–3 mm.

CMR data readout

Until recently, Turbo-FLASH (fast low angle shot) pulse sequences were most commonly used for perfusion imaging. In this type of pulse sequence, acquisition of each k-line is preceded by a radiofrequency (RF) excitation, which results in a readout duration on the order of 350–450 ms, depending on the number of phase-encoding

Table 7.1 Evolution of MR pulse sequences for myocardial perfusion imaging

Studies	Animal	Human	
		Single-center	Multicenter
1. Magnetization transfer technique	+		
2. Arterial spin labeling	+	+	
3. BOLD imaging	+	+	
4. First-pass techniques			
(i) Extravascular CM			
(a) T1-weighted (Gd-based)			
• Inversion recovery			
– Turbo-FLASH	+	+	
– Keyhole technique	+	+	+
– Steady-state	+		
• Saturation recovery			
– Turbo-FLASH	+	+	
– Hybrid EP	+	+	+
(b) T2*-weighted (Fe/Dy-based)	+	+	
(ii) Intravascular CM			
(a) T2*-weighted (Fe-based)	+	+	
(b) T1-weighted (Gd-based)	+		

BOLD, blood oxygen level-dependent; CM, contrast medium; EP, echo-planar; Fe/Dy, iron/dysprosium; FLASH, fast low-angle shot acquisition; Gd, gadolinium.

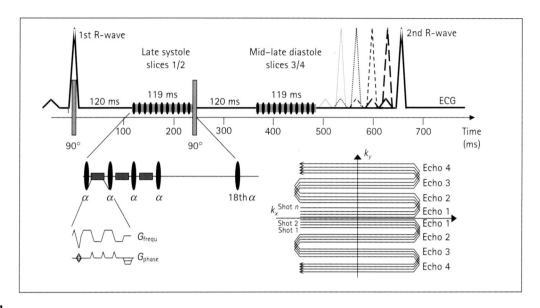

Figure 7.1

Pulse sequence diagram of a hybrid echo-planar perfusion sequence as used in a recent study.[19] A non-slice-selective 90° preparation pulse is followed by a 120 ms delay time. After this delay, a series of 50° α-pulses is played out, with each α-pulse yielding four gradient echoes, i.e. four lines in k-space (as shown for n shots in the lower right corner of the figure). With this sequence, four slices are acquired in an interleaved fashion every two heartbeats. The frequency- and phase-encoding gradients (G_{frequ} and G_{phase}, respectively) are shown in the lower left corner with a rewinder for the phase-encoding gradients and blips at the end of the echo train. With this sequence, signal response is optimized (cf Figure 7.3), while data readout occurs at phases of minimal cardiac motion, i.e. in late systole and mid–late diastole. This approach takes advantage of the fact, that ejection time varies little with increasing heart rate (275 to 235 ms at 80 to 120 beats/min). Further considering isovolumic relaxation, the chances of data acquisition during phase of rapid cardiac motion (early left-ventricular filling) is small even at high heart rates as during hyperemia (represented by the shift of the 2nd R-wave on the ECG). Also, the short acquisition window minimizes the chance of readout of slices 3/4 during atrial contraction (note the position of the P-wave on the ECG).

steps and the duration of TR (which is typically on the order of 5–9 ms).[29–36] In the past few years, the advantage of echo-planar[37–39] or hybrid echo-planar pulse sequences[19,40–42] has become more apparent. In this type of very fast pulse sequence, several k-lines are acquired following one single RF excitation, reducing the TR per k-line to < 2 ms and consequently reducing total acquisition window to 100–150 ms/slice (a schematic of a hybrid echo-planar pulse sequence is given in Figure 7.1). Readout strategies during steady-state conditions of magnetization are characterized by high signal-to-noise ratios (SNR) and have been employed successfully in animal models for monitoring CM first pass through the myocardium.[43]

Magnetization preparations

Traditionally, magnetization preparation, i.e. T1 weighting, was achieved by an inversion recovery (IR) technique that precedes the readout by a 180° inversion pulse. To generate maximum contrast between abnormally and normally perfused myocardium, recovery times on the order of 300–400 ms (to readout of central k-space lines) are required to set precontrast myocardial signal slightly above zero.[29–36,44] Thus, combining this IR preparation scheme with a Turbo-FLASH readout results in a total data acquisition window of 650–750 ms/slice. To shorten the delay time, partial saturation schemes were used, with preparation flip angles of 45°–60°.[40,42] However, this limits the dynamic range of the signal response.[41] To increase the number of slices being imaged per cardiac cycle, a single preparation pulse may be utilized to prepare an entire stack of slices. However, with this approach, recovery time and consequently CM sensitivity vary for each slice. Thus, signal change is dependent not only on CM wash-in but also on the slice acquisition order, i.e. slice position. Alternatively, the readout is prepared by a 90° saturation pulse to render the sequence heart-rate-independent, and is combined with recovery times on the order of 100–150 ms to gain more signal.[41] When combined with a hybrid echo-planar readout, the data acquisition window can be as short as 240 ms/slice.[19] This speed allows for multislice data acquisition, which is crucial for assessment of extent of disease, while the sampling rate remains high, i.e. a complete stack of images is acquired every 1–2 heartbeats. A modification of a saturation recovery preparation has been proposed in which the entire myocardium experiences the saturation preparation except for that portion of tissue that is immediately imaged after preparation. With this scheme, the time period for readout of slice *n* is utilized to prepare slice *n* + 1, and so on, i.e. the acquisition window equals the preparation time.[45] This approach enables acquisitions of up to seven slices every two heartbeats, up to a heart rate of 115 beats/min.

Contrast media

T1-shortening extravascular gadolinium chelates are most commonly used for MR first-pass perfusion imaging. These CM are injected as a bolus in a peripheral (antecubital) or central vein in dosages of 0.025–0.15 mmol/kg body weight at rates of 3–8 ml/s. At higher dosages, T2* effects become more prominent and CM first pass induces a signal drop in blood pool and myocardium when monitored with T2-weighted pulse sequences.[46,47] In order to minimize variability in input, the use of a power injector for CM administration is recommended.

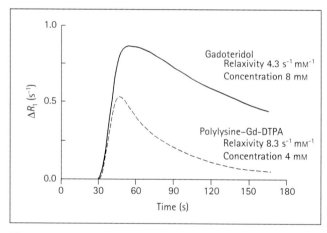

Figure 7.2
Examples of first-pass signal intensity–time curves for intravascular (polylysine–Gd-DTPA) and extravascular (gadoteridol) contrast medium (CM) measured in isolated canine septa at 4.7 T. Both CM boluses (3 ml each) were administered to the septa at a flow rate of 16 ml/min during adenosine-induced hyperemia. Signal was calculated from free induction decays collected every 351.2 ms following an adiabatic 90° RF pulse (for details, see reference 72). Note the considerably lower myocardial signal response for the intravascular CM compared with the extravascular compound (curves are not smoothed). For this comparison, CM concentrations of 4 and 8 mM were chosen to take into account the different relaxivities of the two compounds. The lower signal response for the intravascular CM suggests slow water exchange between intravascular and interstitial compartment. (Modified from Judd et al,[72] from Magn Res Med 1995; 33:215–23[72] with permission from John Wiley & Sons, Inc.)

In addition to the type and dose of CM and the type of pulse sequence used for magnetization preparation and readout, also water exchange rates between the various tissue components determine the signal response in the myocardium (see below). Gadolinium chelates bound to large molecules such as albumin, polylysine, or dendrimers have been extensively assessed in animal preparations in order to use kinetic models assuming restriction of CM to the intravascular compartment. However, several studies indicate that water exchange may not justify such models (see below). Since myocardial signal response is limited for intravascular compared with extravascular CM, SNR decreases, a fact known to reduce test performance.[41,48,49] Examples of typical myocardial signal intensity–time curves during first pass of an extravascular and intravascular T1-shortening CM are given in Figure 7.2. Fewer studies have tested the feasibility of extravascular dysprosium chelates[50,51] and intravascular ultrasmall superparamagnetic iron oxide CM[52] for evaluation of myocardial perfusion by monitoring T2* effects. However, for these CM, changes in T2* are affected by susceptibility, vessel geometry, and distance between vessels, thus favoring measurements of CM concentrations by T1 techniques.

Factors influencing myocardial signal response

In first-pass perfusion studies, signal change in the myocardium during CM wash-in is related to changes in myocardial CM concentration. However, myocardial signal at a given CM concentration varies considerably, depending upon imaging parameters such as magnetization preparation (preparation flip angle), delay time between preparation and readout, readout flip angle, trajectories within *k*-space during readout, and others. The influence on signal intensities in phantoms of various preparation flip angles, delay times, and readout flip angles for a given hybrid echo-planar pulse sequence are shown in Figure 7.3. By reduction of the preparation flip angle together with a shorter delay time, the acquisition duration per slice can be reduced considerably, allowing for better cardiac coverage, but is traded for a reduced contrast-to-noise ratio. A study comparing extended cardiac coverage versus enhanced CM sensitivity has shown the importance of adequate CM sensitivity, i.e. adequate signal increase.[41] An example illustrates the image quality that is achieved by changing relevant imaging parameters (Figure 7.4).[41] The extended coverage approach with an increase in signal of ~80% performed significantly worse than the approach with a signal increase of ~200%. Ideally, perfusion data would be evalu-

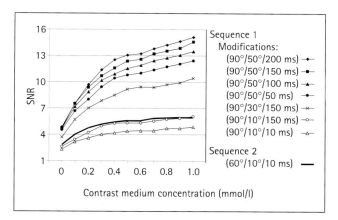

Figure 7.3

The signal behavior for various perfusion pulse sequences is shown here on phantoms (saline doped with Gd-DTPA). The effect of different preparation times in combination with the saturation recovery approach (modifications of sequence 1: preparation flip angle 90°, readout flip angle 50°) is represented by the filled symbols. Sequence 2, providing extended cardiac coverage (preparation flip angle 60°, readout flip angle 10°, preparation time 10 ms) yielded an increase in signal-to-noise ratio (SNR) of 2.77 at 0.5 mmol/l of Gd-DTPA versus saline. By varying the preparation time in the saturation recovery approach (modifications of sequence 1) between 50 and 150 ms yielded a 2.3- to 2.8-fold increase in SNR in comparison with sequence 2. The parameters in parentheses represent preparation flip angle, readout flip angle, and preparation time, respectively. (Reproduced from Bertschinger et al. J Magn Res Imaging 2001; 14:556–62[41] with permission from John Wiley & Sons, Inc.)

ated by dedicated algorithms rather than by subjective reading. Whenever signal responses are compared with a normal database, any change in relevant imaging parameters should be followed by establishing a corresponding normal database. Although the acquisition of perfusion data by CMR is quite robust, these technical considerations illustrate that myocardial signal response is sensitive to imaging parameters, and substantial work with respect to standardization of MR perfusion imaging is needed to allow for a consistent application of this technique at different sites.

Estimates of myocardial perfusion from first-pass data

In first-pass studies, visual assessment of myocardial CM wash-in has been shown to detect hypoperfused myocardium supplied by stenosed coronary arteries.[36,44,53] However, identification of hypoperfused myocardium by observer-independent calculation of perfusion measures would be highly desirable.

Parameters linked to tissue perfusion

Many parameters linked to tissue perfusion have been investigated in animal and human studies in the past few years. Peak signal intensity,[29,30,42,54] signal change over time (slope),[19,21,33–35,41,54,55] arrival time, time to peak signal, mean transit time,[54–57] area under the signal intensity–time curve,[43] and others can be calculated from signal intensity–time curves. For upslope data, a close correlation with microsphere perfusion measurements has been shown in animal models,[55] and the upslope parameter is frequently used in clinical studies as a semiquantitative measure of perfusion.[19,33,35,54] Further, the upslope calculation uses the initial portion of the signal intensity–time curve lasting a few seconds only, which reduces the sensitivity of this parameter for motion (most patients are able hold their breath for this time period) as well as for CM recirculation. To obtain some measure of input, myocardial upslope data are often divided by the upslope of signal in the left ventricular blood pool.[19,21,34,35,41] Clearly, this approach to input correction is suboptimal, and may fail in situations with substantial variations in hemodynamic state, as might occur between rest and stress studies or in an attempt to compare upslope data of a patient with severe reduction in left ventricular function with a normal database consisting of hearts with preserved function. For these conditions, more appropriate input correction strategies would be needed and a quantification of perfusion would solve the problem (see below). In a recent study, myocardial upslope of signal intensity during hyperemia (divided by the upslope in the left-ventricular blood pool) was calculated in 32 sectors per heart (8 sectors per slice) and was compared with a normal database of upslope values.[19] This approach allowed color-coding of CM wash-in in a parametric map that displays hypoperfused areas in an observer-independent fashion. An example of a parametric map acquired in a patient with double-vessel disease is given in Figure 7.5.[19] Figure 7.6 gives another example where MR perfusion imaging documented successful stent implantation into the right coronary artery with normal perfusion in all myocardial segments post intervention. These examples illustrate the capability of MR perfusion imaging to detect CAD and furthermore to assess revascularization procedures.

In order to run algorithms reliably on CMR data, sources of artifacts should be eliminated or corrected for whenever possible. One problem arises from the receiver coil sensitivity, which decreases with increasing coil distance. Consequently, signal intensity change in the posterior parts of the heart is less than in the anterior parts. While attenuation artifacts encountered in SPECT imaging are difficult to correct for,[5] Figure 7.7 demonstrates one easy way in CMR to correct for signal loss with

(a)

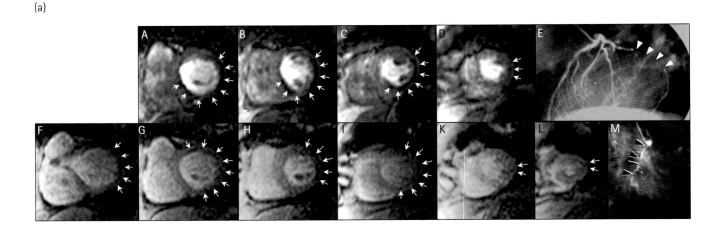

(b)

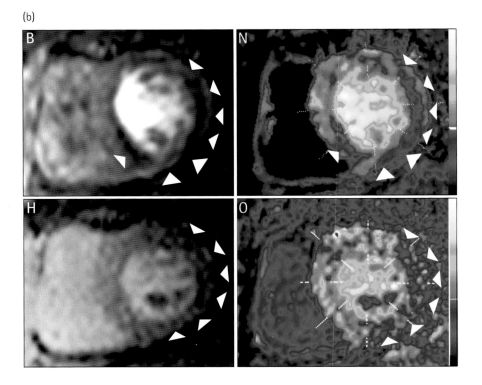

Figure 7.4

(a) Delineation of perfusion deficits is demonstrated for two different perfusion sequences (sequence 1: A–D; sequence 2: F–L) in a patient with a severe proximal stenosis in the left circumflex coronary artery (E, arrowheads) and several stenoses in the right coronary artery (M, arrowheads). Sequence 1 applies a 90° saturation preparation followed by 120 ms delay time; the readout flip angle is 50°. These parameters allow for acquisition of four slices (A–D) every 1.2 s. Sequence 2 acquires the same slices (G–K) but additionally a more basal (F) and apical (L) slice at a comparable sampling rate (1.2 s). Faster acquisition of sequence 2 (identical to sequence 2 in Figure 7.3, thick line) is achieved by a 60° preparation pulse followed by a short delay time of only 10 ms; the readout flip angle is 10°. Both strategies demonstrate a perfusion deficit in the inferolateral wall (arrows on MR images at peak effect of bolus). The delineation of the perfusion deficit is considerably improved on images aquired with sequence 1. Note the transmural distribution of the perfusion abnormality in the center of the defect, with restriction to the subendocardial layer at its borders.

(b) Representative examples of parametric maps (N/O) demonstrate contrast medium wash-in kinetics for slices B/H, respectively. On these parametric maps, linear upslope data above/below the threshold (mean of controls minus 1.75 SD, indicated by the white line on the color bar) are encoded in shades of red and blue, respectively. The quality of data acquired with sequence 1 allowed automatic generation of parametric maps (N) that differentiate subendocardial from transmural perfusion deficits (small and large arrowheads in N, respectively), whereas parametric maps of data acquired with sequence 2 were less reliable and noisy (O). (Reproduced from Bertschinger et al. J Magn Res Imaging 2001; 14:556–62[41] with permission from John Wiley & Sons, Inc.)

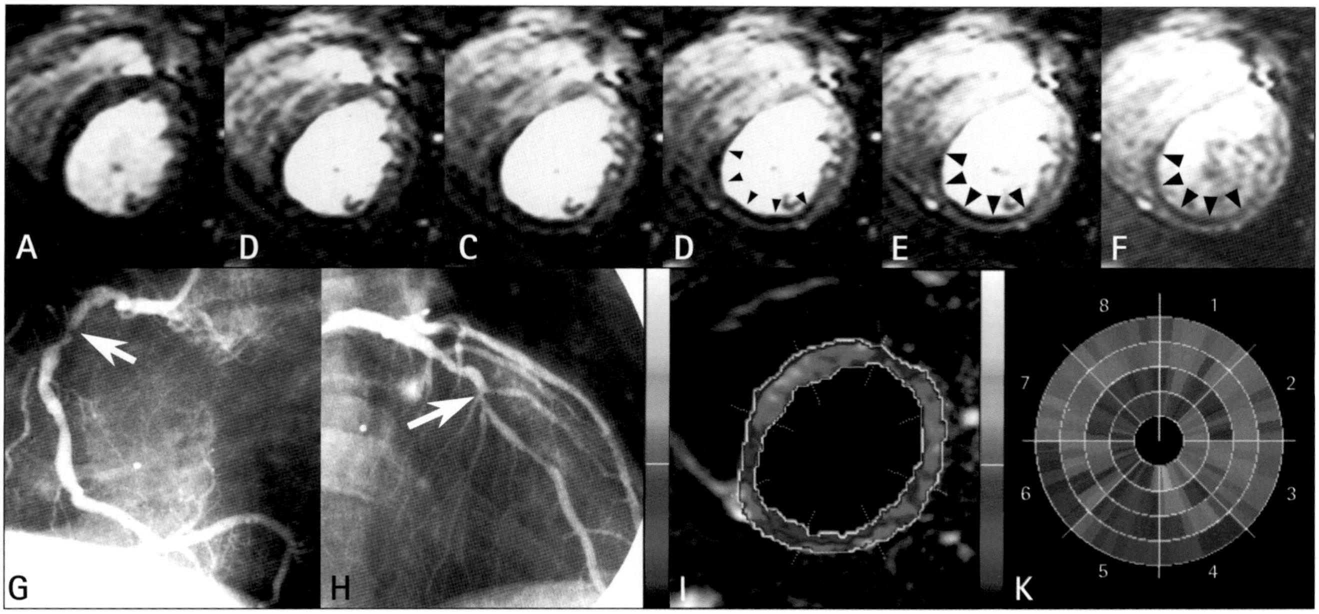

Figure 7.5

In this patient with a stenosis of the right coronary artery (RCA; arrow in G), the transit of contrast medium through the left ventricular myocardium during hyperemia (time resolution 4 slices every 1.2 s) demonstrates delayed wash-in in the subendocardium of sectors 4–6 (arrowheads in D–F). In the corresponding pixelwise parametric slope map (I), the perfusion deficit is demonstrated as a blue area (the color encoding is the same as in Figure 7.4 N/O). In J, a polar map represents perfusion in the subendocardium (with the apex located in the center of the map, and the anterior, lateral, inferior, and septal wall represented by sectors 1, 3, 5, and 6–8, respectively). The subendocardial perfusion deficit in the right coronary artery territory extends from base to apex, whereas the perfusion deficit in the anterior and septal wall (sectors 1, 7, and 8) extends from the midventricular level to the apex (slices 3 and 4), corresponding to the stenosis in the mid-portion of the left anterior descending coronary artery (arrow in H). (Reproduced from Schwitter et al. Circulation 2001; 103:2230–5.[19])

increasing coil distance, namely calculation of relative signal changes by dividing absolute signal change by the baseline precontrast signal intensities. In this patient, who had a stent implantation into the left anterior descending coronary artery, the MR perfusion study demonstrated reduced septal perfusion (due to stent implantation, which compromised septal branches).

Prior to any signal intensity–time curve generation, the perfusion dataset should be corrected for cardiac motion induced by either diaphragmatic drift and/or breathing.[58–60] In this regard, assessment of hyperemic perfusion alone (and not considering resting perfusion to calculate CFR) appears advantageous for detection of hemodynamically significant coronary stenoses, since co-registration of rest and hyperemic scans is avoided.

Absolute quantification of perfusion

In addition to correction of data for coil sensitivity and motion, a quantitative approach also requires conversion of signal intensities into CM concentrations[61] in order to

allow for input correction. A prerequisite for such a conversion is an accurate mathematical description of the signal intensity–CM concentration relationship over the full range of CM concentrations occuring in blood pool and myocardium during first-pass conditions.[62–65] Once signal intensities have been converted into CM concentrations, different models may be applied to calculate flow. Modifications of the basic tracer kinetic model proposed by Kety[66] are widely used to calculate the unidirectional influx constant K_i for diffusion of CM over the capillary membrane (in ml/min/g), where $K_i = EF$, with E being the unidirectional extraction fraction in the first pass and F being flow. While some investigators determine K_i at rest and during hyperemia to calculate a perfusion index or CFR (assuming no relevant change in E for resting and hyperemic conditions),[67,68] others have demonstrated considerable changes in E for different myocardial states.[69]

Since the effect of a CM is measured indirectly through water relaxation, diffusion of water molecules between intravascular and extravascular compartments may modify the MR signal response during first pass. Simulation studies by Larsson and co-workers[70] suggest that water exchange between intravascular and extravascular compartments only minimally affects K_i when using a low bolus of an extravascular CM (≤ 0.1 mmol/kg body

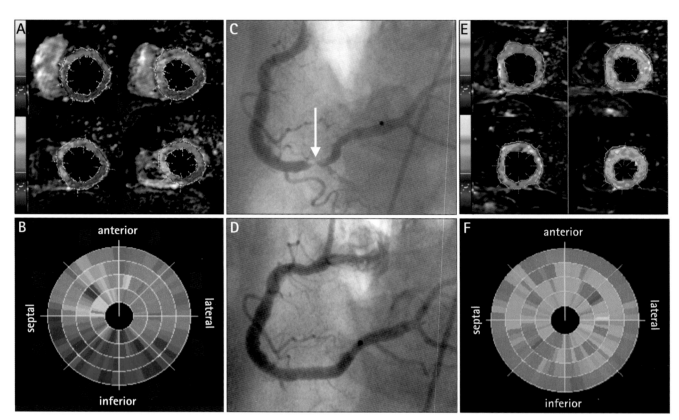

Figure 7.6
In a 66-year-old patient with episodes of chest pain during exercise and at rest, MR perfusion imaging demonstrates a perfusion deficit in the inferior wall during hyperemia (parametric slope maps in A; polar map of the subendocardium in B; color encoding as in Figures 7.4 and 7.5; for pulse sequence details, see reference 19). Subsequent conventional X-ray coronary angiography confirmed stenosis of the right coronary artery (arrow in C), and a stent placement was successfully performed in the same session (D). Repeat MR perfusion imaging was performed before discharge of the patient, and documented normal perfusion in all myocardial segments (E, F).

weight and assuming $E \geqslant 0.3$), but substantially affects signal generated by intravascular CM. However, other investigators have found relevant modification of signal for both intra- and extravascular CM in experimental studies.[71-74]

Depending on model assumptions, the robustness of parameter estimates may vary considerably particularly in the presence of noise. While some simulations have demonstrated regional blood volume and E to be most sensitive to noise when determined from extravascular CM data,[48] other simulations have found regional blood volume estimates to be most reliable when derived from intravascular CM data.[75] To our knowledge, the usefulness of quantitative approaches to prospectively detect CAD in humans has not yet been performed.

Some studies calculating absolute measures of perfusion have used intravascular CM.[64,65,75] Models for intravascular CM should take into account proton exchange rates[70,71,74,76] between the vascular and extravascular bed, leakage of CM in territories of ischemia,[77,78] and vascular architecture.[79] At present, the value of a quantita-

tive approach with intravascular CM for the detection of CAD in humans is not known.

Diagnostic performance of MR perfusion imaging

Animal studies

The feasibility of myocardial first-pass MR perfusion imaging to detect coronary artery stenoses has been demonstrated repeatedly in experimental models.[29,47,51] In addition, experimental settings offer the possibility to directly compare perfusion estimates calculated from MR data with radiolabeled microsphere measurements, which is the generally accepted standard of reference. Table 7.2 provides an overview of animal studies in which extravascular CM, intravascular CM, and spin labeling techniques were compared with microsphere measurements. Excellent agreement was obtained for a spin labeling technique; however, these results were obtained in a non-beating preparation at 4.7 T.[24] Other techniques demonstrated somewhat weaker agreement, with correlation coefficients ranging from 0.70 to 0.91.[43,55,57,80] In several studies, slope or 1/MTT (inverse of the mean transit time) were derived from γ-variate fits of signal intensity–time curves.[55,57,80] Wilke and co-workers[64,65] have even demonstrated the possibility of quantifying perfusion in absolute measures of ml/min/g when applying sophisticated kinetic models to the MR data. However, a 95% confidence interval of ±82%[64] indicates that the sensitivity of this technique might be inadequate at present to detect subtle changes in perfusion. So far, the sensitivity and specificity of a quantitative approach for the detection of ischemia in an unselected patient population has not been determined.

Human studies

While IR techniques have generally been employed in animal studies,[29,30,43,47,55,57,64,71,80,81] different preparation schemes have been used in humans, including IR,[31–37,44,48,53,54,56,63,67,68] saturation recovery,[19,21,41,49,76] 60° preparation,[40] notch pulse preparation,[45] and T2* preparation.[50,52] Many of these studies were to show the feasibility of these various approaches, and therefore were

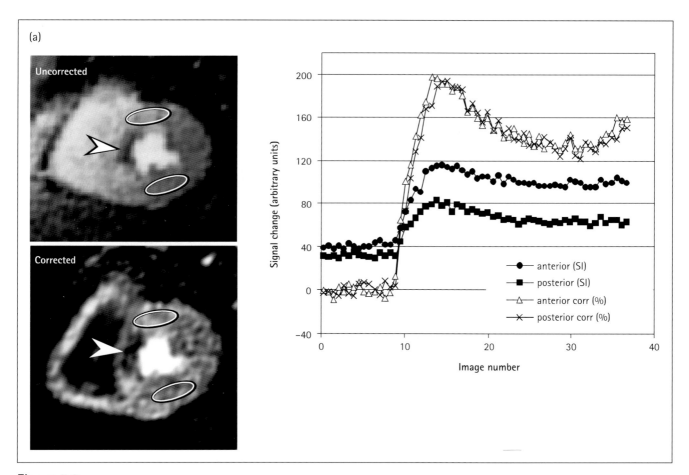

Figure 7.7

In a 47-year-old patient, atypical chest pain developed 2 months after successful stent implantation into a stenosis of the left anterior descending coronary artery (LAD). (a) MR perfusion imaging demonstrates a perfusion deficit in the septal wall during hyperemia on an uncorrected MR image (arrowhead) at the peak effect of the contrast medium bolus (pulse sequence: saturation recovery, hybrid echo-planar readout, acquisition of 3 slices/heartbeat, 0.1 mmol/kg body weight Gd-DTPA-BMA). Uncorrected signal intensity–time curves (closed symbols) of the anterior and posterior walls (ellipses on MR images) show reduced peak signal in the posterior parts of the heart. Dividing first-pass data by baseline signal intensities (precontrast) yields the percentage signal increase, and results in identical signal responses for the two regions of interest irrespective of coil distance (open symbols). In conventional X-ray coronary angiography, the LAD stent showed no stenosis (c) but had compromised take-off of septal branches, and consequently contrast medium injection into the right coronary artery (RCA) demonstrated collateralization of the septum (arrows in c).

Continued on next page

(b)

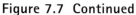

(c)

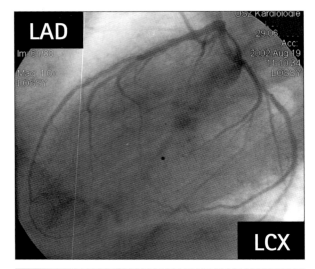

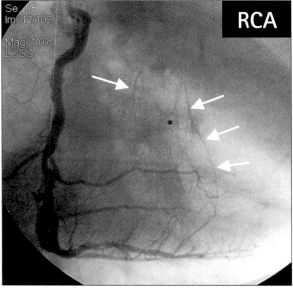

Figure 7.7 Continued

(b) A ^{99m}Tc-tetrofosmin single-photon emission computed tomography (SPECT) hyperemic study showed a perfusion deficit in the septal wall, in agreement with the MR study (arrowheads on long-axis view), but reduced tracer uptake was also noted in the posterior wall in both rest and hyperemic SPECT studies (arrows on short-axis views). CMR did exclude perfusion abnormalities in the inferior wall, and conventional X-ray coronary angiography confirmed normal RCA and left circumflex coronary artery (LCX). Both CMR and invasive left-ventricular angiography showed normal inferior wall motion at rest. Thus, this example demonstrates problematic attenuation in SPECT imaging and an easy approach to correct for coil sensitivity in MR perfusion imaging.

performed in healthy volunteers[40,50,52,76] or in highly selected patient populations with a priori knowledge of coronary anatomy.[32,45,68] Table 7.3 summarizes clinical studies in unselected patient populations where sensitivity and specificity for detection of CAD is reported (including studies with $n \geq 7$). Studies in the mid-1990s aimed at a multislice approach. However, either sensitivity[34] or specificity[44] in these multislice studies were low, which might be explained primarily by hardware limitations at that time. When calculating CFR in various vascular territories, a considerably better performance was reported by Al-Saadi and co-workers,[35] although CM was injected into the right atrium and data acquisition was limited to a single slice. Further improvements in hardware allowing for fast hybrid echo-planar readout and replacing an IR preparation by a more time-efficient

saturation recovery preparation enabled data acquisition in a multislice mode.[19,41] In this study, CM was injected into a peripheral vein and a high diagnostic accuracy of a single hyperemic set of subendocardial data was demonstrated.[19]

Outlook

Some improvements in scanner hardware and coils will certainly occur in the future. Also, the potential advantages of systems operating at 3 T await future studies. In addition, the potential advantages of parallel imaging approaches[82,83] and/or steady-state free precession techniques[43] will be evaluated.

Table 7.2 Experimental validation studies of MR perfusion imaging

Ref	n	Animal	Model	CM (injection site)	Stress	MR approach	Analysis	Reference	Corr r
64	7	Dogs	Stenosis	Intravascular polylysine–Gd-DTPA (left atrium)	Adenosine	IR Turbo-FLASH	Multiple pathway axially distributed model (ml/min/g)	Micro	$\pm 0.82^{a}$
80	7	Dogs	Stenosis	Intravascular polylysine–Gd-DTPA (left atrium)	Dobutamine	IR Turbo-FLASH	γ-variate fit: ratio, slope	Micro	0.77
57	5	Pigs	Stenosis	Intravascular iron oxide particles (left atrium)	Adenosine	IR Turbo-FLASH (at 0.5 T)	γ-variate fit: 1/MTT	Micro	0.70
55	3	Dogs	Occlusions, stenosis	Extravascular Gd-DTPA (left atrium)	Dipyridamole	IR Turbo-FLASH	γ-variate fit: 1/MTT, slope	Micro	0.78 0.66
76	8	Pigs	Occlusions	Extravascular Gd-DTPA (right atrium)	Adenosine	SR Turbo-FLASH	Fermi function: ratio, $R_{F}(0)$	Micro	0.88
43	12	Dogs	Occlusions, stenosis	Extravascular gadoteridol (right atrium)	Adenosine	IR TrueFISP	Ratio, AUC	Micro	0.93
24	3	Rabbits	Occlusions, non-beating heart (Langendorff)	—	—	Spin labeling (at 4.7 T)	$1/T1_{app}$	Micro	0.91–0.97
25	6	Pigs	—	—	Adenosine	Spin labeling alternating IR–EPI	$1/T1_{app}$	Micro	0.83

All studies were performed on 1.5 T systems unless otherwise noted. ^{a}95% confidence interval.
AUC, area under the signal intensity–time curve; EPI, echo-planar imaging; FISP, fast imaging with steady-state precession; FLASH, fast low-angle shot acquisition; IR, inversion recovery; micro, radiolabeled microspheres; MTT, mean transit time; $R_{F}(0) = F$ (the impulse response amplitude represents the relative measure of perfusion); ratio, ischemic/normal region; SR, saturation recovery; $T1_{app}$, apparent T1 of myocardium in the presence of flow.

Table 7.3 Performance of CAD detection by MR perfusion imaging in humans ($n \geqslant 7$)

Ref	n	Acquisition	CM	Rest	Stress	Analysis	Reference standard	Sensitivity (%)	Specificity (%)	AUC
53	14	IR/single	Gd-DTPA	+	Dip	Visual	QCA ($\geqslant 70\%$)	83[a]	100[a]	—
34	8	IR/multi	Gd-DOTA	+	Dip	Upslope	QCA ($\geqslant 80\%$)	65[b]	76[b]	—
44	46	IR/multi	Gadoteridol	+	Dip	Visual	^{201}Th/^{99m}Tc scinti	89	44	—
41	24	SR/multi	Gd-DTPA-BMA	−	Dip	Upslope$_{trans}$	QCA ($\geqslant 50\%$)	82	73	0.76
35	34	IR/single	Gd-DTPA	+	Dip	Upslope CFR	QCA ($\geqslant 75\%$)	90	83	—
19	57	SR/multi	Gd-DTPA-BMA	−	Dip	Upslope$_{subendo}$	QCA ($\geqslant 50\%$)	87	85	0.91
19	43	SR/multi	Gd-DTPA-BMA	−	Dip	Upslope$_{subendo}$	^{13}NH$_3$-PET (CFR)	91	94	0.93

[a] Comparison on a regional basis (5 segments/heart evalutated). [b]Comparison on a regional basis (48 segments/heart evaluated).
AUC, area under the receiver–operator curve; Dip, dipyridamole; IR, inversion recovery; SR, saturation recovery; single, single-slice; multi, multislice; QCA, quantitative coronary angiography (diameter reduction); ^{13}NH$_3$-PET(CFR), coronary flow reserve calculated from positron emission tomography data (threshold: CFR< 1.7); scinti, scintigraphy; Upslope$_{trans}$ and Upslope$_{subendo}$, upslope data derived from full wall thickness and subendocardial layer, respectively; Upslope CFR, coronary flow reserve calculated from upslope data (ratio of slope: hyperemia/rest).

In parallel with these efforts, the promising results from single-center studies[19] need confirmation in multicenter trials. These trials (some of which are currently ongoing) will help to position MR perfusion imaging with respect to other noninvasive imaging techniques such as SPECT, stress echocardiography, and PET. Further, such multicenter trials will provide data for quality assessment and standardization of MR perfusion studies. These aspects of MR perfusion imaging are of paramount importance when one bears in mind the strong dependence of test performance on imaging parameters.[41,49] Once multicenter trials have confirmed the robustness and accuracy of MR perfusion imaging, this technique will be combined with functional and viability tests[11] to generate a powerful one-stop-shop for risk stratification of patients with known or suspected CAD, and furthermore, in patients selected for treatment, this type of CMR examination will also monitor the effects of therapeutic interventions.

References

1. Smith SC Jr, Dove JT, Jacobs AK, et al. ACC/AHA Guidelines for Percutaneous Coronary Intervention (revision of the 1993 PTCA guidelines) – executive summary: a report of the American College of Cardiology/American Heart Association task force on practice guidelines (Committee to Revise the 1993 Guidelines for Percutaneous Transluminal Coronary Angioplasty) endorsed by the Society for Cardiac Angiography and Interventions. Circulation 2001; 103:3019–41.

2. Iskander S, Iskandrian AE. Risk assessment using single-photon emission computed tomographic technetium-99 m sestamibi imaging. J Am Coll Cardiol 1998; 32:57–62.

3. Ladenheim ML, Pollock BH, Rozanski A, et al. Extent and severity of myocardial hypoperfusion as predictors of prognosis in patients with suspected coronary artery disease. J Am Coll Cardiol 1986; 7:464–71.

4. Gibbons RJ, Chatterjee K, Daley J, et al. ACC/AHA/ACP–ASIM Guidelines for the Management of Patients with Chronic Stable Angina: a report of the American College of Cardiology/American Heart Association Task Force on Practice Guidelines (Committee on Management of Patients With Chronic Stable Angina). J Am Coll Cardiol 1999; 33:2092–197.

5. Hendel RC, Berman DS, Cullom SJ, et al. Multicenter clinical trial to evaluate the efficacy of correction for photon attenuation and scatter in SPECT myocardial perfusion imaging. Circulation 1999; 99:2742–9.

6. Taillefer R, DeDuey EG, Udelson JE, et al. Comparative diagnostic accuracy of Tl-201 and Tc-99m sestamibi SPECT imaging (perfusion and ECG-gated SPECT) in detecting coronary artery disease in women. J Am Coll Cardiol 1997; 29:69–77.

7. Gould KL, Kirkeeide RL, Buchi M. Coronary flow reserve as a physiologic measure of stenosis severity. J Am Coll Cardiol 1990; 15:459–74.

8. Ellis S, Alderman E, Cain K, et al. Prediction of risk of anterior myocardial infarction by lesion severity and measurement method of stenoses in the left anterior descending coronary distribution: a CASS registry study. J Am Coll Cardiol 1988; 11:908–16.

9. Ellis S, Alderman EL, Cain K, et al. Morphology of left anterior descending coronary territory lesions as a predictor of anterior myocardial infarction: a CASS registry study. J Am Coll Cardiol 1989; 13:1481–91.

10. Ledru F, Theroux P, Lesperance J, et al. Geometric features of coronary artery lesions favoring acute occlusion and myocardial infarction: a quantitative angiographic study. J Am Coll Cardiol 1999; 33:1353–61.

11. Kim RJ, Fieno DS, Parrish TB, et al. Relationship of MRI delayed contrast enhancement to irreversible injury, infarct age, and contractile function. Circulation 1999; 100:1992–2002.

12. Werns SW, Walton JA, Hsia HH, et al. Evidence of endothelial dysfunction in angiographically normal coronary arteries of patients with coronary artery disease. Circulation 1989; 79:287–91.

13. Muzik O, Duvernoy C, Beanlands RS, et al. Assessment of diagnostic performance of quantitative flow measurements in normal subjects and patients with angiographically documented coronary artery disease by means of nitrogen-13 ammonia and positron emission tomography. J Am Coll Cardiol 1998; 31:534–40.

14. Demer LL, Gould KL, Goldstein RA, et al. Assessment of coronary artery disease severity by positron emission tomography. Comparison with quantitative arteriography in 193 patients. Circulation 1989; 79:825–35.

15. Uren NG, Melin JA, De Bruyne B, et al. Relation between myocardial blood flow and the severity of coronary artery stenosis. N Engl J Med 1994; 330:1782–8.

16. Di Carli M, Czernin J, Hoh CK, et al. Relation among stenosis severity, myocardial blood flow, and flow reserve in patients with coronary artery disease. Circulation 1995; 91:1944–51.

17. Sambuceti G, Parodi O, Marcassa C, et al. Alterations in regulation of myocardial blood flow in one-vessel coronary artery disease determined by positron emission tomography. Am J Cardiol 1993; 72:538–43.

18. Picano E, Parodi O, Lattanzi F, et al. Assessment of anatomic and physiological severity of single-vessel coronary artery lesions by dipyridamole echocardiography. Comparison with positron emission tomography and quantitative arteriography. Circulation 1994; 89:753–61.

19. Schwitter J, Nanz D, Kneifel S, et al. Assessment of myocardial perfusion in coronary artery disease by magnetic resonance: a comparison with positron emission tomography and coronary angiography. Circulation 2001; 103:2230–5.

20. Keijer JT, van Rossum AC, Wilke N, et al. Magnetic resonance imaging of myocardial perfusion in single-vessel coronary artery disease: implications for transmural assessment of myocardial perfusion. J Cardiovasc Magn Reson 2000; 2:189–200.

21. Panting JR, Gatehouse PD, Yang GZ, et al. Abnormal subendocardial perfusion in cardiac syndrome X detected by cardiovascular magnetic resonance imaging. N Engl J Med 2002; 346:1948–53.

22. Li D, Dhawale P, Rubin PJ, et al. Myocardial signal response to dipyridamole and dobutamine: demonstration of the BOLD effect using a double-echo gradient-echo sequence. Magn Reson Med 1996; 36:16–20.

23. Atalay MK, Reeder SB, Zerhouni EA, Forder JR. Blood oxygenation dependence of T1 and T2 in the isolated, perfused rabbit heart at 4.7 T. Magn Reson Med 1995; 34:623–7.

24. Reeder SB, Atalay MK, McVeigh ER, et al. Quantitative cardiac perfusion: a noninvasive spin-labeling method that exploits coronary vessel geometry. Radiology 1996; 200:177–84.

25. Poncelet BP, Koelling TM, Schmidt CJ, et al. Measurement of human myocardial perfusion by double-gated flow alternating inversion recovery EPI. Magn Reson Med 1999; 41:510–19.

26. Wendland MF, Saeed M, Lauerma K, et al. Endogenous susceptibility contrast in myocardium during apnea measured using gradient recalled echo planar imaging. Magn Reson Med 1993; 29:273–6.

27. Belle V, Kahler E, Waller C, et al. In vivo quantitative mapping of cardiac perfusion in rats using a noninvasive MR spin-labeling method. J Magn Reson Imaging 1998; 8:1240–5.

28. Prasad PV, Burstein D, Edelman RR. MRI evaluation of myocardial perfusion without a contrast agent using magnetization transfer. Magn Reson Med 1993; 30:267–70.

29. Saeed M, Wendland MF, Sakuma H, et al. Coronary artery stenosis: detection with contrast-enhanced MR imaging in dogs. Radiology 1995; 196:79–84.

30. Schwitter J, Saeed M, Wendland MF, et al. Assessment of myocardial function and perfusion in a canine model of non-occlusive coronary artery stenosis using fast magnetic resonance imaging. J Magn Reson Imaging 1998; 9:101–10.

31. Manning WJ, Atkinson DJ, Grossman W, et al. First-pass nuclear magnetic resonance imaging studies using gadolinium-DTPA in patients with coronary artery disease. J Am Coll Cardiol 1991; 18:959–65.

32. Lauerma K, Virtanen KS, Sipila LM, et al. Multislice MRI in assessment of myocardial perfusion in patients with single-vessel proximal left anterior descending coronary artery disease before and after revascularization. Circulation 1997; 96:2859–67.

33. Matheijssen NA, Louwerenburg HW, van Rugge F, et al. Comparison of ultrafast dipyridamole magnetic resonance imaging with dipyridamole sestaMIBI SPECT for detection of perfusion abnormalities in patients with one-vessel coronary artery disease: assessment by quantitative model fitting. Magn Reson Med 1996; 35:221–8.

34. Eichenberger AC, Schuiki E, Kochli VD, et al. Ischemic heart disease: assessment with gadolinium-enhanced ultrafast MR imaging and dipyridamole stress. J Magn Reson Imaging 1994; 4:425–31.

35. Al-Saadi N, Nagel E, Gross M, et al. Noninvasive detection of myocardial ischemia from perfusion reserve based on cardiovascular magnetic resonance. Circulation 2000; 101:1379–83.

36. Sensky PR, Jivan A, Hudson NM, et al. Coronary artery disease: combined stress MR imaging protocol one-stop evaluation of myocardial perfusion and function. Radiology 2000; 215:608–14.

37. Edelman RR, Li W. Contrast-enhanced echo-planar MR imaging of myocardial perfusion: preliminary study in humans. Radiology 1994; 190:771–7.

38. Schwitter J, Debatin JF, von Schulthess GK, McKinnon GC. Normal myocardial perfusion assessed with multishot echo-planar imaging. Magn Reson Med 1997; 37:140–7.

39. Schwitter J, Sakuma H, Saeed M, et al. Very fast cardiac imaging. Magn Reson Imaging Clin North Am 1996; 4:419–32.

40. Ding S, Wolff SD, Epstein FH. Improved coverage in dynamic contrast-enhanced cardiac MRI using interleaved gradient-echo EPI. Magn Reson Med 1998; 39:514–19.

41. Bertschinger KM, Nanz D, Buechi M, et al. Magnetic resonance myocardial first-pass perfusion imaging: parameter optimization for signal response and cardiac coverage. J Magn Reson Imaging 2001; 14:556–62.

42. Kraitchman DL, Chin BB, Heldman AW, et al. MRI detection of myocardial perfusion defects due to coronary artery stenosis with MS-325. J Magn Reson Imaging 2002; 15:149–58.

43. Klocke FJ, Simonetti OP, Judd RM, et al. Limits of detection of regional differences in vasodilated flow in viable myocardium by first-pass magnetic resonance perfusion imaging. Circulation 2001; 104:2412–16.

44. Walsh EG, Doyle M, Lawson MA, Blackwell GG, Pohost GM. Multislice first-pass myocardial perfusion imaging on a conventional clinical scanner. Magn Reson Med 1995; 34:39–47.

45. Slavin GS, Wolff SD, Gupta SN, Foo TK. First-pass myocardial perfusion MR imaging with interleaved notched saturation: feasibility study. Radiology 2001; 219:258–63.

46. Saeed M, Wendland MF, Yu KK, et al. Dual effects of gadodiamide injection in depiction of the region of myocardial ischemia. J Magn Reson Imaging 1993; 3:21–9.

47. Wendland MF, Saeed M, Masui T, et al. Echo-planar MR imaging of normal and ischemic myocardium with gadodiamide injection. Radiology 1993; 186:535–42.

48. Larsson HB, Fritz Hansen T, Rostrup E, et al. Myocardial perfusion modeling using MRI. Magn Reson Med 1996; 35:716–26.

49. Muhling OM, Dickson ME, Zenovich A, et al. Quantitative magnetic resonance first-pass perfusion analysis: inter- and intra-observer agreement. J Cardiovasc Magn Reson 2001; 3:247–56.

50. Sakuma H, O'Sullivan M, Lucas J, et al. Effect of magnetic susceptibility contrast medium on myocardial signal intensity with fast gradient-recalled echo and spin-echo MR imaging: initial experience in humans. Radiology 1994; 190:161–6.

51. Wendland MF, Saeed M, Masui T, et al. First pass of an MR susceptibility contrast agent through normal and ischemic heart: gradient-recalled echo-planar imaging. J Magn Reson Imaging 1993; 3:755–60.

52. Panting JR, Taylor AM, Gatehouse PD, et al. First-pass myocardial perfusion imaging and equilibrium signal changes using the intravascular contrast agent NC100150 injection. J Magn Reson Imaging 1999; 10:404–10.

53. Hartnell G, Cerel A, Kamalesh M, et al. Detection of myocardial ischemia: value of combined myocardial perfusion and cineangiographic MR imaging. AJR 1994; 163:1061–7.

54. Keijer JT, van Rossum AC, van Eenige MJ, et al. Magnetic resonance imaging of regional myocardial perfusion in patients with single-vessel coronary artery disease: quantitative comparison with [201]thallium-SPECT and coronary angiography. J Magn Reson Imaging 2000; 11:607–15.

55. Wilke N, Simm C, Zhang J, et al. Contrast-enhanced first pass myocardial perfusion imaging: correlation between myocardial blood flow in dogs at rest and during hyperemia. Magn Reson Med 1993; 29:485–97.

56. Keijer JT, van Rossum A, van Eenige M, et al. Semiquantitation of regional myocardial blood flow in normal human subjects by first-pass magnetic resonance imaging. Am Heart J 1995; 130:893–901.

57. Lombardi M, Jones RA, Westby J, et al. Use of the mean transit time of an intravascular contrast agent as an exchange-insensitive index of myocardial perfusion. J Magn Reson Imaging 1999; 9:402–8.

58. Holland AE, Goldfarb JW, Edelman RR. Diaphragmatic and cardiac motion during suspended breathing: preliminary experience and implications for breath-hold MR imaging. Radiology 1998; 209:483–9.

59. McConnell MV, Khasgiwala VC, Savord BJ, et al. Prospective adaptive navigator correction for breath-hold MR coronary angiography. Magn Reson Med 1997; 37:148–52.

60. Chuang ML, Chen MH, Khasgiwala VC, et al. Adaptive correction of imaging plane position in segmented k-space cine cardiac MRI. J Magn Reson Imaging 1997; 7:811–14.

61. Wedeking P, Sotak CH, Telser J, et al. Quantitative dependence of MR signal intensity on tissue concentration of Gd(HP-DO3A) in the nephrectomized rat. Magn Reson Imaging 1992; 10:97–108.

62. Fritz-Hansen T, Rostrup E, Larsson HB, et al. Measurement of the arterial concentration of Gd-DTPA using MRI: a step toward quantitative perfusion imaging. Magn Reson Med 1996; 36:225–31.

63. Larsson HB, Stubgaard M, Sondergaard L, Henriksen O. In vivo quantification of the unidirectional influx constant for Gd-DTPA diffusion across the myocardial capillaries with MR imaging. J Magn Reson Imaging 1994; 4:433–40.

64. Wilke N, Kroll K, Merkle H, et al. Regional myocardial blood volume and flow: first-pass MR imaging with polylysine–Gd-DTPA. J Magn Reson Imaging 1995; 5:227–37.

65. Kroll K, Wilke N, Jerosch Herold M, et al. Modeling regional myocardial flows from residue functions of an intravascular indicator. Am J Physiol 1996; 271:H1643–55.

66. Kety S. The theory and application of the exchange of inert gas in lung and tissues. Pharmacol Rev 1951; 3:1–41.

67. Fritz-Hansen T, Rostrup E, Sondergaard L, et al. Capillary transfer constant of Gd-DTPA in the myocardium at rest and during vasodilation assessed by MRI. Magn Reson Med 1998; 40:922–9.

68. Cullen JH, Horsfield MA, Reek CR, et al. A myocardial perfusion reserve index in humans using first-pass contrast-enhanced magnetic resonance imaging. J Am Coll Cardiol 1999; 33:1386–94.

69. Tong CY, Prato FS, Wisenberg G, et al. Measurement of the extraction efficiency and distribution volume for Gd-DTPA in normal and diseased canine myocardium. Magn Reson Med 1993; 30:337–46.

70. Larsson HB, Rosenbaum S, Fritz Hansen T. Quantification of the effect of water exchange in dynamic contrast MRI perfusion measurements in the brain and heart. Magn Reson Med 2001; 46:272–81.

71. Wendland MF, Saeed M, Yu KK, et al. Inversion recovery EPI of bolus transit in rat myocardium using intravascular and extravascular gadolinium-based MR contrast media: dose effects on peak signal enhancement. Magn Reson Med 1994; 32:319–29.

72. Judd RM, Atalay MK, Rottman GA, Zerhouni EA. Effects of myocardial water exchange on T1 enhancement during bolus administration of MR contrast agents. Magn Reson Med 1995; 33:215–23.

73. Judd RM, Reeder SB, May Newman K. Effects of water exchange on the measurement of myocardial perfusion using paramagnetic contrast agents. Magn Reson Med 1999; 41:334–42.

74. Donahue KM, Burstein D, Manning WJ, Gray ML. Studies of Gd-DTPA relaxivity and proton exchange rates in tissue. Magn Reson Med 1994; 32:66–76.

75. Neyran B, Janier MF, Casali C, et al. Mapping myocardial perfusion with an intravascular MR contrast agent: robustness of deconvolution methods at various blood flows. Magn Reson Med 2002; 48:166–79.

76. Wilke N, Jerosch HM, Wang Y, et al. Myocardial perfusion reserve: assessment with multisection, quantitative, first-pass MR imaging. Radiology 1997; 204:373–84.

77. Dauber IM, VanBenthuysen KM, McMurtry IF, et al. Functional coronary microvascular injury evident as increased permeability due to brief ischemia and reperfusion. Circ Res 1990; 66:986–98.

78. Svendsen JH, Bjerrum PJ, Haunso S. Myocardial capillary permeability after regional ischemia and reperfusion in the in vivo canine heart. Effect of superoxide dismutase. Circ Res 1991; 68:174–84.

79. Weisskoff RM, Chesler D, Boxerman JL, Rosen BR. Pitfalls in MR measurement of tissue blood flow with intravascular tracers: Which mean transit time? Magn Reson Med 1993; 29:553–8.

80. Kraitchman DL, Wilke N, Hexeberg E, et al. Myocardial perfusion and function in dogs with moderate coronary stenosis. Magn Reson Med 1996; 35:771–80.

81. Saeed M, Wendland MF, Lauerma K, et al. First-pass contrast-enhanced inversion recovery and driven equilibrium fast GRE imaging studies: detection of acute myocardial ischemia. J Magn Reson Imaging 1995; 5:515–23.

82. Pruessmann KP, Weiger M, Scheidegger MB, Boesiger P. SENSE: sensitivity encoding for fast MRI. Magn Reson Med 1999; 42:952–62.

83. Weiger M, Pruessmann KP, Boesiger P. Cardiac real-time imaging using SENSE. SENSitivity Encoding scheme. Magn Reson Med 2000; 43:177–84.

8

CMR of myocardial viability

Anja Wagner, Heiko Mahrholdt, Louise Thomson, Udo Sechtem, Raymond J Kim, Robert M Judd

Introduction

Heart failure caused by coronary artery disease (CAD) is a leading cause of death in the developed countries of the world.[1] The detection of residual myocardial viability in patients with left-ventricular (LV) dysfunction in the setting of CAD is important in planning management, because revascularization of dysfunctional but viable myocardium can improve ventricular function and long-term survival.[2–4] Noncontractile but viable myocardium may result from acute, subacute, or chronic reduction in myocardial perfusion, and is frequently described as stunned or hibernating. Both terms refer to reversible ventricular contractile impairment; however, hibernation is defined by the presence of concomitant reduction of perfusion and contractility, whereas stunning is characterized by persistent contractile impairment after there has been complete return of myocardial perfusion. Stunning has been observed in multiple clinical situations, including unstable angina,[5] exercise-induced ischemia,[6] cardiac surgery[7] (after use of cardioplegic solution), and early following successful reperfusion of acute myocardial infarction.[8] Hibernation is thought to arise in states of chronically reduced myocardial perfusion. It is believed to represent an adapted state in which contractile function is diminished in order to match the decreased supply of substrates and O_2 to the myocardium.

The emphasis placed on the detection of viable myocardium can be justified in terms of the influence of myocardial viability on patient outcome in terms of morbidity and mortality. In the setting of acute LV dysfunction, several studies have shown that prognosis is worse when there is myocardial necrosis than when the myocardial dysfunction is reversible.[9,10] Furthermore, management may be determined by the degree of myocardial viability. Stunned (viable) myocardium may be at risk from further ischemic insult in the presence of a significant coronary stenosis following reperfusion therapy,[9,11] and thus the demonstration of viability in a dysfunctional region may justify early revascularization.

The prognosis in a patient with chronic LV dysfunction may be improved by revascularization if there is sufficient viable myocardium to permit remodeling and recovery of contractile function. Conversely, there is evidence to suggest that revascularization for patients with left ventricular dysfunction and predominantly nonviable myocardium is unlikely to improve outcome and may increase mortality.[12] In addition to the decision to revascularize, the determination of the extent of viable myocardium may be valuable in selecting patients most likely to benefit from medical therapy that can modulate ventricular remodeling.[11]

Definition of myocardial viability

In CAD, the definition of myocardial viability is directly related to that of myocardial infarction, given that infarction is defined as loss of viability. Myocardial infarction

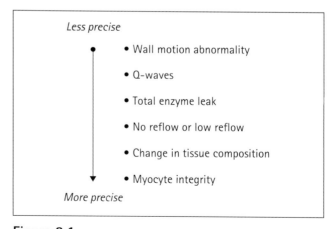

Figure 8.1
Clinical and physiological markers to determine the size of infarction. (Adapted from Kaul S. Circulation 1998; 98:625–7[13] with permission from Lippincott Williams and Wilkins.)

<table>
<tr><td colspan="2">**Table 8.1 Definitions of myocardial viability**</td></tr>
</table>

Table 8.1 Definitions of myocardial viability

Clinical
- Improvement in contraction after revascularization
- Improvement in contraction with low-dose dobutamine
- Absence of a fixed thallium defect
- Presence of glucose uptake
- Reduced perfusion
- Preserved wall thickness and/or thickening

Histologic
- Presence of living myocytes

(Reproduced from Herz 2000; 25:417–30.)

can be detected by a variety of clinical markers that vary in their ability to define the extent of myocardial necrosis. In his review on this subject, Kaul[13] ranked these markers from least to most precise (Figure 8.1) and noted that the critical defining event of infarction, and therefore the loss of viability, is myocyte death. All ischemic events prior to cell death are, at least theoretically, reversible by adequate reperfusion. The presence or absence of cell death can be established by light microscopy, by electron microscopy, or by the use of histologic stains such as triphenyltetra-zolium chloride (TTC).[14] Testing for myocardial viability

by microscopy or histologic staining is obviously not practical in a clinical setting. Accordingly, other means of defining viability have developed based on parameters that can be measured noninvasively (Table 8.1). It is important to recognize, however, that these techniques all provide indirect evidence for viability and that the ultimate proof of the presence of viable myocardium is through demonstration of the presence of living myocytes.

Current noninvasive techniques to assess myocardial viability

Noninvasive imaging techniques for determining myocardial viability include [18F]fluorodeoxyglucose positron emission tomography (FDG-PET), thallium-201 or technetium-99m single-photon emission computed tomography (^{201}Tl-SPECT, ^{99m}Tc-SPECT), and low-dose dobutamine echocardiography (Table 8.1). Myocardial viability is therefore defined in terms of myocardial glucose metabolism (FDG uptake), cellular membrane integrity (thallium redistribution SPECT), mitochondrial function (^{99m}Tc-sestamibi SPECT), or the presence of contractile reserve (dobutamine echo).

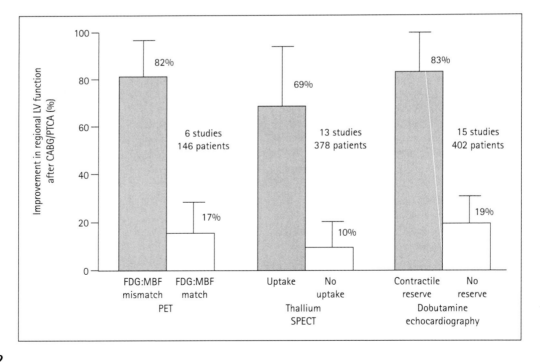

Figure 8.2
Likelihood of improved regional LV function after revascularization by coronary artery bypass graft (CABG) or percutaneous transluminal coronary angioplasty (PTCA), based on noninvasive methods to detect viable myocardium: positron emission tomography (PET), thallium single-photon emission computed tomography (SPECT), and dobutamine echocardiography. Data are pooled from 34 studies involving over 900 patients. The ranges of values reported from the individual studies are indicated by the error lines. The shaded bars represent the positive predictive value and the open bars represent the inverse of the negative predictive value. (Reprinted from Bonow RO. Circulation 1996; 94:2674–80[38] with permission from Lippincott Williams and Wilkins.)

The ability of PET, SPECT, or dobutamine echocardiography to predict recovery of regional LV function following myocardial revascularization is similar (Figure 8.2). Dobutamine echocardiography and PET imaging with metabolic tracers appear to have greater specificity compared with SPECT imaging, while SPECT has greater sensitivity. This translates into a high positive predictive value (82%) for PET and dobutamine echocardiography compared with Tl-SPECT (69%), but higher negative predictive value for SPECT (90%) compared with both PET (83%) and dobutamine echocardiography (81%), as indicated in Figure 8.2. Understanding the differences between these modalities and the inherent difficulties in studying 'recovery after revascularization' helps to explain these observations regarding the accuracy of noninvasive tests.

The process of hibernation in chronically underperfused myocardium involves a continuum of downregula-tion of myocyte metabolism that eventually leads to a reduction in functional myofibrillar elements and de-differentiation of cells.

PET, SPECT and echocardiography assess different indirect markers of cellular viability. In hibernating myocardium, there is potential for a sufficient loss of contractile elements to lead to loss of contractile reserve by echocardiography; however cellular integrity may be maintained and therefore SPECT may be positive for viability.[15] Other important influences include the adequacy of revascularization, the degree of microvascular disease or occurrence of perioperative ischemic events, the timing of revascularization relative to the duration of hibernation, and the timing of the noninvasive assessment of recovery of LV function following revascularization. All of these factors potentially influence the observed recovery of function and thus the observed sensitivity and

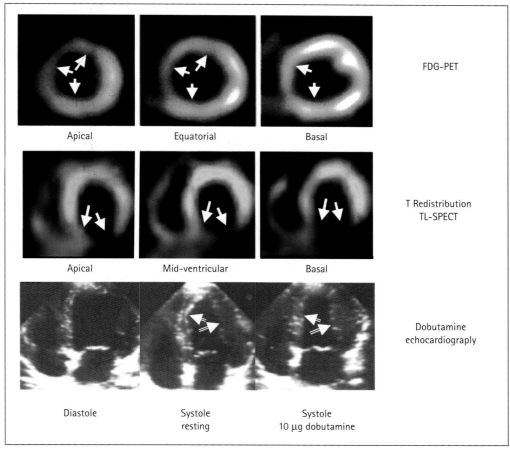

| Apical | Equatorial | Basal | FDG-PET |

| Apical | Mid-ventricular | Basal | T Redistribution TL-SPECT |

| Diastole | Systole resting | Systole 10 µg dobutamine | Dobutamine echocardiography |

Figure 8.3

Examples of [18F]-fluorodeoxyglucose (FDG)-PET (upper panel), thallium redistribution SPECT (middle panel) and dobutamine echocardiography (lower panel) images for the assessment of myocardial viability in three different patients. In the upper panel, there is FDG activity throughout the ventricle, indicating preserved metabolic activity and viability of the entire myocardium. There is a severe inferolateral perfusion defect on the redistribution Tl-SPECT images, consistent with regional absence of viability (arrows). The dobutamine echocardiography demonstrates increased systolic thickening of myocardium with low-dose ionotropic stimulation, indicating viability of these myocardial segments (arrows in middle and right lower panel). None of the techniques, however, can accurately assess the transmural extent of infarction.

specificity of the noninvasive test that is being used to predict recovery.

There are also limitations with each test itself. SPECT is susceptible to attenuation artifacts, and the routine clinical use of PET is limited by high costs. Dobutamine stress echocardiography has the inherent disadvantage that suboptimal or nondiagnostic images occur in up to 15% of patients.[16] Endocardial delineation may be poor in basal lateral and apical segments, and optimal display and interpretation of segments requires a long training period and remains user-dependent[17] (Figure 8.3).

SPECT and PET have limited spatial resolution compared with magnetic resonance imaging (MRI). This leads to the use of a binary determination of viability within a myocardial region, since these modalities cannot assess the transmural extent of infarction across the ventricular wall[18] (see also Figure 8.3). This chapter will outline the advantages of cardiovascular magnetic resonance (CMR) imaging techniques to distinguish between viable and nonviable myocardium and to assess the transmural extent of the infarct.

Magnetic resonance spectroscopy

The hallmark of viable myocardium is the presence of high energy phosphates within the cell. As phosphorus-31 (^{31}P) magnetic resonance spectroscopy (MRS) is the only available technique capable of observing high-energy phosphates noninvasively in vivo, it can be employed to detect and quantify this sign of life within a myocardial region. Yabe et al[19] evaluated patients with significant left anterior descending (LAD) artery stenosis who had reversible and irreversible thallium defects on exercise-redistribution SPECT. MR spectra were localized by one-dimensional chemical shift imaging in a sagittal plane. The volume of interest in this study was on the order of 30 cm^3. Quantification of spectra was done by using hexamethylphosphoric triamide (HMPT) as the reference standard. Representative spectra from the three groups are shown in Figure 8.4. Phosphocreatine content was significantly lower in patients with LAD stenosis compared with normal controls, but did not differentiate between those individuals with thallium redistribution (viable) and those without redistribution (nonviable). The ATP concentration, however, was only reduced in patients without thallium redistribution. This study demonstrated that quantitative MRS measurements are possible in patients with CAD and that MRS can provide information about the presence of myocardial viability. Nevertheless, the technique described by Yabe et al cannot be applied clinically, because volumes of interest likely consists of

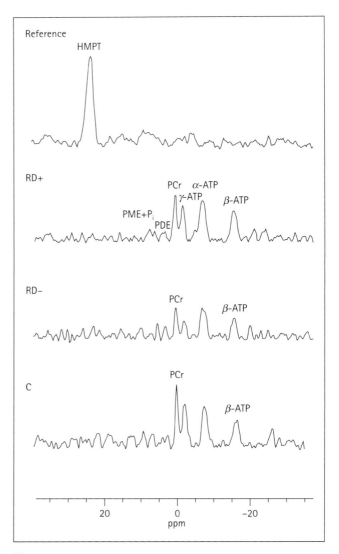

Figure 8.4
^{31}P-MR spectra of control (C) and typical patients with (RD+) and without (RD−) redistribution on 3-hour post-exercise Tl-SPECT images. The RD− patient had a lower myocardial phosphocreatine (PCr) content compared with the RD+ patient and the normal control person. Moreover, the RD+ patient had a lower PCr content than the normal control person. HMPT, hexamethylphosphoric triamide (used as the standard for quantification); PME = phosphomonoesters; P$_i$, inorganic phosphate; PDE, phosphodiesters. (Reprinted from Yabe et al. Circulation 1995; 92:15–23[19] with permission from Lippincott Williams and Wilkins.)

mixtures of scar, normal, and ischemically injured viable myocardium.

Proton spectroscopy (^{1}H-MRS) has higher sensitivity than ^{31}P-MRS and is able to detect the total pool of phosphorylated plus unphosphorylated creatine in both skeletal and cardiac muscle. ^{1}H-MRS theoretically offers a 20-fold improvement in sensitivity over ^{31}P-MRS of phosphorylated creatine. This is due to the inherently higher sensitivity of proton spectroscopy, the higher concentration of total creatine, and the higher proton content in the creatine N-methyl resonance at 3.0 ppm. Consequently, ^{1}H-MRS allows metabolic interrogation of small voxels (< 10 ml) in all regions of the LV that can be performed at the magnetic field strengths of many clinical CMR systems. ^{31}P-MRS, in contrast, is limited by its large voxel size and can only interrogate the anterior wall. As the entire ventricle can be examined by ^{1}H-MRS, comparison of viable and nonviable tissue is possible within the same patient. Thus, the patient can serve as his own control. Bottomley and Weiss[20] were the first to employ proton spectroscopy in patients with remote myocardial infarction (longer than 1 month). In a dog model, they established that enzymatic degradation of creatine in heart extracts resulted in the complete disappearance of the proton N-methyl resonance peak at 3.0 ppm. This study showed for the first time that it is possible to measure creatine within myocardial regions small enough to make this technique clinically useful. Further work is needed to establish the usefulness of creatine measurements by ^{1}H-MRS as compared with established imaging techniques. Assessment of the transmural extent of the infarct appears to be beyond the reach of a spectroscopic approach.

Sodium and potassium imaging

Living myocytes maintain an ionic gradient between the intracellular and extracellular space, and this can be used as another indicator of myocardial viability. Cannon et al[21] showed that sodium-23 (^{23}Na) image intensities were elevated following acute infarction in ex vivo dog hearts and that these elevations were related to increased sodium content measured by flame photometry. Kim et al[22,23] showed that ^{23}Na-MR could be used to measure infarct size and distinguish between reversible and irreversible ischemic injuries in an in vivo dog model. The mechanism responsible for this distinction was thought to be the equilibration of intracellular sodium concentration [Na$^+$] (normally 10–15 mM) with extracellular [Na$^+$] (145 mM) in irreversibly injured myocytes due to their failure to maintain ionic homeostasis (Figure 8.5). More recently, Fieno et al[24] studied the potential of direct MR imaging of potassium-39 (^{39}K) to examine viability, and reported that potassium image intensities were reduced in irreversibly injured regions secondary to loss of intracellular potassium. From a physiologic perspective and in the narrow context of myocardial viability, ^{23}Na- and ^{39}K-MR imaging appear to be similar in demonstration of loss of myocyte integrity due to irreversible injury.

The primary limitation of metabolic CMR to date is that the MR signal is extremely small compared with the proton signal associated with water. Ignoring differences in relaxation times, the MR signals associated with ^{31}P, creatine, ^{23}Na, and ^{39}K are 10^4–10^6 times smaller than the proton signal associated with water. Although judicious selection of imaging parameters based on differences in relaxation times can partially alleviate this deficit,[25] small MR signals generally result in poor spatial resolution and long imaging times. For ^{31}P, for example, the small MR signal generally limits the examination of creatine phosphate and ATP to voxels several cubic centimeters in size, and often precludes examination of the posterior region of the heart.

CMR techniques assessing viability by observing wall thickness and contractile function

Myocardial wall thickness can be accurately defined using CMR and cine imaging techniques that allow visualization of wall thickness in diastole and systole. The formation of a myocardial scar is associated with loss of volume in the necrosed region and subsequent thinning of the myocardial wall at the scar site. CMR studies have demonstrated that the total wall thickness of a chronic transmural myocardial infarct is usually < 6 mm.[26] The hypothesis that thinned and akinetic myocardium represents chronic scarring has been tested by comparing CMR findings with PET and SPECT in identical myocardial regions.[27,28] Thinning of an infarct region may occur early, even in the absence of transmural necrosis. This is especially seen in large anterior myocardial infarcts. The consequence is an increase in the circumferential extent of the infarcted segment, known as infarct expansion.[29] This situation may also be associated with complete absence of wall thickening at rest early after the acute event, despite the presence of some viability. Observing only anatomy and function of the LV at rest may not detect residual viability. However, even a small amount of wall thickening in a region of interest indicates the presence of residual contracting cells and hence of viable myocardium.

Dobutamine stress CMR

If no wall thickening is present or the amount of wall thickening is so small as to leave serious doubt about the potential for recovery of regional ventricular function, inotropic stimulation by dobutamine infusion can be employed with cine imaging to assess residual viability

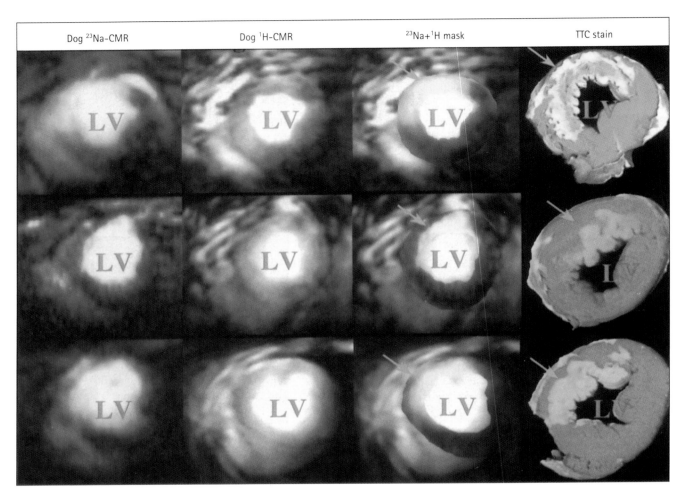

Figure 8.5
LV short-axis cross-sections of three different dog hearts (rows). The leftmost column shows in vivo ^{23}Na-CMR using a light–dark scale in which increasing brightness reflects higher ^{23}Na signal. The second column shows ^{1}H-CMR at the same location, for delineation of anatomy. In the third column, there is a composite ^{23}Na–^{1}H image, in which endocardial and epicardial borders of LV myocardium are defined by ^{1}H images and used to directly superimpose myocardial ^{23}Na image intensities. In the rightmost column, the corresponding postmortem TTC-stained slices (right ventricles removed before staining) are displayed. Note the visual correlation between myocardial regions with elevated ^{23}Na image intensity and the histologically defined infarction. (Reprinted from Kim et al. Circulation 1999; 100:185–92[22] with permission from Lippincott Williams and Wilkins.)

(Figure 8.6).[30] Due in part to the direct analogy with dobutamine echocardiography, dobutamine CMR enjoys a large body of clinical evidence supporting the hypothesis that the technique yields useful information about myocardial viability. The clinical implementation of this approach involves the acquisition of at least two sets of cine MR images: one before and one during intravenous administration of low-dose (5–10 μg/kg/min) dobutamine. In a manner directly analogous to dobutamine echocardiography, cine images before and during dobutamine are inspected side-by-side in order to detect changes in wall thickening.

The tremendously improved temporal resolution of new fast gradient-echo CMR sequences such as FLASH, True-FISP, FFE, and FIESTA permits the capture of cine loops displaying the beating heart, therefore allowing quantitative assessment of wall motion. End-diastolic and end-systolic still frames with well-defined endocardial and epicardial borders make the quantification of chamber volumes and myocardial wall thickness relatively easy[31] (Figure 8.7). The advent of fast sequences make it feasible to acquire breathhold cine images in multiple short-axis and two long-axis imaging planes at rest and with dobutamine infusion (5 and 10 μg/kg/min) within ~30 min. As a result of the advances in imaging speed and quality, a number of CMR protocols have been developed for the assessment of myocardial viability.

First reports of the use of CMR assessment of contractile reserve were published more than a decade ago. In 1995, Dendale et al[32] studied 24 patients early after acute

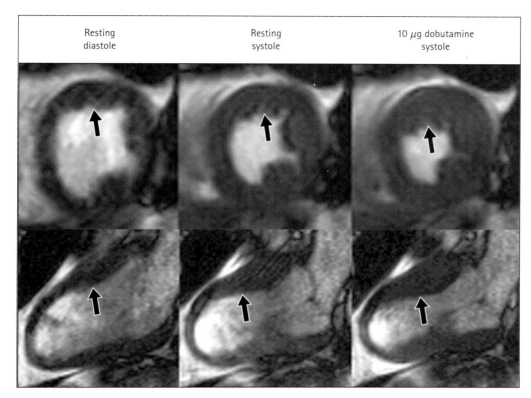

| Resting diastole | Resting systole | 10 μg dobutamine systole |

Figure 8.6
Dobutamine stress CMR study of a 69-year-old male patient after myocardial infarction in the LAD territory. The distal anteroapical myocardium is thinned and does not thicken at rest or with low-dose dobutamine – consistent with absent viability. There is, however, residual myocardial viability of the hypokinetic mid-anterior wall, where contractile function improves after administration of low-dose dobutamine (see arrows). (Adapted from Wagner et al. Magn Reson Imaging Clin North Am 2003; 11:49–66 with permission from Elsevier Science.)

myocardial infarction with low-dose dobutamine CMR and echocardiography using quantitative assessment of wall motion for both imaging modalities. Concordance between echocardiography and CMR in identifying viable and nonviable segments was 81%. With recovery of wall thickening after revascularization taken as the gold standard, studies have shown the positive and negative predictive value of dobutamine CMR to range from 100% to 89% and 73% to 94%, respectively.[33,34]

Baer et al[35] compared conventional dobutamine CMR and dobutamine transesophageal echocardiography (TEE) with the standard of normalized FDG uptake on PET images for detection of viable myocardium. The sensitivity and specificity of these techniques were similar (dobutamine TEE sensitivity 77%, specificity 94%; dobutamine CMR sensitivity 81%, specificity 100%). Therefore, when considering the choice of technique for assessment of viability, parameters such as availability and patient acceptance become important considerations.

Widespread clinical use of dobutamine CMR has been hindered by the need for rapid imaging; however, another important practical disadvantage of dobutamine CMR relates to the risk of administering a dobutamine infusion to a patient in the magnet. Positive inotropic stimulation in patients with CAD is intrinsically associated with the risk of eliciting an ischemic event, and the position of the patient within the magnet impairs physician–patient interaction. In addition, the diagnostic utility of ECG monitoring is diminished due to the ECG waveform being directly altered by the magnetic field. However, despite the small but finite risk, a number of groups have reported successful use of low-dose dobutamine CMR in patients with CAD, and it should be noted that successful use of cine CMR during much higher dobutamine dosages has been described for the detection of ischemia.[16,36]

Analogous to the limitations of dobutamine echocardiography in detecting viability, dobutamine CMR can potentially underestimate the extent of viable myocardium and does not allow the assessment of the transmural extent of myocardial infarction. The data from the dobutamine echocardiography literature suggest that, compared with ^{201}Tl-SPECT, the use of contractile reserve as an approach to detect myocardial viability will have higher specificity but reduced sensitivity.[37–39] The reduced sensitivity may relate to the development of ischemia at even low levels of inotropic stress, and/or to the pathophysiology of hibernating myocardium itself in which cellular dedifferentiation may occur with dropout of myofibrillar units.[40] In both cases, viable myocardium would be unable to respond to inotropic stimulation.

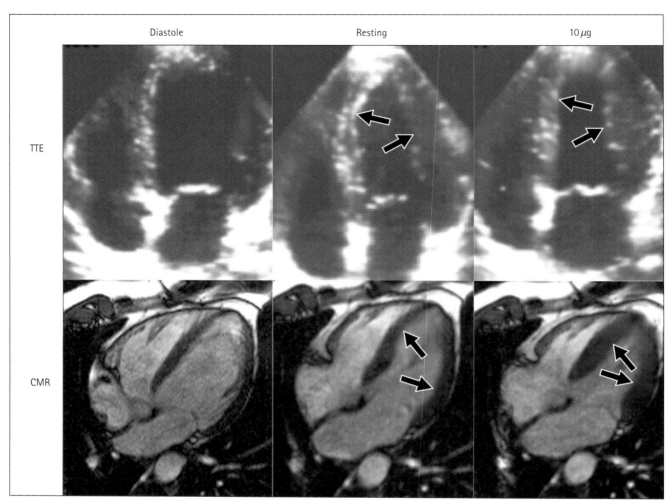

Figure 8.7
Direct comparison of low-dose dobutamine transthoracic echocardiography (TTE) and low-dose dobutamine CMR to assess viability in septal and lateral walls after myocardial infarction in the same patient. Both techniques are capable of visualizing an improvement in wall motion after dobutamine infusion (see arrows) as a sign of residual viability in the areas of interest. (Reprinted from Marholdt H, Wagner A, Judd RM, et al. In: Textbook of Echocardiography (Picano E, ed). Berlin: Springer-Verlag, 2002: Chapter 35; pp 403–19.)

CMR techniques assessing viability using delayed contrast hyperenhancement

Relaxation agents such as gadolinium chelates (gadopentate, gadodiamide, and gadotetriole) are large molecules that rapidly diffuse from the intravascular compartment into the interstitium and remain in the extracellular space. Relaxation agents decrease both the longitudinal relaxation time (T1) and the transverse relaxation time (T2) of water protons within the same compartment as the contrast agent. At clinical doses, the effect on T1 is greatest and results in increased signal intensities on T1-weighted images.

Therefore, most CMR pulse sequences for assessment of contrast enhancement patterns are designed to make image intensities a strong function of T1 (T1-weighted images).

Early studies have been performed using T1-weighted ECG-gated spin-echo images (see SE and TSE panels of Figure 8.8) in which one k-space line was acquired in each cardiac cycle. Because the duration of the cardiac cycle (~800 ms) was comparable to myocardial T1, the resulting images were T1-weighted. Using this approach, myocardial infarction was found in animal studies and in humans,[41,42] and nontransmural infarction was visualized by Dendale et al[34] and Yokota et al.[43]

New CMR techniques

There have been a number of technical improvements in CMR in recent years, one of the most important being the use of k-space segmentation. The acquisition of multiple k-space lines of data during each cardiac cycle[44] has reduced imaging times to the point where images can usually be acquired within a single breathhold. This advance has resulted in improved image quality and improved tolerability of imaging, and has increased the application of CMR to clinical practice.

Advances in imaging pulse sequences to allow increased T1 weighting of images have been particularly important in imaging for myocardial viability. The preparation of the magnetization prior to image acquisition by the use of an inversion pulse significantly increases the degree of T1 weighting in the images. This type of segmented inversion recovery pulse sequence (segmented IR Turbo-FLASH) was recently compared with nine other CMR pulse sequences for depiction of zones of necrotic myocardium in a dog model of myocardial infarction (Figure 8.8).[45]

Image intensities in 'hyperenhanced' regions using T1 spin-echo sequences were 50–100% higher than in normal regions. A much higher contrast between necrotic and normal myocardium was achieved by using the segmented inversion recovery pulse sequence with the inversion time set to null signal from normal myocardium. This sequence resulted in a differential of intensities between normal and hyperenhanced myocardium of ~1000% in animals[45] – a 10-fold increase in the degree of image contrast compared with the conventional spin-echo sequence.

Figure 8.9 shows this optimized segmented inversion recovery sequence in more detail. In order to minimize cardiac motion, the images are acquired in diastole by using a trigger delay. The magnetization of the heart is prepared by a nonselective 180°-inversion pulse to increase T1 weighting. The inversion delay time (TI), which is defined as the time between this 180° pulse and the centre of acquisition of the segmented k-space lines (lines 1–23 in Figure 8.9) is chosen such that the magnetization of normal myocardium is near its zero-crossing, ensuring that normal myocardium will appear as dark as possible.

The higher image quality of the optimized segmented inversion recovery sequence translates into improved diagnostic capabilities. While many previous studies of contrast-enhanced CMR using conventional spin-echo

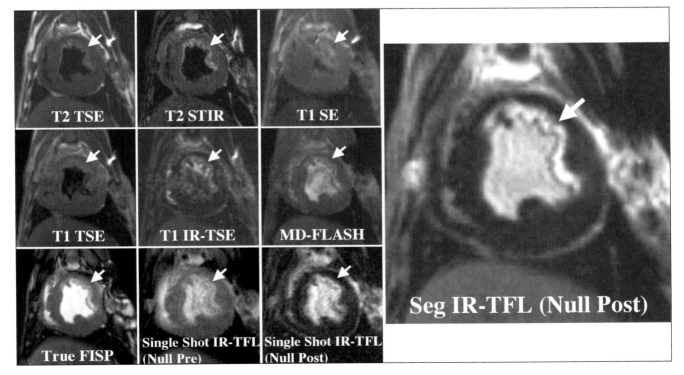

Figure 8.8
Contrast-enhanced images at one short-axis location in the same heart using 10 different CMR techniques. The segmented inversion recovery technique (large image) produced the clearest delineation of the hyperenhanced region (arrows). (Reproduced from Simonetti et al. Radiology 2001; 218:215–23[45] with permission from the Radiological Society of North America.)

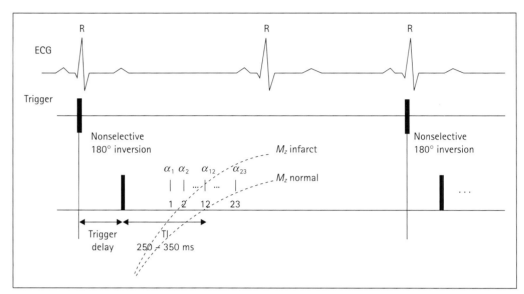

Figure 8.9
Timing diagram for the segmented inversion recovery turbo-FLASH sequence with TI set to null normal myocardium after contrast agent administration. (Adapted from Simonetti et al. Radiology 2001; 218:215–23[45] with permission from the Radiological Society of North America.)

sequences showed that acute myocardial infarction can be detected as a hyperenhanced region, the patients studied typically had large infarcts. The transmural extent of smaller infarcts could often not be evaluated due to limited resolution in spin-echo[42,46–48] images. Two studies attempted to distinguish between transmural and subendocardial hyperenhancement in patients with known infarction using contrast-enhanced spin-echo techniques.[34,43] Nontransmural involvement was visualized in both studies; however Dendale et al[34] found that 15 (27%) of 56 infarct segments had no visible hyperenhancement, and Yokota et al[43] did not observe hyperenhancement in 6 (13%) of 44 patients with documented infarction. The infarcts that were missed were generally small, with normal wall motion at rest[34] and lower peak creatine kinase levels.[43] This reported inability to detect smaller infarcts may have been due to limitations in conventional spin-echo imaging, with its requirement for image acquisition over several minutes during free breathing. Partial-volume effects due to motional averaging over the respiratory cycle, image artifacts due to respiratory motion, and modest T1 weighting due to limited choices for repetition time can all contribute to decreased ability to detect small regions of hyperenhanced myocardium. Conversely, small regions of subendocardial infarction can been visualized with high accuracy using the new segmented IR Turbo-FLASH techniques described above.[49,50]

Delayed enhancement in acute and chronic myocardial infarction

Contrast hyperenhancement has been clearly demonstrated to occur acutely and chronically after myocardial infarction in animal models of infarction and in patients.

Kim et al[50] scanned dogs 1–3 days following reperfused or nonreperfused coronary artery occlusion, and demonstrated hyperenhancement in histologically confirmed sites of infarction. Simonetti et al[45] studied patients with recent myocardial infarction. Eighteen consecutive patients were scanned 19 ± 7 days after enzymatically documented myocardial infarction. In all patients, myocardial hyperenhancement was observed within the appropriate infarct-related artery (IRA) perfusion territory. Figure 8.10 demonstrates six representative examples from this study.

Whereas acute infarcts are characterized by necrotic myocytes, the hallmark of chronic infarcts is the presence of dense collagenous scar. However, despite these underlying structural differences, chronic infarcts also hyperenhance. Kim et al[50] scanned dogs eight weeks after myocardial infarction, when infarct healing had progressed. Figure 8.11 shows an example of a dog with an 8-week-old infarct, in which the hyperenhanced region observed in vivo is clearly associated with a dense collagenous scar defined histologically postmortem. Using high-resolution ex vivo imaging, the regions of hyperenhancement observed in chronic infarcts appeared identical to the infarcted regions defined histologically (Figure 8.12).[50]

Wu et al[49] systematically evaluated whether chronic infarcts in patients hyperenhance using segmented inversion recovery Turbo-FLASH imaging. Patients were enrolled at the time of acute infarction (defined by elevated creatine kinase levels) and had CMR several months later. To assess the specificity of the findings, contrast CMR was also performed in patients with nonischemic idiopathic cardiomyopathy and in healthy volunteers. For patients with chronic myocardial infarction, there were a

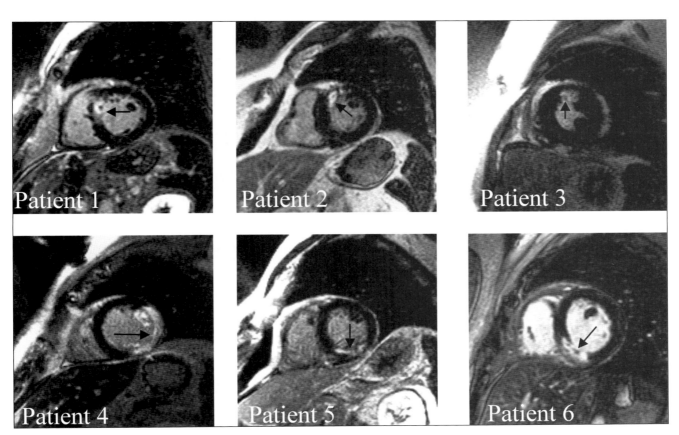

Figure 8.10
Short-axis images in six patients with acute myocardial infarction. The arrows point to the hyperenhanced region, which was in the appropriate infarct-related artery perfusion territory. (Adapted from Simonetti et al. Radiology 2001; 218:215–23[45] with permission from the Radiological Society of North America.)

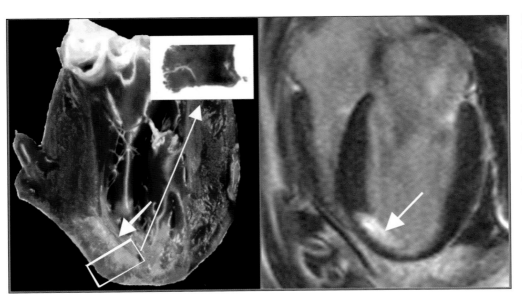

Figure 8.11
In vivo contrast-enhanced images of a dog with an 8-week-old myocardial infarction (right). Despite replacement of necrotic myocytes with dense collagenous scar (blue region of trichrome staining, inset in left panel), hyperenhancement is still observed. (Adapted from Kim Circulation 1999; 100:1992–2002[50] with permission from Lippincott Williams and Wilkins.)

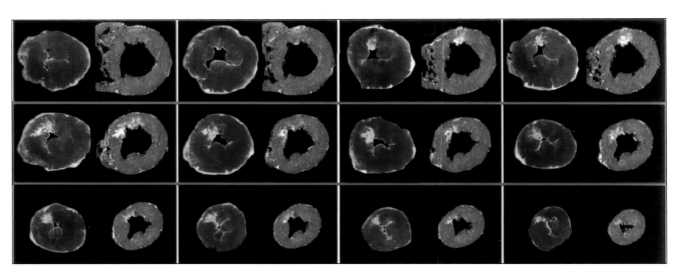

Figure 8.12
Comparison of ex vivo high-resolution contrast-enhanced MR images (right), with acute myocardial necrosis defined histologically by TTC staining (left). (Reprinted from Kim et al. Circulation 1999; 100:1992–2002[50] with permission from Lippincott Williams and Wilkins.)

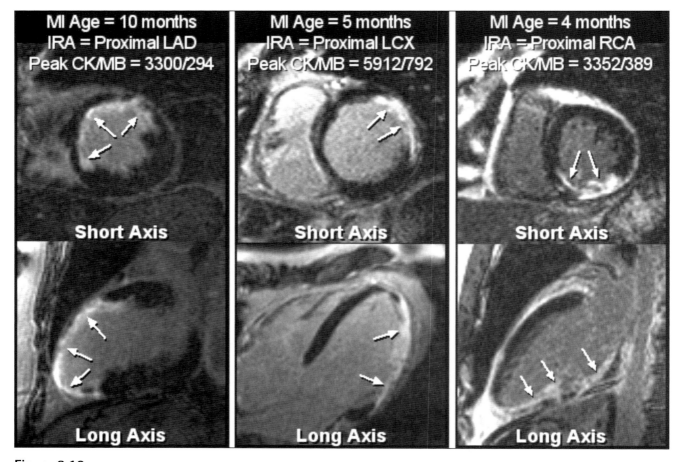

Figure 8.13
Typical short- and long-axis views of three patients with large transmural hyperenhancement in different coronary artery territories. (Reprinted Wu et al. Lancet 2001; 357:21–8[49] with permission from Elsevier Science.)

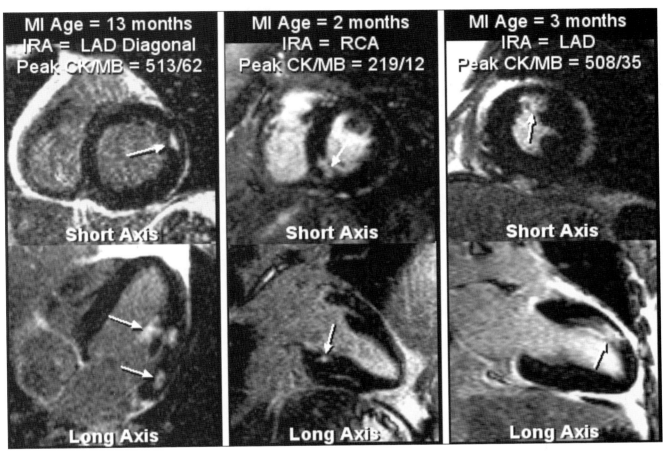

Figure 8.14
Typical short- and long-axis views of three patients with minor CK-MB elevations and small regions of hyperenhancement in different coronary artery territories. (Reprinted from Wu et al. Lancet 2001; 357:21–8[45] with permission from Elsevier Science.)

variety of sizes of hyperenhanced regions observed, ranging from large fully transmural hyperenhanced regions extending over several short-axis slices to small subendocardial hyperenhanced regions, only visible in a single view. Figure 8.13 demonstrates typical short- and long-axis views of three patients with large regions of transmural hyperenhancement in varying coronary artery territories. Figure 8.14 shows views of three patients with minor creatine kinase MB isoenzyme (CK-MB) elevations and small nontransmural regions of hyperenhancement. For each patient, hyperenhancement was in the appropriate IRA territory. None of the 20 patients with nonischemic dilated cardiomyopathy or the 11 normal volunteers exhibited hyperenhancement, resulting in a specificity of 100%. The sensitivities of contrast CMR for the detection of healed infarction were 91% and 100% in groups with 3-month-old and 14-month-old infarcts, respectively. Recently, Klein et al[51] compared contrast-enhanced CMR with the gold standard of FDG-PET and also provided convincing data showing that areas of

hyperenhancement corresponded to regions of chronic infarction defined by PET (Figure 8.15).

Delayed enhancement in reversible ischemic injury

It has been debated whether hyperenhancement occurs solely in necrotic myocardium or whether regions submitted to a period of ischemia ('area at risk') may also hyperenhance. To address this question, Fieno et al[52] used histologic TTC staining of myocardium from animals with induced infarction to define the area of necrosis (middle left panel of Figure 8.16). Fluorescent microparticles had been injected into the left atrium during the time of coronary occlusion in order to define the area at risk (lower left panel of Figure 8.16). It was demonstrated that the area at risk surrounds the infarcted region, but does

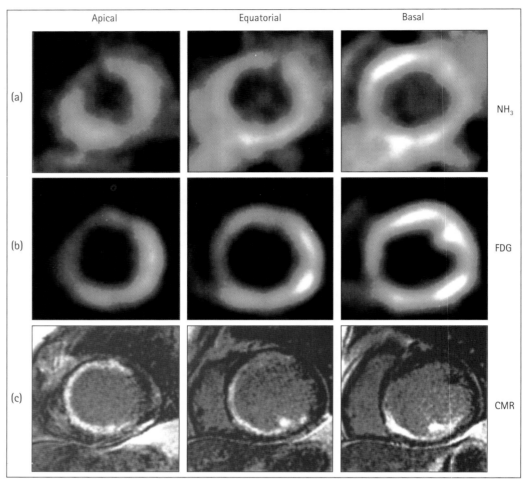

Figure 8.15
(a, b) Short–axis views (apical, equatorial, and basal) of a PET viability study with assessment of rest perfusion (NH₃) and glucose metabolism (FDG). (c) CMR images in corresponding slices showing hyperenhancement. Note that in segments with reduced perfusion and metabolism, there is an increased signal in MRI. Because of better spatial resolution in CMR, distinction can be made between transmural, subendocardial, and papillary defects. The border between enhanced and normal areas is distinct. (Reprinted from Klein et al. Circulation. 2002; 105:162–7.)

not exhibit hyperenhancement on high-resolution ex vivo MR images with a spatial resolution of 500 µm × 500 µm × 500 µm (upper left panel of Figure 8.16). Light microscopy of this area at risk (but not infarcted) showed normal myocyte architecture (middle right panel of Figure 8.16).

Kim et al[50] took two separate experimental approaches within each animal to examine whether areas of reversible ischemia hyperenhance. One coronary artery was instrumented with a hydraulic occluder for the study of transient ischemia.[50] Myocardial infarction was induced in a remote territory by permanent occlusion of a second coronary artery. The animals were examined by CMR 3 days after this procedure, with cine images being acquired before, during, and after a 15 min inflation of the reversible occluder.[53,54] Both regions associated with infarction and regions associated with severe but reversible ischemic injury showed abnormal wall thickening. Hyperenhancement was only seen in infarct regions and did not occur at sites of severe but reversible ischemic injury. When these same animals were scanned 8 weeks later, wall thickening had returned to normal in the region of severe but reversible ischemic injury.[50] Histologic examination performed in a subset of animals at 8 weeks

revealed infarction in the territory subtended by the permanently occluded artery, but no evidence of infarction was found distal to the reversible occluder.

On the basis of these animal studies, it can be concluded that acute and chronic myocardial infarctions hyperenhance on contrast CMR and that the spatial extent of hyperenhancement correlates closely with the spatial extent of histologically defined myocardial necrosis.[49,50,52] Additionally, regions of myocardium at risk, which are subjected to severe transient ischemia, do not hyperenhance.

Mechanism of late contrast enhancement

The cellular-level mechanism responsible for delayed gadolinium (Gd) contrast hyperenhancement has still not been fully elucidated. An important physiologic fact, however, should be remembered: normal myocardial tissue volume is predominately intracellular (~75% of the water space).[55] Since extracellular contrast medium is excluded from this space, the volume of distribution of

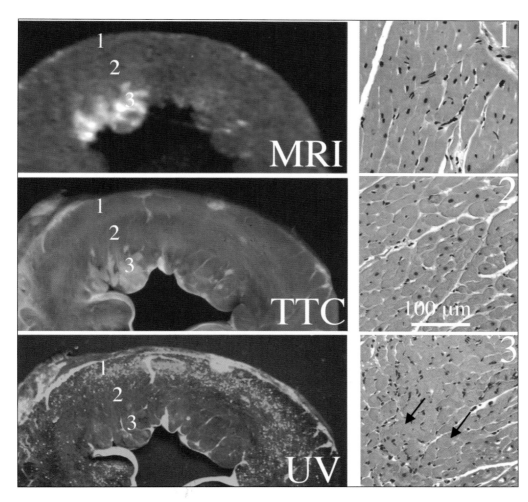

Figure 8.16
Comparison of CMR hyperenhancement (upper left panel), TTC staining (middle left panel) and the myocardium at risk (region without fluorescent microparticles (lower left panel), in an animal with a 1-day-old reperfused infarction. Light-microscopy views of region 1 (not at risk, not infarcted), region 2 (at risk but not infarcted), and region 3 (infarcted) are shown in the right panels. Arrows point to contraction bands. (Reprinted from Fieno et al. J Am Coll Cardiol 2000; 36:1985–91[52] with permission from the American College of Cardiology Foundation.)

contrast medium in normal myocardium is quite small (~25% of the water space), and one could consider viable myocytes as actively excluding contrast medium. One possible mechanism of delayed hyperenhancement is that in acutely infarcted regions, the myocyte membranes are ruptured, allowing the MR contrast agent to passively diffuse into the intracellular space, resulting in an increased tissue-level contrast agent concentration. The loss of sarcolemmal membrane integrity is thought to be very closely related to cell death,[53,54,56] and the idea that an event specific to cell death relates to hyperenhancement would explain the strong spatial relationship of CMR hyperenhancement to necrosis.[50] Extracellular MR contrast agents, such as Gd-DTPA, are excluded from the myocyte's intracellular space by intact sarcolemmal membranes.[57,58] As intact sarcolemmal membranes are present in viable myocardium, this would explain the lack of hyperenhancement of myocardial regions containing living myocardial cells.

Unlike acute infarcts, which are characterized by necrotic myocytes, chronic infarcts are characterized by a dense collagenous scar. At a cellular level, the interstitial space between collagen fibers may be significantly greater than the interstitial space between densely packed living myocytes, characteristic of normal myocardium. Rehwald et al[59] demonstrated that the increased volume of distribution of the contrast agent in scar (compared with normal myocardium) results in a higher concentration of the contrast agent, lowered T1, and consequent hyperenhancement of scar regions.

The mechanism of the lack of hyperenhancement in regions of severe but reversible ischemic injury may be directly related to the mechanism of hyperenhancement in acute infarcts, i.e. it may relate to the integrity of the myocyte membrane. Despite the many effects on the myocyte of severe but reversible ischemic injury, the sarcolemmal membrane remains intact[53,56] and therefore presumably continues to exclude the MR contrast agent from the intracellular space. In this setting, the volume of distribution of the contrast agent in regions of severe but reversible ischemic injury would be expected to remain similar to that of normal myocardium, and no hyperenhancement of these regions would be observed.

Technical considerations in image interpretation

Technical issues may play a role in the interpretation of in vivo MR images. For example, the 'partial-volume' effect can play a role whenever the spatial resolution of the in vivo image is too poor to adequately represent the complex three-dimensional nature of the pathophysiology. However, even with adequate spatial resolution, partial-volume effects can occur with pulse sequences that require long acquisition times (minutes) due to respiratory and/or other subject motion.

Another complexity is the observation that large acute infarcts often exhibit a region of hypoenhancement that is almost always completely surrounded by a larger region of hyperenhancement. The appearance of these hypoenhanced regions by CMR has been related to the 'no-reflow' phenomenon.[60,61] The dark region towards the endocardial core of the infarct visible in the first image of Figure 8.17 corresponds to a 'no-reflow' region that is characterized by substantially reduced perfusion, thought to be due to damage or obstruction at the microcirculatory level that apparently impedes penetration of the MR contrast agent into the core of the infarct. Since flow in these regions is low but not zero, these regions appear dark initially, but as contrast accumulates they slowly become hyperenhanced, as seen in Figure 8.17. Accordingly, the hypoenhanced 'no-reflow' regions should be included in the measurement of infarct size.

Any question regarding the reproducibility of hyperenhancement in acute and chronic myocardial infarction has been largely resolved by the series of studies outlined above. Some debate has persisted, however, regarding the temporal stability of hyperenhancement and whether the spatial extent of hyperenhancement could change depending on the delay after contrast administration before imaging is performed.[62] Imaging within 5 min of contrast injection may not allow adequate contrast agent delivery to the myocardium from the blood pool, and imaging more than 30–40 min after contrast injection will decrease image quality due to contrast washout.

The studies described above[45,49] were conducted using segmented inversion recovery CMR with continuous adjustment of the inversion time in order to null the myocardium. Mahrholdt et al[63] recently showed that within this time window (10–30 min after injection), the size of infarcts as determined by contrast-enhanced CMR does not change (Figure 8.18a) and that the reproducibility of the CMR measurement of infarct size compares favorably with that of ^{99m}Tc-MIBI-SPECT. The discrepancy between this finding and the concerns raised by some authors[62] may relate to details of the CMR technique itself and the pharmacokinetics of the contrast agent.

As discussed earlier, the primary effect of the MR contrast agent is to shorten the myocardial longitudinal relaxation time T1, and the underlying physiology results in a situation where T1 is shortened more in infarcted regions than in normal myocardium. While these regions of shortened T1 (infarcts) can be visualized using traditional T1-weighted CMR techniques, regional differences in image intensities are greatest when an inversion pulse is used.[58] For correct implementation, however, the inversion time (the delay between the inversion pulse and data collection) must be manually selected to null signal from normal myocardial regions. The inversion time needed to null signal from normal myocardium varies from patient to patient as a function of dose, and also varies with time after contrast administration due to contrast agent pharmokinetics.[58] Weinmann et al[58] studied the pharmacokinetics of Gd-DTPA in humans for doses of 0.1 and 0.25 mmol/kg. The solid line in Figure 8.18b shows a monoexponential fit to their data interpolated to a dose of 0.125 mmol/kg (the dose used by Mahrholdt et al). The plasma concentration of the MR contrast agent decreased by a factor of ~2.4 between 3 and 40 min post contrast. This decrease in contrast agent concentration will increase myocardial T1 and will require a corresponding increase in the CMR inversion time to appropriately null normal myocardium. Because interstitial concentrations of Gd-DTPA in the myocardium depend primarily upon plasma concentrations, the correct CMR inversion time can be estimated from basic physical principles (e.g. at 1 min, 0.125 mmol/kg dose, $\Delta 1/T1 = 0.96$ mmol/l $\times 4.5$/s/mmol/l $\times 0.30$\{extracellular space\} = 1.29/s; T1 = 1/(1.29 + 1/0.8 \{precontrast T1\}) = 392 ms; inversion time to null normal myocardium = (392)(ln 2) = 272 ms). The dashed line in

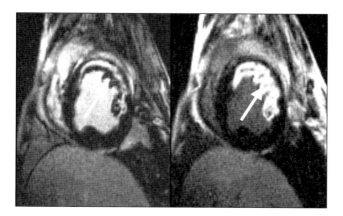

Figure 8.17
The 'no-reflow' phenomenon revealed by contrast-enhanced CMR. The 'no-reflow' zones are almost always completely surrounded by larger regions of hyperenhancement, and, importantly, slowly become hyperenhanced as repeated images are acquired at the same location over time. Labels refer to the time after administration of contrast media. (Adapted from Kim RJ, Choi K, Judd RM. In: Cardiovascular CMR and MRA (Higgins C, ed). Philadelpia: Lippincott Williams & Wilkins, 2002:224 with permission from Lippincott Williams and Wilkins.)

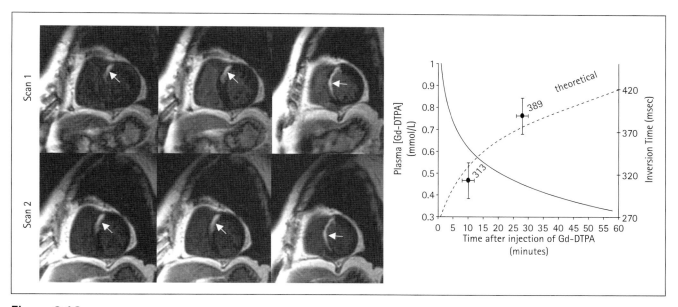

Figure 8.18

(a) The upper and lower panels of CMR images show short-axis views of two CMR studies acquired in the same patient to test the reproducibility of contrast-enhanced MRI infarct detection. The presence, location, and size of the hyperenhanced region were similar in both CMR scans. The first CMR scan was 9 min post contrast whereas the second was performed by a different scanner operator 32 min post contrast.

The graph to the right of the figure displays a monoexponential fit of the serum contrast agent concentration (left-hand vertical axis) as a function of time after contrast administration compared with the corrected CMR inversion time (right-hand vertical axis). (Modified from Mahrholdt et al. Circulation 2002; 106:2322–7.[63])

Figure 8.18b depicts the correct inversion times that are needed for the CMR technique to account for the pharmacokinetics of the MR contrast agent. The changes in inversion times selected by the scanner operators of Mahrholdt's study[63] (filled circles) were similar to those expected based on the pharmacokinetics of the contrast agent (dotted line). Due to this physiologic background, the clinical user of a CMR late enhancement technique should always keep in mind that the longer one waits after contrast administration, the longer the inversion time should be to obtain appropriate contrast between normal and hyperenhanced myocardium. The basic premise is not that infarcted regions have a constant and short T1 (which is obviously untrue in vivo) but that T1 is always shorter in regions of scar compared with normal myocardium. At all timepoints, the longest inversion time should be selected in which normal myocardium is nulled in order to not mistakenly null regions with shorter T1 than normal myocardium.

trast enhancement with perfect registration of myocardial regions. While regions with 76–100% transmural extent of hyperenhancement are often akinetic or dyskinetic, in general, the relationship between the transmural extent of infarction and wall motion is complex, and contrast enhancement patterns are frequently discordant with ventricular motion. This observation emphasizes the fact that contrast enhancement and wall motion reflect different physiologic processes, and suggests that the combination of both cine and contrast CMR is important in the evaluation of ischemic heart disease. Combination CMR in the acute setting might be used to distinguish between myocardial infarction (hyperenhanced, with or without contractile dysfunction), stunned myocardium (not hyperenhanced, but with contractile dysfunction), and normal myocardium (not hyperenhanced, with normal function). Likewise, in the chronic setting, the combination of cine and contrast CMR could be used to identify myocardial scar, hibernating myocardium, and normal myocardium.

Combining cine and contrast CMR for routine assessment of viability

The combination of cine and contrast CMR in an imaging protocol allows easy comparison of wall motion and con-

Clinical applications

CMR can be used to assess viability in acute and chronic clinical settings. Immediately after infarction, myocardial viability can be defined in order to aid management decisions regarding revascularization or in order to assess the degree of myocardial salvage after thrombolysis or percutaneous therapy. For the chronic setting, viability assessment is critical when there is LV dysfunction and a question regarding the potential benefit of revascularization.

Myocardial viability in the acute setting

Hillenbrand et al[64] demonstrated in an animal model that the transmural extent of infarction defined by contrast-enhanced CMR predicts myocardial salvage after acute myocardial infarction. The LAD coronary artery was occluded in 15 animals for either 45 min, 90 min, or permanently. Cine and contrast-enhanced CMR were performed 3 days after the procedure and cine CMR was also performed at 10 and 28 days after the procedure. The transmural extent of hyperenhancement on day 3 was related to future improvement in both wall thickening score and absolute wall thickening at 10 and 28 days ($p < 0.0001$ for each). For example, of the 415 segments on day 3 that were dysfunctional and had less than 25%

transmural hyperenhancement, 362 (87%) improved by day 28. Conversely, no segments (0 of 9) with 100% hyperenhancement improved. The transmural extent of hyperenhancement on day 3 was a better predictor of improvement in contractile function than occlusion time ($p < 0.0001$).

Similar predictive values were recently obtained in a patient study.[65] Twenty-four patients who presented with their first myocardial infarction and were successfully revascularized underwent cine and contrast-enhanced CMR of their hearts within 7 days of the peak MB band of creatine kinase (CK-MB). Cine CMR was repeated 8–12 weeks later. A total of 524 of 1571 segments (33%) were dysfunctional on the initial scan. Improvement in segmental contractile function on the follow-up scan was inversely related to the transmural extent of infarction measured on the initial scan ($p < 0.001$). Improvement in global contractile function, as assessed by ejection fraction and mean wall thickening score, was not predicted by peak CK-MB ($p = 0.66$) or by total infarct size, as defined by CMR ($p = 0.70$). The best predictor of global improvement was the extent of dysfunctional myocardium that was not infarcted or had infarction comprising < 25% of LV wall thickness ($p < 0.005$ for ejection fraction, $p < 0.001$ for mean wall thickening score). The accuracy of contrast-enhanced CMR in predicting improvement of

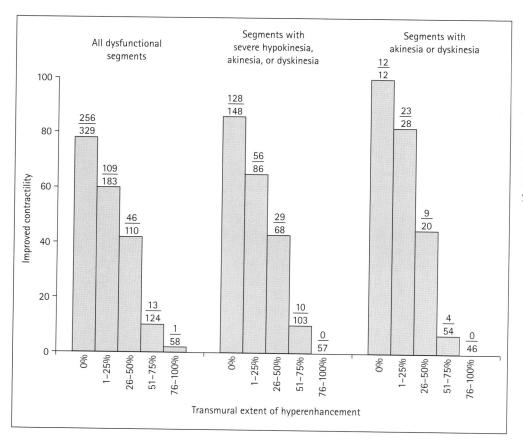

Figure 8.19
The relationship between the transmural extent of hyperenhancement prior to revascularization and the likelihood of increased contractility after revascularization. (Reprinted from Kim et al. N Engl J Med 2000; 343:1445–53[67] with permission from the Massachusetts Medical Society.)

regional myocardial function in patients after acute myocardial infarction was recently confirmed by Gerber et al,[66] including 20 patients who underwent contrast-enhanced CMR at 4 days and again at 7 months after acute infarction.

Myocardial viability in the chronic setting

Kim et al[67] demonstrated that contrast CMR is able to identify reversible myocardial dysfunction in patients with chronic LV dysfunction. Cine and contrast CMR were performed in 50 consecutive patients before they underwent coronary revascularization by percutaneous transluminal coronary angioplasty (PTCA) or coronary artery bypass graft. Cine CMR was repeated ~11 weeks after revascularization to assess changes in regional wall motion. It was shown that the likelihood of functional improvement of all segments was inversely correlated to the transmural extent of hyperenhancement (Figure 8.19): 256 of 329 segments (78%) with no hyperenhancement improved, whereas only 1 of 58 segments with > 75% hyperenhancement improved. The same relationship between the transmural extent of hyperenhancement and contractile improvement was found for segments with severe hypokinesia at baseline and in segments with akinesia or dyskinesia at baseline ($p < 0.001$ for both). On a patient-by-patient basis, it was shown that an increasing extent of dysfunctional but viable myocardium before revascularization correlated with greater improvements in both the mean wall motion score ($p < 0.001$) and the ejection fraction after revascularization ($p < 0.001$).

The relationship between the transmural extent of viability and the likelihood of functional improvement found in this study strongly suggests that it is not useful to rely on a single cutoff value of transmural extent to predict functional improvement. For example, a cutoff value of 25% transmural extent of hyperenhancement had positive and negative predictive values for functional improvement of 71% and 79%, respectively, for all dysfunctional regions and 88% and 89% for akinetic or dyskinetic regions. While these predictive accuracies compare favorably with those reported previously using other imaging modalities,[68] the full diagnostic information available by contrast CMR is not utilized. For example, if the hyperenhanced region has a transmural extent of 75%, there is a 100% negative predictive value for no recovery of function following revascularization.

Figure 8.20a shows a cine and contrast-enhanced CMR study of a patient with reversible dysfunction who had severe hypokinesia of the anteroseptal wall (arrows). The area of the wall motion abnormality did not hyperenhance, representing viable myocardium, and, as expected, the contractility improved after revascularization (Figure 8.20b). However, Figure 8.21a, illustrates a patient with irreversible dysfunction who had akinesia of the anterolateral wall (arrows). This region was hyperenhanced, indicating the presence of a nearly transmural infarct. There was no improvement in contractility following revascularization (Figure 8.21b).

Contrast CMR has advantages over the other imaging modalities used to assess viability. With contrast CMR, myocardial regions are not interpreted in a binary fashion as either viable or nonviable, because the transmural extent of viable myocardium is directly visualized. Knowledge of the transmural extent of viability is helpful in predicting functional improvement, and may also improve our understanding of the underlying pathophysiologic influences on functional improvement in individuals and in differing states of ventricular dysfunction. This point is illustrated by the study by Kim et al,[67] in which the average extent of hyperenhancement across the ventricular wall was 10% ± 7% for all dysfunctional segments that improved with revascularization and 41% ± 14% for those that did not improve ($p < 0.001$). This result, consistent with previous studies that have analyzed needle biopsy specimens taken during bypass surgery,[69,70] indicates that significant myocardial viability can be present without subsequent functional improvement. These data underscore the importance of differentiating between the current clinical 'gold standard' definition of myocardial viability, namely improvement in wall motion after revascularization, and the actual definition, namely the presence of living myocytes (see Figure 8.1), and also serve to demonstrate the importance of combining cine CMR with contrast-enhanced CMR in the assessment of viability.

Evolving applications of contrast CMR

Contrast CMR provides information about the presence and extent of myocardial infarction that potentially leads to evolution of current clinical practice. For the first time, it is possible to routinely assess the transmural extent of myocardial infarction and to identify small subendocardial infarcts. CMR demonstration of the transmural extent of the infarction allows reassessment of the complex relationship between infarction and contractile function. CMR is uniquely sensitive for infarct detection, and this technology applied in at-risk populations may lead to changes in our understanding of the frequency of myocardial damage.

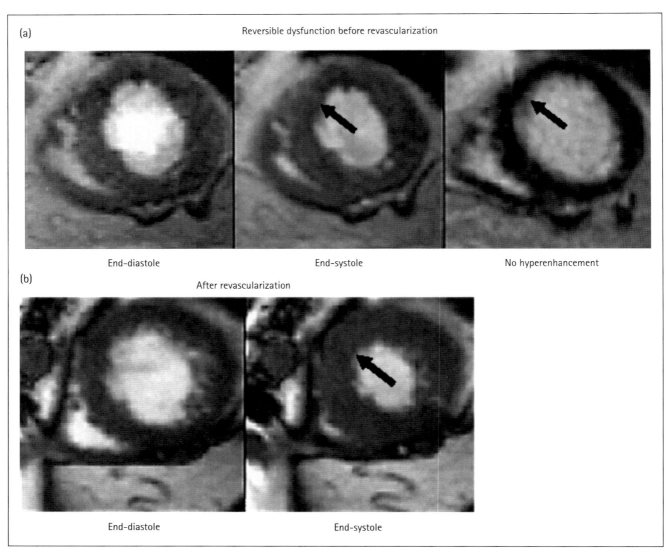

Figure 8.20
(a) Cine and contrast-enhanced FLASH CMR study of a patient with reversible dysfunction who had severe hypokinesia of the anteroseptal wall (arrows). The region with wall motion abnormality did not hyperenhance prior to revascularization, indicating the presence of viable myocardium. (b) As expected, the contractility in this region improved after revascularization. (Reprinted from Mahrholdt et al. Dtsch Med Wochenschr 2002; 127:1001–8 with permission from Georg Thieme Verlag, Stuttgart, Germany.)

Contrast CMR detects infarcts in regions of normal wall motion

While myocardial infarction is often associated with impaired contractile function, the relationship between infarction and contractile function is complex. For example, Lieberman et al[71] demonstrated that sizing of myocardial infarcts based on contractile function results in an overestimation of infarct size[72–75] due to a 'threshold phenomenon' caused by a 'disproportionate role of the subendocardial layer of the myocardium in overall wall thickening'.[76,77] Accordingly, the spatial extent of contrac-

tile dysfunction may be larger than the spatial extent of the infarct itself. It is important to recognize, however, that many of the studies supporting the concept of infarct overestimation based on contractile function were performed prior to the development of concepts such as 'myocardial stunning',[74,77–79] which complicates interpretation of the available data.

However, recent data suggest that the spatial extent of contractile dysfunction may be smaller than that of the infarct itself, resulting in an underestimation of infarct size. For example, Wu et al[49] studied a population of patients with chronic infarction and found that 25% of all

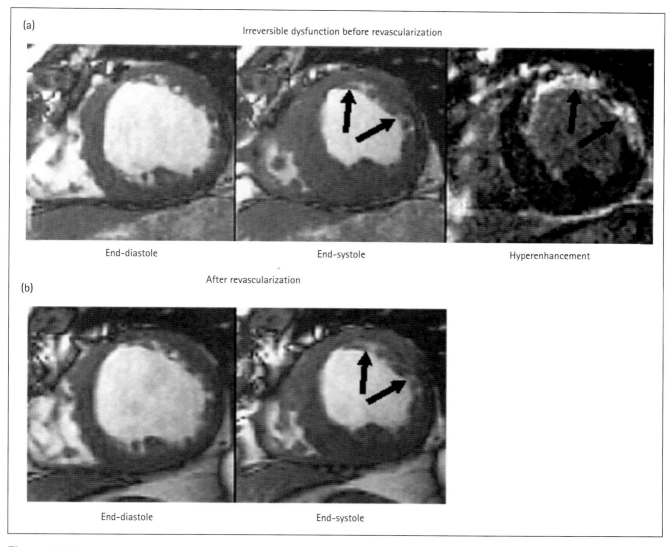

Figure 8.21
(a) Cine and contrast-enhanced FLASH CMR study of a patient with irreversible dysfunction of the anterolateral wall (arrows). This region was hyperenhanced, indicating the presence of transmural infarction and scar prior to revascularization. (b) The contractility of the wall did not improve after revascularization. (Reprinted from Mahrholdt et al. Dtsch Med Wochenschr 2002; 127:1001–8 with permission from Georg Thieme Verlag, Stuttgart, Germany.)

segments exhibiting CMR evidence of subendocardial infarction (62 of 250) had normal wall motion. Until recently, the literature reporting the relationship between wall thickening and transmural extent of infarction was predominantly in patients with acute[72,73,75–77] myocardial injury, and the relationship had not been established in patients with chronic infarction. Mahrholdt et al[80] systematically evaluated this question using contrast-enhanced CMR to examine the transmural extent of infarction and cine CMR to assess contractile function in the same imaging session. Mahrholdt et al.[80] studied patients with chronic myocardial infarction who had cardiac enzyme

confirmation of infarction at least five months previously and catheterization showing single vessel disease with an open artery (Figure 8.22). It was demonstrated that in the setting of reperfused chronic MI, the transmural extent of infarction approaches 50% of wall thickness before contractile dysfunction can be systematically identified. Thus it can be concluded that contractile function alone cannot be used to rule out chronic myocardial infarction (Figure 8.23).

These results underscore that the relationship of contractile function and the transmural extent of the infarct is complex. Infarct size can be overestimated by using

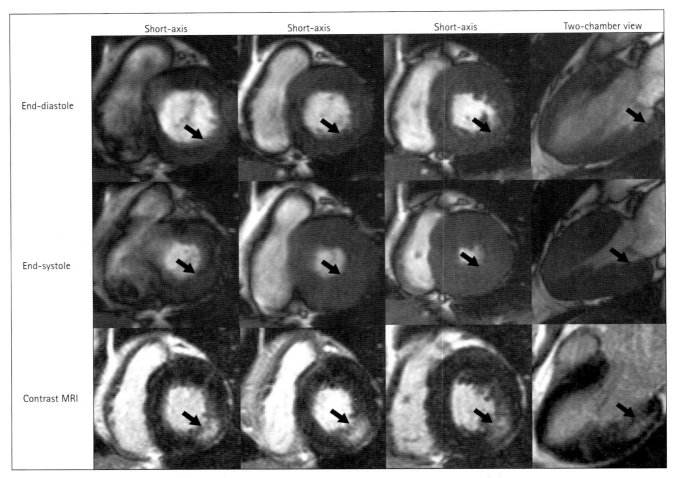

Figure 8.22
Cine and contrast-enhanced MR images from a patient with known myocardial infarction in the circumflex area (by enzymes and catheter findings). Despite the clearly visible inferior lateral myocardial infarction (see black arrows in lower panel), there is no wall motion abnormality present (arrows in upper panels). (Modified from Mahrholdt et al. Dtsch Med Wochenschr 2002; 127:1001–8 with permission from Georg Thieme Verlag, Stuttgart, Germany.)

contractile function as an indicator in the acute setting.[68,71,81] The work presented by Wu et al[49] and Mahrholdt et al[80] demonstrated that systematic underestimation of infarct size is possible in a chronic setting. These findings imply that without biochemical evidence of infarction or significant wall thinning, imaging techniques that define infarction as regionally impaired contractile function may systematically miss patients with subendocardial chronic infarcts.

Contrast CMR detects subendocardial infarcts that are missed by routine SPECT

Routine segmented inversion recovery turbo-FLASH imaging provides a voxel size about 1.4 mm × 1.9 mm × 6.0 mm (0.016 cm^3). This is > 50-fold improved compared with SPECT (10 mm × 10 mm × 10 mm (1 cm^3) full-width at half-maximum).[82,83] To evaluate if CMR can detect subendocardial infarcts that are missed by SPECT, Wagner et al[84] performed contrast-enhanced CMR and routine clinical SPECT examinations in 91 patients. CMR and SPECT images were scored for the presence, location, and transmural extent of infarction. To compare each imaging modality with a gold standard, in vivo contrast-enhanced CMR and SPECT images were also acquired in 12 animals with myocardial infarction and 3 animals without infarction. In the animal studies, infarction was defined by histochemical staining (Figure 8.24).

In the animals, both contrast-enhanced CMR and SPECT detected all segments with nearly transmural infarction (> 75% transmural extent of the LV wall by histology). CMR also identified 100 of the 109 segments (92%) with subendocardial infarction (< 50% transmural

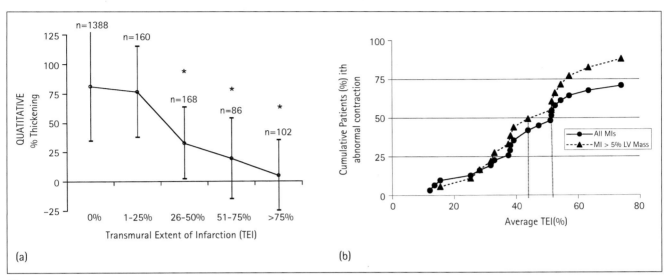

(a)   (b)

Figure 8.23

Panel A summarises the segmental results for all subjects from the work of Mahrholdt et al. The TEI is expressed in quartiles (e.g. none, 1–25%, etc), error bars represent SD. All Groups marked * are statistically different from 0% (p < 0.05). Panel B summarizes the results by patient as opposed to segmentally. The cumulative percent with abnormal contraction was defined as all subjects minus those with completely normal contraction. For all MI's the TEI reached 53% before half of the patients had abnormal function (right-hand dotted line) and for patients with MI > 5% LV the TEI reached 43% before half of the patients had abnormal function (left-hand dotted line). (Reprinted from Mahrholdt et al. J Am Coll Cardiol 2003; 42:505–12.)

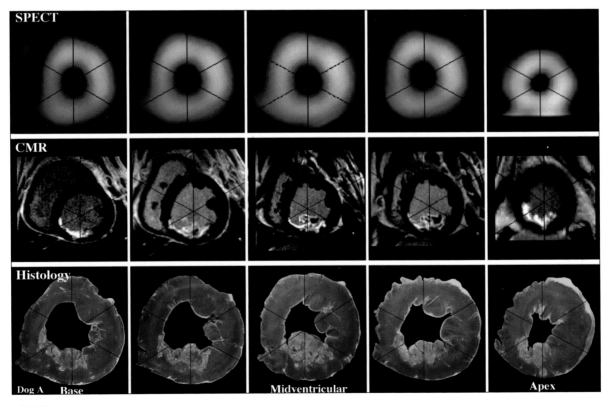

Figure 8.24

Typical appearance of myocardium in one animal with a medium-sized infarct, with corresponding SPECT images (top), MR images (middle), and histologic slices (bottom) displayed. Slices are arranged from base to apex, starting left and advancing to right. A 30-segment model was used for analysis of the dog images. Five short-axis views were divided into six circumferential segments and analyzed in a 30-segment model. (Reprinted from Wagner et al. Lancet 2003; 361:374–9[84] with permission from Elsevier Science.)

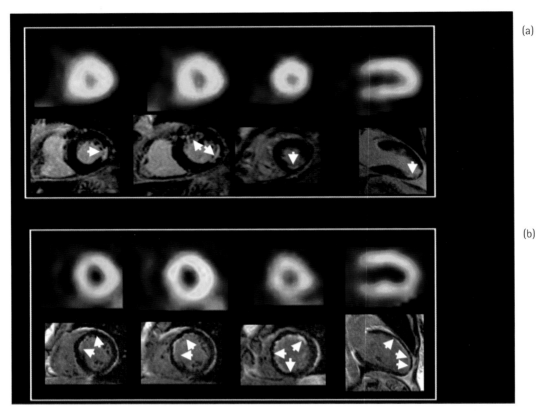

Figure 8.25
Short-axis views of rest [201]TI-SPECT (a) and contrast-enhanced CMR (b) in two patients with subendocardial infarcts. The rest SPECT studies in these two patients were reported as normal, whereas the contrast-enhanced MR images revealed subendocardial infarction. (a) Patient B: creatine kinase 513 IU/l; occluded left circumflex coronary artery, and history of an older anteroseptal infarct with angioplasty and stent-implantation in the left anterior descending coronary artery. (b) Patient C: No history of an acute event or recognized infarction; 90% stenosis of the LAD coronary artery. (Reprinted from Wagner et al. Lancet 2003; 361:374–9[84] with permission from Elsevier Science.)

extent of the LV wall by histology), whereas SPECT identified 31 (28%). Both SPECT and CMR showed a high specificity for the detection of infarction (97% and 98%, respectively). In the 91 patients, all segments with nearly transmural infarction (> 75% of the thickness of the LV wall defined by contrast-enhanced CMR) were also interpreted as infarction in the SPECT images. However, of the 181 segments with subendocardial infarction (< 50% transmural extent of the LV wall defined by CMR), 85 (47%) were not detected by SPECT. On a per-patient basis, six (13%) subjects with subendocardial infarcts visible by CMR had no evidence of infarction by SPECT (Figure 8.25).

Thus, it can be concluded that while SPECT and CMR detect transmural myocardial infarcts at similar rates, CMR systematically detects subendocardial infarcts that are missed by SPECT. Further investigation is needed to determine the prognostic significance of these subendocardial infarcts, which can be only detected by CMR.

Detection of previously unrecognized myocardial infarction

It is estimated that 30–40% of all myocardial infarcts occur without recognition by the patient or the physician.[85–87] This finding is based on the appearance of new Q-waves on annual 12-lead ECGs. However, since non-Q-wave infarcts are not included in these estimates, one can assume that the incidence of unrecognized infarcts is likely to be underestimated.

For example Kim et al[88] assessed 100 patients with contrast CMR who had been referred for coronary angiography but in whom there was no history of previous myocardial infarction and who had no prior revascularization. Hyperenhancement was present in 57 (57%) patients and Q-waves were found in 14%. Accordingly, unrecognized myocardial infarction was found at approximately a fourfold higher rate by CMR than 12-lead ECG.

The risk associated with unrecognized myocardial infarcts defined by ECG is substantial, with long-term mortality comparable to that of recognized infarction in populations such as the Frammingham study population.[85–87] Whether the same high risk exists for patients with an unrecognized myocardial infarction diagnosed by contrast-enhanced MRI is currently unknown.

Summary

The 'gold standard' definition of myocardial viability is the presence of living myocytes. Existing clinical techniques to evaluate viability include ^{201}Tl- and ^{99m}Tc-MIBI-SPECT, FDG-PET, and dobutamine echocardiography.

The signals from high-energy phosphates by ^{31}P-MRS, creatine by ^{1}H-MRS, and intracellular potassium by ^{39}K-MRS are all directly related to the presence of living myocytes, but the intrinsically low MR signal limits spatial resolution and typically precludes examination of the posterior wall of the heart. The magnitude of the ^{23}Na signal is greater and allows generation of images comparable in quality to those of nuclear medicine. Nevertheless, image quality for ^{23}Na-MRI remains significantly worse than that of ^{1}H-MRI.

Myocardial viability can be examined by ^{1}H-CMR either by (1) low-dose dobutamine combined with cine CMR; or (2) contrast-enhanced CMR using routine clinically approved agents. Dobutamine CMR detects myocardial viability in a manner directly analogous to dobutamine echocardiography, and has been shown to have at least comparable sensitivity and specificity. This approach, however, defines viability indirectly as regions with dobutamine-recruitable intropic reserve. Contrast-enhanced CMR defines myocardial viability in a manner analogous to histochemical staining, and data in animals suggest that regions without 'delayed hyperenhancement' contain living myocytes independent of contractile function. Data in humans demonstrate that regions of contractile dysfunction by cine CMR but without hyperenhancement by contrast-enhanced CMR recover contractile function when adequately revascularized in both the acute and chronic settings. In routine clinical practice, examining myocardial viability using contrast-enhanced CMR is preferred over low-dose dobutamine cine CMR because the examination is easier and safer to perform and the transmural extent of viable myocardium can be visualized directly.

Emerging data suggest that contrast-enhanced CMR also provides useful clinical information not normally associated with myocardial viability, such as the detection of myocardial infarcts in regions of normal contractile function, the detection of subendocardial infarcts missed by routine perfusion SPECT, and the assessment of unrec- ognized myocardial infarction. The prognostic value of this information is currently unknown and under investigation.

Acknowledgements

This work was supported by grants from the Deutsche Forschungsgemeinschaft (AW), the Robert Bosch Foundation (HM), the NIH R01-HL64726 (RJK), and the NIH R01-HL63268 and KO2-HL04394 (RMJ).

References

1. Gheorghiade M, Bonow RO. Chronic heart failure in the United States: a manifestation of coronary artery disease. Circulation 1998; 97:282–9.

2. Hammermeister KE, DeRouen TA, Dodge HT. Variables predictive of survival in patients with coronary disease. Selection by univariate and multivariate analyses from the clinical, electrocardiographic, exercise, arteriographic, and quantitative angiographic evaluations. Circulation 1979; 59:421–30.

3. Harris PJ, Harrell FE, Lee KL, et al. Survival in medically treated coronary artery disease. Circulation 1979; 60:1259–69.

4. Mock MB, Ringqvist I, Fisher LD, et al. Survival of medically treated patients in the Coronary Artery Surgery Study (CASS) registry. Circulation 1982; 66:562–8.

5. Nixon JV, Brown CN, Smitherman TC. Identification of transient and persistent segmental wall motion abnormalities in patients with unstable angina by two-dimensional echocardiography. Circulation 1982; 65:1497–503.

6. Kloner RA, Allen J, Cox TA, et al. Stunned left ventricular myocardium after exercise treadmill testing in coronary artery disease. Am J Cardiol 1991; 68:329–34.

7. Breisblatt WM, Stein KL, Wolfe CJ, et al. Acute myocardial dysfunction and recovery: a common occurrence after coronary bypass surgery. J Am Coll Cardiol 1990; 15:1261–9.

8. Touchstone DA, Beller GA, Nygaard TW, et al. Effects of successful intravenous reperfusion therapy on regional myocardial function and geometry in humans: a tomographic assessment using two-dimensional echocardiography. J Am Coll Cardiol 1989; 13:1506–13.

9. Anselmi M, Golia G, Cicoira M, et al. Prognostic value of detection of myocardial viability using low-dose dobutamine echocardiography in infarcted patients. Am J Cardiol 1998; 81:21G–28G.

10. Picano E, Sicari R, Landi P, et al. Prognostic value of myocardial viability in medically treated patients with global left ventricular dysfunction early after an acute uncomplicated myocardial infarction: a dobutamine stress echocardiographic study. Circulation 1998; 98:1078–84.

11. Previtali M, Fetiveau R, Lanzarini L, et al. Prognostic value of myocardial viability and ischemia detected by dobutamine stress echocardiography early after acute myocardial infarction treated with thrombolysis. J Am Coll Cardiol 1998; 32:380–6.

12. Allman KC, Shaw LJ, Hachamovitch R, Udelson JE. Myocardial viability testing and impact of revascularization on prognosis in patients with coronary artery disease and left ventricular dysfunction: a meta-analysis. J Am Coll Cardiol 2002; 39:1151–8.

13. Kaul S. Assessing the myocardium after attempted reperfusion: Should we bother? Circulation 1998; 98:625–7.

14. Fishbein MC, Meerbaum S, Rit J, et al. Early phase acute myocardial infarct size quantification: validation of the triphenyl tetrazolium chloride tissue enzyme staining technique. Am Heart J 1981; 101:593–600.

15. Schwarz ER, Schaper J, vom Dahl J, et al. Myocyte degeneration and cell death in hibernating human myocardium. J Am Coll Cardiol 1996; 27:1577–85.

16. Nagel E, Lehmkuhl HB, Bocksch W, et al. Noninvasive diagnosis of ischemia-induced wall motion abnormalities with the use of high-dose dobutamine stress MRI: comparison with dobutamine stress echocardiography. Circulation 1999; 99:763–70.

17. Hoffmann R, Lethen H, Marwick T, et al. Analysis of interinstitutional observer agreement in interpretation of dobutamine stress echocardiograms. J Am Coll Cardiol 1996; 27:330–6.

18. Bache RJ, Schwartz JS. Effect of perfusion pressure distal to a coronary stenosis on transmural myocardial blood flow. Circulation 1982; 65:928–35.

19. Yabe T, Mitsunami K, Inubushi T, Kinoshita M. Quantitative measurements of cardiac phosphorus metabolites in coronary artery disease by ^{31}P magnetic resonance spectroscopy. Circulation 1995; 92:15–23.

20. Bottomley PA, Weiss RG. Non-invasive magnetic-resonance detection of creatine depletion in non-viable infarcted myocardium. Lancet 1998; 351:714–18.

21. Cannon PJ, Maudsley AA, Hilal SK, et al. Sodium nuclear magnetic resonance imaging of myocardial tissue of dogs after coronary artery occlusion and reperfusion. J Am Coll Cardiol 1986; 7:573–9.

22. Kim RJ, Judd RM, Chen EL, et al. Relationship of elevated ^{23}Na magnetic resonance image intensity to infarct size after acute reperfused myocardial infarction. Circulation 1999; 100:185–92.

23. Kim RJ, Lima JA, Chen EL, et al. Fast ^{23}Na magnetic resonance imaging of acute reperfused myocardial infarction. Potential to assess myocardial viability. Circulation 1997; 95:1877–85.

24. Fieno DS, Kim RJ, Rehwald WG, Judd RM. Physiological basis for potassium (^{39}K) magnetic resonance imaging of the heart. Circ Res 1999; 84:913–20.

25. Parrish TB, Fieno DS, Fitzgerald SW, Judd RM. Theoretical basis for sodium and potassium MRI of the human heart at 1.5 T. Magn Reson Med 1997; 38:653–61.

26. Dubnow MH, Burchell HB, Titus JL. Postinfarction ventricular aneurysm. A clinicomorphologic and electrocardiographic study of 80 cases. Am Heart J 1965; 70:753–60.

27. Baer FM, Smolarz K, Jungehulsing M, et al. Chronic myocardial infarction: assessment of morphology, function, and perfusion by gradient echo magnetic resonance imaging and ^{99m}Tc-methoxy-isobutyl-isonitrile SPECT. Am Heart J 1992; 123:636–45.

28. Baer FM, Voth E, Schneider CA, et al. Comparison of low-dose dobutamine-gradient-echo magnetic resonance imaging and positron emission tomography with [^{18}F]fluorodeoxyglucose in patients with chronic coronary artery disease. A functional and morphological approach to the detection of residual myocardial viability. Circulation 1995; 91:1006–15.

29. Pirolo JS, Hutchins GM, Moore GW. Infarct expansion: pathologic analysis of 204 patients with a single myocardial infarct. J Am Coll Cardiol 1986; 7:349–54.

30. Dendale P, Franken PR, van der Wall EE, de Roos A. Wall thickening at rest and contractile reserve early after myocardial infarction: correlation with myocardial perfusion and metabolism. Coron Artery Dis 1997; 8:259–64.

31. Sechtem U, Baer FM, Voth E, et al. Assessment of Viability by MR-Techniques. Dordrecht: Kluwer, 1996:211–36.

32. Dendale PA, Franken PR, Waldman GJ, et al. Low-dosage dobutamine magnetic resonance imaging as an alternative to echocardiography in the detection of viable myocardium after acute infarction. Am Heart J 1995; 130:134–40.

33. Sandstede JJ, Bertsch G, Beer M, et al. Detection of myocardial viability by low-dose dobutamine cine MR imaging. Magn Reson Imaging 1999; 17:1437–43.

34. Dendale P, Franken PR, Block P, et al. Contrast enhanced and functional magnetic resonance imaging for the detection of viable myocardium after infarction. Am Heart J 1998; 135:875–80.

35. Baer FM, Voth E, LaRosee K, et al. Comparison of dobutamine transesophageal echocardiography and dobutamine magnetic resonance imaging for detection of residual myocardial viability. Am J Cardiol 1996; 78:415–19.

36. Zoghbi WA, Barasch E. Dobutamine MRI: A serious contender in pharmacological stress imaging? Circulation 1999; 99:730–2.

37. Beller GA. Comparison of ^{201}Tl scintigraphy and low-dose dobutamine echocardiography for the noninvasive assessment of myocardial viability. Circulation 1996; 94:2681–4.

38. Bonow RO. Identification of viable myocardium. Circulation 1996; 94:2674–80.

39. Perrone-Filardi P, Pace L, Prastaro M, et al. Assessment of myocardial viability in patients with chronic coronary artery disease. Rest–4-hour–24-hour ^{201}Tl tomography versus dobutamine echocardiography. Circulation 1996; 94:2712–19.

40. Ausma J, Schaart G, Thone F, et al. Chronic ischemic viable myocardium in man: aspects of dedifferentiation. Cardiovasc Pathol 1995; 4:29–37.

41. de Roos A, Doornbos J, van der Wall EE, van Voorthuisen AE. MR imaging of acute myocardial infarction: value of Gd-DTPA. AJR 1988; 150:531–4.

42. de Roos A, van Rossum AC, van der Wall E, et al. Reperfused and nonreperfused myocardial infarction: diagnostic potential of Gd-DTPA-enhanced MR imaging. Radiology 1989; 172:717–20.

43. Yokota C, Nonogi H, Miyazaki S, et al. Gadolinium-enhanced magnetic resonance imaging in acute myocardial infarction. Am J Cardiol 1995; 75:577–81.

44. Edelman RR, Wallner B, Singer A, Atkinson DJ, Saini S. Segmented turboFLASH: method for breath-hold MR imaging of the liver with flexible contrast. Radiology 1990; 177:515–21.

45. Simonetti OP, Kim RJ, Fieno DS, et al. An improved MR imaging technique for the visualization of myocardial infarction. Radiology 2001; 218:215–223.

46. Eichstaedt HW, Felix R, Danne O, et al. Imaging of acute myocardial infarction by magnetic resonance tomography (MRT) using the paramagnetic relaxation substance gadolinium-DTPA. Cardiovasc Drugs Ther 1989; 3:779–88.

47. Lima JA, Judd RM, Bazille A, et al. Regional heterogeneity of human myocardial infarcts demonstrated by contrast-enhanced MRI. Potential mechanisms. Circulation 1995; 92:1117–25.

48. Van Rossum AC, Visser FC, Van Eenige MJ, et al. Value of gadolinium-diethylenetriamine pentaacetic acid dynamics in magnetic resonance imaging of acute myocardial infarction with occluded and reperfused coronary arteries after thrombolysis. Am J Cardiol 1990; 65:845–51.

49. Wu E, Judd RM, Vargas JD, et al. Visualisation of presence, location, and transmural extent of healed Q-wave and non-Q-wave myocardial infarction. Lancet 2001; 357:21–8.

50. Kim RJ, Fieno DS, Parrish TB, et al. Relationhip of MRI delayed contrast enhancement to irreversible injury, infarct age, and contractile function. Circulation 1999; 100:1992–2002.

51. Klein C, Nekolla SG, Bengel FM, et al. Assessment of myocardial viability with contrast-enhanced magnetic resonance imaging: comparison with positron emission tomography. Circulation 2002; 105:162–7.

52. Fieno DS, Kim RJ, Chen EL, et al. Contrast-enhanced magnetic resonance imaging of myocardium at risk: distinction between reversible and irreversible injury throughout infarct healing. J Am Coll Cardiol 2000; 36:1985–91.

53. Jennings RB, Schaper J, Hill ML, et al. Effect of reperfusion late in the phase of reversible ischemic injury. Changes in cell volume, electrolytes, metabolites, and ultrastructure. Circ Res 1985; 56:262–78.

54. Whalen DA, Hamilton DG, Ganote CE, Jennings RB. Effect of a transient period of ischemia on myocardial cells. I. Effects on cell volume regulation. Am J Pathol 1974; 74:381–97.

55. Polimeni PI. Extracellular space and ionic distribution in rat ventricle. Am J Physiol 1974; 227:676–83.

56. Reimer KA, Jennings RB. Myocardial ischemia, hypoxia and infarction. In: The Heart and Cardiovascular System (Fozzard HA, et al eds). New York: Raven Press, 1992; 1875–973.

57. Koenig SH, Spiller M, Brown RD 3rd, Wolf GL. Relaxation of water protons in the intra- and extracellular regions of blood containing Gd(DTPA). Magn Reson Med 1986; 3:791–5.

58. Weinmann HJ, Brasch RC, Press WR, Wesbey GE. Characteristics of gadolinium-DTPA complex: a potential NMR contrast agent. AJR 1984; 142:619–24.

59. Rehwald WG, Fieno DS, Chen EL, et al. Myocardial magnetic resonance imaging contrast agent concentrations after reversible and irreversible ischemic injury. Circulation 2002; 105:224–9.

60. Rochitte CE, Lima JA, Bluemke DA, et al. Magnitude and time course of microvascular obstruction and tissue injury after acute myocardial infarction. Circulation 1998; 98:1006–14.

61. Judd RM, Lugo-Olivieri CH, Arai M, et al. Physiological basis of myocardial contrast enhancement in fast magnetic resonance images of 2-day-old reperfused canine infarcts. Circulation 1995; 92:1902–10.

62. Oshinski JN, Han HC, Ku DN, Pettigrew RI. Quantitative prediction of improvement in cardiac function after revascularization with MR imaging and modeling: initial results. Radiology 2001; 221:515–22.

63. Mahrholdt H, Wagner A, Holly TA, et al. Reproducibility of chronic infarct size measurements by contrast enhanced MRI. Circulation 2002; 106:2322–7.

64. Hillenbrand HB, Kim RJ, Parker MA, et al. Early assessment of myocardial salvage by contrast-enhanced magnetic resonance imaging. Circulation 2000; 102:1678–83.

65. Choi K, Kim RJ, Gubernikoff G, et al. The transmural extent of acute myocardial infarction predicts long term improvement in contractile function. Circulation 2001; 104:1101–7.

66. Gerber BL, Garot J, Bluemke DA, et al. Accuracy of contrast-enhanced magnetic resonance imaging in predicting improvement of regional myocardial function in patients after acute myocardial infarction. Circulation 2002; 106:1083–9.

67. Kim RJ, Wu E, Rafael A, et al. The use of contrast-enhanced magnetic resonance imaging to identify reversible myocardial dysfunction. N Engl J Med 2000; 343:1445–53.

68. Kloner RA, Parisi AF. Acute myocardial infarction: diagnostic and prognostic applications of two-dimensional echocardiography. Circulation 1987; 75:521–4.

69. Maes A, Flameng W, Nuyts J, et al. Histological alterations in chronically hypoperfused myocardium. Correlation with PET findings. Circulation 1994; 90:735–45.

70. Dakik HA, Howell JF, Lawrie GM, et al. Assessment of myocardial viability with 99mTc-sestamibi tomography before coronary bypass graft surgery: correlation with histopathology and postoperative improvement in cardiac function. Circulation 1997; 96:2892–8.

71. Lieberman AN, Weiss JL, Jugdutt BI, et al. Two-dimensional echocardiography and infarct size: relationship of regional wall motion and thickening to the extent of myocardial infarction in the dog. Circulation 1981; 63:739–46.

72. Force T, Kemper A, Perkins L, et al. Overestimation of infarct size by quantitative two-dimensional echocardiography: the role of tethering and of analytic procedures. Circulation 1986; 73:1360–8.

73. Sakai K, Watanabe K, Millard RW. Defining the mechanical border zone: a study in the pig heart. Am J Physiol 1985; 249:H88–94.

74. Armstrong WF. 'Hibernating' myocardium: asleep or part dead? J Am Coll Cardiol 1996; 28:530–5.

75. Weiss JL, Bulkley BH, Hutchins GM, Mason SJ. Two-dimensional echocardiographic recognition of myocardial injury in man: comparison with postmortem studies. Circulation 1981; 63:401–8.

76. Myers JH, Stirling MC, Choy M, et al. Direct measurement of inner and outer wall thickening dynamics with epicardial echocardiography. Circulation 1986; 74:164–72.

77. Homans DC, Pavek T, Laxson DD, Bache RJ. Recovery of transmural and subepicardial wall thickening after subendocardial infarction. J Am Coll Cardiol 1994; 24:1109–16.

78. Dilsizian V, Rocco TP, Freedman NM, et al. Enhanced detection of ischemic but viable myocardium by the reinjection of thallium after stress-redistribution imaging. N Engl J Med 1990; 323:141–6.

79. Afridi I, Kleiman NS, Raizner AE, Zoghbi WA. Dobutamine echocardiography in myocardial hibernation. Optimal dose and accuracy in predicting recovery of ventricular function after coronary angioplasty. Circulation 1995; 91:663–70.

80. Mahrholdt H, Wagner A, Choi K, et al. Contrast MRI detects subendocardial infarcts in regions of normal wall motion. Circulation 2001; 104(Suppl 2):341 (abst).

81. Weintraub WS, Hattori S, Agarwal JB, et al. The relationship between myocardial blood flow and contraction by myocardial layer in the canine left ventricle during ischemia. Circ Res 1981; 48:430–8.

82. Kuikka J, Yang J, Kiliainen H. Physical performance of Siemens E.Cam gamma camera. Nucl Med Commun 1998; 19:457–62.

83. Garvin AA, James J, Garcia EV. Myocardial perfusion imaging using single-photon emission computed tomography. Am J Card Imaging 1994; 8:189–98.

84. Wagner A, Mahrholdt H, Holly TA, et al. MRI detects subendocardial infarcts which are missed by SPECT. Lancet 2003; 361:374–9

85. Kannel WB, Abbott RD. Incidence and prognosis of unrecognized myocardial infarction. An update on the Framingham study. N Engl J Med 1984; 311:1144–7.

86. Sigurdsson E, Thorgeirsson G, Sigvaldason H, Sigfusson N. Unrecognized myocardial infarction: epidemiology, clinical characteristics, and the prognostic role of angina pectoris. The Reykjavik Study. Ann Intern Med 1995; 122:96–102.

87. Nadelmann J, Frishman WH, Ooi WL, et al. Prevalence, incidence and prognosis of recognized and unrecognized myocardial infarction in persons aged 75 years or older: The Bronx Aging Study. Am J Cardiol 1990; 66:533–7.

88. Kim H, Wu E, Meyers SN, et al. Prognostic significance of unrecognized myocardial infarction detected by contrast enhanced MRI. Circulation 2002; in press.

9

Coronary magnetic resonance angiography

Debiao Li, Vibhas Deshpande

Introduction

Coronary artery disease is the leading cause of death in both men and women in the USA and the Western world. Cardiac catheterization with contrast-enhanced coronary artery angiography is currently the standard test for the assessment of coronary artery disease, on the basis of which treatment decisions such as interventional procedures (bypass, stent, and angioplasty) or medical therapy are made. More than one million diagnostic cardiac catheterizations are performed in the USA each year. Cardiac catheterization is an invasive procedure with certain risks of mortality and morbidity, and costs more than $3 billion each year in the USA alone. Furthermore, its capability of determining the functional significance of coronary artery stenosis is limited. Although semiquantitative techniques based on the conventional angiogram exist for estimating the flow restriction caused by coronary stenosis,[1] nutritive myocardial perfusion cannot be directly evaluated.

Despite the availability of various screening tests, including echocardiographic, radionuclide, and ultrasound approaches, a substantial minority of patients referred for coronary angiography have no significant coronary artery disease.[2,3] There is a clear need for a noninvasive, cost-effective, and reliable method of directly detecting functionally significant coronary artery disease (defined as a reduction in the luminal diameter of at least 50%) in the high-prevalence population. Ideally, those who show no evidence of coronary abnormality in such a screening test will be spared the risk and high cost of conventional angiography. The ideal examination should provide both anatomical and functional information about the heart, and could be useful in assessing postinterventional procedure results as well.

Magnetic resonance imaging (MRI) is an attractive screening technique for coronary artery disease because it is noninvasive, does not require ionizing radiation or iodinated contrast media, can provide hemodynamic information in addition to vascular morphology, can

provide three-dimensional (3D) structural data, and may be significantly less expensive than conventional angiography. The MR techniques for the evaluation of vascular anatomy, collectively known as magnetic resonance angiography (MRA), have become routine clinical tests in the head and neck, abdomen, and extremities. However, MRA of coronary arteries is a more challenging task. A number of factors have hindered its progress. These include the motion of the heart during cardiac and respiratory cycles, the highly tortuous course and the small size of coronary arteries, and the adjacency of coronary arteries to epicardial fatty tissues, atrial appendages, coronary veins, and major blood pools, which have little natural image contrast with coronary arteries. The spatial displacement of coronary arteries during each heartbeat and respiratory cycle is on the order of several centimeters. The proximal coronary arteries have calibers in the range of 2–4 mm and rarely exceed 5 mm in normal humans.[2,4] Distal portions of coronary arteries and branch vessels are even smaller. As a result, the visualization of coronary arteries requires elimination or significant reduction of motion effects during cardiac and respiratory cycles, high-resolution volumetric coverage of the region of interest, background signal suppression, and optimal image processing and display methods.

Brief history of coronary MRA

Early attempts of assessing the patency of coronary artery bypass grafts and visualizing native coronary arteries (late 1980s)

Due to technical limitations (in both hardware and software) at the time, early efforts at visualizing coronary arteries had only marginal success.[5–9] Therefore, early attempts to image coronary arteries focused on detecting the patency of coronary artery bypass grafts (CABGs), since these usually have relatively large lumens and a more direct course, and are less mobile than native coronary arteries. The goal of these studies was to visualize the lumen in axial images at multiple anatomical levels of the grafts and to detect the presence of flow. ECG-triggered spin-echo and gradient-echo cine techniques were used. Flowing blood manifests as a signal void in spin-echo images and appears hyperintense in gradient-echo cine images. Composite data from six studies show that 172 of 188 CABGs that were identified as patent on the basis of selective coronary angiography were determined correctly as patent (sensitivity 91%), and 68 of 86 CABGs were classified correctly as occluded (specificity 79%).[10–15] False-positive assessments of CABG patency were caused by metal hemostatic clips resembling signal void of flowing blood in spin-echo images, or a pericardial collection of air or fluid, or native coronary arteries and veins.[10] False-negative assessments of CABG patency were caused by the remaining intraluminal signal of slow flow in stenotic CABGs in spin-echo imaging.[10,15] These studies could not quantify the degree of stenosis because they did not visualize the whole length of the CABG, and patent but stenotic CABGs may mimic normal grafts.

Early attempts to visualize native coronary arteries used ECG-gated spin-echo,[6,16] two-dimensional (2D)[8,9] and 3D gradient-echo cine,[17] and echo-planar imaging[18] sequences. Spin-echo images depict the rapid flowing blood in coronary arteries as a dark signal if blood moves out of the imaging plane between the 90° and 180° radiofrequency (RF) pulses. With previous knowledge of the anatomy of the coronary arteries gained from conventional angiography, Paulin et al[6] were able to identify the orifices and the proximal portions of both left and right coronary arteries.

Gradient-echo sequences show the vessel lumen as a bright signal because of the inflow-enhancement effect. Fresh blood moving into the imaging plane between sequence repetitions has full magnetization and creates a larger signal than stationary tissues because the magnetization of stationary tissues become progressively reduced after each sequence repetition. Four-dimensional (three spatial axes and one temporal axis) data were acquired using a 2D gradient-echo cine sequence at multiple axial positions and multiple timeframes during the cardiac cycle.[8,9] Images were then displayed in rapid succession in temporal or spatial series,[9] or as projections after removal of adjacent blood pools.[8] Three-dimensional volume imaging in conjunction with retrospective ECG gating generated continuous slices in one scan.[17] However, the imaging time for each scan was very long (~30 min). To reduce imaging time, echo-planar imaging (EPI) techniques were introduced, which collected raw data needed for image reconstruction with one single RF pulse, result-

ing in an imaging time ranging between 40 and 100 ms.[18] This freezes the motion of the heart, and thus image blur caused by cardiac and respiratory motion was eliminated. Low signal-to-noise ratio (SNR), low spatial resolution, and image artifacts caused by resonance frequency offset are major problems for EPI.

These early techniques and studies were not able to visualize coronary arteries consistently, because heart motion caused by respiration was not eliminated or fully compensated for, images were not acquired along coronary artery axes in oblique planes, the total imaging time was very long, and image reformatting either was not attempted because of the thick slices or suffered from misregistration between sequentially acquired slices due to patient motion. Therefore, the coronary arteries were not consistently visualized in their entirety, motion-related image artifacts were routinely present, and the spatial resolution was relatively low. It was difficult to make disease diagnosis based on these images.

2D breathhold coronary artery imaging with segmented data acquisition (early 1990s)

A major advance in coronary MRA came with the ability to acquire a segment of k-space data within each heartbeat.[19–21] In this scheme, multiple phase-encoding lines of the raw data for an image (instead of one line per cardiac cycle with the conventional cine method) are acquired during mid-diastole of each heartbeat when the heart has little motion. This method reduced the number of cardiac cycles required to acquire the raw data for image reconstruction. As a result, a single slice was acquired within a single breathhold, freezing the respiratory motion. In addition, images were acquired in oblique planes along the axes of coronary arteries, allowing the visualization of a large portion of a coronary artery in a slice. The acquisition of a 2D slice within a single breathhold became possible with the availability of higher gradient magnitudes and shorter gradient switching times in MRI systems at the time.

Using the 2D breathhold method, Edelman et al[20] consistently visualized all four major coronary arteries (LM, left main; LAD, left anterior descending; LCX, left circumflex; and RCA, right coronary artery) and some major branches. Another important technical advancement was the improved field homogeneity, which permitted consistent suppression of the signal from epicardial fat that surrounds proximal portions of coronary arteries and their major branches.[22–24] Lipid tissue has a shorter T1 than muscle and blood, and tends to have a stronger signal than blood in coronary arteries with a T1-weighted gradient-echo sequence. Fat and water have different resonance frequencies (~220 Hz at 1.5 T). A frequency-selective prepulse (typically with a 90° flip angle) that excites only the fat signal, followed by gradient spoiling, was applied to suppress the fat signal before water signal acquisition. Other improvements included the use of a surface coil to enhance SNR and an image-editing algorithm to eliminate the overlapping chambers to generate a maximum-intensity projection from multiple slices.[25]

Despite the relatively low spatial resolution, there was a good correlation between the MRI-estimated proximal coronary artery diameter and that measured from conventional angiography. Preliminary clinical trials demonstrated early promise of this 2D single-slice breathhold data acquisition scheme.[26,27] An overall sensitivity and specificity of 97% and 70% were noted in 39 patients. However, further studies revealed the pitfalls of the technique.[28] The major problem was that only one slice was acquired per breathhold. Because the course of the coronary artery is highly tortuous, multiple partially overlapping slices are required to assess the integrity of a coronary artery in separate breathholds. Nevertheless, patients may not be able to suspend their breath at exactly the same position. Potential position misregistration between adjacent slices may cause misinterpretation of a segment of the artery out of the imaging plane as stenosis, or vice versa. In addition, the large number of breathholds required per imaging session placed a large burden on patients. Finally, the spatial resolution (on the order of $2 \times 1 \times 4$ mm^3) was inadequate for accurate disease diagnosis.

Another 2D imaging technique for coronary MRA developed in the early 1990s is interleaved spiral data space scanning.[21] Spiral readouts have good flow properties and higher imaging efficiency and SNR than the conventional rectilinear data acquisition scheme. With this technique, the acquisition window per cardiac cycle was short, minimizing cardiac motion effects. In addition, higher flip angle was used to improve SNR because of the application of a small number of RF pulses per cardiac cycle. The major problem is potential image artifacts caused by resonance frequency offset in the presence of field inhomogeneities.

3D coronary artery imaging (since early 1990s)

Although 2D methods have continued to be used for coronary artery imaging up to today, they have gradually been replaced by 3D imaging. In principle, 3D imaging can overcome many of the problems associated with 2D methods. The advantages of 3D imaging include the acquisition of thin and contiguous slices so that image processing can be performed, a high SNR, and less operator dependence compared with 2D imaging because the orientation of the imaging volume is less critical. 3D imaging of coronary arteries was first attempted without respiratory motion compensation.[24,29–31] Respiratory gating with navigator echoes was then used to reduce respiratory motion effects.[4,32]

The milestones in 3D coronary artery imaging include the initial use of respiratory gating with navigator echoes, volume-targeted imaging with breathhold, contrast-enhanced coronary artery imaging, navigator-echo-guided real-time slice correction, and TrueFISP coronary artery imaging. These will be presented in detail in the following sections. It should be pointed out that each new stage of coronary artery imaging was accompanied by improvements in the hardware and software of the imaging systems.

Respiratory motion compensation for coronary MRA

The major challenge for coronary artery imaging is to overcome the effects of coronary motion during the cardiac and respiratory cycles. The effect of coronary motion during a cardiac cycle is removed by data acquisition during mid-diastole, when the heart motion is minimal. This is accomplished by synchronizing data acquisition to the ECG signal. The effect of respiratory motion poses the major obstacle for coronary artery imaging. In this section, methods used for respiratory motion reduction other than breathhold are reviewed.

Motion artifacts

In MRI, there are motion artifacts other than just blurring of the moving object itself. This is due to the fact that in MRI the raw data in k-space is the Fourier transform of the image. After data collection, the actual image is obtained by performing an inverse Fourier transform on the raw data. This process dictates that the object to be imaged needs to remain constant during the entire imaging process. If this condition is not satisfied, i.e. if the structure to be imaged changes position from the time one part of the k-space is acquired to the time another part of the k-space is acquired, this structure will not be reconstructed correctly and image artifacts will result. For periodic physiological motion such as heartbeat and respiration, the image artifacts include image blurs as expected, but also image ghosts, which are periodic replicas of the moving anatomical structures superimposed on nonmoving structures. In 2D and 3D Fourier transform imaging, the frequency encoding is obtained quickly compared with physiological motion (heartbeat and respiration). Therefore, no obvious motion artifacts will occur in this direction. However, in the remaining directions where phase encoding is performed, this ghosting artifact will occur when the object moves during data acquisition.

Techniques that compensate for respiratory motion can be separated in two groups. In the first, the respiratory ordered phase-encoding method will remove or limit the effect of the ghosting, but will not remove image blur, or prevent loss of resolution. In the second group, the respiratory gating techniques limit both ghosting and blurring. Therefore, respiratory gating techniques are of greater importance and will be discussed more thoroughly.

Respiratory ordered phase encoding

Ghosting artifacts are caused by the periodicity of tissue motion. These artifacts can be eliminated by destroying periodicity of the motion effect in the raw data within *k*-space. This can be accomplished by ordering the acquisition of phase-encoding lines to match the amplitude of the respiratory motion. This method is referred to as respiratory ordered phase encoding (ROPE).[33,34] If the moving structure is not within the region of interest and the goal is to remove the interference of the ghosts of moving objects with the stationary tissue, or if a simple loss of resolution in the moving structure is acceptable, the ROPE technique will help reduce image ghosts.

Because the ROPE technique does not remove the image blur caused by the respiratory motion of coronary arteries, this technique itself is not sufficient for respiratory motion artifact reduction for coronary MRA. However, the same basic principle is used to limit ghosting effects induced by cardiac motion when multiple phase-encoding steps are collected within one cardiac cycle. These phase-encoding steps are re-ordered such that the periodic variations within *k*-space are eliminated in a technique referred to as segmented *k*-space acquisition.[19,20,35,36]

Respiratory gating

Similar to ECG triggering, where data acquisition is synchronized to the heartbeat, the respiratory wave can also be monitored and used to control the timing of data acquisition or to determine the data used for image reconstruction. The basic principle of respiratory gating is that data are used for image reconstruction only when the res-

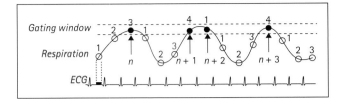

Figure 9.1
Schematic diagram of coronary MRA with respiratory gating. Only data obtained when the respiratory signal is within the gating window are used for image reconstruction (solid circles). Data are collected during diastole of each cardiac cycle through ECG triggering. The numbers below the respiratory signal (*n*, *n* + 1, ...) are phase encoding lines; the numbers above the respiratory signal (1, 2, ...) are the acquisitions for each phase encoding line.

piration signal falls within a certain range, the gate window, as illustrated in Figure 9.1. Therefore, respiratory gating will lengthen the total imaging time because effectively no data are collected during the remaining part of the respiratory cycle. In general, motion artifacts are reduced more with a narrower gate window, which also results in longer imaging time. Thus, it is important to collect data within the most consistent respiratory position in the breathing cycle. This is usually the relaxed position at the end of expiration. In principle, if the heart returns to exactly the same position during each respiratory cycle, the respiration can be frozen and reconstructed images will be free of respiration effects.

Techniques to obtain a respiratory signal
Abdominal belt

Initially, a reference for the respiratory motion was obtained by placing a belt containing a displacement transducer around the upper abdomen.[37,38] Thereby, the anterior–posterior displacement of the abdomen was determined. The disadvantage of this technique is that the belt does not give the absolute displacement value of the respiratory motion. In addition, the correlation between the abdominal respiratory motion and the actual motion of the coronary arteries is variable for each individual.

Navigator echoes

A more direct and absolute measurement of respiration-induced motion can be obtained by the use of navigator echoes, as illustrated in Figure 9.2. This technique was first developed to monitor respiratory motion to improve abdominal MRI,[39–41] and was later successfully applied for respiratory gating of coronary MRA.[4,32,42–45] Typically the

(a)   (b)

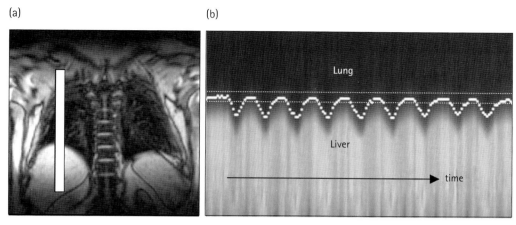

Figure 9.2

Tracking respiratory motion with navigator echoes. (a) The coronal image on the left shows the column of tissue excited by the navigator echo. (b) The resulting temporal display of multiple navigator echoes, showing diaphragmatic motion. The boundary between liver (high signal in the lower portion of the image) and lung (low signal in the upper portion of the image) is marked with thick lines and the range of motion accepted for image reconstruction is indicated by dotted lines.

motion of the diaphragm in the superior–inferior (SI) direction is tracked, assuming that the SI motion of the diaphragm is synchronized to the heart (and coronary artery) motion caused by the respiration.

With the navigator echo technique, the MR signal of a beam is measured, using frequency encoding along the long axis of the beam. After data acquisition, a one-dimensional (1D) Fourier transform is performed, and a 1D image along the beam is created. When this beam is placed over a structure that moves during respiration along the direction of the beam, this motion can be measured by tracking a marker in the beam (typically a boundary between high and low signal intensities). These navigator echoes should have a spatial resolution along the beam of ≤ 1 mm in order to detect the motion of the heart with adequate resolution. These one-dimensional images can be obtained within 10–20 ms, thereby showing real-time information of the respiratory motion. There are two methods to obtain such a beam for a navigator image: the spin-echo method and the 2D selective excitation method.

The first method to obtain a navigator echo is by using different slice selection gradients for the 90° and 180° pulses.[39] The spin echo is then formed by the intersection of the two different slices of the RF pulses. The advantage of this method is the relatively simple implementation. The disadvantage is that the high excitation flip angles used could result in magnetization saturation of the entire two slices within the object. The 90° and 180° pulses could saturate the blood magnetization and reduce the coronary artery signal if they cut across the heart. This interference with imaging the coronary arteries limits the flexibility to position the navigator beam.

A more flexible way of implementing the navigator echo is using a 2D selective excitation.[46] By modulation of both the RF pulse shape and gradient during the RF pulse, only the signal within a pencil beam will be excited. This allows the use of lower excitation angles and a greater flexibility to position the beam without interfering with data acquisition.

The next question is the positioning of this navigator beam in order to obtain the best motion signal for respiratory gating of the coronary MRA. From motion studies of the heart, it is known that the major component of respiratory motion is in cranio-caudal direction.[43] Most studies up to now have used the dome of the diaphragm to detect the cranio-caudal motion. The sharp interface between liver and lung results in a clear edge on the navigator echo image.

The use of diaphragmatic displacement for respiratory gating is based on the assumption that the motion detected from the navigator echo is correlated with that of the coronary arteries. Wang et al[43] studied this relationship by acquiring images with breathholds at different timeframes of the respiratory cycle. A close correlation was found.

Intuitively, left diaphragmatic motion should correlate more closely to heart motion than right diaphragmatic motion, although the differences appeared to be insignificant in the study by Korin et al.[41] Practically, when a spin-echo technique is used to acquire navigator echoes, it is difficult in some subjects to place the 90° and 180° pulses on the left side without intersecting the heart because of the proximity of the heart to the chest wall. In these cases, the navigator echo beam had to be placed in the right side of the thoracic space.

The interference of the navigator echo pulses with the heart is not a problem if a 2D excitation pulse is used to create the navigator echo. This type of navigator can be placed on the heart itself, and therefore allows a more direct measure of the coronary artery motion. When the navigator beam is in an oblique orientation, the craniocaudal motion of the heart can be determined by correcting for the beam angulation.

Various methods have been used to determine the respiratory motion from navigator echoes, including edge detection,[4] cross-correlation,[39,42,47] and least squares methods.[40,48] The edge detection method uses a signal intensity threshold to determine the edge of the object. Usually a low-pass filter is first applied to the navigator echo to remove spikes in the data before edge detection. Both the correlation and least squares methods compare the current navigator echo profile with a range of shifts to a reference profile. With the correlation method, the shift that results in the maximal correlation between the current and the reference profiles is taken as the estimated displacement between the current position and reference position. With the least squares method, the shift with the smallest squared difference between the current and reference profiles is taken as the estimated displacement.

Algorithms used for respiratory gating

During each heartbeat, after a trigger delay time, a navigator echo is first acquired, followed by the collection of a segment of the raw data of the coronary MRA in mid-diastole. These data are accepted for eventual reconstruction if the position of the respiration as determined by the navigator falls within the gating window. The measurement is repeated n times before the next segment of the raw data is measured. There are a number of approaches to performing the actual respiratory gating. The approaches are broadly classified based on when these decisions are made, and how the number of repetitions n and the gating window are determined.

Prospective gating[42,44,48]

In this approach, the decision to accept or reject the data is made in real time, based on a gating window that is chosen at the start of the scan. The collection of each segment of data is repeated until it is found to lie within the gating window. The number of repetitions n is variable for each segment of data and depends on the breathing pattern. This guarantees that all data used for image reconstruction are within the gating window. The disadvantage is that the gating window has to be determined at

the start of the scan and remains fixed, without taking into consideration the actual breathing pattern during the data acquisition process. On one hand, this may result in prolonged imaging time if the gating window is too narrow and/or there is a significant change of breathing pattern or bulk motion of the subject during imaging. On the other hand, if the gating window is too wide, the resultant image will be suboptimal in terms of motion artifact removal.

Retrospective gating[4,32]

In this approach, the decision to accept the data is made after all the data is acquired. Therefore, the gating window can be chosen after the acquisition, allowing the flexibility of changing this window at the time of image reconstruction after taking into consideration the actual breathing pattern during data acquisition. By reconstructing multiple sets of images at different gating windows, coronary arteries can be visualized at different phases of the breathing cycle. In addition, for multiple overlapping scans, the same center positions of the gating window can be used retrospectively to register the slabs. The disadvantage of the method is that the number of repetitions is fixed and has to be determined prior to data acquisition. This will result in an unequal number of repetitions for different segments of data used in image reconstruction, reducing the time efficiency of the method.

With this method, the acquisition of each segment of data is repeated n times in n consecutive heartbeats, so that the total imaging time of the segment will be greater than the duration of a respiratory cycle. Assuming a respiratory period of 3–4 s, five acquisitions of each segment of the data (in five heartbeats) will ensure full coverage of the respiratory cycle. If the subject has a long respiratory cycle or an erratic breathing pattern, the number of repetitions for the collection of each segment of data will need to be increased, resulting in a relatively long imaging time, especially for a 3D scan.

Diminishing variance algorithm (DVA)

The third approach to respiratory gating is a hybrid method between the prospective and retrospective approaches, referred to as the diminishing variance algorithm.[49] In this scheme, the entire data space is first covered in a sequential mode. At the end of the first pass of k-space, a histogram is constructed. Subsequently, the data segment that is farthest from the center of the histogram is reacquired and the histogram is updated. This process is repeated until certain stopping criteria are reached.

A multicenter study including seven institutions and 109 subjects was undertaken to evaluate the accuracy of navigator-echo-guided coronary MRA among patients with suspected coronary disease.[3] In all cases, coronary MRA was performed within 14 days before X-ray angiography. Similar to the breathhold approach, the first step is the localization of the coronary arteries. The first localizing scan (~1 min) employed a multistack and multislice, segmented gradient-echo sequence for localization of the heart and diaphragm in the three orthogonal planes (transverse, sagittal, and coronal). From the coronal data set, a navigator-gated 3D segmented echo-planar localizer scan with 40 slices (~2 min) was collected around the base of the heart to cover the region extending from the apex of the left ventricle to the pulmonary artery.[90] This allowed identification of the course of the major right and left coronary arteries. With the use of a three-point planscan tool, a plane through the major axis of the proximal and middle segments of the right coronary artery was prescribed.

After localization of the coronary arteries, high-resolution scans were performed on a targeted volume. Coronary MRA was performed with the use a 3D segmented *k*-space gradient-echo sequence (FLASH) with navigator-echo-guided real-time slice correction during free breathing. To enhance the contrast between the coronary arteries and the surrounding epicardial fat and myocardium, a frequency-selective fat-suppression prepulse and a T2-weighted magnetization preparation scheme were applied. For the RCA, a double-oblique 3D volume was imaged with use of the coordinates prescribed by the three-point planscan tool. For the LM, LAD, and LCX coronary arteries, a double-oblique transverse 3D volume with anterior–posterior and left–right angulations (5° each) was imaged with the volume centered on the origin of the LM coronary artery (as defined from the second localization scan). The navigator echo was collected on the right hemidiaphragm.[87] The gating window used for the navigator was 5 mm at the end of expiration, with a correction factor of 0.6. The typical imaging parameters included TR/TE = 7.7/2.2 ms, FOV = 360×360 mm^2, an acquisition matrix size of 360×512, an in-plane resolution of 1.0×0.7 mm^2, 8 lines acquired per heartbeat, 10 slices per 3D slab (interpolated to 20), and a slice thickness of 3.0 mm (interpolated to 1.5 mm). The time required for each scan was on the order of 10–15 min. The study was conducted on 1.5 T systems (Gyroscan ACS-NT, Phillips Medical Systems, Best, the Netherlands) equipped with Power-Trak 6000 gradients (23 mT/m and 219 μs rise time).

Seven coronary artery segments were evaluated: the LM artery and the proximal and middle segments of the LAD artery (0 to 2 cm and 2 to 4 cm), the LCX artery (0 to 1.5 cm and 1.5 to 3.0 cm), and the RCA (0 to 2 cm and 2 to 5 cm). Eighty-four percent (636/759) of the proximal and middle coronary artery segments in MR images had diagnostic image quality. In these segments, 78 (83%) of 94 clinically significant lesions were detected by MRA. The results of the study are given in Table 9.1. Overall, coronary MRA had an accuracy of 72% (95% confidence interval 63–81%) in diagnosing coronary artery disease. The sensitivity, specificity, and accuracy for patients with disease of the LM coronary artery or three-vessel disease were 100%, 85%, and 87%, respectively. The negative predictive values for any coronary artery and for left main artery or three-vessel disease were 81% and 100%, respectively. Two examples of coronary artery stenosis detection using this method are shown in Figure 9.16.

A high sensitivity, negative predictive value, and overall accuracy for using MRA to detect coronary artery disease, especially in subjects with LM disease or three-vessel disease, was found in this prospective, multicenter study. Its high negative predictive value suggests that it may have a role in ruling out clinically significant coronary disease in patients who are candidates for X-ray angiography. In this study, on the basis of negative coronary MRA, X-ray angiography could have been avoided in 18 subjects. All patients with LM coronary artery or three-vessel disease were identified as having clinically significant coronary artery disease. These data support the use of coronary MRA to identify (or rule out) LM or three-vessel disease reliably. This study also reveals that MRA has a relatively low positive predictive value, meaning a substantial number of false-positive diagnoses. Further technical advances are required to enhance spatial resolution and reduce image artifacts to reduce false-positive observations.

Coronary MRA with free breathing and real-time slice correction allows longer imaging time and higher SNR and spatial resolution than breathhold imaging. However, it is prone to incomplete motion compensation or prolonged imaging time with inconsistent breathing patterns or diaphragmatic position drifting.[91] Methods have been proposed to overcome this problem.[92–94] Another issue is the selection of the imaging slice correction factor based on diaphragmatic position shift. A factor of 0.6 is commonly used to correct motion in the superior–inferior direction;[43] however, a lower factor was observed in the work by Keegan et al.[95]

To further reduce imaging time, TrueFISP has been used to acquire coronary artery images during free breathing.[67] A volunteer example is shown in Figure 9.17. Because of the use of a shorter TR (3.1 ms), the imaging time was only 60 s.

Imaging techniques under development

In addition to the three major techniques introduced above, which have undergone extensive clinical testing,

Table 9.1 Diagnostic accuracy of coronary magnetic resonance angiography to detect stenoses of ≥ 50%.

Variable	Left main coronary artery	Left anterior descending coronary artery	Left circumflex coronary artery	Right coronary artery	Any coronary artery disease (consensus/site reading)[a]	Left main coronary artery or three-vessel disease (consensus/site reading)[a]
No. of true positives	81	31	49	43	18/25	74/75
No. of true negatives	4	29	8	37	56/51	16/15
No. of false positives	2	4	7	3	4/7	0/1
No. of false negatives	9	29	21	17	25/18	13/10
Prevalence (%)	6	41	19	40	59	15
Sensitivity (%)	67	88	53	93	93 (88–98)/88 (82–94)	100 (97–100)/94 (89–99)
Specificity (%)	90	52	70	72	42 (32–52)/58 (48–68)	85 (78–92)/88 (82–94)
Accuracy (%)	89	65	67	80	72 (63–81)/75 (67–83)	87 (81–93)/89 (83–95)
Positive predictive value (%)	30	56	29	69	70 (61–79)/75 (67–83)	54 (44–64)/58 (48–68)
Negative predictive value (%)	98	86	86	94	81 (73–89)/77 (69–85)	100 (97–100)/99 (95–100)

[a] Values in parentheses are 95% confidence intervals.
(Reproduced from Kim et al. N Engl J Med 2001; 345:1863–9[3] with permission from the Massachusetts Medical Society.)

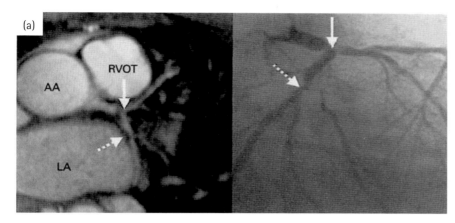

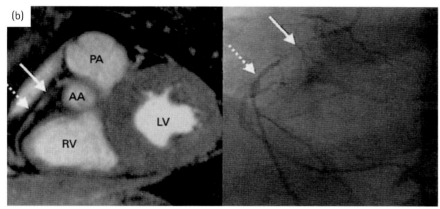

Figure 9.16
Coronary angiography in a 53-year-old man with exertional chest pain. (a) Coronary MRA (left) and a corresponding X-ray coronary angiogram (right) indicating a severe lesion at the bifurcation of the LAD and the LCX, involving the LM (solid arrows), and a more distal focal stenosis of the LCX (broken arrows). (b) Coronary MRA (left) and a corresponding X-ray image (right) indicating two stenoses of the proximal (solid arrows) and middle (broken arrows) RCA. AA, ascending aorta; LA, left atrium; RVOT, right ventricular outflow tract; PA, pulmonary artery; RV, right ventricle; LV, left ventricle. (Reproduced from Kim et al. N Engl J Med 2001; 345:1863–9[3] with permission from the Massachusetts Medical Society.)

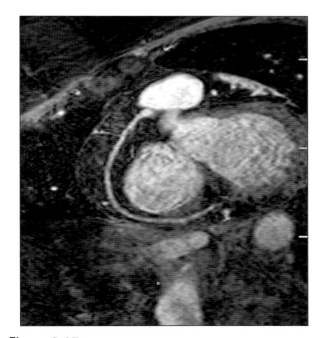

Figure 9.17
Image of RCA acquired with 3D TrueFISP during free breathing and navigator-echo-guided slice correction.

many other techniques currently under development offer great potentials to further improve coronary MRA. Some of these techniques and advances will be introduced briefly in this section.

Coronary MRA with radial sampling

Radial k-space acquisition (projection reconstruction, PR) techniques offer several advantages over rectilinear Fourier imaging and are particularly useful for cardiac imaging applications. Principally, radial acquisitions allow a relative tradeoff between SNR and number of acquired lines (views) rather than the tradeoff between resolution or FOV and number of acquired phase encode lines inherent to Fourier techniques. Some degree of streak artifact and loss of SNR has been deemed an acceptable tradeoff for the desirable isotropic resolution of PR images.[96] An undersampled PR technique incorporating TrueFISP has been used recently for coronary artery imaging.[97] With a relatively small number of lines, coronary artery images

(a)   (b)   (c)

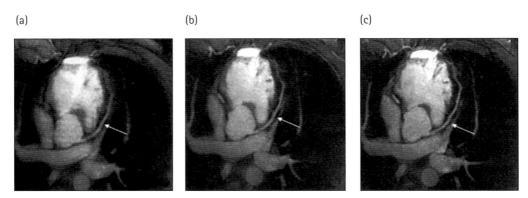

Figure 9.18
Targeted maximum-intensity projection images of the LAD (solid arrow) of a single volunteer using 3D projection reconstruction TrueFISP. Imaging parameters for this image set are (a) 93 views/partition asymmetric, (b) 123 views/partition asymmetric, and (c) 153 views/partition asymmetric. Notice the improvement in image sharpness and vessel delineation as the number of views per partition was increased from 93 to 123 between images (a) and (b). Images (b) and (c) appear very similar. Each of these images was acquired with a 1.0 × 1.0 mm² isotropic in-plane voxel size. (Reproduced from Larson et al. Magn Reson Med 2002; **48**:594–601[97] with permission from John Wiley & Sons, Inc.)

with isotropic in-plane resolution of 1 × 1 mm² were obtained (Figure 9.18).

Free-breathing black-blood coronary MRA

All the techniques discussed above create bright-blood images in which blood in the arteries has higher signal intensity than surrounding tissues. These techniques have certain limitations, including difficulty in accurately quantifying luminal stenosis, especially in the presence of complex flow at and near severe stenoses.[98] Metallic implants such as clips and sternal wires may also cause image artifacts. A spin-echo dark-blood approach has been proposed to overcome these problems. This technique uses a dual-inversion magnetization preparation scheme to suppress the signal of blood that moves into the imaging plane between the preparation pulses and data acquisition. The data acquisition sequence is a fast spin-echo technique. Navigator echoes are used for real-time slice correction as in bright-blood MRA. Promising results have been demonstrated using this technique.[98,99] Two examples are given in Figure 9.19. Further patient studies are required to verify the utility of this approach. Similar techniques have been used for vessel wall imaging to detect and characterize plaques.[100–102]

Accelerated coronary MRA with parallel data acquisition

A new imaging paradigm has emerged in the last few years in which multicomponent detection arrays are used to perform some fraction of image data acquisition in parallel. These techniques tend to fall into two general categories: SMASH (simultaneous acquisition of spatial

(a)   (b)

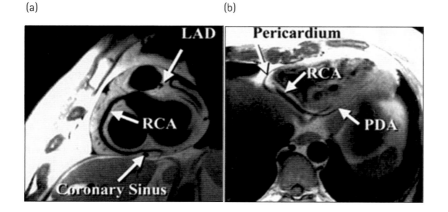

Figure 9.19
Free-breathing black-blood coronary MRA in a healthy adult subject (fast spin-echo, interecho spacing 5.2 ms, repetition time two cardiac cycles, echo time 25 ms, echo train length 23). (a) Double-oblique MRA depicting the RCA and a perpendicular view of the left anterior descending coronary artery (LAD) and the coronary sinus. (b) Transverse MRA depicting the distal RCA and proximal posterior descending coronary artery (PDA). (Reproduced from Stuber et al. Radiology 2001; **219**:278–83[98] with permission from the Radiological Society of North America.)

(a)

T2prep

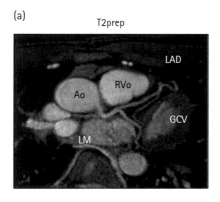

(b)

Bracco B22956

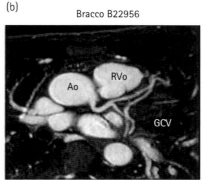

Figure 9.20
Multiplanar reformatted (a) baseline T2Prep image and (b) B22956-enhanced IR image. Improved vessel delineation of the LM, LAD, LCX, and GCV can be appreciated visually. B22956 is a gadolinium-based blood pool agent from Bracco Imaging SpA, Milan. GCV, great cardiac vein. (Reproduced from Huber et al. Magn Reson Med 2003; 49:115–21[111] with permission from John Wiley & Sons, Inc.)

harmonics)[103] and SENSE (sensitivity encoding).[104] SMASH operates primarily in *k*-space, while SENSE operates primarily in the image domain. These techniques have the potential to accelerate the imaging speed by a factor of two or more. Investigations are in progress to assess the feasibility of applying these techniques to coronary artery imaging.

Coronary MRA with spiral acquisitions

While 3D thin-slab coronary MRA has traditionally been performed using a Cartesian acquisition scheme, spiral *k*-space data acquisition offers several potential advantages.[21,105,106] Spiral acquisitions were found to be superior to the Cartesian scheme with respect to SNR, CNR, and image quality.[107,108] Further clinical evaluations are required to define the utility of this technique.

Coronary MRA with blood pool contrast agents

Newly developed blood pool contrast agents offer great potential for improving SNR and spatial resolution in coronary MRA.[65,72,109–111] These agents stay in the blood pool much longer and have a greater T1 relaxivity than the conventional extracelluar contrast agents in current clinical use. Several blood pool agents are currently in various stages of clinical trials for coronary artery imaging. These agents maintain a much longer and greater T1-shortening effect than conventional extracelluar agents and allow for blood signal enhancement with data acquisition during free breathing, when the imaging time is on the order of 10 min[111] (Figure 9.20). They have enabled coverage of the entire heart with a free-breathing scan.[110] All major coronary arteries and their relationship with

cardiac chambers have been visualized with volume rendering (Figure 9.21).

Coronary MRA at 3.0 T

Current limitations on the SNR and spatial resolution of coronary MRA at 1.5 T can be improved by imaging at higher field strengths. In theory, SNR is directly related to the strength of the static magnetic field. Three-tesla systems have recently been approved for clinical use. Improved SNR and resolution are expected in these systems. Despite many technical challenges with coronary MRA at 3 T, promising results have been shown using the same technique as at 1.5 T[112] (Figure 9.22).

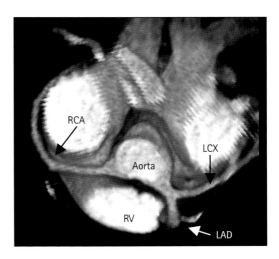

Figure 9.21
Volume rendering of images acquired from a pig with 0.10 mmol/kg blood pool agent Gadomer-17 (SHL 643A; Schering, Berlin), using a 3D respiratory-gated segmented gradient-echo sequence (TR/TE = 4.0/1.5). Major coronary arteries and their spatial relationship with cardiac structures are clearly delineated. (Reproduced from Li et al. Radiology 2001; 218:670–8[110] with permission from the Radiological Society of North America.)

(a)   (b)

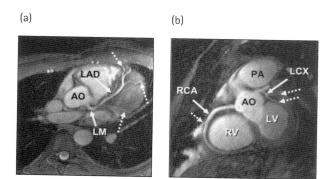

Figure 9.22
Example of coronary MRA obtained in the (a) left and (b) right coronary arterial systems. (a) displays the LM and LAD together with smaller-diameter branching vessels (dotted arrows), obtained with a voxel size of $0.6 \times 0.6 \times 3.0$ mm³. (b) was obtained with a $0.7 \times 1.0 \times 3.0$ mm³ voxel size, and shows the RCA together with the proximal LCX. RV, right ventricle; PA, pulmonary artery; AO, ascending aorta. (Reproduced from Stuber et al. Magn Reson Med 2002; 48:425–9[112] with permission from John Wiley & Sons, Inc.)

Other imaging techniques

Other coronary MRA techniques include interactive imaging,[113–116] breathing autocorrection with spiral interleaves,[117] echo-planar imaging,[52,118–120] diminished variance algorithm with navigator echo,[49,121] multiple breathhold imaging with a respiratory feedback monitor[51] or real-time slice following,[122] free breathing with retrospective respiratory gating[4,32,123,124] or adaptive motion correction,[125] hybrid ordered phase encoding for improved respiratory artifact reduction,[92,93] and vessel tracking.[126] While some of these techniques have been replaced by new methods, others continue to improve.

Discussion and conclusions

Significant progress has been made in coronary MRA in the last decade, in both technical developments and initial clinical testing. With current MR techniques, it is now possible to consistently visualize proximal and middle portions of major coronary artery branches with a spatial resolution of 1.5 mm³ in healthy volunteers and patients with coronary artery disease. MRA has a high negative predictive value and may be useful for ruling out clinically significant coronary artery disease in proximal portions of coronary arteries (LM or three-vessel disease) in patients referred to conventional angiography.[3] It is ideally suited for depicting anomalous coronary arteries. Although clinical studies are encouraging (sensitivity 68–94% and specificity 57–97%)[3,63,74,123,124,127–130] MRA alone is not yet adequate for routine diagnosis of coronary artery disease. The major limitations include relatively low spatial resolu-

tion, lack of stenosis quantification, failure to depict distal and branch vessels consistently, variability of image quality (depending on machine, user, and patient), technical failures in some subjects, and poor positive predictive values.

Technically, both breathhold and free-breathing approaches are likely to be useful in coronary artery imaging.[131] TrueFISP imaging is a highly promising method for data acquisition, but further refinements of the techniques are necessary. The major challenges are to overcome the effects of respiratory motion and to improve spatial resolution, SNR, and consistency of image quality. Another important area of further investigation regards the processing and display of coronary artery images.[132,133] Currently, disease diagnosis is done by assessing original images. Improved image reformatting and processing methods will be helpful.

An alternative approach to minimally invasive coronary artery imaging is multislice computed tomography, which has shown promising results.[134,135] Advantages of this technique include higher speed and higher resolution than MRI. However, it requires ionizing radiation and iodinated contrast media. Difficulties in stenosis detection may arise if there are high densities of calcifications. Image artifacts may mimic stenoses if the data are reconstructed at a suboptimal time in the cardiac cycle. The main advantage of MRI is the ability to potentially obtain a comprehensive test on the coronary artery disease in the same sitting, including morphological, functional, hemodynamic, and metabolic information. With further improvements, coronary MRA will become an important part of this comprehensive examination.

Acknowledgement

This work was supported in part by US National Institutes of Health Grant HL38698.

References

1. Edelman RR, Manning WJ, Gervino E, Li W. Flow velocity quantification in human coronary arteries with fast, breath-hold MR angiography. J Magn Reson Imaging 1993; 3:699–703.

2. Manning WJ, Edelman RR. Magnetic resonance coronary angiography. Magn Reson Q 1993; 9:131–51.

3. Kim WY, Danias PG, Stuber M, et al. Coronary magnetic resonance angiography for the detection of coronary stenoses. N Engl J Med 2001; 345:1863–9.

4. Hofman MBM, Paschal CB, Li D, et al. MRI of coronary arteries: 2D breath-hold versus 3D respiratory gated acquisition. J Comput Assist Tomogr 1995; 19:56–62.

5. Alfidi RJ, Masaryk TJ, Haacke EM, et al. MR angiography of peripheral, carotid, and coronary arteries. AJR 1987; 149:1097–109.

6. Paulin S, von Schulthess GK, Fossel E, et al. MR imaging of the aortic root and proximal coronary arteries. AJR 1987; 148:665–70.

7. Vered Z, Kenzora J, Gutierrez F. Noninvasive evaluation of the left main coronary artery in man with magnetic resonance imaging. Am J Noninvas Cardiol 1990; 4:154–8.

8. Cho ZH, Mun CW, Friedenberg RM. NMR angiography of coronary vessels with 2D planar image scanning. Magn Reson Med 1991; 20:134–43.

9. Dumoulin CL, Souza SP, Darrow RD, Adams WJ. A method of coronary MR angiography. J Comput Assist Tomogr 1991; 15:705–10.

10. White RD, Caputo GR, Mark AS, et al. Coronary artery bypass graft patency: noninvasive evaluation with MR imaging. Radiology 1987; 164:681–6.

11. Rubinstein RI, Askenase AD, Thickman D, et al. Magnetic resonance imaging to evaluate patency of aortocoronary bypass grafts. Circulation 1987; 76:786–91.

12. White RD, Pflugfelder PW, Lipton MJ, Higgins CB. Coronary artery bypass grafts: evaluation of patency with cine MR imaging. AJR 1988; 150:1271–4.

13. Jenkins JPR, Love HG, Foster CJ, et al. Detection of coronary bypass graft patency as assessed by magnetic resonance imaging. Br J Radiol 1987; 61:2–4.

14. Aurigemma GP, Reichek N, Axel L, et al. Noninvasive determination of coronary artery graft patency by cine magnetic resonance imaging. Circulation 1989; 80:1595–602.

15. Frija G, Schouman-Claeys E, Lacombe P, et al. A study of coronary artery bypass graft patency using MR imaging. J Comput Assist Tomogr 1989; 13:226–32.

16. Lieberman JM, Botti RE, Nelson AD. Magnetic resonance imaging of the heart. Radiol Clin North Am 1984; 22:847–58.

17. Lenz GW, Haacke EM, White RD. Retrospective cardiac gating: a review of technical aspects and future directions. Magn Reson Imaging 1989; 7:445–55.

18. Stehling M, Chapman B, Howseman A, et al. Real-time NMR imaging of coronary vessels. Lancet 1987; 2:964–5.

19. Burstein D. MR imaging of coronary artery flow in isolated and in vivo hearts. J Magn Reson Imaging 1991; 1:337–46.

20. Edelman RR, Manning WJ, Burstein D, Paulin S. Coronary arteries: breath-hold MR angiography. Radiology 1991; 181:641–3.

21. Meyer CH, Hu BS, Nishimura DG, Macovski A. Fast spiral coronary artery imaging. Magn Reson Med 1992; 28:202–13.

22. Edelman RR, Chien D, Atkinson DJ, Sandstrom J. Fast time-of-flight MR angiography with improved background suppression. Radiology 1991; 179:867–70.

23. Manning WJ, Li W, Boyle NG, Edelman RR. Fat-suppressed breath-hold magnetic resonance coronary angiography. Circulation 1993; 87:97–104.

24. Li D, Paschal CB, Haacke EM, Adler LP. Coronary arteries: three-dimensional MR imaging with fat saturation and magnetization transfer contrast. Radiology 1993; 187:401–6.

25. Edelman RR, Manning WJ, Pearl J, Li W. Human coronary arteries: projection angiograms reconstructed from breath-hold two-dimensional MR images. Radiology 1993; 187:719–22.

26. Manning WJ, Li W, Edelman RR. A preliminary report comparing magnetic resonance coronary angiography with conventional angiography. N Engl J Med 1993; 328:828–32.

27. Pennell DJ, Bogren HG, Keegan J, et al. Assessment of coronary artery stenosis by magnetic reesonance imaging. Heart 1996; 75:127–33.

28. Duerinckx AJ, Urman MK. Two-dimensional coronary MR angiography: analysis of initial clinical results. Radiology 1994; 193:731–8.

29. Paschal CB, Haacke EM, Adler LP, Finelli DA. Magnetic resonance coronary artery imaging. Cardiovasc Intervent Radiol 1992; 15:23–31.

30. Paschal CB, Haacke EM, Adler LP. Three-dimensional MR imaging of the coronary arteries: preliminary clinical experience. J Magn Reson Imaging 1993; 3:491–500.

31. Stillman AE, Wilke N, Li D, et al. Ultrasmall superparamagnetic iron oxide to enhance MRA of the renal and coronary arteries: studies in human patients. J Comput Assist Tomogr 1996; 20:51–5.

32. Li D, Kaushikkar S, Haacke EM, et al. Coronary arteries: three-dimensional MR imaging with retrospective respiratory gating. Radiology 1996; 201:857–63.

33. Bailes DR, Gilderdale DJ, Bydder GM, et al. Respiratory ordered phase encoding (ROPE): a method for reducing respiratory motion artifacts in MR imaging. J Comput Assist Tomogr 1985; 9:835–8.

34. Haacke EM, Patrick JL. Reducing motion artifacts in two-dimensional Fourier transform imaging. Magn Reson Med 1986; 4:359–76.

35. Chien D, Atkinson DJ, Edelman RR. Strategies to improve contrast in TurboFLASH imaging: reordered phase encoding and k-space segmentation. J Magn Reson Imaging 1991; 1:63–70.

36. Atkinson D, Edelman R. Cineangiography of the heart in a single breath-hold with a segmented TurboFLASH sequence. Radiology 1991; 178:357–60.

37. Runge VM, Clanton JA, Partain CL, James AE Jr. Respiratory gating in magnetic resonance imaging at 0.5 tesla. Radiology 1984; 151:521–3.

38. Ehman RL, McNamara MT, Pallack M, et al. Magnetic resonance imaging with respiratory gating: techniques and advantages. AJR 1984; 143:1175–82.

39. Ehman RL, Felmlee JP. Adaptive technique for high-definition MR imaging of moving structures. Radiology 1989; 173:255–63.

40. Felmlee JP, Ehman RL, Riederer SJ, Korin HW. Adaptive motion compensation in MRI: accuracy of motion measurement. Magn Reson Med 1991; 18:207–13.

41. Korin HW, Ehman RL, Riederer SJ, et al. Respiratory kinematics of the upper abdominal organs: a quantitative study. Magn Reson Med 1992; 23:172–8.

42. Sachs TS, Meyer CH, Hu BS, et al. Real-time motion detection in spiral MRI using navigators. Magn Reson Med 1994; 32:639–45.

43. Wang Y, Riederer SJ, Ehman RL. Respiratory motion of the heart: kinematics and the implications for spatial resolution of coronary MR imaging. Magn Reson Med 1995; 33:713–19.

44. Oshinski JN, Hofland L, Mukundan S, et al. Two-dimensional coronary MR angiography without breath holding. Radiology 1996; 201:737–43.

45. McConnell MV, Khasgiwala VC, Savord BJ, et al. Comparison of respiratory suppression methods and navigator locations for MR coronary angiography. AJR 1997; 168:1369–75.

46. Pauly J, Nishimura D, Macovski A. A *k*-space analysis of small-tip-angle excitation. J Magn Reson 1989; 81:43–56.

47. Liu Y, Riederer SJ, Rossman PJ, et al. A monitoring, feedback, and triggering system for reproducible breath-hold MR imaging. Magn Reson Med 1993; 30:507–11.

48. Wang Y, Rossman PJ, Grimm RC, et al. Navigator-echo-based real-time respiratory gating and triggering for reduction of respiratory effects in 3D coronary imaging. Radiology 1996; 198:55–60.

49. Sachs TS, Meyer CH, Irarrazabal P, et al. The diminishing variance algorithm for real-time reduction of motion artifacts in MRI. Magn Reson Med 1995; 34:412–22.

50. Wang Y, Christy PS, Korosec FR, et al., Coronary MRI with a respiratory feedback monitor: the 2D imaging case. Magn Reson Med 1995; 33:116–21.

51. Wang Y, Grimm RC, Rossman PJ, et al. 3D coronary MR angiography in multiple breath-holds using a respiratory feedback monitor. Magn Reson Med 1995; 34:11–16.

52. Wielopolski PA, Manning WJ, Edelman RR. Single breath-hold volumetric imaging of the heart using magnetization-prepared 3D segmented echo-planar imaging. J Magn Reson Imaging 1995; 5:403–10.

53. Wielopolski PA, van Geuns RJ, de Feyter PJ, Oudkerk M. Breath-hold coronary MR angiography with volume-targeted imaging. Radiology 1998; 209:209–19.

54. Wielopolski PA, van Geuns RJ, de Feyter PJ, Oudkerk M. Coronary arteries. Eur Radiol 2000; 10:12–35.

55. Li D, Carr JC, Shea SM, et al. Coronary arteries: magnetization-prepared contrast-enhanced three-dimensional volume-targeted breath-hold MR angiography. Radiology 2001; 219:270–7.

56. Brittain JH, Hu BS, Wright GA, et al. Coronary angiography with magnetization-prepared T$_2$ contrast. Magn Reson Med 1995; 33:689–96.

57. Botnar RM, Stuber M, Danias PG, et al. Improved coronary artery definition with T2-weighted, free-breathing, three-dimensional coronary MRA. Circulation 1999; 99:3139–48.

58. Goldfarb JW, Edelman RR. Coronary arteries: breath-hold, gadolinium-enhanced, three-dimensional MR angiography. Radiology 1998; 206:830–4.

59. Zheng J, Li D, Bae KT, et al. Three-dimensional gadolinium-enhanced coronary MR angiography: initial experience. J Cardiovasc Magn Reson 1999; 1:33–41.

60. Kessler W, Laub G, Achenbach S, et al. Coronary arteries: MR angiography with fast contrast-enhanced three-dimensional breath-hold imaging-initial experience. Radiology 1999; 210:566–72.

61. Sakuma H, Goto M, Nomura Y, et al. Three-dimensional coronary magnetic resonance angiography with injection of extracellular contrast medium. Invest Radiol 1999; 34:503–8.

62. Wang Y, Winchester PA, Yu L, et al. Breath-hold three-dimensional contrast-enhanced coronary MR angiography: motion-matched *k*-space sampling for reducing cardiac motion effects. Radiology 2000; 215:600–7.

63. Carr JC, Tahieri H, Shea SM, et al. MR angiography of the coronary arteries using magnetization-prepared contrast-enhanced breath-hold volume targeted imaging (MPCE-VCATS): initial clinical experience. In: Proceedings of the 86th Scientific Assembly and Annual Meeting, Radiological Society of North America. Chicago, 2000:285.

64. Hofman MB, Henson RE, Kovacs SJ, et al. Blood pool agent strongly improves 3D magnetic resonance coronary angiography using an inversion pre-pulse. Magn Reson Med 1999; 41:360–7.

65. Stuber M, Botnar RM, Danias PG, et al. Contrast agent-enhanced, free-breathing, three-dimensional coronary magnetic resonance angiography. J Magn Reson Imag 1999; 10:790–9.

66. Carr JC, Simonetti OP, Bundy JM, et al. Cine MR angiography of the heart with segmented true fast imaging with steady-state precession. Radiology 2001; 219:828–34.

67. Spuentrup E, Bornert P, Botnar RM, et al. Navigator-gated free-breathing three-dimensional balanced fast field echo (TrueFISP) coronary magnetic resonance angiography. Invest Radiol 2002; 37:637–42.

68. Li W, Stern JS, Mai VM, et al. MR assessment of left ventricular function: quantitative comparison of fast imaging employing steady-state acquisition (FIESTA) with fast gradient echo cine technique. J Magn Reson Imaging 2002; 16:559–64.

69. Oppelt A, Graumann R, Fischer H, et al. FISP: a new fast MRI sequence. Electromedica 1986; 3:15–18.

70. Deshpande VS, Shea SM, Laub G, et al. 3D magnetization-prepared True-FISP: A new technique for imaging coronary arteries. Magn Reson Med 2001; 46:494–502.

71. Deimling M, Heid O. Magnetization prepared trueFISP imaging. In: Proceedings of the Society for Magnetic Resonance in Medicine, San Francisco, 1994:495.

72. Li D, Dolan B, Walovitch RC, Lauffer RB. Three-dimensional MR imaging of coronary arteries using an intravascular contrast agent. Magn Reson Med 1998; 39:1014–18.

73. Bundy JM, Simonetti OP, Laub G, Finn JP. Segmented TrueFISP cine imaging of the heart. In: Proceedings of the International Society for Magnetic Resonance in Medicine, 7th Annual Meeting, Philadelphia, 1999:1282.

74. McCarthy RM, Deshpande VS, Shea SM, et al. 3D magnetization-prepared True FISP: initial clinical evaluation of a new MR technique for imaging coronary arteries In: Proceedings of the Radiological Society of North America Annual Meeting, Chicago, 2001:1469.

75. Deshpande VS, Shea SM, Chung YC, et al. Improving spatial resolution of breath-hold 3D True-FISP imaging of coronary arteries using asymmetric sampling. J Magn Reson Imaging 2002; 15:473–8.

76. Nishimura DG, Vasanawala S. Analysis and reduction of the transient response in SSFP imaging. In: Proceedings of the International Society for Magnetic Resonance in Medicine, 8th Annual Meeting, Denver, 2000:301.

77. Deshpande VS, Chung YC, Zhang Q, et al. Reduction of transient signal oscillations in True-FISP using a linear flip angle series magnetization preparation. Magn Reson Med 2003; 49:151–7.

78. Deshpande VS, Shea SM, Li D. Artifact reduction in True-FISP imaging of the coronary arteries by adjusting imaging frequency. Magn Reson Med 2003; 49:803–9.

79. Shea SM, Deshpande VS, Chung YC, Li D. 3D True-FISP imaging of the coronary arteries: improved contrast with T2-preparation. J Magn Reson Imaging 2002; 15:597–602.

80. Deshpande VS, Shea SM, Li D. Contrast-enhanced coronary artery imaging using 3D TrueFISP. Magn Reson Med 2003; 50:570–7.

81. Manning WJ, Li W, Cohen SI, et al. Improved definition of anomalous left coronary artery by magnetic resonance coronary angiography. Am Heart J 1995; 130:615–17.

82. McConnell MV, Ganz P, Selwyn AP, et al. Identification of anomalous coronary arteries and their anatomic course by magnetic resonance coronary angiography. Circulation 1995; 92:3158–62.

83. Post JC, van Rossum AC, Bronzwaer JGF, et al. Magnetic resonance angiography of anomalous coronary arteries. Circulation 1995; 92:3163–71.

84. Klessen C, Post F, Meyer J, et al. Depiction of anomalous coronary vessels and their relation to the great arteries by magnetic resonance angiography. Eur Radiol 2000; 10:1855–7.

85. Bunce NH, Lorenz CH, Keegan J, et al. Coronary artery anomalies: assessment with free-breathing three-dimensional coronary MR angiography. Radiology 2003; 227:201–8.

86. Oshinski JN, Hofland L, Dixon WT, Pettigrew RI. Magnetic resonance coronary angiography using navigator echo gated real-time slice following. Int J Card Imaging 1998; 14:191–9.

87. Stuber M, Botnar RM, Danias PG, et al. Submillimeter three-dimensional coronary MR angiography with real-time navigator correction: comparison of navigator locations. Radiology 1999; 212:579–87.

88. Manke D, Bornert P, Nehrke K, et al. Accelerated coronary MRA by simultaneous acquisition of multiple 3D stacks. J Magn Reson Imaging 2001; 14:478–83.

89. Bogaert J, Kuzo R, Dymarkowski S, et al. Coronary artery imaging with real-time navigator three-dimensional turbo-field-echo MR coronary angiography: initial experience. Radiology 2003; 226:707–16.

90. Stuber M, Botnar RM, Danias PG, et al. Double-oblique free-breathing high resolution three-dimensional coronary magnetic resonance angiography. J Am Coll Cardiol 1999; 34:524–31.

91. Taylor AM, Jhooti P, Wiesmann F, et al. MR navigator-echo monitoring of temporal changes in diaphragm position: implications for MR coronary angiography. J Magn Reson Imaging 1997; 7:629–36.

92. Jhooti P, Wiesmann F, Taylor AM, et al. Hybrid ordered phase encoding (HOPE): an improved approach for respiratory artifact reduction. J Magn Reson Imaging 1998; 8:968–80.

93. Bunce NH, Jhooti P, Keegan J, et al. Evaluation of free-breathing three-dimensional magnetic resonance coronary angiography with hybrid ordered phase encoding (HOPE) for the detection of proximal coronary artery stenosis. J Magn Reson Imaging 2001; 14:677–84.

94. Nguyen TD, Ding G, Watts R, Wang Y. Optimization of view ordering for motion artifact suppression. Magn Reson Imaging 2001; 19:951–7.

95. Keegan J, Gatehouse P, Yang GZ, Firmin D. Coronary artery motion with the respiratory cycle during breath-holding and free-breathing: implications for slice-followed coronary artery imaging. Magn Reson Med 2002; 47:476–81.

96. Peters DC, Korosec FR, Grist TM, et al. Undersampled projection reconstruction applied to MR angiography. Magn Reson Med 2000; 43:91–101.

97. Larson AC, Simonetti OP, Li D. Coronary MRA with 3D undersampled projection reconstruction TrueFISP. Magn Reson Med 2002; 48:594–601.

98. Stuber M, Botnar RM, Kissinger KV, Manning WJ. Free-breathing black-blood coronary MR angiography: initial results. Radiology 2001; 219:278–83.

99. Stuber M, Botnar RM, Spuentrup E, et al. Three-dimensional high-resolution fast spin-echo coronary magnetic resonance angiography. Magn Reson Med 2001; 45:206–11.

100. Fayad ZA, Fuster V, Fallon JT, et al. Noninvasive in vivo human coronary artery lumen and wall imaging using black-blood magnetic resonance imaging. Circulation 2000; 102:506–10.

101. Fayad ZA, Fuster V. Clinical imaging of the high-risk or vulnerable atherosclerotic plaque. Circ Res 2001; 89:305–16.

102. Kim WY, Stuber M, Bornert P, et al. Three-dimensional black-blood cardiac magnetic resonance coronary vessel wall imaging detects positive arterial remodeling in patients with nonsignificant coronary artery disease. Circulation 2002; 106:296–9.

103. Sodickson DK, Manning WJ. Simultaneous acquisition of spatial harmonics (SMASH) – fast imaging with radiofrequency coil arrays. Magn Reson Med 1997; 38:591–603.

104. Pruessmann KP, Weiger M, Scheidegger MB, Boesiger P. SENSE: sensitivity encoding for fast MRI. Magn Reson Med 1999; 42:952–62.

105. Bornert P, Aldefeld B, Nehrke K. Improved 3D spiral imaging for coronary MR angiography. Magn Reson Med 2001; 45:172–5.

106. Yang PC, McConnell MV, Nishimura DG, Hu BS. Magnetic resonance coronary angiography. Curr Cardiol Rep 2003; 5:55–62.

107. Bornert P, Stuber M, Botnar RM, et al. Direct comparison of 3D spiral vs. Cartesian gradient-echo coronary magnetic resonance angiography. Magn Reson Med 2001; 46:789–94.

108. Taylor AM, Keegan J, Jhooti P, et al. A comparison between segmented k-space FLASH and interleaved spiral MR coronary angiographys seqences. J Magn Reson Imaging 2000; 11:394–400.

109. Johansson LO, Nolan MM, Taniuchi M, et al. High resolution magnetic resonance coronary angiography of the entire heart using a new blood-pool agent, NC100150 injection: comparison with invasive x-ray angiography in pigs. J Cardiovasc Magn Reson 1999; 1:139–43.

110. Li D, Zheng J, Weinmann HJ. Contrast-enhanced MR imaging of coronary arteries: comparison of intra- and extravascular contrast agents in swine. Radiology 2001; 218:670–8.

111. Huber ME, Paetsch I, Schnackenburg B, et al. Performance of a new gadolinium-based intravascular contrast agent in free-breathing inversion-recovery 3D coronary MRA. Magn Reson Med 2003; 49:115–21.

112. Stuber M, Botnar RM, Fischer SE, et al. Preliminary report on in vivo coronary MRA at 3 tesla in humans. Magn Reson Med 2002; 48:425–9.

113. Hardy CJ, Darrow RD, Pauly JM, et al. Interactive coronary MRI. Magn Reson Med 1998; 40:105–11.

114. Hardy CJ, Saranathan M, Zhu Y, Darrow RD. Coronary angiography by real-time MRI with adaptive averaging. Magn Reson Med 2000; 44:940–6.

115. Nayak KS, Pauly JM, Yang PC, et al. Real-time interactive coronary MRA Magn Reson Med 2001; 46:430–5.

116. Sussman MS, Stainsby JA, Robert N, et al. Variable-density adaptive imaging for high-resolution coronary artery MRI Magn Reson Med 2002; 48:753–64.

117. Hardy CJ, Zhao L, Zong X, et al. Coronary MR angiography: respiratory motion correction with BACSPIN. J Magn Reson Imaging 2003; 17:170–6.

118. Yang GZ, Burger P, Gatehouse PD, Firmin DN. Locally focused 3D coronary imaging using volume-selective RF excitation. Magn Reson Med 1999; 41:171–8.

119. Botnar RM, Stuber M, Danias PG, et al. A fast 3D approach for coronary MRA. J Magn Reson Imaging 1999; 10:821–5.

120. Deshpande VS, Wielopolski PA, Shea SM, et al. Coronary artery imaging using contrast-enhanced 3D segmented EPI. J Magn Reson Imaging 2001; 13:676–81.

121. Sachs TS, Meyer CH, Pauly JM, et al. The real-time interactive 3-D-DVA for robust coronary MRA. IEEE Trans Med Imaging 2000; 19:73–9.

122. Shea SM, Kroeker RM, Deshpande VS, et al. Coronary artery imaging: 3D segmented *k*-space data acquisition with multiple breath-holds and real-time slab following. J Magn Reson Imaging 2001; 13:301–7.

123. Muller MF, Fleisch M, Kroeker R, et al. Proximal coronary artery stenosis – three-dimensional MRI with fat saturation and navigator echo. J Magn Reson Imaging 1997; 7:644–51.

124. Woodard PK, Li D, Haacke EM, et al. Detection of coronary stenoses on source and projection images using three-dimensional MR angiography with retrospective respiratory gating: preliminary experience. AJR 1998; 170:883–8.

125. Wang Y, Ehman RL. Retrospective adaptive motion correction for navigator-gated 3D coronary MR angiography. J Magn Reson Imaging 2000; 11:208–14.

126. Foo TK, Ho VB, Hood MN. Vessel tracking: prospective adjustment of section-selective MR angiographic locations for improved coronary artery visualization over the cardiac cycle. Radiology 2000; 4:283–9.

127. Sardanelli F, Molinari G, Zandrino F, Balbi M. Three-dimensional, navigator-echo MR coronary angiography in detecting stenoses of the major epicardial vessels, with conventional coronary angiography as the standard of reference. Radiology 2000; 214:808–14.

128. van Geuns RJ, Wielopolski PA, de Bruin HG, et al. MR coronary angiography with breath-hold targeted volumes: preliminary clinical results. Radiology 2000; 217:270–7.

129. Regenfus M, Ropers D, Achenbach S, et al. Noninvasive detection of coronary artery stenosis using contrast-enhanced three-dimensional breath-hold magnetic resonance coronary angiography. J Am Coll Cardiol 2000; 36:44–50.

130. Regenfus M, Ropers D, Achenbach S, et al. Comparison of contrast-enhanced breath-hold and free-breathing respiratory-gated imaging in three-dimensional magnetic resonance coronary angiography. Am J Cardiol 2002; 90:725–30.

131. Foo TK, Saranathan M, Hardy CJ, Ho VB. Coronary artery magnetic resonance imaging: a patient-tailored approach. Top Magn Reson Imaging 2000; 11:406–16.

132. Etienne A, Botnar RM, Van Muiswinkel AM, et al. 'Soap-bubble' visualization and quantitative analysis of 3D coronary magnetic resonance angiograms. Magn Reson Med 2002; 48:658–66.

133. Cline HE, Thedens DR, Irarrazaval P, et al. 3D MR coronary artery segmentation. Magn Reson Med 1998; 40:697–702.

134. Achenbach S, Giesler T, Ropers D, et al. Detection of coronary artery stenoses by contrast-enhanced, retrospectively electrocardiographically-gated, multislice spiral computed tomography. Circulation 2001; 103:2535–8.

135. Nieman K, Oudkerk M, Rensing BJ, et al. Coronary angiography with multi-slice computed tomography. Lancet 2001; 357:599–603.

10

CMR evaluation of cardiac valvular disease

Craig H Scott, Victor A Ferrari, Christine H Lorenz

Introduction

The cardiac valves are small, rapidly moving structures that perform the vital function of controlling blood flow in the heart. Without valves, the heart would not be able to generate pressure, and thus forward flow. Echocardiography is the best noninvasive imaging technology to diagnose valve pathology due to its ability to resolve the leaflets with sufficient spatial and temporal resolution to evaluate valve morphology and function. Cardiac magnetic resonance imaging (CMR) can also successfully evaluate heart valve function using comparable techniques. In addition, CMR is uniquely suited to evaluate the effects of valvular disease on left- and right-ventricular function; however, this topic is addressed elsewhere in this book.

The purpose of this chapter is to discuss heart valve function and dysfunction as well as findings associated with valvular disease, to compare echocardiography with CMR techniques, and to provide strategies to allow the user to optimize the evaluation of cardiac valves using CMR. A review of basic valve anatomy and function will be given first, followed by a description of echocardiography and CMR techniques. An understanding of certain fundamental echocardiographic principles is crucial before attempting to image valvular function using CMR methods.

Cardiac valves in the normal heart

This section discusses normal heart valve function. Pathologic changes in the valves or in the heart alter the relationships introduced below, and will be discussed later in this chapter.

There are four cardiac valves: tricuspid, pulmonic, mitral, and aortic. The tricuspid and mitral valves start as a single valve early in development, but divide into two valves when the heart septates. These valves are referred to as the atrioventricular (AV) valves. The AV valves are connected to the papillary muscles, which are attached to the ventricles via the chordae tendineae. As the heart contracts, the papillary muscles shorten, tightening the valve apparatus and preventing the valves from bulging backward into the atria. The pulmonic and aortic valves also form after the division of the truncus arteriosus into the aorta and pulmonary artery. These valves are referred to as the ventriculoarterial (VA) valves as defined by their position, or the semilunar valves by their configuration. The VA valve leaflets are supported by struts that are attached to the intima of the great vessels.

The following considerations are important:

- The entire cardiac output must traverse each valve in sequence. If there is no shunting present, the same average flow crosses each valve per minute.
- The AV valves are larger (4–6 cm^2) than the VA valves (3–4 cm^2).
- When the valves are open, the pressure between the two chambers (for the AV valves, the atria and ventricles; for the VA valves, the ventricles and the great vessels) can be assumed to be the same.
- Any valve will open with only a slight pressure increase in the direction of flow, and will remain closed as long as there is a greater downstream pressure.

These principles will have greater significance in the discussion of valve pathology.

Basic imaging concepts

Two-dimensional echocardiography

The echocardiographic image is created by scanning an ultrasound beam (2–4 MHz for chest wall or transthoracic echocardiography (TTE)) through a sector, then detecting the echoes from the beam as they reflect from various interfaces in the body. A two-dimensional image can be constructed using the direction of the beam and the time it takes for the echo to return to the transducer. The spatial and temporal resolution of the echocardiographic image is limited by three principles: the speed of sound, its frequency, and the attenuation properties of the structures to be imaged. The temporal resolution of the image is related to the speed of sound. Since the speed of sound is finite, and since the echo machine must wait for the deepest signal to return before sending out another pulse, it can only produce a finite number of images per second. Fortunately, physics allows for >30 frames/s, which provides excellent temporal resolution. Spatial resolution is dependent on the frequency of the ultrasound beam. Unfortunately, as the beam frequency increases, more attenuation occurs (less of the original beam returns to the transducer), thereby reducing the practical depth of imaging. Frequencies between 2 and 4 MHz are used with TTE, while frequencies of 7 MHz can be used with transesophageal echo (TEE) probes. Greater frequency and decreased attenuation are the main reasons TEE images are clearer and can resolve smaller structures. Because of the way in which the image is constructed using scan lines, the lateral resolution decreases with increasing depth for both TTE and TEE, but is constant along a single scan line in the depth direction.

Doppler imaging

The Doppler principle as applied to ultrasound states that an object moving toward or away from an ultrasound source will change the frequency of the reflected sound proportional to the speed of the object relative to the source. The most common application of the Doppler principle in echocardiography is to determine the velocity and direction of flowing blood. Doppler imaging produces a signal only if the flow, or a vector of the flow, is moving toward or away from the transducer. Laminar flow perpendicular to the transducer cannot be evaluated using Doppler imaging. There are two versions of Doppler imaging: continuous-wave (CW) and pulsed-wave (PW) imaging. Both methods have strengths and drawbacks. PW Doppler can determine the velocity even in a very small area, akin to a 'velocity biopsy', but is limited to velocities under ~ 1 m/s. Above this value (known as the Nyquist limit), the signal becomes aliased, and its velocity and direction cannot be accurately assessed. CW Doppler has no velocity limit (in the physiologic range), and can quantify the magnitude and direction of the velocity along a line, but cannot determine the depth from which the velocity signal originated. Spectral Doppler produces a graph of velocity versus time for either PW or CW (Figure 10.1).

The brightness of the graph at a particular timepoint denotes the power of the signal at that velocity. A brighter

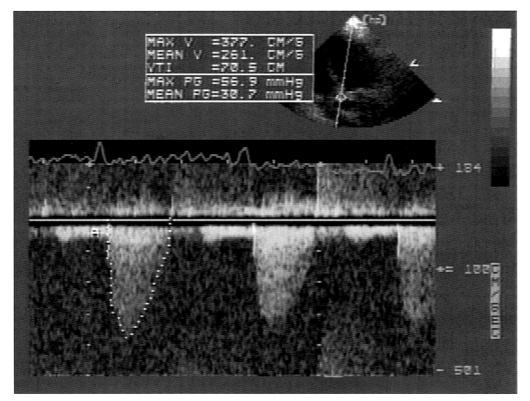

Figure 10.1
Continuous-wave Doppler echocardiographic display in a patient with aortic stenosis from the apical five-chamber view. The graphic depicts the relationship between velocity (in cm/s) on the vertical axis and time (in s) on the horizontal axis. By tracing the velocity envelope, the peak and mean transvalvular gradients (56.9 and 30.7 mmHg, respectively), as well as the velocity–time integral, VTI (70.5 cm), may be calculated. These values are important in determining the degree of valvular stenosis in addition to quantifying the valve area – an important parameter used in decisions regarding valve replacement.

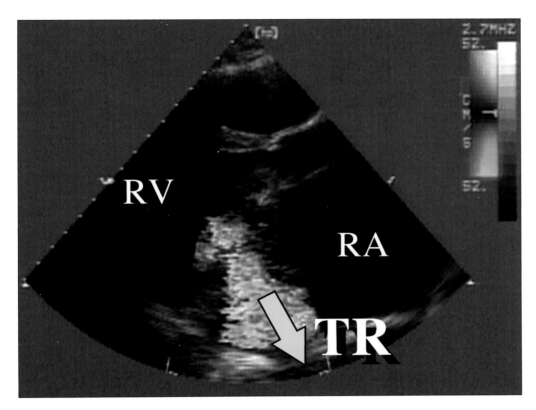

Figure 10.2
Color Doppler image of a patient with moderate–severe tricuspid regurgitation (TR). The severely dilated right atrium (RA) and the moderately dilated right ventricle (RV) are identified. The direction of the eccentric regurgitant flow from the valve plane to the dome of the RA is shown by the arrow. The turbulent flow is encoded by green and yellow, while more laminar flow would be identified by blue and red.

tracing indicates that more of the blood signal is flowing at that specific velocity. Color Doppler uses the PW method to map the velocities in a given area and display those velocities using pseudocolors. The more advanced color maps can display the slower laminar flow, usually coded as red and blue, while coding the faster, usually turbulent, flows that exceed the Nyquist limit as yellow and green: even though their absolute velocity or direction cannot be determined, the presence of turbulence can be detected and displayed, thereby depicting regurgitant and stenotic flow as jets of rapidly moving blood (Figure 10.2).

Magnetic resonance imaging

CMR of the valves requires careful attention to imaging parameters. Adequate CMR is a balance between image contrast and spatial and temporal resolution. Increasing one parameter usually results in a decrease of the others. Typically, MR images of the heart must be gated to acquire enough signal to make a usable image, and to demonstrate flows relative to the cardiac cycle. Imaging small structures such as normal valve leaflets is difficult because cardiac motion is only relatively consistent. The heart does not return to its exact starting point with each beat due to variations in filling and small changes in the R–R interval introduced by respiration and changes in sympathetic tone. The mechanics of respiration (the

motion of the diaphragm) also introduces variation. The combination of a small structure 1 mm thick moving inconsistently over a several centimeter-long path and an imaging technique with a slow 'shutter speed' makes CMR of the valves especially challenging.

Fortunately, MR images can be formed in different ways, each with specific strengths and weaknesses. MR images are created by manipulating the magnetic gradients and radiofrequency (RF) pulses in such a way as to encode the different areas of the image so they can be localized in three dimensions (slice-select, frequency, and phase directions). The pulse sequence, a programmed variation of the 3D magnetic field and modulated RF energy, can change the appearance of the image, highlighting different aspects. The most commonly used pulse sequences for cardiac applications include the spin-echo and gradient-echo techniques.

The conventional spin-echo (CSE) method produces images where no signal returns from areas with moving blood; therefore, the cardiac chambers and vessels appear black. Tissue signal is dependent on the relative proton concentration. The sequence is made up of two RF pulses. Changing the time between the pulses, also known as the echo time (TE), changes the image: if TE >40 ms, there is greater contrast between blood and tissue, while if TE < 20 ms, there is less motion artifact and more signal, so for imaging valvular heart disease, the best balanced image is acquired using a TE = 20–40 ms. This technique can acquire multiple slices, but not multiple frames, so may be best used for scout images to plan other acquisitions. Newer methods, known as fast spin-echo (FSE) techniques, allow image acquisitions that have high contrast between blood and tissue, as in CSE images, but may be acquired in significantly less time. These techniques produce high-quality images of the valves and permits assessment of valvular morphology.[1]

Gradient-echo techniques depict laminar blood flow with a bright signal intensity and turbulent blood flow as dark. Tissue contrast is lower than in CSE sequences, but the images can be collected rapidly through systole, allowing cine or motion images to be acquired. Gradient-echo images can be optimized in various ways. Acquisition of multiple image lines can shorten image acquisition to one breathhold. TE can be increased to allowing the visualization of turbulent jets and facilitate quantification of regurgitation or stenosis.

Echo-planar imaging can be applied to both spin-echo and gradient techniques. It increases temporal resolution by acquiring all image lines after one pulse, but is technically challenging to implement and requires higher-strength gradient magnets. The images can be distorted by inhomogeneities of the magnetic field caused by metallic implants, such as clips or prosthetic heart valves. Echo-planar imaging holds promise for valve evaluation, but is not used commonly for clinical studies.

Velocity mapping techniques allow for blood flow quantification. Information about velocity is encoded in the phase of the detected MR signal. This information can be incorporated into an image, allowing the CMR equivalent of color Doppler imaging but with less of a directional limit and no aliasing velocity[2] (Figure 10.3)

With present techniques, it is possible to reform real-time analysis of the CMR signal with image rates up to 6 frames/s, which is close to color Doppler echocardiography, which can have frame rates of 6–15 frames/s, depending on the machine settings and capabilities.

Color flow CMR compares well with color Doppler echocardiography, providing similar results. However, it does not fully image the regurgitant jet close to the valve. High flow velocities do not image as well, because spins moving through the plane may not be fully excited, while spins moving within the plane may move too far during readout.

CMR velocity mapping relies on the fact that moving blood carries with it the RF frequency shifts from a different area of the image, and is therefore out of phase with the RF frequencies of the 'local' tissue. Two phase maps are acquired: a reference phase map and a velocity-encoded phase map. Subtraction of these two maps reduces artifacts and results in a usable velocity map. This map can be oriented within the imaging plane in the frequency and/or phase directions, which provides an image similar to echocardiogram color Doppler or through the plane (orthogonal to the plane) in the slice-selection direction. Turbulent flow (which is common in valve pathology) will cause signal loss if TE is long. If TE is shortened to 3.6 ms, velocities up to 6 m/s can be measured without loss of signal.[3] The limits of shortening echo time are dependent on the capabilities of the CMR system. Few jets of stenosis or regurgitation exceed 6 m/s, which would require a 144 mmHg pressure difference to be present, which only occurs in very unusual circumstances, such as dynamic left-ventricular outflow obstruction due to asymmetric septal hypertrophy of the left ventricle.

Doppler echocardiography can also provide an assessment of cardiac diastolic performance by measuring the velocity and pattern of AV valve inflow. CMR can provide similar information using velocity mapping to detect the relatively slow flow of AV valve inflow.[4]

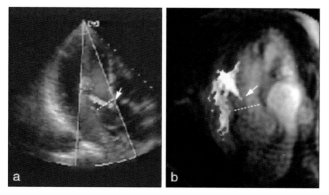

Figure 10.3
Color flow Doppler ultrasound image from the apical long axis view of a patient with aortic regurgitation (AR) (a) and corresponding real-time color flow MR images (b). The arrows point to the AR jets, and the dotted lines indicate the aortic valve plane. (Adapted from Nayak et al. Magn Reson Med 2000; 43:251–8.[2])

Fluid dynamics

The use of a few fluid dynamics principles permits the calculation of valve areas that are too small to resolve even with high-resolution imaging. These methods also facilitate the estimation of pressure differences between chambers and the determination of the severity of regurgitation. Fluid dynamic evaluation relies on velocity information, which can be acquired through echo Doppler or CMR velocity mapping; therefore, these concepts apply to both imaging modalities.

The continuity equation

The continuity equation states that an incompressible fluid flowing through a closed pipe must accelerate if the

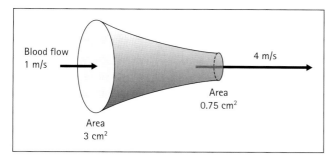

Figure 10.4
Cone-shaped model of the left-ventricular outflow tract (LVOT) in aortic stenosis, with a depiction of the stenotic valve to the right and the origin of the LVOT to the left. The blood flow entering the cone on the left must equal the flow exiting the cone to the right; therefore, the continuity equation can be used to solve for the area of the stenotic valve (typically the unknown parameter in clinical applications).

pipe narrows. In other words, flow past any point in the pipe must be the same:

$$A_1 V_1 = A_2 V_2, \qquad \text{where flow = cross-sectional area } (A) \times \text{ average velocity } (V).$$

If we model the left-ventricular outflow tract (LVOT) and proximal aorta as a round pipe (Figure 10.4), then any degree of aortic stenosis will result in an acceleration of the flow from the beginning of the LVOT to the narrowest part of the valve. Blood is essentially incompressible; therefore, the model is practical from a physiological standpoint.[5]

PW Doppler acquired from the apical views or CMR velocity mapping in either the long or the short axis can measure the velocity just below the aortic valve, while 2D imaging can determine the diameter of the LVOT. The area of the LVOT can be determined using

$$A = \pi r^2 = \pi d^2/4, \qquad \text{where } r \text{ is the radius and } d \text{ is the diameter of the LVOT.}$$

Alternatively, the cross-sectional LVOT area can be measured directly from the short-axis images at this location.

CW Doppler or CMR velocity mapping with short echo times can measure the rapid velocity flow at the valve orifice. Given that the stenosis is limited to the valve, the maximum velocity occurs at this location. CW cannot determine the location of the maximum-velocity jet, but it can determine its velocity profile. The CMR velocity map can be acquired in the short- or long-axis plane, provided that the region of greatest velocity is present in the image plane. Therefore, we have three values for the continuity equation:

$$A_1 = \pi \, (\text{LVOT diameter})^2/4,$$
$$V_1 = \text{PW Doppler velocity at the LVOT},$$
$$V_2 = \text{CW Doppler velocity at the valve};$$

thus, the aortic valve area A_2 can be calculated as

$$A_2 = A_1 V_1 / V_2.$$

The continuity equation can also be used to measure the mitral valve area. A_1 and V_1 are measured at the LVOT in the same fashion as aortic stenosis measurements, but the V_2 measurement is taken at the stenotic mitral valve using the CW Doppler or CMR velocity mapping. Since the LV inflow and outflow must be the same per beat (in the absence of aortic regurgitation), the continuity equation may still be applied.

The modified Bernoulli equation

The modified Bernoulli equation states that, assuming a small regurgitant orifice between two chambers at different pressures, the velocity of fluid flowing from the high-pressure chamber to the low-pressure chamber (and ignoring viscosity and flow acceleration of the fluid) is given by the equation

$$\frac{\rho V^2}{2} = \Delta p,$$

i.e. $$V = \sqrt{2\Delta p / \rho} \,,$$

where Δp is the difference in pressure and V is the maximum velocity of the fluid (of mass density ρ) traversing the small orifice. Note that as long as the orifice is small, the velocity is related only to the pressure, not to the size of the orifice. This relationship does not apply if the orifice is large compared with the size of the chambers, which occasionally occurs with severe or torrential tricuspid regurgitation, and which limits its use in pulmonary artery (PA) pressure estimation under these conditions.

This relationship between pressure and velocity is quite useful in valvular pathology. Regurgitant jet orifices tend to be quite small, on the order of 1 mm² or less. Fortunately, small degrees of tricuspid valve regurgitation (TR) are quite common, occurring in ~60% of patients having echocardiograms. TR meets the criterion for application of the modified Bernoulli equation: two chambers (right atrium (RA) and right ventricle (RV)) at different pressures during systole with a small orifice between. Therefore, if we assume an RA pressure, and there is no pulmonic stenosis, we can estimate the pressure in the pulmonary artery, and assess patients for pulmonary hypertension without invasive catheterization:

PA pressure (mm Hg) = 4 (peak TR velocity)²

+ RA pressure (estimated),

where the unit conversions for mass density and other variables have been performed.

The modified Bernoulli equation can also be used to estimate the gradient across any stenotic valve or prosthetic valve, or between the ventricles in the case of a ventricular septal defect.

The pressure half-time measurement

The pressures in the cardiac chambers vary throughout the cardiac cycle. In the case of mitral stenosis, for example, the pressure in the left atrium (LA) remains elevated throughout diastole because the small mitral orifice does not allow for adequate volume to empty from the LA in a timely manner. Since the pressure remains high, the velocity of flow across the mitral value also remains elevated for longer than normal. Therefore, a measurement of the slope (rate of decline) of the mitral inflow velocity can estimate the degree of mitral stenosis. The pressure half-time is the time it takes for the pressure to fall to 50% of its original value, or roughly 70% of the original velocity (by the modified Bernoulli equation). The mitral valve area is therefore given as

mitral valve area (cm^2) = 220/pressure half-time (s),

where 220 is an empirically determined value and corrects for the units. This measurement is semiquantitative and can be impacted upon by coexisting disease, such as aortic regurgitation, which will increase the pressure in the LV during diastole, thus decreasing the pressure half-time and resulting in an overestimation of the mitral valve area.

Deceleration slope

A similar principle to pressure half-time can be used to qualitatively estimate the degree of aortic regurgitation (AR). If the AR is minimal, the pressure will fall slowly in the aorta as distal run-off occurs in diastole. If there is a significant amount of AR, the central aortic pressure will drop more quickly and the LV pressure will rise as blood flows into the LV across both the mitral (normal, antegrade) and aortic (abnormal, retrograde) valves during diastole. Thus, the velocity of the AR jet will decrease more quickly in severe AR. By extension, the deceleration slope will be shallow in mild AR but steep in severe AR. Like pressure half-time, however, the deceleration slope can be affected by factors such as the rate of distal run-off or coexisting mitral regurgitation.

PISA (proximal isovelocity surface area)

The degree of regurgitation can be estimated in several ways: the absolute area or volume of the regurgitant jet, the area or volume of the jet relative to the area of the chamber, the regurgitant orifice area, or the reversal of flow caused by the regurgitation at some upstream or downstream point. A recent technique known as the proximal isovelocity surface area (PISA) method calculates the regurgitant orifice area by taking advantage of the anatomy and the aliasing velocity of the PW color Doppler image. Further description is beyond the scope of this chapter, but Enriquez-Sarano et al[6] have described the clinical relevance of this measurement.

Review

Velocity imaging is essential to the assessment of stenosis and regurgitation, but its limitations must be considered. The combination of spectral and color displays of PW and CW Doppler echocardiography allow us to circumvent many of the limitations described above regarding these techniques. CMR velocity mapping is also a powerful tool for evaluating cardiac valve function and is less limited than echocardiography with respect to direction and maximum velocity. By using velocity imaging in combination with the continuity and modified Bernoulli equations, the pressure half-time measurement, and deceleration slopes, the degree of valvular stenosis and regurgitation of all four cardiac valves may be semiquantitatively or quantitatively estimated.

Optimizing CMR of heart valves

CMR provides accurate assessment of flow velocities and anatomic measurements as well as hemodynamic parameters, comparable to echocardiographic techniques. However, just as in echocardiography, certain limitations and quality control measures must be considered in order to obtain reproducible results.

In general, these technical factors may be classified into two categories: the location of the measurement, and the scan parameters. Measurement in the correct location is required to avoid problems such as structures moving through the imaging slice, phase offset errors due to imaging far from the isocenter, and measuring obliquely relative to the flow direction. Scan parameters must be chosen to provide a satisfactory assessment of the valve and its potential range of transvalvular velocities. These parameters include an appropriate TE for minimizing signal loss, a maximum encoded velocity value (VENC) in the expected range relative to the valve pathology, adequate temporal resolution to avoid undersampling of velocities, and adequate coverage of the cardiac cycle (retrospective vs prospective triggering).[7–9]

Since the critical parameters vary depending on the valve being studied and the desired hemodynamic measurement, we will describe these features together with the associated valve disorder.

For qualitative assessment of valve disease, it is important to recognize that the type of sequence used, and the imaging parameters used (especially TE), strongly influence the appearance of jets. Conventional gradient-echo cine sequences are sensitive to dephasing from local turbulence and therefore, produce larger signal voids compared with newer fast imaging techniques. However, the apparent size of a jet (and thus severity of regurgitation or stenosis) is related to TE, with a longer TE resulting in more dephasing and thus more signal loss from a given jet. The newer steady-state imaging sequences (bFFE, TrueFISP, and FIESTA)[10–12] are inherently less sensitive to flow disturbances, and thus may mask mild valve disease. On the other hand, they can be more useful for depicting the high-velocity core of a stenotic jet. Real-time imaging approaches allow rapid evaluation of valves interactively, but care must be taken to assure adequate signal and temporal resolution.[13] In general, for qualitative assessment, a standard protocol should be established to assure consistency in interpretation.

For all valve examinations, the scout images described below are a prerequisite to identify the correct imaging planes.

Standard localization[14]

1. Transverse (axial) rapid scout images from the aortic arch to the level of the diaphragm.
2. Two-chamber scout bisecting the apex and mitral valve plane.
3. Two short-axis scouts at the mitral valve plane and at the midventricular level to demonstrate the orientation of the aortic outflow tract.
4. True four-chamber, LVOT and two-chamber cine acquisitions

Quality control issues in CMR of valvular disease

As mentioned in the protocols above, the accuracy of the measurements are dependent on selecting the correct temporal resolution, VENC, and slice position. In addition, it is important to measure at the isocenter of the magnet to avoid unwanted phase offsets due to eddy currents. Measurements are often corrected via the scanner manufacturer's software for gradient-induced phase offsets (Maxwell term correction[15]). Further correction can be done on a patient-to-patient basis by acquiring a reference phase map with the same parameters in a uniform phantom. Nonetheless, it is important at each imaging center to gain a level of confidence in the measurements and an estimation of the degree of accuracy one can expect. It is recommended that internal consistency controls be performed wherever possible. For example:

1. Does the stroke volume determined from LV volume changes during systole match that determined from an aortic flow measurement?
2. Do the flow volumes in the left and right pulmonary arteries sum to the volume in the main pulmonary artery?
3. In the absence of shunt, does the pulmonary artery stroke volume match the aortic stroke volume?

Variations in both the image acquisition technique and the image analysis may contribute to errors. It is important that that users be aware of these potential pitfalls when performing flow measurements with MRI.

Valvular stenosis – principles

Stenosis of the cardiac valves is caused by aging, as well as a number of other disease processes. For example, aortic stenosis can be the result of a congenital bicuspid valve in a younger population, while the elderly have so-called 'senile' calcific disease. Rheumatic disease can also result in aortic stenosis. Membranes that obstruct flow can be found below the aortic valve in the LVOT (subaortic) or in the aorta above the aortic valve (supravalvular) resulting in stenosis, but do not result in obstruction of the valve itself. This finding (elevated transaortic gradient in the setting of normal leaflet motion) is a feature of a sub- or supravalvular obstruction, and must be excluded in patients presenting for evaluation. Mitral stenosis is usually caused by rheumatic valve disease as a result of streptococcal infection(s) earlier in life, and carcinoid tumors of the lung can produce serotonin and similar substances that cause valve dysfunction and stenosis. Rheumatic disease can also affect the tricuspid valve, but spares the pulmonic valve. Tricuspid stenosis is also seen with carcinoid tumors of the gastrointestinal tract. Most pulmonic stenosis is congenital and is not uncommonly associated with syndromes, such as tetralogy of Fallot. See Table 10.1 for more information.

Regardless of the cause, stenosis results in more important hemodynamic changes when the valve area is reduced to 2 cm². Symptoms tend to be mild, and exercise tolerance may be affected. Valves with smaller areas will develop gradients or increased resistance to flow, while valves <1 cm² can result in clinical symptoms at rest or with minimal exertion.

Table 10.1 Causes of valvular stenosis

Aortic	Mitral	Tricuspid	Pulmonic

Rheumatic
Senile calcific
Bicuspid/congenital
Sub/supravalvular membranes
	Rheumatic
	Anorexigen use
	Pulmonary carcinoid
		Rheumatic
		Gastrointestinal carcinoid
			Congenital:
			  subvalvular, valvular,
			  supravalvular

Table 10.2 Qualitative and quantitative definitions of valvular stenosis

Quantitative (area in cm^2)	Qualitative
>2.0	Sclerosis
1.5–2.0	Mild stenosis
1.0–1.5	Moderate stenosis
<1.0 (0.7–1.0)[a]	Severe stenosis[a]
(<0.7)	Critical stenosis[a]

[a] Critical stenosis is reserved for the aortic valve only. All other valves are considered severe if the valve area is <1.0.

Valve area can be qualitatively and quantitatively classified using invasive and noninvasive techniques. While each valve has a different normal area, their stenotic areas can be qualitative grouped as shown in Table 10.2.

Valve area is related to valve gradient through Ohm's law, which states that the pressure gradient across a stenotic valve will increase linearly with increases in flow:

$$\Delta p = FR,$$

where $\Delta p =$ is the change in pressure across the valve, F is the flow (or cardiac output), and R is the resistance, which is inversely proportional to the valve area. Therefore, as cardiac output increases, stenotic gradients rise. This is one of the reasons why patients with stenosis develop symptoms, or have worsening of symptoms, with exertion.

In general, the degree of stenosis at a given timepoint is considered to be relatively constant. However, valves are composed of biological tissue, and can deform with increased pressure. Therefore, the valve area may actually increase slightly at higher cardiac outputs. Conversely, in patients with decreased ventricular function, gradients will be low; however, cardiac output is also low, thereby masking significant stenosis. This underestimation of stenosis, usually of the aortic valve, is most commonly noted during cardiac catheterization using the flow-dependent Gorlin equation to estimate valve area. Conversely, the continuity equation is independent of flow and will therefore correctly identify stenosis in a low-flow state. The modified Bernoulli equation will indicate the low gradient appropriately as well.

Stenosis results in both cardiac and vascular remodeling. Stenosis causes gradients that tend to increase pressure proximal to the stenotic valve. This is a stimulus for dilatation of the atria, and concentric hypertrophy (wall thickening without a change in chamber dimensions) of the ventricles. This increased pressure can be transmitted back to the proximal valve or chamber; for example, mitral stenosis can increase LA pressure, thereby increasing RV pressure, and resulting in RV hypertrophy. Table 10.3 lists the major changes in anatomy that occur with stenotic valves.

Imaging valvular stenosis

Valve disease can modify the appearance and the function of the valve as well as altering blood flow and heart chamber size, function and wall thickness (Table 10.3). Valves can be described as thickened, calcified, or with reduced mobility and leaflet pliability. Noninvasive flow and gradient measurements can provide additional functional information. Finally, stenosis causes structural

Table 10.3 Anatomic changes as a result of valvular stenosis

Aortic	Mitral	Tricuspid	Pulmonic
Aortic poststenotic dilation	Left-atrial enlargement	Inferior/superior vena caval dilatation	Right-ventricular hypertrophy and enlargement
Left-ventricular hypertrophy	Pulmonary hypertension	Hepatic enlargement/congestion	
	Right-ventricular hypertrophy	Peripheral edema	

changes to the heart, with pressure-related changes in the chamber proximal (upstream) to the stenosis. If that chamber is a ventricle, hypertrophy will result, while atria tend to dilate. This is unlike regurgitation, which is a volume load to the upstream chamber and causes dilatation of both the atria and ventricles. In the case of aortic stenosis, the rapidly flowing jet increases shear in the proximal aorta and may result in poststenotic dilatation of the proximal segment of the aorta. Imaging protocols and interpreters must take these changes into account.

CMR has not been highly successful in studying valve morphology – due in part to limitations in spatial and temporal resolution. The problems are technical in origin: the heart moves through the chest with respiration; the AV valve plane moves toward and away from the LV apex during systole and diastole, respectively; and the valves themselves have displacements of 1–2 cm during the cardiac cycle, This somewhat chaotic movement makes the use of gated acquisitions challenging. A large body of research has focused on the attempt to increase the speed of acquisition, without sacrificing spatial resolution. In 1998, a Task Force of the European Society of Cardiology published guidelines for the use of CMR for cardiac valve assessment. Its conclusions were that echocardiography should be more commonly used for the assessment of valve morphology in stenosis, except for some specific disease states: supravalvular pulmonic and aortic stenosis.[16] This is not to say that CMR cannot assess other aspects of valvular stenosis, but rather that echocardiography was adequate for initial screening and assessment, and was widely available. Quantification of aortic[17] and mitral[18] stenosis using CMR velocity mapping has been compared with Doppler- or catheterization-based valve area assessments with favorable results. Calcification of the aortic valve and root is commonly seen in senile aortic stenosis, and can be identified using gradient-echo CMR.[19]

Since the Task Force report, however, other studies using new techniques have shown promise in assessment of valve morphology: black-blood CMR techniques, using a double inversion recovery fast spin-echo sequence with breathholding techniques, identified three leaflets in 85% of subjects and at least two leaflets in 97%. They were easily able to differentiate normal from bicuspid or thickened valves[1] (Figure 10.5).

Black-blood CMR improves valve morphology assessment by eliminating artifacts due to moving and static blood, and complements cine gradient-echo techniques, which can image valve calcification. The breathhold technique significantly reduces imaging time while maintaining the benefits of a T1-weighted method (high blood–tissue contrast).

Velocity mapping can also be used to determine valve area. One study measured the valve area by performing velocity mapping at the level of the aortic valve, then measuring the area of the velocity map.[20] This is akin to using the planimetry method for determining valve area in echocardiography. This method has potential limitations: partial-volume effects occur between the valve and the blood pool if the voxel size is too large (too many voxels are half valve and half blood flow, resulting in a systematic error in velocity information), and these partial-volume effects worsen as the orifice gets smaller. Hamilton[21] showed that there must be at least 16 pixels across the orifice to keep the error due to partial-volume effects to <10%. In order to achieve this resolution given a valve area of 0.7 cm,[2] the diameter of the orifice would be ~1 cm; therefore, the voxel dimension would have to be smaller than 0.63 mm in order to minimize the partial-volume effect, which translates to a 16 cm field of view with a 256 × 256 acquisition. The next assumption is that the flow pattern is not parabolic but plug in configuration (Figure 10.6). If only voxels with velocities >50% of

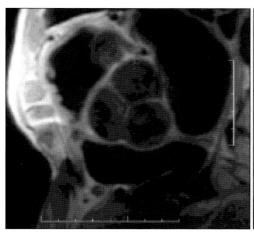 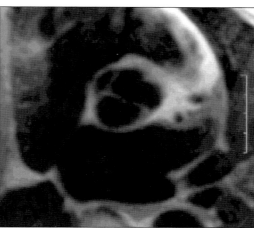

(a)   (b)

Figure 10.5
Fast spin-echo images for the normal (a) and bicuspid (b) aortic valves. (Modified from Arai et al. J Magn Reson Imag 1999; 10: 771–7.[1])

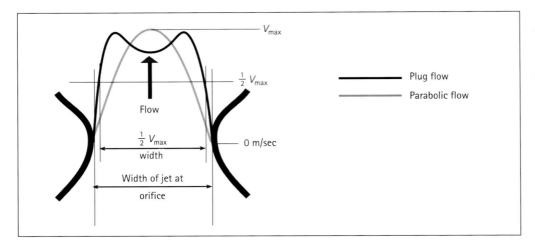

Figure 10.6
Comparison of velocity profiles in plug versus parabolic flows in aortic stenosis.

maximum are included, and since plug flow tends to normalize the velocity profile across the orifice, ignoring the lower velocities excludes more partial-volumed pixels, thus increasing the accuracy.[22] Bicuspid aortic valve disease can also be discerned by velocity-mapping the orifice.[1]

Cardiac output (CO) can be quantified by velocity mapping using these assumptions, with high correlation between CMR and invasive determinations. CO has important prognostic value and helps to confirm the determined gradients and valve area. It can be measured in the distal ascending aorta or the pulmonary artery before the bifurcation. For imaging simplicity in the case of aortic stenosis, CO may be measured at the valve plane, although the flow pattern may make analysis more difficult.[20]

Mitral stenosis results in an increase in LA pressure and causes a gradient to form between the LA and LV. The result is that diastolic filling, which is usually rapid and biphasic, becomes prolonged, with increased and sustained gradients throughout diastole. As the degree of mitral stenosis worsens, the end-systolic mitral inflow gradient increases and the end-diastolic gradient increases to an even greater extent, thus the slope of the pressure gradient over the course of diastole. Determination of diastolic velocities across the stenotic mitral valve allow determination of this slope, and the valve area is given by the pressure half-time equation as well as the peak valve gradient using the modified Bernoulli equation. CMR phase shift velocity mapping using a reduced echo time (3.6 ms) to allow imaging of turbulent flow has been used to determine mitral and aortic stenosis peak gradients[3] (Figure 10.7). This technique permits in-plane and through-plane velocity measurements, which is useful for valves with complicated anatomy where planimetry of the valve area is difficult.

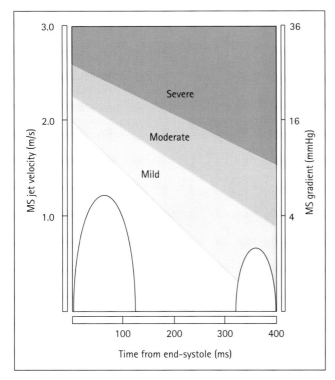

Figure 10.7
Effect of severity of mitral stenosis (MS) on diastolic gradient. Pressure half-time echo-cordiographic methods and CMR techniques correlate well with larger transvalvular gradients.

Valvular regurgitation – principles

Valvular regurgitation results from multiple disease processes. Regurgitation is caused by valve destruction (e.g. due to endocarditis or trauma) or by dysfunction due to gradual deterioration of a bicuspid aortic valve or myxomatous degeneration of the mitral valve. It may also occur as a result of loss of support structures, such as in aortic dissection with resultant aortic insufficiency, or due

Table 10.4 Causes of valvular regurgitation			
Aortic	*Mitral*	*Tricuspid*	*Pulmonic*
Endocarditis	Endocarditis	Physiologic	Physiologic
Rheumatic	Rheumatic	Endocarditis	Congenital
Hypertension	Myxomatous degeneration	Rheumatic	Pulmonary hypertension
Bicuspid/congenital	Marfan syndrome	Right-ventricular biopsy	
Aortic dissection	Systemic hypertension	Pulmonary hypertension	
	Left-ventricular chamber dilation	Deceleration injury	
	Deceleration injury		

to dilatation of the LV, which results in mitral insufficiency. Rheumatic valve disease can cause reduction in leaflet pliability resulting in stenosis, but also results in regurgitation when the valve closes improperly or the valve coaptation is distorted or compromised. Table 10.4 lists the most common causes of valvular regurgitation.

Unlike stenosis, there is no universally accepted numeric value for determination of the degree of regurgitation. Qualitative assessments (mild, moderate, severe) are typically used clinically. The tricuspid and pulmonic valves have small degrees of regurgitation during normal function in most patients. The common occurrence (~ 60% of patients) of TR means that in many cases where assessment of pulmonary hypertension is needed, the TR velocity can estimate the pressure adequately. The one case where the relationship does not hold is in very severe, or torrential, TR. The modified Bernoulli equation assumes that the orifice between the chambers is small, but if it is large, then the velocity is lower, and thus underestimates the actual gradient.

The velocity of the jet itself is not helpful in determining the severity of regurgitation: the jet velocity is solely dependent on the pressure difference between the two chambers if the regurgitant orifice is small. However, measurement of other parameters can assist in quantifying regurgitation. Valvular orifice area can be calculated with the PISA method. The volume of the regurgitation can be assessed in 2D and 3D velocity mapping. This allows for calculation of the regurgitant fraction:

regurgitant fraction = regurgitant volume/stroke volume,

which can be directly measured by CMR techniques. The deceleration slope can also be used to quantify regurgitation, and is typically used for AR. Small amounts of AR cause little change in the central arterial pressure during diastole, while severe AR will cause a drop in aortic pressure and a rise in diastolic ventricular pressure. Therefore, the slope of the diastolic AR jet will be steeper as AR worsens.

Regurgitation causes a volume load to the proximal chamber as well as the chamber in the direction of flow.

AR causes dilatation and hypertrophy of the LV due to regurgitation and increased preload. AR can also dilate the aorta, because the stroke volume has to be greater in order to maintain cardiac output, and rheologic factors (shear stress, etc.) result in trophic changes at the endothelial level. A similar event occurs with mitral regurgitation. The LA dilates because of the volume and pressure increase, and the LV dilates as well because of the extra volume present on the subsequent beat. In order to move the larger volume in a similar amount of time, the filling velocity must increase. Finally, severe regurgitation can cause reversal of forward flow in parts of the circulation. AR is considered severe if flow reverses in the distal aortic arch and/or abdominal aorta during diastole. Severe AR can even cause diastolic mitral regurgitation, when the pressure in the LV rises rapidly due to the large regurgitant volume. This extra volume load in the LV can actually reverse the direction of mitral flow across an open mitral valve (diastolic mitral regurgitation), or cause the valve to close prematurely. Also, severe mitral regurgitation can reverse flow in the pulmonary veins, which are normally filling the LA during systole. These associated findings in the setting of valvular disease are useful in quantifying (or confirming) the degree of regurgitation. With time, aortic and mitral regurgitation can cause irreversible cardiac dilatation and decreased atrial and ventricular function.

Imaging valvular regurgitation

Valvular diseases that result in regurgitation will modify the appearance of the valve as well as changing blood flow direction and heart chamber size, function, and wall thickness. (Table 10.5). Regurgitant valves can prolapse, be eroded by endocarditis, or undergo thickening and fibrosis by rheumatic disease. As in stenotic lesions, non-invasive flow and gradient measurements can provide useful information. Regurgitation is a volume load to the proximal chamber and causes dilatation of both atria and ventricles; therefore, imaging must focus not only on the

Table 10.5 Chronic changes as a result of valvular regurgitation

Aortic	Mitral	Tricuspid	Pulmonic
Eccentric left-ventricular hypertrophy (wall thickening plus chamber enlargement)	Left-atrial enlargement Pulmonary hypertension Right-ventricular hypertrophy	Inferior/superior vena caval dilation Hepatic enlargement/congestion Peripheral edema	Right-ventricular dilatation

regurgitant jet, but also on its effects on cardiac and extracardiac structure and function.

CMR can image regurgitation in various ways. Since regurgitation is typically turbulent, owing to the high pressure and relatively small regurgitant orifice, dephasing of spins will occur in certain pulse sequences, such as conventional cine MR acquisitions. In these sequences, blood will typically appear bright, but turbulence will cause dephasing and a signal void in the territory of the jet. Cine MR flow void size has been compared with color Doppler echocardiography-derived mitral regurgitant area,[23] with the CMR flow void method consistently having smaller areas. Velocity mapping can also be used to demonstrate regurgitant jets – again because of their turbulence and high velocities. By applying the modified Bernoulli equation, we can calculate jet velocity given a known pressure difference. For example, if the LA pressure were 20 mmHg and the systolic systemic pressure 120 mmHg, the difference (100 mmHg) would result in a jet with a 5 m/s maximum velocity (100 mmHg = $4 \times (5 \text{ m/s})^2$). AR has a velocity of ~4 m/s, while tricuspid regurgitation velocity in the normal patient at sea level is ~2 m/s. It is possible to combine phase-acquired velocity mapping with a color display similar to the color Doppler display, and by only displaying jets with velocities higher than, for example 1.5 m/s, or coloring higher velocities differently, regurgitant jets may be highlighted. Accurate placement of the imaging plane and velocity mapping can allow for assessment of reversal of flow seen in severe regurgitation.

Changes in chamber size, wall thickness, and global and regional function can be accurately assessed using CMR. Cine MR in the LV short- and long-axis views provides excellent qualitative and quantiative information regarding anatomy and function. CMR is presently considered the gold standard for volumetric assessment,[24] and end-diastolic and end-systolic volumes permit calculation of ejection fraction and stroke volume.

There are special considerations regarding the accurate quantification of regurgitant volumes. Quantification of regurgitation can be based on regurgitant volume or fraction; however, if only a single valve is significantly regurgitant and no intracardiac shunt is present, then assessment of LV and RV stroke volumes can be used to calculate regurgitant volume. Further, if only one valve in the left or

one valve in the right heart are regurgitant, then the ventricular stroke volume can be compared with the velocity profiles measured in the great vessels, and these results have been favorably compared with Doppler echocardiography measurements of pulmonic regurgitation.[25]

AR can be quantified by using a single phase-velocity-encoded slice at or below the level of the coronary ostia, perpendicular to the aorta. This method works well for the aortic valve, because the valve plane is relatively stationary during diastole, and therefore during the period the regurgitation is occurring.[26] As the imaging plane moves distally in the aorta, aortic compliance introduces inaccuracies in the measurement – resulting in a decrease in measured regurgitant volume by up to 70% in mild AR and 30% in severe AR.[27] Also, coronary flow may account for as much as 14% of reverse flow in the ascending aorta during diastole.[28] If the imaging plane is too close to the valve, blood acceleration will interfere with the measurement. Nineteen patients and four normal volunteers were studied with this technique and the results compared with echo- or angiographically-derived estimates of AR.[27] The two methods agreed, with some overlap at the moderate–severe or severe grades. One advantage is that this method is not affected by regurgitation of other heart valves. Phase velocity mapping with accurate imaging plane position has an accuracy >90% and equally high intra- and inter-observer variability.[20] Volumetric calculations compared with phase velocity mapping also show reasonable correlations (the accuracy in 89% for regurgitant fraction and 84% for regurgitant volume). Recently, methods for correction of through-plane motion with respect to calculating regurgitant volumes have been proposed, and further experience is being accumulated.[29]

Anatomic imaging is helpful in determining the cause of the regurgitation. CMR excels at imaging the great vessels. It has been proven efficacious in AR due to endocarditis and aortic dissection from hypertension or Marfan syndrome. Spin-echo MR can determine the size and shape of aortic aneurysms from any cause, and in cases of endocarditis with mycotic aneurysm, CMR may be superior to TEE.[30] In patients with Marfan syndrome, CMR is the imaging technique of choice due to its ability to accurately measure aortic root size and distensibility, and to repeat these measures without the use of invasive procedures or ionizing radiation.[31] In fact, CMR may be able to identify a subset of Marfan patients who have aortic root asymmetry that may predispose to dissection even before the root has dilated.[32] CMR is the gold standard for imaging aortic dissection, with the highest sensitivity and specificity of any imaging technique.

Unfortunately, mitral valve functional imaging is much less conducive to a single-slice method due to through-plane motion. Newer slice-following methods, which adjust the imaging plane to compensate for the longitudinal through-plane motion have improved upon this technical problem.[29] Finally, atrial fibrillation is common in patients with significant mitral regurgitation. The control volume method, which is a generalization of the continuity equation, utilizes a 3D velocity data acquisition centered on the regurgitant orifice.[33] A control volume containing only the regurgitation is then drawn, allowing for any variant anatomy and excluding LV outflow. The method has been successfully tested in vitro, in a phantom that simulates mitral valve systolic motion.[34] In order to be successful, the control volume must track the motion of the mitral valve, which has yet to be applied in vivo.

Prosthetic heart valves

Most heart valve prostheses contain some metal components, which commonly have paramagnetic properties. This characteristic causes a local disturbance of the magnetic field around the device, which, while preventing direct imaging of the device itself, does not significantly affect the flow profile created by the device. This profile can be detected downstream of the prosthesis and thus permits assessment of valvular function. An in vitro and in vivo study of bileaflet mechanical heart valves was able to determine downstream flow velocity profiles in normal valves and in subjects without symptoms.[35] The valve disturbed the image within one valve diameter from the prosthesis using a free induction decay acquired echo sequence, which minimized flow artifact by shortening echo time and image acquisition.[36] Unlike normal ascending aortic flow (which is similar to plug flow), downstream to a bileaflet prosthesis, flow has two distinct peaks, which can have twice the velocity of the trough between them.[37] Aortic wall shear forces may be affected by these rapid eccentric jets, resulting in focal dilatation of the aorta, especially if the prosthesis is not seated perpendicular to the aortic walls.

Another important point is that heart valve function and position are not appreciably affected by CMR and may be performed safely,[38] allowing assessment of

secondary findings, such as cardiac function and wall thickness.

Echocardiography can be somewhat limited in the assessment of prosthetic valves due to the inability of sound to penetrate the metal and carbon fiber elements that make up mechanical valves. However, TEE can adequately assess valve function and diagnose endocarditis in most patients. Only rarely can mechanical prosthetic valve function not be fully assessed by echocardiography; however, in patients with contraindications to TEE, fluoroscopy of the valve leaflets or CMR are other alternatives.

The next section will focus on the practical aspects of imaging the cardiac valves, and will provide information useful for clinical imaging of valvular function.

CMR sequences
The aortic valve

Evaluation of the aortic valve with CMR includes a description of the valve morphology, the degree of stenosis or regurgitation, and LV size and function. The assessment of LV function is discussed elsewhere in this book. One approach to imaging the aortic valve is described below:

- *Step 1:* From the LVOT cine images[14], acquire a second set of cine images in a perpendicular orientation, which depicts a coronal view of the LV outflow tract (Figure 10.8a,b).
- *Step 2:* To visualize the valve en face in order to verify the number of leaflets, acquire another cine view at the level of the aortic valve, using both the coronal and LVOT views to guide placement of the imaging slice (Figure 10.9a,b). The valve will move through the imaging plane during systole, but in most cases the leaflets can be visualized. If further evaluation is required, a black blood turbo spin-echo technique can be used in the same slice plane for visualization of the valve leaflets[1].
- *Step 3:* The aortic valve area may be estimated by calculating the pressure gradient using the modified Bernoulli equation, or by using the continuity equation.[39] For estimation of the peak velocity at the valve plane, it is important to determine the direction of the flow jet through the valve, since many jets are eccentric. The direction of the jet can usually be appreciated from the two previously acquired cine views of the outflow tract. In some rare cases, it may be necessary to acquire yet another cine view bisecting the jet in one of these views. Real-time imaging is an emerging technique that can also be used to evaluate flow patterns as shown in Figure 10.10.[13] Cine phase contrast flow imaging may then be performed with encoding in

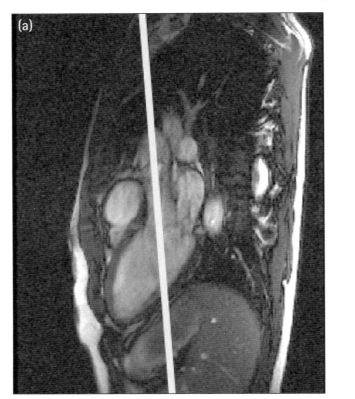

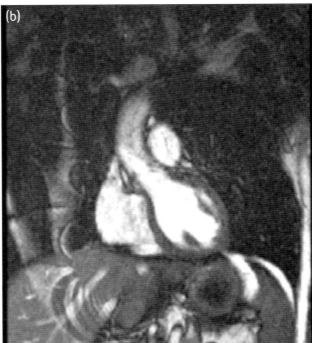

Figure 10.8
(a) Left-ventricular outflow tract view, showing slice position for oblique coronal view of the aortic outflow tract. (b) Resulting view from slice placement shown in (a).

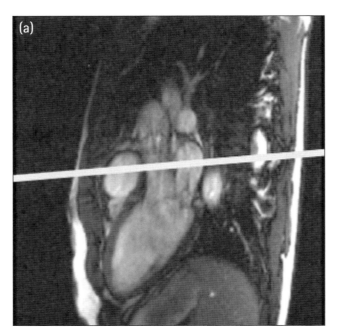

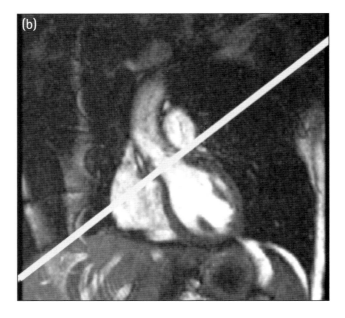

Figure 10.9
Slice position for acquiring en face view of the aortic valve.

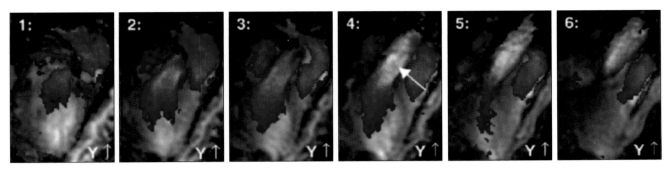

Figure 10.10
Real-time color-encoded flow images in contiguous planes. (Adapted from Nayak and Hu. Magn Reson Med 2003; 49:188–92.[13])

either the through-plane or the in-plane direction. For through-plane measurement, assure that the slice is placed perpendicular to the jet, just above the aortic valve (Figure 10.11; the arrow indicates the direction of the flow jet and the line indicates the slice location). TE should be as short as possible, and temporal resolution should be ≤30 ms to avoid underestimation of the peak velocity. Spatial resolution should 1–2 mm in-plane and 5–6 mm through-plane to minimize partial-volume effects. VENC should be set to 500 to 600 cm/s to avoid aliasing. For in-plane flow measurements, assure that the field of view is rotated so that the jet direction is along the readout direction in the image (along the direction of the arrow in Figure 10.11).

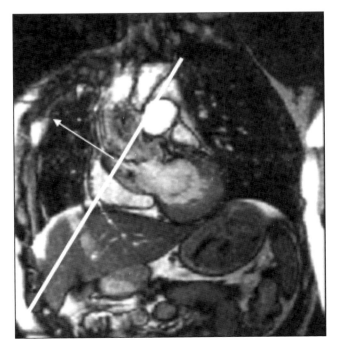

Figure 10.11
Oblique coronal view of aortic stenosis jet. The arrow indicates the direction of the jet and the line indicates the slice position perpendicular to the jet. (Image courtesy of Dr Anna John, Royal Brompton Hospital, London.)

- *Step 4:* Once the acquisition is complete, the peak velocity can be determined using single-pixel interrogation or small ROI interrogation of the images throughout time to find the maximum velocity. This velocity can then be used in the modified Bernoulli equation to estimate the peak pressure gradient.[39] Adequate temporal resolution is essential in making flow measurements. Figure 10.12 illustrates the importance of adequate temporal resolution in making flow measurements. The curve in Figure 10.12a has a temporal resolution of 55 ms while the curve in Figure 10.12b has a temporal resolution of 22 ms. One can readily see that poor temporal resolution can result in undersampling of the early systolic period and underestimation of the peak velocity. Alternatively, to use the continuity equation, one can make an additional flow measurement below the valve in the outflow tract.
- *Step 5:* For AR, the slice position should be parallel to the valve, at the valve plane (at end-diastole) or just above the valve plane as shown in Figure 10.13. It is not critical to be perpendicular to the regurgitant jet in this case, since the flow volume, not the peak velocity, will be measured. The VENC can normally be in the range of 200–300 cm/s without resulting in aliasing. TE should be minimized, and the temporal resolution should be ≤30 ms. In this case, since flow during diastole is important, it is important to use retrospective triggering in order to assure that data are acquired over the entire cardiac cycle.
- *Step 6:* To evaluate the severity of aortic regurgitation, the regurgitant volume or regurgitant fraction can be estimated. By planimetering the flow field across the aortic valve throughout the cardiac cycle, one can plot the average velocity versus time as shown in Figure 10.14. The forward volume can be determined as the area under the positive part of the flow curve. The regurgitant volume can be determined as the area under the negative part of the flow curve from ES to the end of the cardiac cycle (Figure 14). The regurgitant fraction is then the ratio of the reverse to the forward flow volume.

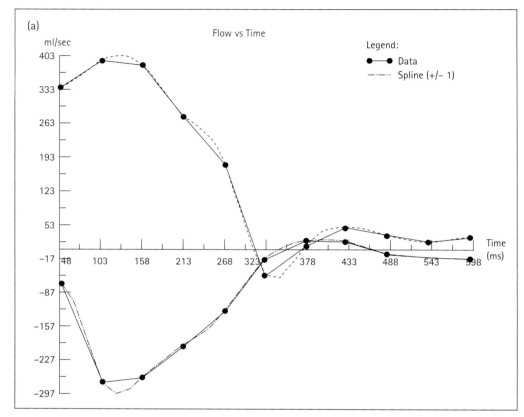

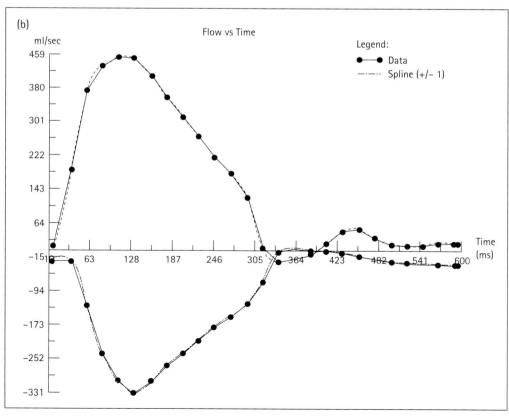

Figure 10.12
Flow-versus-time curves:
(a) temporal resolution of
55 ms; (b) temporal
resolution of 22 ms. Poor
temporal resolution can
result in missing the peak in
early systole and thereby
underestimating the peak
velocity.

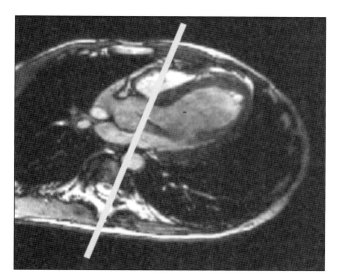

Figure 10.13
Slice positioning for aortic regurgitation. The slice is placed parallel to the valve plane.

The mitral valve

The mitral valve is especially difficult to assess due to its geometry and its motion during the cardiac cycle. However, estimates of mitral regurgitant volume can be made when the measurement of the mitral valve inflow is combined with measurement of aortic valve outflow (assuming no AR). For mitral stenosis, measurement of the peak inflow velocity and inflow area can also be made.

- *Step 1:* Starting with four-chamber and LVOT cine series, one can identify the location of the mitral leaflets throughout the cardiac cycle. For mitral stenosis, one can place a flow imaging slice perpendicular to the mitral leaflets at the narrowest region (Figure 10.15). Temporal resolution should be <30 ms, and the VENC should initially be 200–300 ms, but may need to be increased to avoid aliasing in the case of severe stenosis. The resulting flow curve from a small ROI or single pixel in the inflow region shows the E- and A-waves analogous to Doppler echocardiography measurements (Figure 10.16).
- *Step 2:* For mitral regurgitation, a two-step acquisition is required. First, an aortic flow acquisition is required, with the flow-imaging slice above the valve as shown in Figure 10.17. VENC can be 150–200 cm/s.
- *Step 3:* The next acquisition is at the mitral valve plane. The acquisition may be planned at end-diastole across the mitral annulus on an LVOT cine or four-chamber cine series (Figure 10.18). Flow encoding can normally be between 150 and 300 cm/s. Only flow during

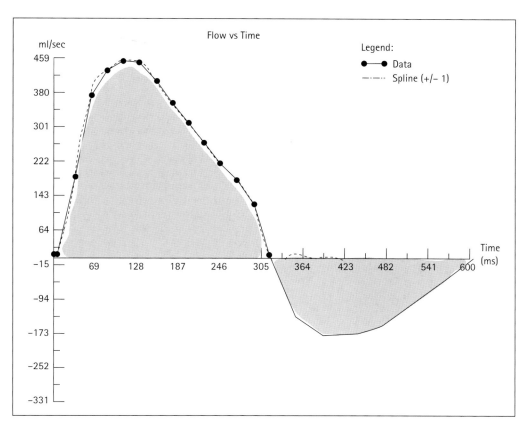

Figure 10.14
Demonstration of aortic regurgitation. The area under the curve from ED to ES (positive flow values) is the forward stroke volume and the area under the curve from ES to ED (negative flow values) is the regurgitant volume.

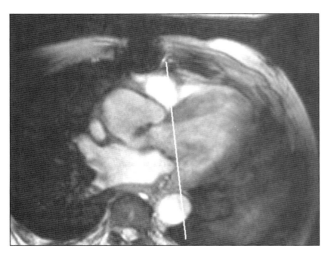

Figure 10.15
Slice positioning for mitral stenosis evaluation with a flow-imaging slice perpendicular to the mitral leaflets at the narrowest region.

diastole will be measured, therefore, aliased flow in systole due to the regurgitant jet can be ignored.

- *Step 4:* Determination of regurgitant fraction combines the forward stroke volume across the aortic valve and the inflow through the mitral valve. The amount of blood that crosses the mitral valve during diastole minus the amount that crosses the aortic valve during systole is the regurgitant volume (assuming no aortic

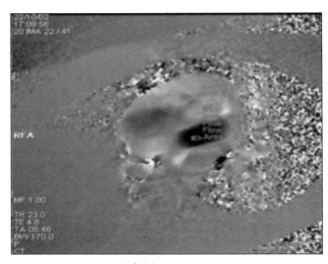

(a)

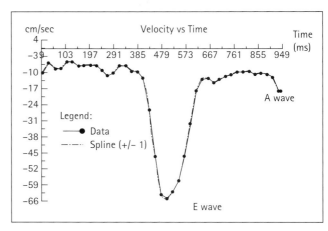

(b)

Figure 10.16
The resulting flow curve (b) from a small ROI or a single pixel in the inflow region (a) shows the E- and A-waves analogous to echocardiography.

regurgitation). The regurgitant fraction is thus the regurgitant volume divided by the forward stroke volume. For the mitral acquisition, it is important to ignore systole where motion of the mitral valve plane is artifactually identified as velocity through the valve, and begin planimetering the mitral valve flow area only in diastole.

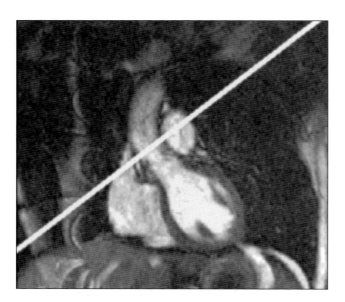

Figure 10.17
The first step in the evaluation of mitral regurgitation, with a flow acquisition imaging slice above the aortic valve.

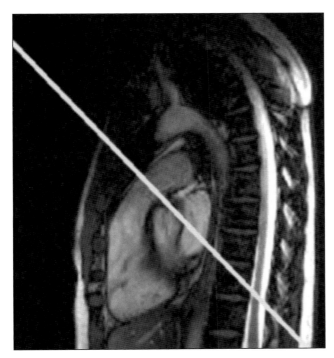

Figure 10.18
The second step in the evaluation of mitral regurgitation, with a flow imaging acquisition across the mitral annulus.

The tricuspid valve

The tricuspid regurgitant fraction can be determined in a manner similar to the mitral regurgitant fraction, using flow acquisitions of the tricuspid valve and the pulmonary artery. However, for estimating the peak velocity of a tricuspid regurgitant jet, CMR is imprecise. The direction of the jet is often difficult to determine, and dephasing in the jet itself results in decreased accuracy.

The pulmonic valve

Additional scout images are required to locate the pulmonic valve.

- *Step 1:* From the initial transverse scout images, select locations showing the bifurcation of the main pulmonary artery with the left and right pulmonary arteries, and the pulmonic valve level in the RV outflow tract (RVOT). Acquire a cine series through the main PA and valve level as shown in Figure 10.19.
- *Step 2:* Using the resulting RVOT cine image, one can generally visualize the location of the pulmonic valve. Compared with the aortic valve, which can usually be seen even in a static image, the pulmonic valve can often only be seen in a cine loop. If the pulmonary artery is distorted, one may wish to perform another coronal oblique view through the valve as shown in Figure 10.20.
- *Step 3:* To visualize the valve en face, the procedure is the same as for the aorta. Using the two RVOT cines acquired in the last step, one can place a slice parallel to the valve at end-diastole and acquire an additional cine sequence (Figure 10.21).
- *Step 4:* To assess the degree of pulmonic regurgitation, the procedure is analogous to that for the aortic valve. The slice for velocity measurement is placed just above the pulmonic valve at ED as shown in Figure 10.21. The VENC can be set between 200 and 300 cm/s, and the TE should be minimized. The temporal resolution should be ≤30 ms. Again, since measurement during diastole is needed to make a calculation of regurgitant fraction, retrospective triggering is desirable to capture the entire cardiac cycle. Figure 10.22a shows the magnitude image and Figure 10.22b the phase image in systole, with black indicating flow towards the head (PA and Ao) and white indicating flow towards the feet

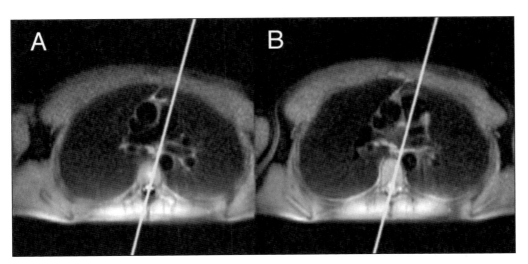

Figure 10.19
Slice placement for a right ventricular outflow tract (RVOT) cine taken on axial localizer images near the pulmonary bifurcation (a) and at the pulmonic valve level (b).

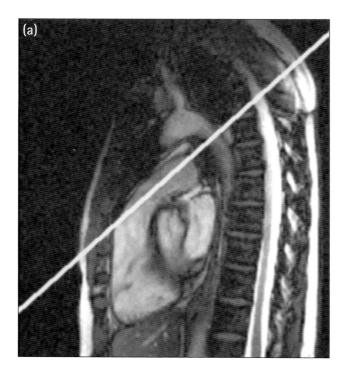

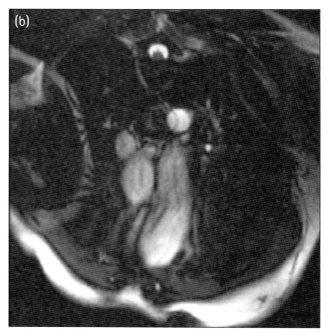

Figure 10.20
RVOT cine (a) and oblique coronal view of pulmonic valve (b) for visualization of the valve plane.

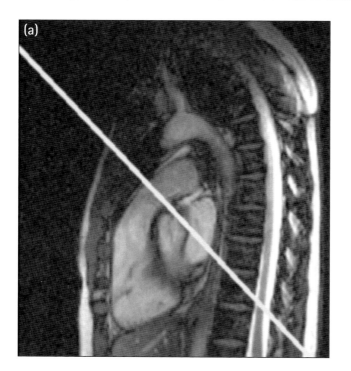

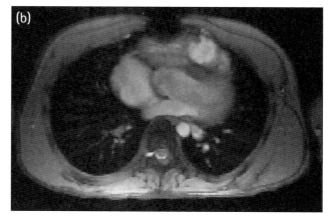

Figure 10.21
Slice positioning on images shown in Figure 10.20 for an en face view of the pulmonic valve.

(descending aorta, Figure 22b). Figure 10.23b shows the phase image in diastole, with regurgitant flow through the pulmonic valve shown in white. Similar to the case for aortic regurgitation, the pulmonic valve flow field can be planimetered, and the resulting flow curve plotted to determine the forward and reverse flow volumes.

- *Step 5:* To assess the degree of pulmonic stenosis, the procedure for estimating the peak velocity for estimation of the pressure gradient is the same as for the aortic valve.

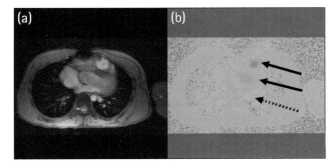

Figure 10.22
Magnitude image (a) and the corresponding phase image (b) in systole, with black indicating flow towards the head (PA and Ao) and white indicating flow towards the feet (descending aorta).

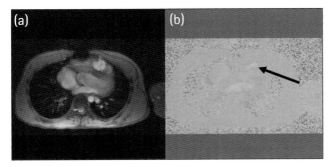

Figure 10.23
Magnitude (a) and phase (b) images shown in diastole, with regurgitant flow through the pulmonic valve shown in white.

Conclusions

CMR techniques for the assessment of valvular disease are evolving. The future will provide more functionality for imaging cardiac structures, especially heart valves. Presently, echocardiography is the accepted technique for evaluation of heart valves, but CMR is an adjunct technique, providing information about congenital abnormalities, the evaluation of valve ring abscesses, and quantitative data on chamber volumes and cardiac function. Future advances in pulse sequences, real-time image formation, and improvements in hardware will accelerate the development of CMR as a tool to evaluate heart valve morphology and function.

References

1. Arai A, Epstein F, Bove K, et al. Visualization of aortic valve leaflets using black blood MRI. J Magn Reson Imag 1999; 10:771–7.

2. Nayak K, Pauly J, Kerr A, et al. Real-time color flow MRI. Magn Reson Med 2000; 43:251–8.

3. Kilner PJ, Manzara CC, Mohiaddin RH, et al. Magnetic resonance jet velocity mapping in mitral and aortic valve disease. Circulation 1993; 87:1239–48.

4. Nakagawa Y, Fujimoto S, Nakano H, et al. Magnetic resonance velocity mapping of normal transtricuspid velocity profiles. Int J Card Imaging 1997; 13:433–6.

5. Skjaerpe T, Hegrenaes L, Hatle L. Noninvasive estimation of valve area in patients with aortic stenosis by Doppler ultrasound and two-dimensional echocardiography. Circulation 1985; 72:810–18.

6. Enriquez-Sarano M, Miller P, Hayes S, et al. Effective mitral regurgitant orifice area: clinical use and pitfalls of the proximal isovelocity surface area approach. J Am Coll Cardiol 1995; 25:703–9.

7. Lotz J, Meier C, Leppert A, et al. Cardiovascular flow measurement with phase-contrast MR imaging: basic facts and implementation. Radiographics 2002; 22:651–71.

8. McCauley T, Pena C, Holland C, et al. Validation of volume flow measurements with phase-contrast MR imaging for peripheral arterial waveforms. J Magn Reson Imaging 1995; 5:663–8.

9. Hangiandreou N, Rossman P, Riederer S. Analysis of MR phase-contrast measurements of pulsatile velocity waveforms. J Magn Reson Imaging 1993; 3:387–94.

10. Slavin G, Saranathan M. FIESTA-ET: high-resolution cardiac imaging using echo-planar steady-state free precession. Magn Reson Med 2002; 48:934–41.

11. Carr J, Simonetti O, Bundy J, et al. Cine MR angiography of the heart with segmented true fast imaging with steady-state free precession. Radiology 2001; 219:828–34.

12. Plein S, Bloomer T, Ridgway J, et al. Steady-state free precession magnetic resonance imaging of the heart: comparison with segmented *k*-space gradient-echo imaging. J Magn Reson Imaging 2001; 14:230–6.

13. Nayak K, Hu B. Triggered real-time MRI and clinical applications. Magn Reson Med 2003; 49:188–92.

14. Lorenz C, Walker E, Morgan V, et al. Normal human right and left ventricular mass, systolic function, and gender differences by cine magnetic resonance imaging. J Cardiovasc Magn Reson 1999; 1:7–21.

15. Bernstein M, Zhou X, Polzin J, et al. Concomitant gradient terms in phase contrast MR: analysis and correction. Magn Reson Med 1998; 39:300–8.

16. Cardiology Task Force of the European Society of Cardiology. Guidelines for the Use of Magnetic Resonance Imaging in the Evaluation of Valvular Heart Disease. Eur Heart J 1998; 19:19–39.

17. Sondergaard L, Hildebrandt P, Lindvig K, et al. Valve area and cardiac output in aortic stenosis: quantification by magnetic resonance velocity mapping. Am Heart J 1993; 126:1156–64.

18. Heidenreich PA, Steffens J, Fujita N, et al. Evaluation of mitral stenosis with velocity-encoded cine-magnetic resonance imaging. Am J Cardiol 1995; 75:365–9.

19. Pucillo AL, Schechter AG, Kay RH, et al. Identification of calcified intracardiac lesions using gradient echo MR imaging, J Comput Assist Tomogr 1990; 14:743–47.

20. Sondergaard L, Staahlberg F, Thomsen C. Magnetic resonance imaging of valvular heart disease. J Magn Reson Imaging 1999; 10:627–38.

21. Hamilton C. Correction of partial volume inaccuracies in quantitative phase contrast MR angiography. Magn Reson Imaging 1994; 12:1127–30.

22. Tang C, Blatter D, Parker D. Correction of partial-volume effects in phase-contrast flow measurements. J Magn Reson Imaging 1995; 5:175–80.

23. Aurigemma G, Reichek N, Schiebler M, et al. Evaluation of mitral regurgitation by cine magnetic resonance imaging. Am J Cardiol 1990; 66:621–5.

24. Bellenger N, Davies L, Francis J, et al. Reduction in sample size for studies of remodeling in heart failure by the use of cardiovascular magnetic resonance. J Cardiovasc Magn Reson 2000; 2:271–8.

25. Rebergen S, Chin J, Ottenkamp J, et al. Pulmonary regurgitation in the late postoperative follow-up tetralogy of Fallot. Volumetric quantitation by nuclear magnetic resonance velocity mapping. Circulation 1993; 88:2257–66.

26. Dulce M, Mostbeck G, O'Sullivan M, et al. Severity of aortic regurgitation: interstudy reproducibility of measurements with velocity-encoded cine MR imaging, Radiology 1992; 185:235–40.

27. Chatzimavroudis GP, Walker PG, Oshinski JN, et al. Slice location dependence of aortic regurgitation measurements with MR. Magn Reson Med 1997; 37:545–51.

28. Bogren H, Klipstein R, Firmin D, et al. Quantitation of antegrade and retrograde blood flow in the human aorta by magnetic resonance velocity mapping. Am Heart J 1989; 117:1214–22.

29. Kozerke S, Schwitter J, Pedersen E, et al. Aortic and mitral regurgitation: Quantification using moving slice velocity mapping. J Magn Reson Imaging 2001; 14:106–12.

30. McCuskey WH, Loehr SP, Smidebush GC, et al. Detection of mycotic pseudoaneurysm of the ascending aorta using MRI. Magn Reson Imaging 1993; 11:1223–6.

31. Adams JN, Brooks M, Redpath TW, et al. Aortic distensibility and stiffness index measured by magnetic resonance imaging. Br Heart J 1995; 73:265–9.

32. Meijboom LJ, Groenink M, van der Wall EE, et al. Aortic root asymmetry in Marfan patients; evaluation by magnetic resonance imaging. Int J Cardiac Imaging 2000; 16:161–8.

33. Walker PG, Oyre S, Pedersen EM, et al. A new control volume method for calculating valvular regurgitation. Circulation 1995; 92:579–86.

34. Walker PG, Houlind K, Djurhuus C, et al. Motion correction for the quantification of mitral regurgitation using control volume method. Magn Reson Med 2000; 43:726–33.

35. Hasenkam JM, Ringgaard S, Houlind K, et al. Prosthetic heart valve evaluation by magnetic resonance imaging. Eur J Cardio-Thorac Surg 1999; 16:300–5.

36. Scheidegger M. FID-acquired-echoes (FAcE): a short echo time imaging method for flow artefact suppression. Magn Reson Imaging 1991; 9:517–24.

37. Botnar R, Nagel E, Scheidegger M, et al. Assessment of prosthetic valve performance by magnetic resonance velocity imaging. Magma 2000; 10:18–26.

38. Shellock F. MR imaging of metallic implants and materials: a compilation of the literature. AJR 1988; 151:811–14.

39. Oshinsky J, Parks W, Markou C, et al. Improved measurement of pressure gradients in aortic coarctation by magnetic resonance imaging. J Am Coll Cardiol 1996; 28:1818–26.

11

CMR in congenital heart disease

Mark A Fogel

Introduction

Cardiac magnetic resonance imaging (CMR) has been around for nearly 20 years and is slowly becoming established in the evaluation of anatomy, physiology and function in congenital heart disease (CHD).[1–30] Presently, the technique is used as an adjunct to other imaging modalities such as echocardiography and angiography; however, in some areas such as vascular rings, it has become the 'gold standard'.[31–34] With the advent of advanced techniques such as fast imaging (e.g. TrueFISP) 'real-time' cine,[35] dark-blood spin-echo,[36] three-dimensional gadolin-

ium,[37] dynamic gadolinium angiography,[38] etc., CMR is poised to become a first-line imaging modality in pediatric cardiology (Figures 11.1 and 11.2).

CMR in CHD takes advantage of many of the specialized CMR techniques discussed in this book. One logical question is why CMR in CHD deserves a special chapter. There are three reasons why this application of CMR stands on its own:

- *Anatomy:* The pre- and postoperative anatomy in CHD is very unlike any found in adult heart disease. For example, atrioventricular, ventriculo-arterial and

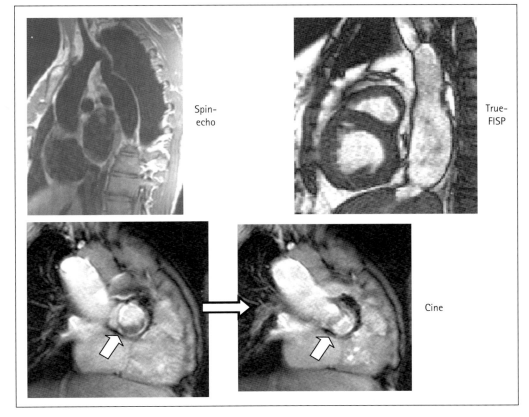

Figure 11.1
Types of two-dimensional CMR for anatomy and morphology. Dark-blood spin echo image (upper left) of a patient with coarctation of the aorta and static TrueFISP image (upper right) of a patient with supero-inferior ventricles (after Fontan operation) are two techniques used to evaluate morphology in CHD. Cine CMR (lower two panels) is also used to determine valve morphology and to confirm anatomy – this patient has a double-outlet right ventricle, and, after a complete repair and cine CMR, demonstrates a bicuspid aortic valve.

Spin-echo

True-FISP

Cine

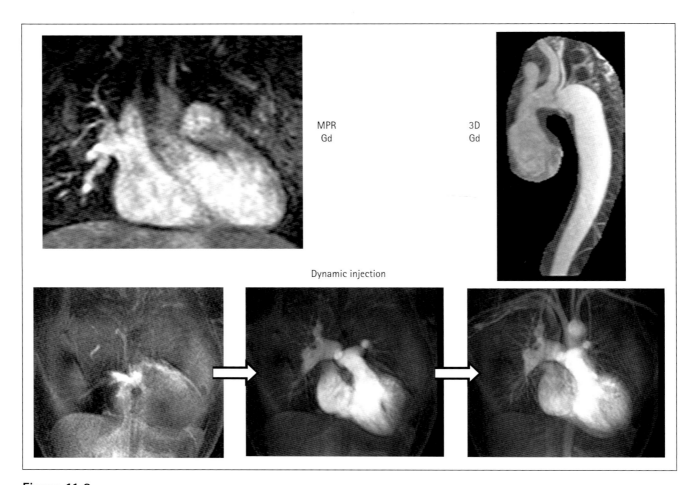

MPR
Gd

3D
Gd

Dynamic injection

Figure 11.2
Types of gadolinium (Gd)-enhanced CMR for anatomy and morphology. The upper left panel represents multiplanar reconstruction (MPR) of a patient with anomalous right pulmonary venous connection to the right superior vena cava. MPR allows a 3D data set to be cut into any 2D plane desired. The upper right panel represents a 3D maximum-intensity projection (MIP) of a patient with interrupted aortic arch who, after a repair, has residual obstruction. The 3D MIP can be rotated in any view to visualize the salient points of the anatomy. The lower three panels represent a 3D subsecond dynamic Gd injection of a patient with transposition of the great arteries after an arterial switch procedure and LaCompte maneuver with bilateral branch pulmonary artery stenosis (left greater than right). Images progress over time (left, little Gd; middle, right heart phase; right, right and left heart phases together). This simulates an angiogram in the catheterization laboratory.

veno-atrial connections can be connected in a dizzying number of ways. Morphology of ventricles and atria play an important role in CHD (e.g. D- versus L-looped ventricles), and the evaluation of conduits and baffles constructed to separate the circulations has little parallel in the adult world. As such, anatomy and morphology must be delineated by CMR in ways that are not required in adult heart disease, and the physician interpreting the study needs to be schooled in the nuances of the anatomy of CHD.

- *Physiology:* In many ways, the unique physiology of CHD is similar to the uniquenss of the anatomy. Evaluation of shunts, for example, plays a critical role in evaluating any disease entity in pediatrics, and yet has little role in the adult world. Ventricular function

in bizarrely shaped ventricles is routine in the practice of CMR in children, and demands unique solutions. Again, CMR must be adapted to fit these needs, and the physician interpreting the study needs to understand the complex physiology.

- *Technical challenges:* In the world of CMR, many tradeoffs are made to allow quicker and simpler imaging. One can obtain spatial resolution at the cost of temporal resolution, and vice versa. This is particularly relevant in children, by the mere fact that they require increased spatial resolution because of their size as well as increased temporal resolution because of their higher heart rates. The tradeoffs that can be performed in adults can only be taken advantage of to a limited degree in children. Furthermore, children under 7–9

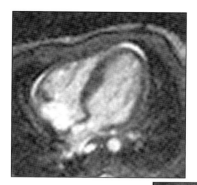

4 chamber

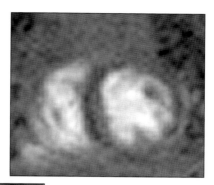

LV short
axis

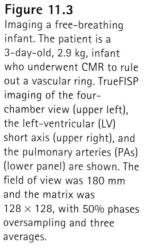

PAs

Figure 11.3
Imaging a free-breathing infant. The patient is a 3-day-old, 2.9 kg, infant who underwent CMR to rule out a vascular ring. TrueFISP imaging of the four-chamber view (upper left), the left-ventricular (LV) short axis (upper right), and the pulmonary arteries (PAs) (lower panel) are shown. The field of view was 180 mm and the matrix was 128 × 128, with 50% phases oversampling and three averages.

years of age usually need to be sedated, which make sequences designed for breathholding useless. Since this is the mainstay of adult CMR, 'workarounds' need to be developed. Therefore, modifications or new approaches to CMR are needed to successfully image children, and the physician performing the scan needs to understand these. An example of imaging a 3-day-old, 2.9 kg, free-breathing infant to rule out a vascular ring is demonstrated in Figure 11.3.

CMR does have its limitations and challenges in CHD. Sedation for young patients to hold still for long periods of time is always a consideration. Even if holding still is not an issue, cooperation may be problematic (e.g. breathholding). In addition, intravascular coils placed via catheter, wires, and clips may all cause artifact problems if they are near the structure of interest. CMR cannot image rapidly moving leaflets of valves and chordae as well as echocardiography can – although with faster sequences and 'slice tracking' technologies, this is becoming less of an issue. Echocardiography is still advantageous if portability to the bedside is necessary, since a critically ill patient would need to be moved the CMR scanner to be imaged. And finally, surgery for CHD may lead the patient to have arrhythmias that may not allow proper data acquisition; other patients may have bizarre T-waves or bundle branch blocks that may not trigger properly. This is also becoming less of an issue now that 'single-shot' CMR images (with the whole image being constructed in one heartbeat) and 'real-time' CMR (with images being constructed continually

without regard to ECG triggering) are a reality. Pacemakers are still a problem, and patients with them usually do not undergo CMR.

This chapter discusses the present state of the art of CMR in CHD and some of the newer techniques available. For simplicity, the imaging techniques discussed will be generic; however, some of the 'lingo' of CMR will be related to the Siemens Medical Systems scanners. The reader should understand that other manufacturers, for the most part, have similar sequences but under a different name.

The chapter is divided into two main parts: CMR for anatomy and then CMR for physiology and function. The future of CMR in CHD will be addressed briefly.

CMR for anatomy in CHD

In most instances, CMR provides all the anatomic information necessary for diagnosis, and may add information that could not have been acquired by other imaging modalities. Nowhere is this more apparent than in older children, adolescents, and adults with CHD, where echocardiographic windows can be poor (limited by acoustic windows and the interposition of lung or bone) and adequate imaging can sometimes be impossible.[9] CMR, however, can obtain data in complex planes or create these complex planes offline using multiplanar reconstruction (MPR) (also called oblique sectioning;[39] see below) (Figure 11.4). The ability of CMR to perform

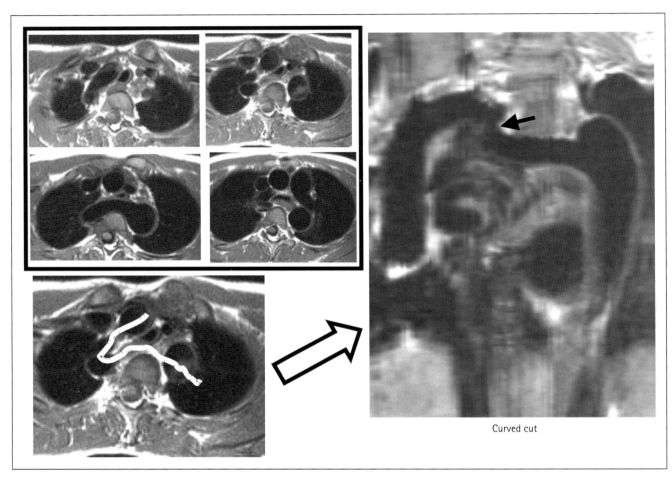

Figure 11.4

Right aortic arch with coarctation and multiplanar reconstruction (MPR). The images demonstrate a right aortic arch with coarctation and a left descending aorta. The boxed upper left four panels are axial images progressing from superior to inferior as the images progress from left to right and top to bottom. The lower left panel in these boxed images demonstrates the aortic arch crossing from the right hemithorax to the left hemithorax. The lower left panel of the figure as a whole shows how MPR is used in a curved cut – the white line is the image plane of a 'curved cut' and the resultant image is demonstrated in the right panel. The coarctation is easily seen in this view (white arrow).

this function is extremely important in CHD, since the presence of cardiovascular abnormalities with bizarre shapes, extra or missing vascular structures, and cardiac malposition all require nonstandard views. In addition, CMR is not subject to artifacts of calcification or patch materials used for surgical reconstruction, which is an important part of the evaluation of the postoperative patient.

It would be ideal to image misshapen cardiovascular structures in CHD in one plane. Various sweeps are performed from different windows in echocardiography[40,41] to view the entire heart and great vessels, leaving the echocardiographer to integrate this information into a three-dimensional (3D) structure, which then needs to be communicated to the patient's physician and surgeon. 3D echocardiography is slowly making headway in creating a picture of the region of interest in one image, but is still cumbersome and not readily available or routine. CMR

takes advantage of its ability to acquire contiguous parallel images to obtain a full-volume data set of the thoracic cardiovascular structures. Offline, the stack of 2D images can then generate a 3D shaded surface display[8,10–12] on the screen of a computer or as a hardcopy. Another way this can be generated is using a gadolinium injection, a volumetric 3D sequence and performing a maximum-intensity projection (MIP). This 3D display can be viewed from any desired angle, sectioned in any plane, and individual structures may be removed to reveal the salient points of the anatomy. This allows the 3D anatomy to be viewed by physician and surgeon in a familiar way, and does not require the ability to integrate the 2D data 'in your head' into a 3D one.

Another 3D mode that also takes advantage of the 'contiguous parallel slice' ability is MPR. Not only can the images be stacked and reformatted in any desired straight plane, they can also be reformatted to any curved plane (the so-called 'curved cut') to visualize tortuous structures in one image (Figure 11.4). This reformatting can be done on any of the sequences used, including the gadolinium-enhanced images.

Morphology is an important stepping stone in the functional analysis of the cardiovascular system and in determining the physiology of the specific lesion. The anatomic information can yield evidence that the functional and physiologic analysis is consistent with the underlying anatomy (e.g. ventricular volume overload in the presence of semilunar valve insufficiency). Similarly, functional and physiologic analysis must be interpreted in light of the prevailing anatomy.

CMR techniques used in imaging anatomy and morphology

With the advent of better coils and faster gradients, as well as improved hardware and software, the number of techniques that are available have greatly increased (Figures 11.1 and 11.2). An in-depth description of how these techniques work is beyond the scope of this chapter; only the briefest overview is given here. The reader is referred to appropriate textbooks for more information.

T1-weighted imaging in multiple forms has been a mainstay of morphologic imaging in CHD for many years: blood is black and signal-poor, while myocardium and blood vessel walls are signal-rich. Presently, this type of imaging can be done in multiple ways. Standard T1 spin-echo imaging takes on the order of 8–10 min to perform a full axial volume set of the thorax, and can have artifacts in the blood pool even with saturation bands placed above and below the imaging slab (although that does help). Turbo T1 spin-echo imaging uses multiple 'echoes' to speed image acquisition at the cost of a decreased number of slices per scan, yet a full axial volume set of the thorax still takes less time than the standard imaging. A newer technique called dark-blood imaging removes artifacts from blood by using a non-selective 180° radiofrequency (RF) pulse (to null-out all signal in the volume) followed immediately by a selective 180° RF pulse in the slice of interest (to get back the signal). The result is a crisp, sharp image relative to the other forms of T1 imaging. Black-blood imaging can be performed with both T1 and T2 weighting (using longer echo times (TE) to aid in 'blackening' the blood), as well as using HASTE sequences. This can be done as a breathhold (where at most four or five images can be obtained in 20 s) or non-breathhold in sedated patients (at the cost of time).

TrueFISP (fast imaging with steady-state precession) imaging is a newer technique where blood is signal-rich

and the myocardium and blood vessel walls have much less signal. It has a high signal-to-noise ratio (SNR) and relies on contrast between the blood pool and the myocardium and blood vessels for delineation of anatomy. The technique itself takes very little time to perform, and a full axial volume set of the thorax can be acquired in under two minutes. It comes in two forms:

- *Single shot*: The entire image is built in less than one heartbeat. This is useful for patients who cannot hold their breath (such as infants) or who have arrhythmias (such as the postoperative patient). The image is acquired in diastole to avoid blurring of the image from systolic motion so a delay from the R-wave of the ECG is usually put in. For patients who cannot hold their breath (e.g. small children under sedation), we have found that three averages gives a crisper picture than one average.
- *Segmented*: The entire image is built in a breathhold but is built up over multiple heartbeats. Similar to the single-shot mode, the image is acquired at the end of the cardiac cycle. We adjust the number of slices acquired to accommodate a 20 s breathhold (usually 10–15 slices).

There are some special circumstances where other non-gadolinium static sequences are advantageous. For example, if a cardiac tumor is present, T2-weighted and STIR sequences may be used to characterize the tumor better and define the borders (Figure 11.5). Addition of fat saturation to some of the sequences can be useful to characterize fatty infiltration of the myocardium (although in our experience, this has not helped in the diagnosis of right-ventricular dysplasia). An example of a patient with a cardiac lipoma with both fat-saturated and non-fat-saturated imaging is shown in Figure 11.6.

We have used dark-blood T2 HASTE sequences with good success to demonstrate morphology (minimize TE and aggressively 'rectangularize' the field of view). Some would advocate using dark-blood TrueFISP for anatomy, although we have found no advantage to this.

Gradient echo cine CMR or cine TrueFISP (see the next section for greater detail) are used to image valves; this can be done en face to determine, for example, whether the patient has a bicuspid aortic valve (Figure 11.1), or can be imaged in long axis. In these techniques, both blood as well as myocardium are signal-intense, but the myocardium is less so than blood. Valves appear signal-poor relative to blood. These techniques are also used to confirm anatomy; for example, what appears to be a stenotic left pulmonary artery in a patient after an arterial switch and LeCompte maneuver for transposition of the great arteries should cause turbulence and loss of signal on cine.

Cine CMR can also obtain static images at various levels of the body (multislice, single-phase), 'labeling'

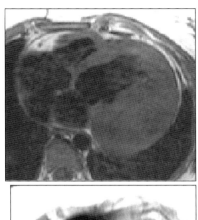

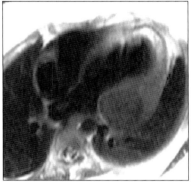

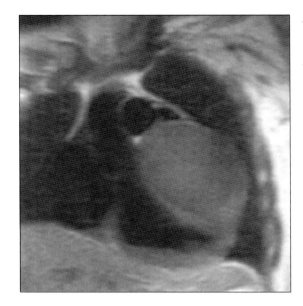

Figure 11.5
Left-ventricular tumor. The top left image is T1-weighted, while the bottom left and right images are T2-weighted. The T2 weighting separates the borders of the tumor and myocardium.

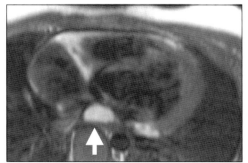

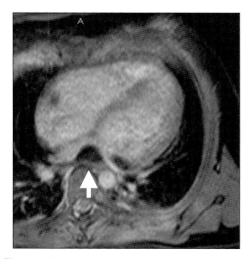

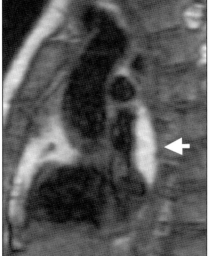

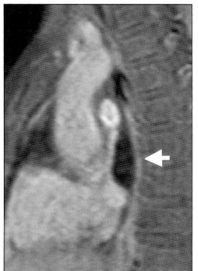

Figure 11.6
Left-atrial lipoma. The top left and the middle images represent T1-weighted images without fat saturation, while the lower left and the right images are flash sequences with fat saturation. Note how the tumor 'disappears' with fat saturation (arrows).

blood-containing structures with high signal intensity. As an example, this blood 'labeling' can be used to find collateral vessels off the aorta in a patient with a cyanotic lesion. This may be used in anticipation of cardiac catheterization with possible coiling or surgery.

Gadolinium-enhanced studies

Injection of gadolinium enhances the magnetic signal from the cardiovascular tree and can take two forms: static and dynamic injections. With static injections, a volumetric data set is obtained during the passage of gadolinium in the structure of interest (e.g. pulmonary arteries or aorta) and can be viewed as either a maximum-intensity projection (MIP) three-dimensionally or can be 'sliced' in any view using MPR. If viewed as an MIP, the volume data set can be rotated in any plane to view the salient features of the anatomy; it can be made into a shaded surface display if that is easier to visualize. If viewed using MPR, just as with static TrueFISP and T1-weighted imaging, any straight or curved plane can be created. Even movies of 'walking through the body' can be created by multiple, contiguous parallel MPR slices run one right after the other.

With dynamic, time resolved injections, the effect is similar to an angiogram in the catheterization laboratory. Gadolinium is injected in a vein and is followed through the heart and great vessels with rapid acquisition of 3D volume data sets with subsecond temporal resolution. The MIP created in these images is made up of multiple slices stacked one upon the other; therefore, each slice can be viewed individually for the presence of gadolinium (unlike in the catheterization lab). This technique is useful in anatomy in confirming shunts and stenotic or dilated vessels.

Scanning protocol

After the patient is lying still in the scanner (and sedated if necessary), initial localizers using TrueFISP are performed in three planes to locate the heart in the chest.

The next set of scans are gated TrueFISP contiguous axial (transverse) images throughout the entire thorax. Occasionally, the upper abdomen needs to be included if heterotaxy or anomalous pulmonary venous connections below the diaphragm are being considered. This is done in the 'single-shot' mode if the patient cannot breathhold or if an arrhythmia is present. If the patient can breathhold, a segmented sequence can be performed.

Technically, in the TrueFISP 'single-shot' mode, we obtain three or more averages, which gives crisper images (although the SNR is not an issue in these sequences). In this mode, the entire thorax can be covered in one scan, which usually takes approximately one minute. For the TrueFISP segmented approach with breathholding, we usually use only one average and limit the number of slices in given scan to limit the breathhold time (usually, 10–15 slices can be obtained for a 15–20 s breathhold). The set of slices is moved by the thickness of the slab to cover the next part of the thorax until the entire chest is imaged. Most of the other parameters are similar to the single shot technique. The whole process of obtaining a full cardiothoracic data set takes under two minutes.

The contiguous axial images are used as an initial evaluation of the cardiovascular anatomy, and are used themselves as localizers to obtain further imaging in the region of interest. If the study is terminated prematurely for whatever reason (e.g. if the patient awakes from sedation, becomes hemodynamically unstable, or there are technical difficulties with the scanner), this set of images can be used for further evaluation of the areas of interest using offline analysis (e.g. multiplanar reconstruction, or 3D shaded surface display).

The next series of images concentrate on the areas of interest. MPR is generally used on the axial images to get the correct angles and slice positions of this next set. If the axial images are unclear or if nothing was previously known about the patient's diagnosis, a set of contiguous coronal (more commonly) and sagittal images (less commonly) are used. Otherwise, the focus is on the salient findings from the axial images by confirming (or elucidating the anatomy) from an orthogonal plane. For example, if right pulmonary artery stenosis is demonstrated on the axial images, a set of off-axis coronal images along the long axis of the right pulmonary artery determines narrowing in the supero-inferior dimension. If a coarctation is suspected, then the 'candy cane' view of the aorta is used to delineate the narrowing in one view.

The choice of what sequence to use for the regions of interest depends on what is needed. If general anatomy is sought, TrueFISP imaging can be performed as in the axial set. If higher-resolution morphology is needed (e.g. ventricular morphology to determine D- or L-looping) or the TrueFISP images are not clear, dark-blood imaging is used.

Cine CMR, including standard FLASH gradient-echo sequences or TrueFISP, is then performed to confirm the diagnosis from the spin-echo images or to visualize valve morphology. If, for example, stenosis of the left-ventricular outflow tract is suspected from the narrowness of the pathway in a patient who has had a double-outlet right-ventricle repair, a cine sequence is performed to observe the loss of signal. As TrueFISP imaging can underestimate signal loss in turbulent regions, we prefer to use standard gradient-echo imaging in these cases.

Cine CMR is also used in determining the minimum and maximum annular size when balloon valvuloplasty or angioplasty is contemplated. If a ventricular septal defect (VSD) is suspected, cine CMR is performed to confirm the diagnosis and measure the size of the hole. Small holes may be missed by the spin-echo images.

In the protocol, functional imaging is then performed, which is the subject of the next section. Finally, the appropriate kind of gadolinium-enhanced imaging is done to assess the 3D nature of the lesion.

Although this is the morphology section, it is important to keep in mind that after the anatomy is defined, functional imaging needs to be performed (next section). For example, evaluation of coarctation of the aorta is not complete without assessment of ventricular hypertrophy, ejection fraction, and cardiac index, which can be performed by CMR with cine (as well as phase-encoded velocity mapping for the cardiac index). The ratio of pulmonary to systemic blood flow is an elementary requirement in the evaluation of a patient with double-outlet right ventricle or a ventricular septal defect, and this can be performed by CMR with phase-encoded velocity mapping.

Before proceeding to the uses of CMR in CHD for morphology, it is helpful to understand the approach to the patient with CHD that needs to be sorted out by the CMR physician. Patients with CHD are usually referred for CMR with a known diagnosis, and specific details need to be addressed by the study. Sometimes, everything needs to be sorted out by CMR. In CHD, no anatomic detail is taken for granted, and a standardized, systematic approach to the cardiovascular system is performed. Using the segmental approach,[42,43] all cardiac segments, intersegmental connections, and the various anomalies that occur in these segments and connections need to be identified. This can certainly be done by CMR, which many times can delineate the anatomy better than echocardiograhy (e.g. crisscross atrioventricular relations).

Major uses of CMR in morphologic evaluation of congenital heart disease

There are a few broad categories for which CMR has found an increasingly important role in morphology in

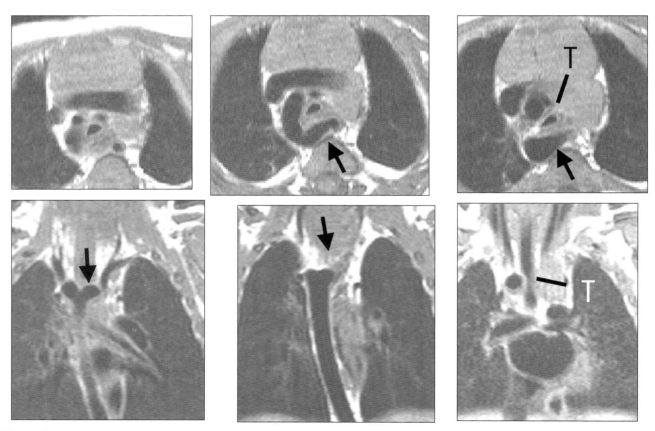

Figure 11.7
Right aortic arch with diverticulum of Kommerell. Axial (top images progress from superior to inferior as images progress from left to right) and coronal spin-echo images (bottom images progress from posterior to anterior as images progress from left to right) demonstrate the ring and diverticulum (arrow) Note how the trachea is compressed (T).

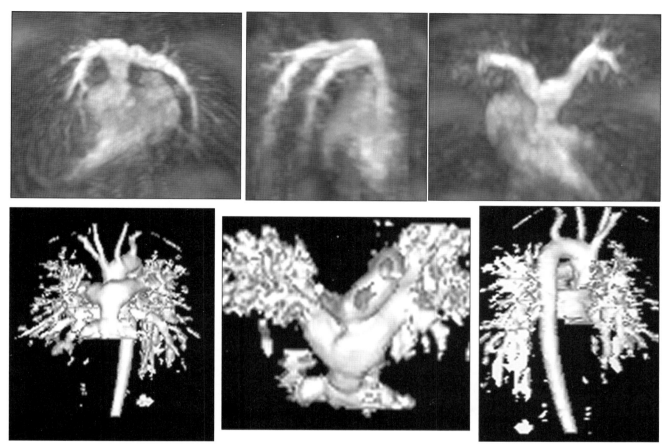

Figure 11.13
Patient with transposition of the great arteries after arterial switch procedure and LaCompte maneuver: 3D gadolinum-enhanced MIP and shaded surface display. The upper panels are the right heart phase of a 3D gadolinium-enhanced MIP from the anterior (left), lateral (middle), and superior (right) aspects of the patient. This demonstrates the 'V' shape of the LaCompte maneuver. The bottom panes are 3D shaded surface displays of the right and left heart phases of a gadolinium injection from the anterior (left), superior (middle), and posterior (right) and aspects of the patient.

the branch PAs crossing each other to reach the contralateral lung in patients with truncus arteriosus. In all cases, CMR can and should be used to delineate size, geometry, and site of origin.

Venous connections

This category is divided into systemic and pulmonary veins, which may be difficult to visualize by echocardiography because of their position in the chest or poor echocardiographic windows. CMR is extremely useful in delineating these connections, both with non-gadolinium and gadolinium-enhanced imaging.

Systemic veins

These anomalies may be isolated lesions and curiosities, such as persistent left superior vena cava draining to the coronary sinus, or these isolated lesions may have marked physiologic consequences, such as when the right or a persistent left superior vena cava connects to the left atrium,[51] causing cyanosis (Figure 11.15). Still other systemic vein anomalies may be associated with intracardiac lesions and will affect the conduct of surgery (all the more reason for CMR pre-evaluation). For example, hypoplastic left heart syndrome and tricuspid atresia are associated with a persistent left superior vena cava, which needs to be either connected to the LPA or ligated if a 'bridging vein' exists during the bidirectional cavo-pulmonary connection surgery.

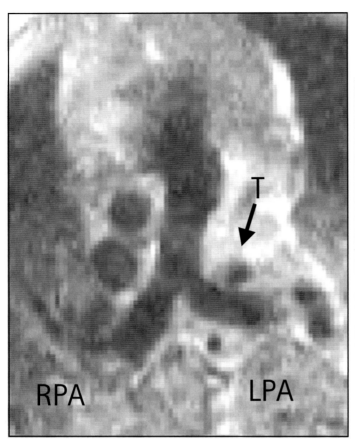
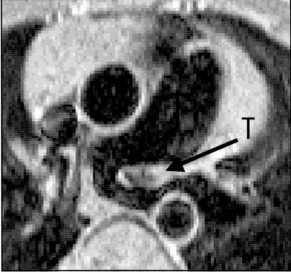

Figure 11.14
Patient with a pulmonary artery sling. The left panel is a spin-echo image of the bifurcation view the pulmonary artery demonstrating the left pulmonary artery (LPA) arising from the right pulmonary artery (RPA) and coursing behind the trachea (T). The right panel demonstrates another patient with the same pathology.

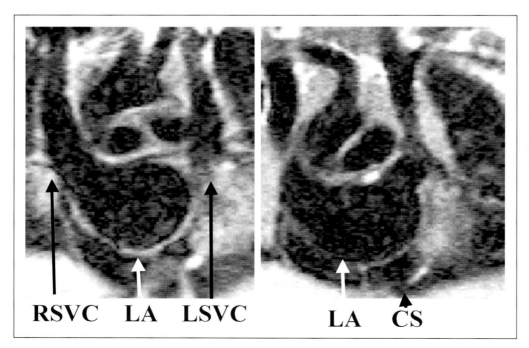

Figure 11.15
Patient with a right superior vena cava (RSVC) connected to the left atrium (LA) and a left superior vena cava (LSVC) connected to the coronary sinus. The two coronal spin-echo images demonstrate the defect, with the left image posterior to the right image.

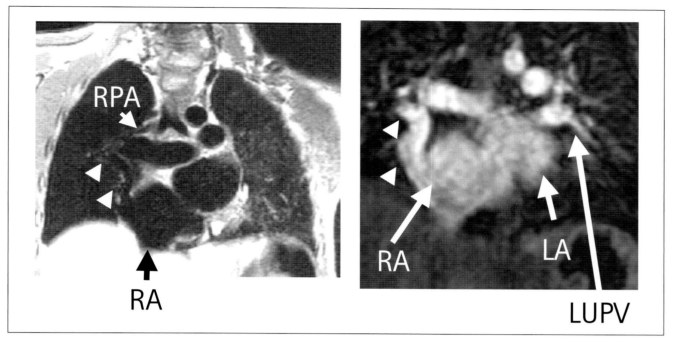

Figure 11.16
Patient with a 'scimitar' pulmonary vein entering into the right atrium (RA) near the inferior vena cava. The two coronal images (spin-echo on left, gadolinium-enhanced MPR on right) demonstrate the defect. Arrowheads point to the anomalous pulmonary vein. LA, left atrium; LUPV, left upper pulmonary vein; RPA, right pulmonary artery.

Since most systemic veins run in a supero-inferior plane, coronal images are obtained after the contiguous axial images, delineating the vein along its long axis. This allows confirmation of the connections, assessment of the size of the vessel, and identification of any areas of stenosis. Gadolinium injections, both static and dynamic, are useful in these lesions. For example, in a right superior vena cava connection to the left atrium, a time-resolved dynamic gadolinium injection will demonstrate contrast in the left side of the heart first when injecting into the right arm.

Pulmonary veins

There are a myriad of pulmonary venous anomalies that have either abnormal connections or stenosis. In total anomalous pulmonary venous connection, all the pulmonary veins connect abnormally to the right atrium, coronary sinus, systemic veins, or a confluence, where they may drain via a vertical vein supracardiac or infradiaphragmatic (e.g. to the inferior vena cava) and may be obstructive (Figures 11.16 and 11.17). They may not even all drain to the same place with the 'mixed venous type'.

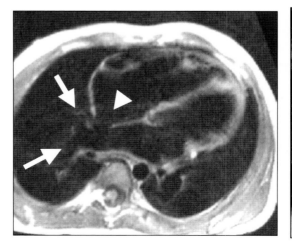

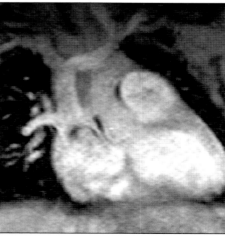

Figure 11.17
Patient with sinus venosus atrial septal defect (ASD) of the superior vena cava type and partial anomalous pulmonary venous connection. The spin-echo image on left demonstrates the ASD by an arrowhead and the anomalous right veins by an arrow. The cine MRI on the right demonstrates the right upper pulmonary vein draining anomalously to the superior vena cava.

There may be individual pulmonary vein atresia or stenosis, or all the pulmonary veins may drain to a confluence and end in a blind pouch with no exit – the so-called atresia of the common pulmonary vein.

Axial images can delineate the pulmonary venous anatomy and can also follow the vertical vein along its course through the thorax or abdomen. Coronal images that cut the individual pulmonary veins in the supero-inferior dimension can then be obtained to confirm the diagnosis. Again, gadolinium injections can aid in this diagnosis.

Extracardiac conduits and baffles

These are key structures in the repair of CHD and are important to evaluate because stenosis or leaks occur.

Echocardiography may be hampered in imaging these structures because they may pass immediately underneath the sternum near the lungs, or may be very posterior in the chest. CMR can usually succeed where echocardiography fails, although there are caveats as well (e.g. artifacts from sternal wires may hamper imaging).

There are multiple kinds of extracardiac conduits:

- *ventriculo-arterial*, such as an RV-to-PA conduit (as in a Rastelli procedure[52] – Figure 11.18), an LV-to-PA conduit[53] (as in a patient with transposition of the great arteries and/or inverted ventricles – Figures 11.19 and 11.20), or an apical LV-to-descending aorta conduit[54] (Figure 11.21);
- *veno-atrial*, such as in a Baffes procedure, which was used in the 1950s to palliate patients with transposition of the great arteries, where the inferior vena cava is ligated and flow channeled via a conduit to the left atrium;

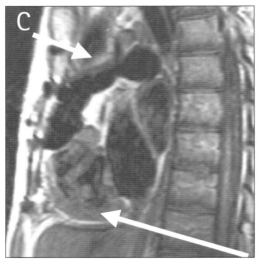
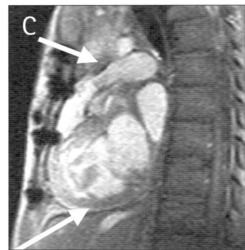

Figure 11.18
Patient with transposition of the great arteries, ventricular septal defect and pulmonic stenosis after a Rastelli procedure. The spin-echo image on the left and the cine on the right demonstrate the right ventricle (RV) to pulmonary artery (PA) conduit part of this surgical repair.

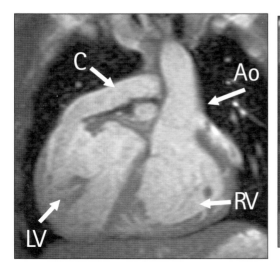
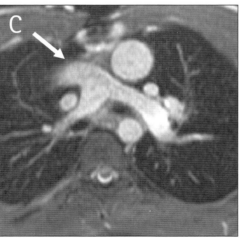

Figure 11.19
Patient with transposition of the great arteries {I,D,D} and pulmonic stenosis after a left ventricle (LV) to pulmonary artery conduit (C). The TrueFISP coronal image on the left demonstrates markedly dilated and hypertrophied ventricles and profiles both outflow tracts and conduit. The TrueFISP image on the right is an axial view of the pulmonary arteries and the conduit insertion into the right pulmonary artery. Ao, aorta; RV, right ventricle.

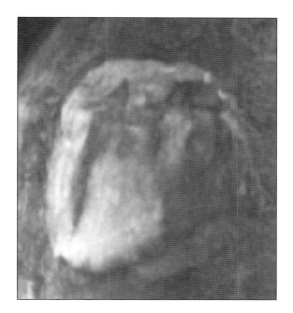
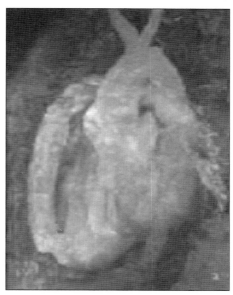

Figure 11.20
Three-dimensional gadolinium-enhanced images of a patient with transposition of the great arteries {S,L,L} and pulmonic stenosis after a left ventricle (LV) to pulmonary artery (PA) conduit. The left panel shows the 'right heart–pulmonary' phase of a static gadolium injection, which demonstrates an apical LV-to-PA conduit. The right panel demonstrates both phases of the injection, including the 'left heart' side.

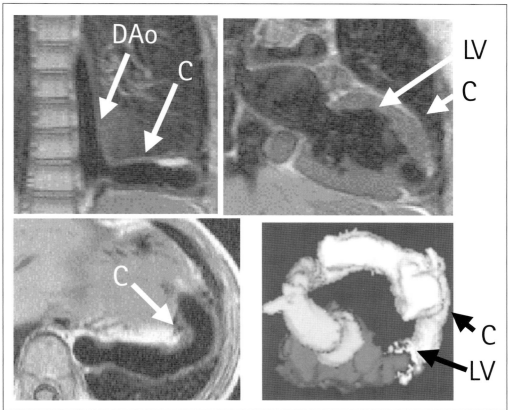

Figure 11.21
Patient with left-ventricular outflow tract obstruction due to a bulboventricular foramen who underwent an apical left ventricle (LV) to descending aortic (DAo) conduit. The upper panels are coronal images demonstrating insertion of the conduit (C) into the LV and DAo. The lower left image is the axial spin-echo view of the conduit. The lower right image is a 3D shaded surface display viewed from the superior aspect of the patient.

- *veno-arterial*, such as an extracardiac conduit for the Fontan procedure,[55] where the inferior vena cava is hooked up to the RPA;
- *arterio-arterial*, such as an ascending-to-descending aortic conduit in the case of coarctation of the aorta or an aortic-to-aortic conduit in the case of reconstructing the heart of thoracopagus conjoined twins who share one heart (Figure 11.22).

Intracardiac baffles (Figures 11.23–11.26) can also be categorized:

- *atrial baffles*, channel venous blood to arteries or the ventricles, such as in the lateral wall tunnel Fontan reconstruction[55] (Figures 11.23 and 11.24), Mustard,[56] and Senning[57] (Figure 11.25) procedures for transposition of the great arteries;

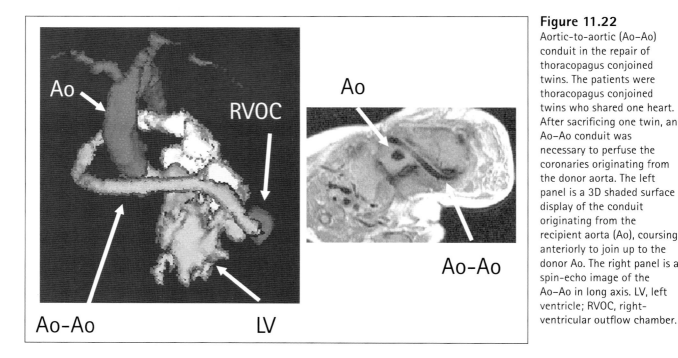

Figure 11.22
Aortic-to-aortic (Ao–Ao) conduit in the repair of thoracopagus conjoined twins. The patients were thoracopagus conjoined twins who shared one heart. After sacrificing one twin, an Ao–Ao conduit was necessary to perfuse the coronaries originating from the donor aorta. The left panel is a 3D shaded surface display of the conduit originating from the recipient aorta (Ao), coursing anteriorly to join up to the donor Ao. The right panel is a spin-echo image of the Ao–Ao in long axis. LV, left ventricle; RVOC, right-ventricular outflow chamber.

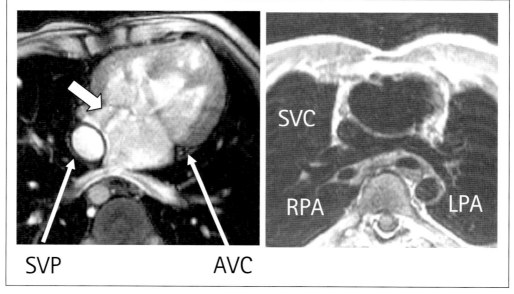

Figure 11.23
Fontan reconstruction. The patient has an L-looped single ventricle with a complete atrioventricular canal (AVC). The left panel is a TrueFISP cine image of the long axis of the heart (what would have been a 'four-chamber view' if four chambers existed). The Fontan baffle (systemic venous pathway, SVC) and AVC are evident, along with flow across the fenestration (white arrow). The panel on the right is an axial view demonstrating the superior vena cava (SVC) to right pulmonary artery (RPA) anastomosis and the left pulmonary artery (LPA) by 2D spin-echo imaging.

- *ventricular baffles*, exemplified by LV blood baffled to the aorta through a ventricular septal defect, such as in the Rastelli procedure[52] (Figure 11.26) or in the repair of double-outlet RV;
- *arterial baffles*, such as the Takeuchi operation[58] in the repair of an anomalous left coronary artery.

Depending on the kind of conduit or baffle, contiguous axial images can be used to follow the conduit and baffle in short axis (as in the Fontan procedure) or to outline its long axis (as in an LV-to-descending aorta conduit). In either case, double oblique angled images are usually necessary to obtain the orthogonal view. It is not always

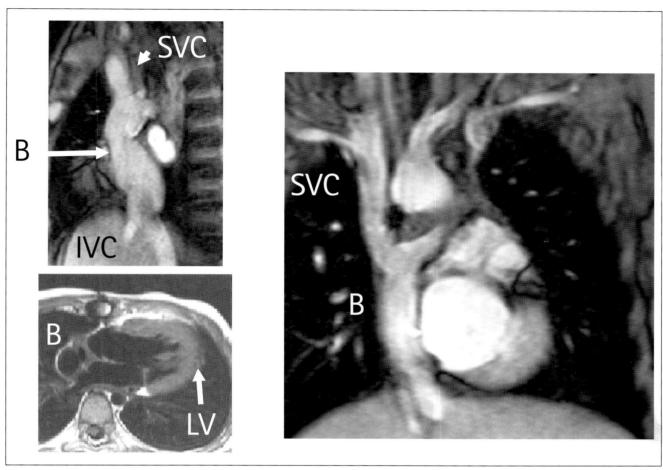

Figure 11.24
Fontan reconstruction. The patient has tricuspid atresia. The upper left panel is a TrueFISP cine image of the Fontan baffle (B) in an off-axis sagittal view, while the right panel is the baffle in an off-axis coronal view. The lower left panel is a spin-echo image of the long axis of the heart (what would have been a 'four-chamber view' if four chambers existed). IVC, inferior vena cava; LV, left ventricle; SVC, superior vena cava.

possible to obtain a long axis view in one image and the CMR physician must be satisfied with 2 or 3 images; in these instances, 3D gadolinium sequences or shaded surface displays are an invaluable part of the study. Stenosis, regurgitation, or leaks across the baffle from one channel to the other can be detected by cine CMR.

Complex spatial relationships

In complex CHD, such as heterotaxy syndrome, the orientation and position of various cardiovascular structures relative to each other and the rest of the body can be sorted out by CMR easier than by other imaging modalities. Besides cardiovascular structures, CMR can demonstrate other related structures that are important to the patient's care, such as the tracheo-bronchial tree (e.g.

bilateral right- or left-sided bronchi), liver (right-sided, left-sided, or midline) and spleen (Is there one?). CMR, in this area, becomes a 'one-stop-shop'. As one may have surmised, 3D imaging and MPR gives the physician a powerful tool with which to analyze the complex geometry.

Axial images are the first series of images to be performed, which can follow the various cardiovascular structures and, in general, yield a first approximation of the anatomy. More scans are obtained in double oblique angles to further delineate the morphology and regions of interest identified on the axial images. For the liver and spleen, as well as for orientation purposes for cardiovascular structures, straight coronal images seem to be the best. Confirmation of certain diagnoses are made using cine CMR.

An example of such complex relationships is in patients who have double-inlet left ventricle[59] and supero-inferior ventricles[60] where the two ventricles (as is implied in the name) are oriented supero-inferiorly instead of

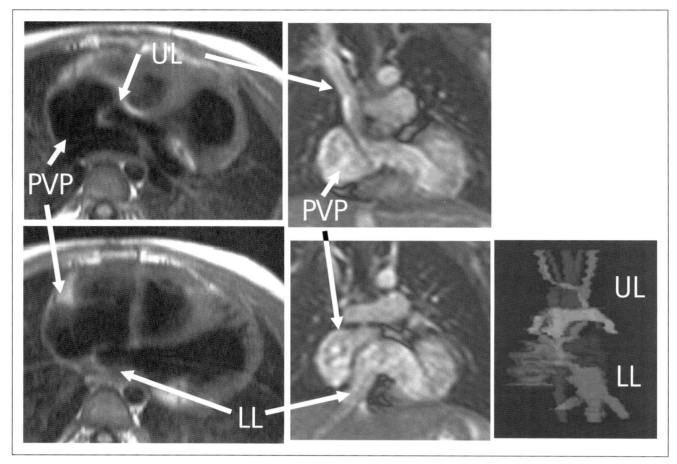

Figure 11.25
Senning operation for transposition of the great arteries. The left panels are spin-echo axial images and the middle panels are TrueFISP static images of the upper limb (UL) and lower limb (LL) of the systemic venous pathway of the Senning baffle. The middle panels demonstrate this reconstruction in long axis. The lower right panel is a 3D shaded surface display of the reconstruction from a posterior view, where the UL and LL can be visualized better. PVP, pulmonary venous pathway.

antero-posteriorly and right-left (Figures 11.27 and 11.28). The ventricular septum lies parallel to the axial plane. When connecting the atria to the ventricles, the atrioventricular valves appear to enter the LV (in the figure, the inferior ventricle). To depict the ventricular relationship, coronal or sagittal images are utilized, while the emptying of blood from both atria into the LV can be demonstrated by off-axis sagittal views (although the standard axial images can show this, but less well).

General morphology and miscellaneous diseases

General morphologic evaluation can also be performed by CMR, although this is not the only imaging modality which can do it. Nevertheless, CMR can be useful in the older child, adolescent, and adult for this, and can add

information not previously known. Furthermore, because of the wide field of view, a single CMR study may serve the purpose of multiple other studies (e.g. heterotaxy syndrome[61,62]).

CMR may also add another dimension to studies of lesions that have been previously performed. For example intracardiac tumors[63] can be characterized by CMR utilizing T1- and T2-weighted images, fat saturation, proton density images, and gadolinium-enhanced images to demarcate the extent of the tumor and its water content (Figures 11.5, 11.6, and 11.29).

CMR for physiology and function in CHD

CMR is becoming the premier imaging modality for those who are serious about the assessment of physiology and

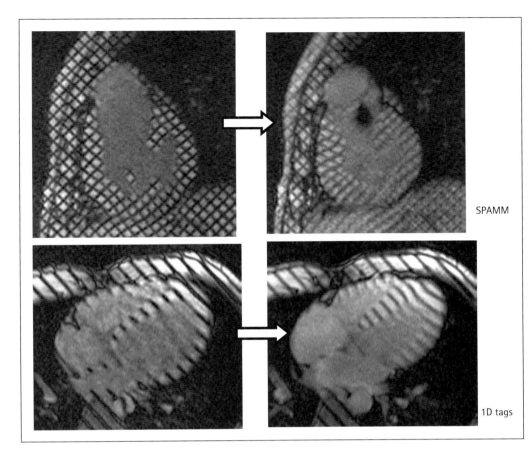

Figure 11.31
Myocardial tagging for function in CHD. The top panels are spatial modulation of magnetization (SPAMM) cine images of a patient with hypoplastic left heart syndrome (ventricular short axis) after a Fontan procedure demonstrating regional myocardial deformation and neoaortic insufficiency (black jet). The left panel is at end-diastole (ED) and the right panel is at end-systole (ES). The lower panels are 1D tagged (stripes) images (four-chamber view) of a patient who underwent CMRI to evaluate for right-ventricular dysplasia. As with the upper panels, the left is at ED and the right is at ES, and the regional deformation of the ventricle can be seen.

CMR sequence, essentially dividing the wall into 'cubes of magnetization'. This can be done in 2D and 3D, in systole and/or diastole, and is used in assessing regional wall motion, thickening (or thinning), and strain. The tags tend to fade as a function of time and with increased temporal resolution (which can be as high as 15 ms); however, there are some algorithms available that can work around these issues at the cost of time.

A second type of myocardial tagging is the 'stripes' (or 1D) method, where spins are saturated in just one set of parallel planes. This type has the same uses as the SPAMM technique.

Blood (bolus) tagging[30,67,68]

Similar to the 'stripes' method of myocardial tagging, this is a gradient-echo sequence that utilizes an RF 'prepulse' to produce saturated spins along a plane across a blood vessel (a signal-poor line on the image). When the tag is placed perpendicular to the flow, blood displaces the band of saturation, whereas stationary structures (e.g. chest wall and spine) maintain the saturation band's original position (Figure 11.32). Each image represents blood displacement between tagging and image acquisition. This technique essentially 'visualizes' the blood velocity profile.

The technique of saturating the spins of the blood can also be used to enhance the visualization of shunts by cine CMR by 'blacking out' the blood (Figure 11.32) on either side of the communication (two runs to visualize right-to-left and left-to-right flow; see below for greater detail).

Dynamic gadolinium (Figure 11.2)

In the morphology section, dynamic, time-resolved gadolinium injections were discussed. The ability of CMR to inject dye and follow it through the heart similar to an angiogram can be used to assess shunt physiology such as a patent ductus arteriosus or a right superior vena cava connection to the left atrium.

Use of CMR in physiology and function

The above techniques can be used in a number of ways clinically as well as experimentally to aid in the elucidation of physiology and function in CHD. This has become

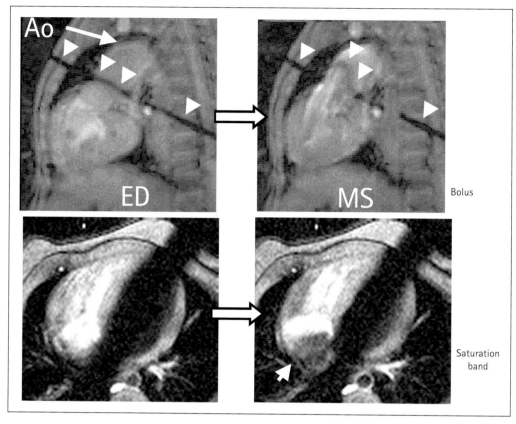

Figure 11.32
Blood tagging for physiology and function in CHD. The top panels are bolus (blood-tagged) cine images of the aorta (Ao) of a patient with a single ventricle after a Fontan procedure, demonstrating the velocity profile in the ascending aorta (Ao). The left panel is at end-diastole (ED) and the right panel is at mid-systole (MS). Arrowheads point to the blood tag and the tag on the stationary structures (chest wall and spine). The lower panels show the four-chamber view of a patient with an atrial–septal communication. A saturation band is placed on the left atrium, destroying all the signal from blood (black on the image), which is seen to cross the atrial septum into the right atrium (the arrow shows left-to-right flow).

even more important as we move from an era of just being able to repair lesions to an era of optimization of repair, longevity of the physiology that is being created, and the quality of life that a patient with CHD will have. Unfortunately, space limitations to do not permit a full discussion on this subject here.

Cine CMR

The three most important functions of this technique are the assessment of global cardiac function, and the evaluation of vessel stenosis and valvar competence.

In the assessement of global function, these sequences are used to obtain ventricular mass, ventricular end-diastolic volume, stroke volume, ejection fraction, and cardiac index. In addition, from a qualitative standpoint, as in echocardiography, single or multiple short-axis views as well as long-axis views of the ventricle can be obtained.

Myocardial thickening and regional wall motion can be grossly visualized in this manner as well. As with echocardiography, dobutamine infusions may be used to enhance the evaluation of myocardium performance in a state of higher workload, although this has yet to catch on in pediatrics.

Accurate assessment of these functional indices is a major strength of cine CMR.[14,19,22,27,69,70] Since CMR can acquire contiguous, parallel, tomographic images, it avoids all major assumptions of ventricular shape, which are required for calculations of volumes and masses in other imaging modalities. Because of this, it has a particular advantage in the highly variable ventricular shapes found in CHD. This technique has been used in the past to evaluate patients with a variety of congenital heart diseases, including single ventricles, tetralogy of Fallot, and transposition of the great arteries.

To obtain ventricular volumes and mass (with subsequent cardiac index and ejection fraction calculations), multiple, contiguous, sets of cine CMR runs are performed through the entire ventricle at the same temporal resolution. The results are multiple full-volume data sets at 15–20 ms intervals. By tracing the endocardial borders on all images at the phase or phases of interest (usually end-diastole and end-systole), ventricular volumes are obtained by multiplying the measured areas by the slice thickness and summing the result (Simpson's rule may also be used). Ventricular mass is obtained by tracing the epicardial borders which measures both ventricular mass and volume and subtracting the chamber volume. Stroke volume and ejection fraction can be then be calculated. Cardiac index is also calculated as the product of the stroke volume and heart rate divided by body surface area.

To assess vessel stenosis and valvar competence, cine CMR visualizes turbulent blood flow by a loss of signal (Figure 11.9). Grading the regurgitation is similar to color Doppler echocardiography. Volumetric assessment of the regurgitant flow may be calculated using phase-encoded velocity techniques alone or in combination with cine CMR techniques (see below in the discussion of phase-encoded velocity). Similarly, valvular stenosis may be detected using cine CMR, and peak velocities may be measured using phase-encoded velocity techniques. Of course, gradients may be calculated utilizing peak velocities as in echocardiography. Examples of CHD lesions where this comes into play are coarctation of the aorta, stenosis of branch pulmonary arteries as may be seen in transposition of the great arteries after a LaCompte maneuver, or Shone's complex.

Phase-encoded velocity mapping

In CHD, blood velocity mapping has a vide variety of applications. For example, in patients with atrial or ventricular septal defects, velocity mapping is useful in determining the ratio of pulmonary to systemic blood flow (Q_p/Q_s).[25] In patients with tetralogy of Fallot as well as the Fontan procedure, an important component to the patient's hemodynamic profile is how much blood is going to each lung; velocity mapping can easily define this by acquiring a phase map over each branch pulmonary artery. The sum of the flows is compared with a phase map across the main pulmonary artery as an internal check. In patients with coarctation of the aorta, quantification of collateral flow may be obtained by placing a phase map over the proximal and distal descending aorta; patients with significant collateral flow will have distal descending aortic flow greater than proximal descending aortic flow.

Semilunar valve insufficiency is found not infrequently in CHD. Patients who have a subaortic membrane or who undergo a transannular patch repair for tetralogy of Fallot, or placement of a valveless conduit all have the same semilunar valve regurgitation physiology. One way to quantify this is the regurgitant fraction, which is easily calculated from a phase map distal to the semilunar valve in question. The area under the curve of the reverse flow relative to the area under the curve of the forward flow multiplied by 100 will give the regurgitant fraction in percent.

In patients with atrioventricular valve insufficiency, such as Ebstein's anomaly, cleft mitral valve (such as in incomplete atrioventricular canal defects), or residual leakage postoperatively, a combination of cine CMR and velocity mapping must be used. Cine CMR is used to measure ventricular volume at end-diastole and end-systole to obtain the total amount of blood ejected by the ventricle, and phase-encoded velocity mapping assesses the amount of forward flow from the ventricle. Alternatively, a velocity map may be placed over the atrioventricular valve in question.

As with echocardiography, velocities obtained from CMR are useful for noninvasive estimates of pressure using the Bernoulli equation. This can be performed with both through-plane and in-plane velocity mapping and is useful in lesions such as coarctation of the aorta, discrete branch pulmonary stenosis, and conduit stenosis.

Further, CMR can provide velocities perpendicular to flow, and in three dimensions, 3D velocities in different regions of a blood vessel or ventricular chamber at a given level may be obtained for use in fluid mechanics of cardiovascular research.

Finally, although it is not in widespread clinical use, myocardial velocimetry, the CMR cousin to Doppler tissue imaging of echocardiography, may be used to assess myocardial wall motion.

Magnetic tagging

With myocardial tagging, regional wall motion may be assessed qualitatively and is used clinically where these questions arise. Examples include single-ventricle systolic function after Fontan procedure, diastolic function in the presence of coarctation, and assessing for RV dysplasia.

Quantitative analysis to assess regional wall strain and wall motion is still labor-intensive. This involves tracking the grid intersections through the phase of interest and creating a triangular grid from the intersections. Regional wall strain and motion can then be quantified using homogeneous strain analysis, which has been performed in pediatrics in patients with single ventricles, transplant patients and patients with transposition of the great arteries after atrial inversion procedures.[16,18,28,29]

With blood tagging, the displacement of the saturation band placed on blood relative to the chest wall and spine allows for calculation of velocity, since the time between saturation band placement and image acquisition is known and the distance of the displacement can be measured. Flow can be calculated with a few assumptions by measuring the area under the saturation band placed on the blood relative to the original position, converting this to a volume, and then dividing this volume by the time between tagging and image acquisition. This has been done in pediatrics in single-ventricle patients who have undergone the Fontan procedure and also in patients who have undergone an aortic-to-pulmonary anastomosis.[30,67]

Dynamic gadolinium

As mentioned above, the ability of CMR to inject dye and follow it through the heart similar to an angiogram can be used to assess shunt physiology. A lesion such as a patent ductus arteriosus, if there is right-to-left flow during part of the cardiac cycle, will demonstrate gadolinium in the descending aorta while the dye is still in the pulmonary arteries. In patients, for example, with a right superior vena cava connection to the left atrium, dye injected in the right arm will 'light up' the left side of the heart first!

The future

CMRI plays a special role in pediatric cardiology from both an anatomic and physiologic/functional standpoint. In addition, there must be a special 'carve-out' for pediatric heart disease in the world of CMRI because of the unique anatomy and physiology as well as the technical challenges which pediatric patients present. This technology should be used in centers that are experienced in both the technical aspects of CMRI in children as well as knowledgeable about all aspects of congenital and acquired heart disease in children.

CMRI has come a long way in the past 20 years but still has a long way to go in terms of development as well as acceptance by pediatric cardiologists, surgeons, and other health care providers of children with heart disease. The many advances that have occurred hold the promise of even better quality imaging as well as greater insights into the pathology of congenital heart disease, however, the potential for further advancement is clear. Real time CMRI for function and blood flow, holographic and multimodality displays (in conjunction with echocardiography and CT scanning) as well as the promise of interventional CMRI are just some examples of the future.

Congenital heart disease is complex; so is pediatric CMRI. It is paradoxical, however, that when CMRI is applied to congenital heart disease, things can become a bit simpler in the right hands.

References

1. Didier D, Higgins CB, Fisher M, et al. Congenital heart disease: Gated magnetic resonance imaging in 72 patients. Radiology 1986; 158:227–35.

2. Fletcher BD, Jacobsteink MD, Nelson AD, et al. Gated magnetic resonance imaging of congenital cardiac malformations. Radiology 1984; 150:137–40.

3. Higgins CB, Byrd BF, Farmer DW, et al. Magnetic resonance imaging in patients with congenital heart disease. Circulation. 1984; 70:851–60.

4. Reed JD, Soulen RL. Cardiovascular MRI: current role in patient management. Radiol Clin North Am 1988; 26:589–606.

5. Link KM, Lesko NM. Magnetic resonance imaging in the evaluation of congential heart disease. Magn Reson Q 1991; 7:173–90.

6. Bank ER. Magnetic resonance of congenital cardiovascular disease. An update. Radiol Clinic North Am 1993; 31:553–72.

7. Fogel MA. Evaluation of ventricular geometry and performance in congenital heart disease utilizing magnetic resonance imaging. Proc SPIE 1994; 2168:195–217.

8. Adams R, Fellows KE, Fogel MA, Weinberg PM. Anatomic delineation of congenital heart disease with 3D magnetic resonance imaging. Proc SPIE 1994; 2168:184–94.

9. Fogel MA, Ramaciotti C, Hubbard AM, Weinberg PW. Magnetic resonance and echocardiographic imaging of pulmonary artery size throughout stages of Fontan reconstruction. Circulation 1994; 90:2927–36.

10. Bornemeier RA, Weinberg PM, Fogel MA. Angiographic, echocardiographic and three-dimensional magnetic resonance imaging of extracardiac conduits in congenital heart disease. Am J Cardiol. 1996; 78:713–17.

11. Fogel MA, Hubbard A, Weinberg PM. A simplified approach for assessment of intracardiac baffles and extracardiac conduits in congenital heart surgery with two- and three-dimensional magnetic resonance imaging. Am Heart J 2001; 142:1028–36.

12. Fogel MA, Baxter B, Weinberg PM, et al. Midterm follow-up of patients with transposition of the great arteries after atrial inversion operation using two- and three-dimensional magnetic resonance imaging. Pediatr Radiol 2002; 32:440–6.

13. Fogel MA, Rychik J, Chin A, et al. Evaluation and follow-up of patients with left ventricular apical to aortic conduits using two- and three-dimensional magnetic resonance imaging and Doppler echocardiography: a new look at an old operation. Am Heart J 2001; 141:630–6.

14. Fogel MA, Hubbard AM, Fellows KE, Weinberg PM. MRI for physiology and function in congenital heart disease: functional assessment of the heart preoperatively and postoperatively. Semin Roentgenol 1998; 33:239–51.

15. Weinberg PM, Hubbard AM, Fogel MA. Aortic arch and pulmonary artery anomalies in children. Semin Roentgenol 1998; 33:262–80.

16. Fogel MA, Weinberg PM, Gupta KB, et al. Mechanics of the single left ventricle: a study in ventricular–ventricular interaction II. Circulation 1998; 98:330–8.

17. Fogel MA, Weinberg PM, Rychik J, et al. Caval contribution to flow in the branch pulmonary arteries of Fontan patients using a novel application of magnetic resonance presaturation pulse. Circulation 1999; 99:1215–21.

18. Donofrio MT, Clark BJ, Ramaciotti C, et al. Regional wall motion and strain of transplanted hearts in pediatric patients using magnetic resonance tagging. Am J Physiol 1999; 277:R1481–7.

19. Fogel MA. Assessment of cardiac function by MRI. Pediatr Cardiol 2000; 21:59–69.

20. Fogel MA, Weinberg PM, Hubbard A, Haselgrove J. Diastolic biomechanics in normal infants utilizing MRI tissue tagging. Circulation 2000; 102:218–24.

21. Eyskens B, Reybrouck T, Bagaert J, et al. Homograft insertion for pulmonary regurgitation after repair of tetralogy of Fallot improves cardiorespiratory exercise performance. Am J Cardiol 2000; 85:221–5.

22. Niezen RA, Helgbing WA, van der Wall EE, et al. Biventricular systolic function and mass studied with MRI imaging in children with pulmonary regurgitation after repair for tetralogy of Fallot. Radiology 1996; 201:135–40.

23. Rebergen SA, Chin JGJ, Ottenkamp J, et al. Pulmonary regurgitaion in the late postoperative follow-up of tetralogy of Fallot. Volumetric quantification by MR velocity mapping. Circulation 1993; 88:2257–66.

24. Rebergen SA, Ottenkamp J, van der Wall EE, et al. Postoperative pulmonary flow dynamics after Fontan surgery: assessment with nuclear magnetic resonance velocity mapping. J Am Coll Cardiol 1993; 21:123–31.

25. Beerbaum P, Korperich H, Barth P, et al. Non-invasive quantification of left-to-right shunt in pediatric patients. Phase-contrast cine magnetic resonance imaging compared with invasive oxymetry. Circulation 2001; 10:2476–82.

26. Gutberlet M, Boeckel T, Hosten N, et al. Arterial switch procedure for d-transposition of the great arteries: quantitative midterm evaluation of hemodynamic changes with cine MR imaging and phase-shift velocity mapping – initial experience. Radiology 2000; 214:467–75.

27. Fogel MA, Weinberg PM, Chin AJ, et al. Late ventricular geometry and performance changes of functional single ventricle throughout staged Fontan reconstruction assessed by magnetic resonance imaging. J Am Coll Cardiol 1996; 28:212–21.

28. Fogel MA, Weinberg PM, Fellows KE, Hoffman EA. A Study in ventricular–ventricular interaction: single right ventricles compared with systemic right ventricles in a dual chambered circulation. Circulation 1995; 92:219–30.

29. Fogel MA, Gupta KB, Weinberg PW, Hoffman EA. Regional wall motion and strain analysis across stages of Fontan reconstruction by magnetic resonance tagging. Am J Physiol 1995; 269:H1132–52.

30. Fogel MA, Weinberg PM, Hoydu A, et al. The nature of flow in the systemic venous pathway in Fontan patients utilizing magnetic resonance blood tagging. J Thorac Cardiovasc Surg 1997; 114:1032–41.

31. Ho V, Prince M. Thoracic MR aortography: imaging techniques and strategies. Radiographics 1998; 18:287–309.

32. Beekman R, Hazekamp M, Sobotka M, et al. A new diagnostic approach to vascular rings and pulmonary slings: the role of MRI. Magn Reson Imaging 1998; 16:137–45.

33. van Son J, Julsrud P, Hagler D, et al. Imaging strategies for vascular rings. Ann Thorac Surg 1994; 57:604–10.

34. Didier D, Ratib O, Beghetti M, et al. Morphologic and functional evaluation of congenital heart disease by magnetic resonance imaging. J Magn Reson Imaging 1999; 10:639–55.

35. Lee VS, Resnick D, Bundy JM, et al. MR evaluation in one breath hold with real-time true fast imaging with steady-state precession. Radiology 2002; 222:835–42.

36. Edelman RR, Chien D, Kim D. Fast selective black blood MR imaging. Radiology 1991; 181:655–60.

37. Roest AAW, Helbing WA, van der Wall EE, de Roos A. Postoperative evaluation of congenital heart disease by magnetic resonance imaging. J Magn Reson Imaging 1999; 10:656–66.

38. Finn JP, Baskaran V, Carr JC, et al. Low-dose contrast-enhanced three-dimensional MR angiography with subsecond temporal resolution – initial results. Radiology 2002; 224:896–904.

39. Hoffman EA, Gnanaprakasam D, Gupta KB, et al. VIDA: an environment for multidimensional image display and analysis. Proc SPIE 1992; 1660:694–711.

40. Snider AR, Serwer GA. Echocardiography in Pediatric Heart Disease. St Louis, MO: Mosby Year Book, 1990: 21–77.

41. Chin AJ. Noninvasive Imaging of Congenital Heart Disease. Armonk NY: Futura, 1994: 7–8.

42. Weinberg PM. Systematic approach to diagnosis and coding of pediatric cardiac disease. Pediatr Cardiol 1986; 7:35–48.

43. Van Praagh R. The segmental approach to diagnosis in congential heart disease. Birth Defects 1972; 8:4–23.

44. Morrow WR, Huhta JC, Aortic arch and pulmonary artery anomalies. In: The Science and Practice of Pediatric Cardiology (Garson A, Bricker JT, McNamara DG, eds.). Philadelphia: Lea & Feibiger, 1997:1421–52.

45. Schuford WH, Sybers RG, Hogan GB. The Aortic Arch and Its Malformations. Springfield, MA: Charles C Thomas, 1974: 41–244.

46. Knight L, Edwards JE. Right aortic arch: types and associated cardiac anomalies. Circulation 1974; 50:1047–51.

47. Lakier JB, Stanger P, Heymann MA, et al. Tetralogy of Fallot with absent pulmonary valve. Circulation 1974; 50:167–74.

48. Van Praagh R, Van Praagh S. The anatomy of comon aorticopulmonary trunk (truncus arteriosus communis) and its embryologic implications. Am J Cardiol 1965; 16:406–25

49. Kutsche LM, Van Mierop LH. Anomalous origin of a pulmonary artery from the ascending aorta: associated anomalies and pathogenesis. Am J Cardiol 1988; 61:850–6.

50. Gumbiner CH, Mullins CE, McNamara DG. Pulmonary artery sling. Am J Cardiol 1980; 45:316–20.

51. Vasquez-Perez J, Frontera-Izquierdo P. Anomalous drainage of the right superior vena cava into the left atrium as an isolated anomaly: rare case report. Am Heart J 1979; 97:89–91.

52. Marcelletti C, Mair DD, McGoon DC, et al. The Rastelli operation for transposition of the great arteries. J Thorac Cardiovasc Surg 1976; 72:427–34.

53. Crupi G, Pillai R, Parenzan L, et al. Surgical treatment of subpulmonary obstruction in transposition of the great arteries by means of a left ventricular–pulmonary artery conduit. J Thorac Cardiovasc Surg 1985; 89:907–13.

54. Norwood WI, Lang P, Castaneda AR, et al. Management of infants with left ventricular outflow obstruction by conduit interposition between ventricular apex and thoracic aorta. J Thorac Cardiovasc Surg 1983; 86:771–6.

55. Fontan F, Baudet E. Surgical repair of tricuspid atresia. Thorax 1971; 26:240–8.

56. Mustard WT. Successful two-stage correction of transposition of the great vessels. Surgery 1964; 55:469–72.

57. Senning A. Surgical correction of transposition of the great vessels. Surgery 1959; 45:966–80.

58. Takeuchi S, Imamura H, Katsumoko K, et al. New surgical method for repair of anomalous left coronary artery from pulmonary artery. J Thorac Cardiovasc Surg 1979; 78:7–11.

59. Anderson RH, Zuberbuhler JR, Hoy SY, et al. Double-inlet left ventricle with rudimentary right ventricle and ventriculoarterial concordance. Am J Cardiol 1883; 52:573–7.

60. Sathe SV, Khanolkar UB, Kaneria VK, et al. Supero-inferior ventricles: report of six cases. Am Heart J 1991; 121:1234–6.

61. Ivemark BI. Implications of agenesis of the spleen in the pathogenesis of conotruncus anomalies in childhood: an analysis of the heart malformations in the splenic agenesis syndrome, with fourteen new cases. Acta Paed Scand 1955; 44(Suppl 104):1–110.

62. Moller JH, Nakib A, Anderson RC, et al. Congenital cardiac disease assoicated with poly-splenia. A developmental complex of bilateral 'left sidedness'. Circulation 1967; 36:789–99.

63. Nadas AS, Ellison RC. Cardiac tumors in infancy. Am J Cardiol 1968; 21:363–6.

64. Sechtem U, Pflugfelder PW, White RD, et al. Cine MRI: potential for the evaluation of cardiovascular function. AJR 1987; 148:239–46

65. Rebergen SA, Niezen RA, Helbing WA, et al. Cine gradient-echo MR imaging and MR velocity mapping in the evaluation of congenital heart disease. Radiographics 1996; 16:467–81

66. Fogel MA, Weinberg PM. Haselgrove J. Non-uniform flow dynamics in the aorta of normal children: a simplified approach to measurement using magnetic resonance velocity mapping study. J Magn Reson Imaging 2002; 15:672–8.

67. Fogel MA, Weinberg PM, Hoydu A, et al. Effect of surgical reconstruction on flow profiles in the aorta using magnetic resonance blood tagging. Ann Thorac Surg 1997; 63:1691–700.

68. Edelman RR, Mattle HP, Kleefield J, et al. Quantification of blood flow with dynamic MR imaging and presaturation bolus tracking. Radiology 1989; 171:551–6.

69. Maddahi J, Crues J, Berman DS, et al. Noninvasive quantification of left ventricular myocardial muscle mass by gated proton nuclear magnetic resonance imaging. J Am Coll Cardiol 1987; 10:682–92.

70. Boxt LM, Katz J. Magnetic resonance imaging for quantification of right ventricular volume in patients with pulmonary hypertension. J Thorac Imaging 1993; 8:92–7.

12

CMR in cardiomyopathy

Sanjay K Prasad, Dudley J Pennell

Introduction

Overview

Cardiomyopathy is an important cause of morbidity and mortality characterized by a group of diseases where there is direct involvement of the heart muscle by the disease process itself. Generally, they are chronic and progressive conditions with impairment of cardiac function.[1] In accordance with the World Health Organization (WHO) classification (Table 12.1),[2] they are divided into four main groups: dilated, hypertrophic, restrictive and arrhythmogenic right ventricular cardiomyopathy. In addition, there are 'specific cardiomyopathies' that are associated with specific cardiac or systemic disorders (amyloid, sarcoid, siderotic) (Table 12.2). The diagnosis of primary cardiomyopathy requires exclusion of other etiological factors.

Cardiovascular Magnetic Resonance (CMR) is well suited to the evaluation of myocardial disease.[3,4] Key advantages include the high spatial resolution and the high contrast between flowing blood and myocardium. Assessment can be multiplanar in 3D, with good anatomical delineation of the apex and right ventricle that can be more difficult to achieve with other more established imaging modalities such as echocardiography. Furthermore, no geometrical assumptions are made regarding the shape of the left or right ventricles. Indeed, in patients with cardiomyopathy, the heart is frequently not ellipsoidal, with distorted morphology due to ventricular dilatation or thickening. CMR provides accurate and reproducible tomographic static and dynamic images of the heart with high temporal and spatial resolution in any desired plane without limitation by the acoustic window,[5] and with excellent reproducibility.[6] Unlike X-ray angiography, CMR is noninvasive and there is no exposure to ionizing radiation.

Table 12.1 Classification of the cardiomyopathies

Type of cardiomyopathy	Description
Dilated	Dilatation and impaired contraction of the left or both ventricles. Caused by familial/genetic, viral and/or immune, alcoholic/toxic, or unknown factors.
Hypertrophic	Left- and/or right-ventricular hypertrophy, often asymmetrical, which usually involves the interventricular septum. Nine sarcoplasmic protein mutations are known, but with variable clinical phenotype.
Restrictive	Restricted filling and reduced diastolic size of either or both ventricles, with normal or near-normal systolic function. Can be primary or associated with other disease such as amyloidosis.
Arrhythmogenic right ventricular	Progressive fibrofatty replacement of the right-ventricular myocardium. Affects left ventricle in 15% of cases during life. Familial disease is common, with two genes already identified.
Unclassified	Diseases that do not fit readily into any category. Examples include mitochondrial disease and fibroelastosis.

Table 12.2 Specific cardiomyopathies

Ischemic	Presents with dilated poorly functioning left ventricle due to ischemic damage from coronary artery disease.
Valvular	Presents as ventricular dysfunction that is out of proportion to the abnormal loading conditions produced by the valvular stenosis and/or regurgitation.
Hypertensive	Presents with left-ventricular hypertrophy with features of cardiac failure due to systolic or diastolic dysfunction.
Inflammatory	Cardiac dysfunction as a consequence of myocarditis.
Metabolic	Wide variety of causes: endocrine abnormalities, glycogen storage disease, metabolic deficiencies (hypokalemia), and nutritional disorders (beri beri).
General systemic disease	Connective tissue disorders and infiltrative diseases such as sarcoidosis and leukemia.
Muscular dystrophies	Duchenne, Becker-type, and myotonic dystrophies.
Neuromuscular disorders	Friedreich's ataxia, Noonan syndrome, and lentiginosis.
Sensitivity and toxic reactions	Includes reactions to alcohol, catecholamines, anthracyclines, irradiation, and others.
Peripartum	Manifest shortly after birth, and may recur with subsequent pregnancies.

Role of CMR

In the assessment of cardiomyopathy, CMR can be used diagnostically to evaluate morphological and functional parameters. Systolic function can be appraised from the vertical long-axis (VLA) and horizontal long-axis (HLA) cines as well as the short-axis cine stack. Diastolic dysfunction is increasingly recognized as abnormal in many patients with cardiomyopathy, as demonstrated in Framingham data.[7] It can occur both in isolation, where it is characterized by features of heart failure but with normal ejection fraction, and in conjunction with systolic dysfunction.[8,9] Recognition is important in view of the increased associated morbidity and mortality.[10] Typical features are abnormal peak filling rates and time–volume curves, deranged ventricular inflow measurements, and dilatation of the left atrium. Diastolic function can be measured using CMR from high-temporal-resolution cine datasets, or using myocardial tagging.

In addition, specific CMR sequences can derive more specific information about myocardial tissue that provides a mechanistic basis for the cardiomyopathy. T1-weighted, dark-blood spin-echo sequences visualize the myocardium with good contrast to adjacent structures such as epicardial fat and ventricular blood. Late enhancement following gadolinium administration can be used to identify any regions of fibrosis or scarring, as well as inflammatory and infiltrative processes. T2-weighted spin-echo sequences also demonstrate infiltrative processes and highlight any myocardial edema or pericardial effusion. CMR T2* sequences can also be used to show siderosis (iron overload) in hemochromatosis and thalassemia. The high degree of accuracy and repro-

ducibility facilitates follow-up and appraisal of therapeutic response. An expanding role is in early detection of phenotypic changes, where the excellent image quality enables family screening in the inherited forms of cardiomyopathy and the opportunity to initiate prompt treatment. For clinical studies, the sample size required is markedly reduced due to the lower variability compared with other imaging modalities.[11]

Dilated cardiomyopathy
Clinical features

Dilated cardiomyopathy (DCM) is the commonest form of cardiomyopathy (~60%). Some variation in nomenclature occurs around the world. In the WHO classification, idiopathic DCM is considered as a final common pathway that is the end-product of myocardial damage due to (1) immunological, (2) viral, metabolic, and cytotoxic effects, and (3) genetic factors.[12] The commonest cause of a dilated heart, however, is the sequelae of coronary artery disease (CAD) and hypertension, known in some countries as ischemic cardiomyopathy. This will be dealt with separately.

The hallmark feature of primary DCM is dilatation, usually of both ventricles, associated with impaired contractile function. There is an increase in the end-diastolic and end-systolic volume indexes, together with a reduction in stroke volume and ejection fraction. Valvular abnormalities can be associated, and include mitral and tricuspid regurgitation due to stretching of the valve ring. Typically, wall thickness is normal so that the LV mass index is increased. Unlike CAD, there is less localized wall motion abnormality and thinning. In the WHO classification, patients with the variant of impaired systolic function and mildly dilated LV are categorized in the *unclassified* cardiomyopathy group.

The incidence of primary DCM is around 5–8 cases per 100 000 population per year. This rate is increasing. It is more prevalent in males and Afro-Caribbeans. It accounts for around 25% of cases of congestive heart failure in the USA.[13] The usual mode of presentation is with symptoms and signs of heart failure. In patients with recent-onset DCM, about 25% will show spontaneous recovery within 12 months. For the remainder, the natural history without treatment is a 5-year mortality rate of 50%.[14]

Macroscopically, there is usually dilatation of all four chambers. Wall thickness is usually normal, although LV hypertrophy may develop as a means of reducing systolic wall stress. Apical thrombi are frequently seen. Coronary arteries are usually normal or show only mild plaque disease that is out of proportion to the degree of ventricular dysfunction. Myocardial biopsy from affected regions typically shows widespread interstitial and perivascular fibrosis, particularly affecting the subendocardial layer. Regions of necrosis and cellular infiltration may be seen.[15]

CMR findings

The initial suggested approach (Table 12.3) is an ECG-gated T1-weighted multislice spin-echo sequence of the entire heart in a transverse plane for anatomical delineation and to exclude any structural abnormalities. Cines, preferably using steady-state free precession (SSFP) sequences,[16] (Figure 12.1) should then be acquired in a VLA and HLA plane to assess overall long-axis function, determine any regional changes, and highlight any valvular abnormalities. A short-axis cine stack using well-established techniques[17,18] provides volumetric data to establish the LV and right-ventricular (RV) end-diastolic and end-systolic volumes, together with the stroke volume and ejection fraction and LV mass. Myocardial tagging can identify regional strain pattern abnormalities and provides quantitative assessment of contractility.

An important aspect of the qualitative assessment is to look for any regional wall motion abnormalities or regional wall thinning that might indicate an ischemic basis as the underlying cause. RV function is normally affected in most cases of non-ischemic dilated cardiomyopathy, but the extent of involvement is variable. Left, atrial (LA) volume can be measured and carries prognostic significance in DCM.[19] Valvular function can be assessed using a combination of flow mapping and measurement of differences in stroke volume between RV and LV. In patients with DCM, this is helpful to measure the extent of mitral regurgitation where surgical repair may improve outcome. Diastolic function can be assessed by a combination of the time–volume inflow curve of the LV and the tagging strain pattern. This technique can be used to follow therapeutic response, including to exercise.[20]

In acute myocarditis, gadolinium enhancement demonstrates patchy and sometimes diffuse patterns of uptake.[21] This reflects early edematous changes. The degree of myocardial enhancement appears to correlate with clinical status and LV function. These abnormalities are also demonstrated using T2-weighted spin-echo sequences.

In studies of late gadolinium enhancement in DCM, fibrosis is absent in ~60% of cases (Figure 12.2).[22] It has been suggested that in the appropriate clinical circumstances, coronary angiography would not be necessary for these patients to exclude coronary disease as the causative factor, because no damage to the myocardial substrate is present. In about a quarter of patients with DCM, there is patchy midwall hyperenhancement that has no correlation with coronary artery territories and that is distinct from

Table 12.3 Dilated cardiomyopathy protocol	
Morphology	*Multislice T1-weighted spin-echo sequence*
Function (cines) and volume	• VLA • HLA • SA stack
Valves	• Gradient-echo cine CMR • Consider flow maps
Contractility	• Tagging sequences in SA stack plus HLA and VLA planes.
Late enhancement	• Uptake of gadolinium in VLA, HLA, and SA planes to detect fibrotic changes and exclude silent infarcts.
VLA, vertical long-axis; HLA, horizontal long-axis; SA, short-axis.	

(a)

(b)

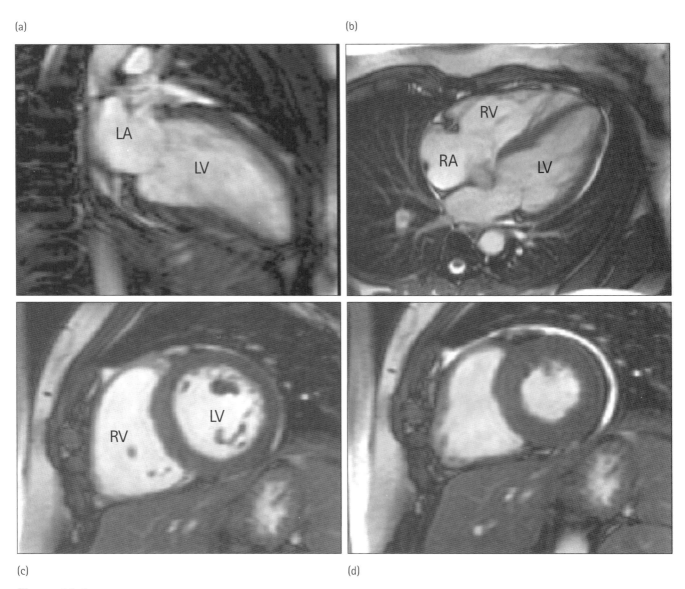

(c)

(d)

Figure 12.1
Measurement of volumes with steady-state free precession (SSFP) cines. SSFP images of cardiac chambers: (a) vertical long-axis; (b) four-chamber view; (c) mid-ventricle short-axis cut in diastole; (d) same mid-ventricle short-axis cut in systole. LV, left ventricle; LA, left atrium; RV, right ventricle; RA, right atrium.

an ischemic pattern (Figure 12.3). This has been shown before in pathological studies, but has not been previously visualized in vivo. The prognostic importance of this finding is unknown, but active investigation into a possible relationship with arrhythmias is underway. Finally, in a small group of about one in seven patients being managed with DCM, the gadolinium-enhancement pattern seen is indistinguishable from infarcts seen in CAD. In these patients, it is likely that the clinical diagnosis is infarction perhaps due to recanalization and a minor residual plaque, which did not present as an acute event and was therefore untreated. Alternatively, thrombosis

may be an explanation. Both would result in global remodeling,[23] and when coronary angiography is performed it appears to be normal, and the label of DCM incorrectly applied. Another possibility is that DCM and coronary disease can occur in tandem, although this explanation does not accord well with the principle of Ockham's razor.

In DCM, CMR can be used to monitor the efficacy of drug treatment.[24] This has been demonstrated in either DCM or heart failure of general causation for growth hormone (Figure 12.4),[25] angiotensin-converting enzyme (ACE) inhibitors,[26] beta-blockers (Figure 12.5),[27,28] and

(a)

(b)

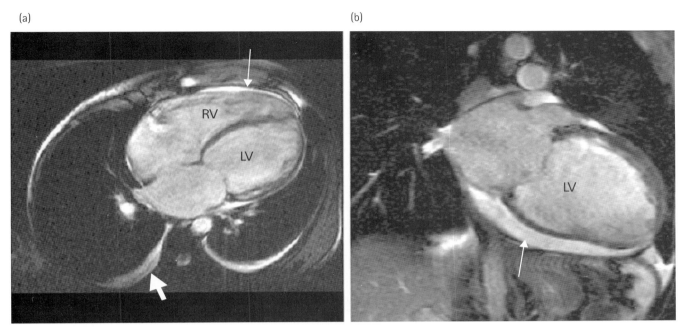

Figure 12.2
Dilated cardiomyopathy. CMR of a patient with idiopathic DCM seen in (a) horizontal long-axis (HLA) and (b) vertical long-axis (VLA) planes. There is marked biventricular dilatation. In addition, a pleural (short arrow) and pericardial (long arrow) effusion are present. Abbreviations as in Figure 12.1. LV, left ventricle; RV, right ventricle.

endothelin antagonists (Figure 12.6).[29] Recently, an important therapeutic option in patients with DCM is the use of resynchronization with pacemakers and the use of implantable cardioverter–defibrillators. At present, CMR is contraindicated in these patients. Work is however, underway to develop CMR-compatible versions of these devices.[30]

Finally, in specialized centers, it has proven possible to measure the myocardial levels of high-energy phosphates in DCM, and show that the phosphocreatine-to-ATP ratio is decreased.[31,32] Patient outcomes are linked to the level of this ratio, and it proved to be more predictive than the ejection fraction or the clinical heart failure class.[33]

Comparison with other techniques

Whilst echocardiographic assessment in DCM provides information on LV abnormalities, in ~15% of cases, the study is suboptimal due to poor acoustic windows. There is often limited information on the RV. Reproducibility and accuracy are also not as good as in CMR.[6] Angiography with LV assessment provides the gold-standard delineation of coronary anatomy, but is not ideal for the definition of the myocardial consequences of ischemic damage, and in addition is invasive and involves ionizing radiation.

Hypertrophic cardiomyopathy
Clinical features

Hypertrophic cardiomyopathy (HCM) is characterized by inappropriate LV hypertrophy in the absence of any obvious cause of hypertrophy (e.g. hypertension or aortic stenosis). There is usually asymmetrical involvement of the interventricular septum, but the clinical phenotype is widely variable. A key functional hallmark is impaired diastolic function. Myocardial function is preserved or hyper-contractile until late in the natural history of the disease, when systolic impairment and ventricular dilatation may be seen. A subset of patients demonstrate dynamic LV outflow tract (LVOT) gradient that can be provoked by stress. Other features include systolic anterior motion of the mitral valve and mitral regurgitation due to the Venturi effect of blood in the LVOT on the mitral valve.

Histologically, there is myocyte disarray and increased fibrosis. HCM is the result of sarcomeric mutational defects, and at least ten gene abnormalities have been identified.[34] The overall prevalence of HCM is about 1 in 500 of the general population. The commonest presentation of de novo cases is shortness of breath or dizziness. Chest pain, presyncope and syncope, and arrhythmias are also seen. Sudden death can be a feature in the familial type of HCM, and can occur even if hypertrophy is not marked particularly in some genotypes such as cardiac troponin T or I gene abnormalities.[35] Typically, the

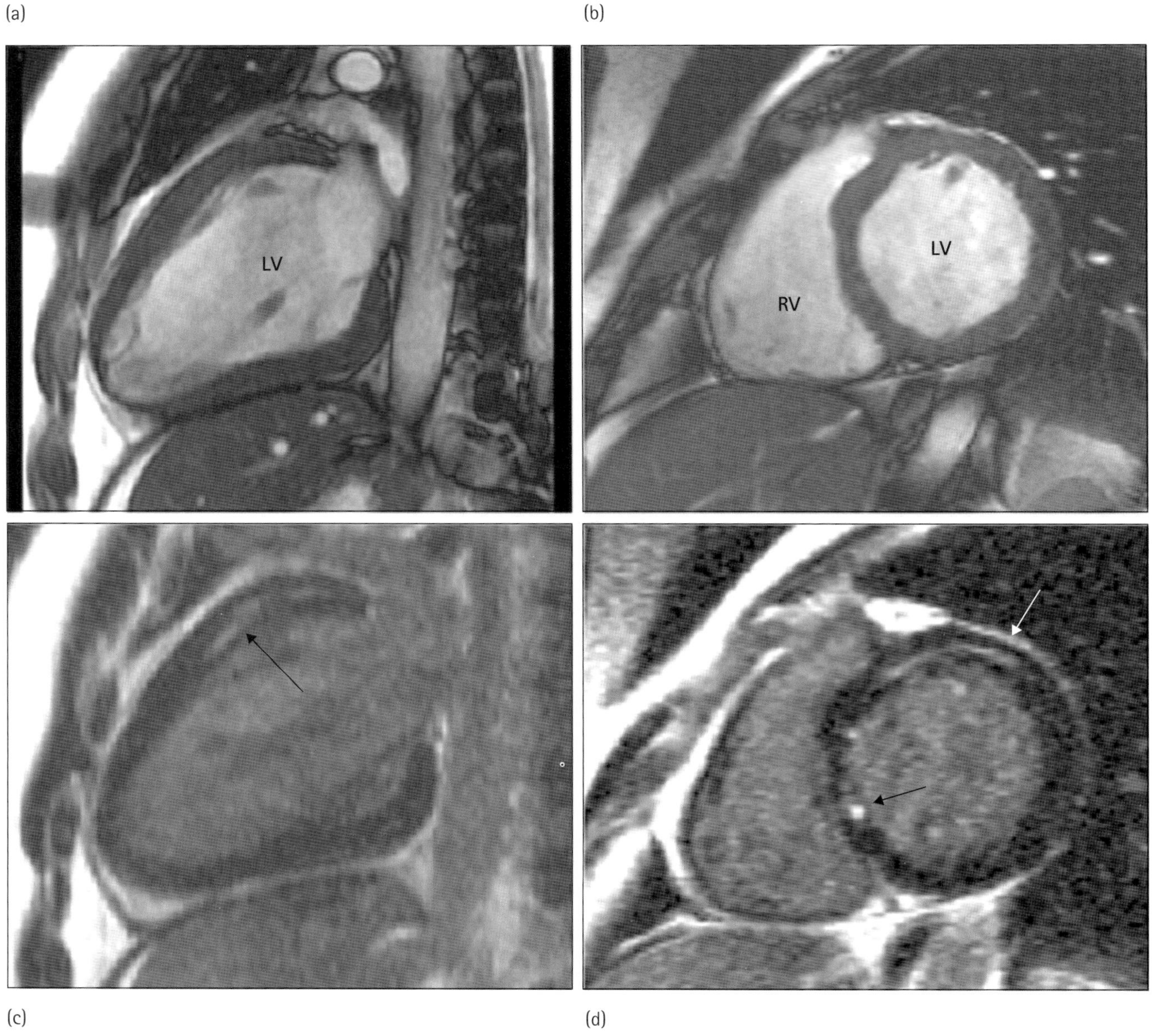

(a)

(b)

(c)

(d)

Figure 12.3

Detection of fibrosis in dilated cardiomyopathy. CMR of a 48-year-old patient with DCM. The vertical long axis is shown pre (a) and post (c) gadolinium. The mid-short-axis cut is also shown pre (b) and post (d) Gd DTPA. There is patchy mid-wall late enhancement that is most obvious in the anterior and septal walls (arrows). The pattern is distinct from fibrosis/scarring seen with ischemic heart disease in that it does not commence in the subendocardial layer and does not necessarily follow the coronary artery perfusion territories. Abbreviations as in Figure 12.1

diagnosis is made by a combination of echocardiography with an abnormal ECG.

CMR in HCM

CMR is extremely useful in the diagnosis of HCM. The whole myocardium and epicardial and endocardial borders can be well visualized, including the apex and inferior walls (Figure 12.7). Apical HCM can be very difficult to assess by echocardiography with poor visualization, but this is not a limitation with CMR (Figure 12.8).[36] Therefore, CMR is ideal for determining the phenotype, and is being applied in proband/relative studies for assessing family risk. CMR is also ideal for cross-sectional gene studies, and longitudinal studies between family members for this reason.[37]

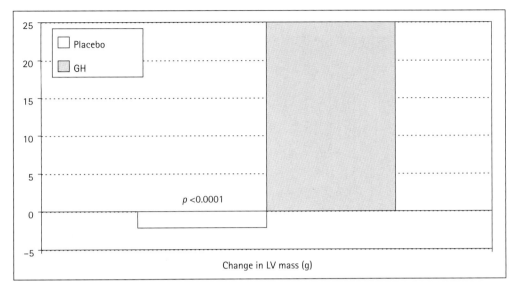

Figure 12.4
Growth (GH) hormone in dilated cardiomyopathy. This CMR study compared 25 patients on placebo with 25 patients on 2 IU/day of GH over 12 weeks. There was a highly significant difference in LV mass response between the groups.

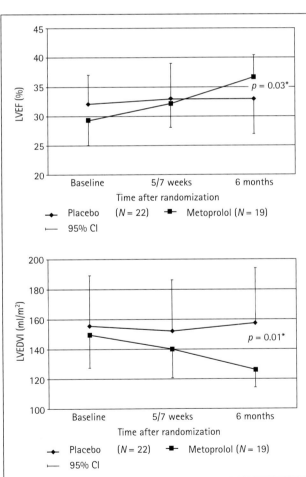

Figure 12.5
Beta-blocker treatment in heart failure. The LV ejection fraction (LVEF) increases and end-diastolic volume index (LVEDVI) decreases in patients with heart failure on beta-blocker therapy compared with placebo, using CMR as the measurement technique in 41 patients.

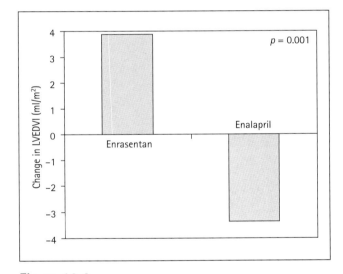

Figure 12.6
Assessment of endothelin antagonists. An endothelin antagonist (enrasentan) was compared with an ACE inhibitor (enalapril) using CMR in asymptomatic NYHA class 1 patients. Enalapril caused a significant reduction in the LV end-diastolic volume index (LVEDVI) compared with an adverse remodelling effect seen with enrasentan.

A recommended CMR protocol is outlined in Table 12.4. Depending on the genotype, there is a heterogeneous pattern of myocardial thickening, with an increase in the end-systolic and end-diastolic wall thickness and the ratio of septal to lateral wall thickness. The overall LV mass may be significantly increased, and both atria may be dilated. Using high-temporal-resolution SSFP cines and appropriate analysis software, the peak filling rate and time to peak filling rate can be established – both act as markers of diastolic function and may reveal

(a)

(b)

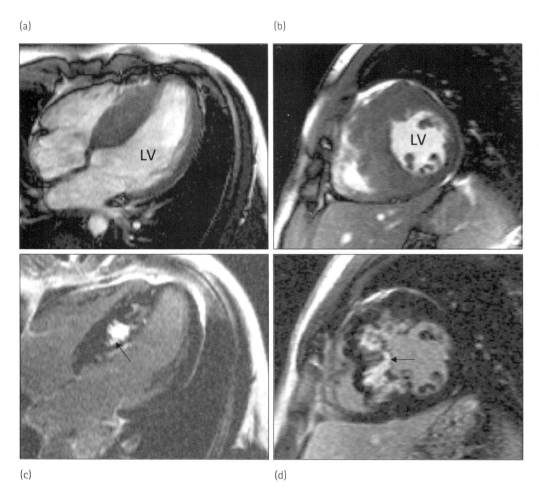

(c)

(d)

Figure 12.7
Hypertrophic cardiomyopathy. HCM with a troponin I mutation. The horizontal long-axis cut is shown pre (a) and post (c) gadolinium. The mid-short-axis cut is also shown pre (b) and post (d) gadolinium. The LV mass was significantly increased, with asymmetric septal hypertrophy. Following Gd-DTPA, patchy scarring was seen in the mid-septum (arrow).

a restrictive filling pattern due to reduced compliance. CMR can aid in the identification of mitral regurgitation and also outflow tract obstruction by identifying a signal void in the jet flow from a narrowed outflow tract and secondly by using velocity mapping proximal and distal to the outflow tract. Tagging patterns show abnormal regional contractility with reduced septal wall motion and impaired radial and circumferential strain patterns.[38] Long-axis function is reduced, and ventricular torsion is usually increased (Figure 12.9).[39]

Late gadolinium enhancement imaging may show areas of increased signal intensity, which can be patchy or diffuse. In one study of 21 asymptomatic or mildly symptomatic patients, 81% of patients were affected,[40] with the main distribution being in hypertrophied regions particularly the RV insertion point. These findings may represent fibrosis, severe myocardial disarray or fibrosis from small-vessel myocardial ischemia. The presence of enhancement was associated inversely with regional contraction, and positively with regional hypertrophy. Other work has

shown that patients with gadolinium uptake are at increased risk of cardiac events.[41] In younger patients (<40 years), the extent of gadolinium uptake is linked to risk factors for sudden cardiac death (Figure 12.10). In older patients (>40 years), the extent of gadolinium is linked to progression to heart failure (Figure 12.11). Further insights into the ventricular physiology in HCM have been obtained from perfusion studies demonstrating that the absolute coronary blood flow rate per gram of myocardial mass and the vasodilator flow reserve are significantly lower in patients with HCM than with normal healthy subjects.[42] Work is in progress to determine if these findings have clinical benefit in determining the functional severity of disease state in a patient and also the prognosis.

CMR has been used to assess the therapeutic response to interventions such as septal ablation (Figure 12.12).[43,44] The size and location of induced infarction, reduction in outflow tract obstruction, and longitudinal reduction in LV mass can be readily determined. The role of CMR in early detection of phenotypic abnormalities is

(a)   (b)

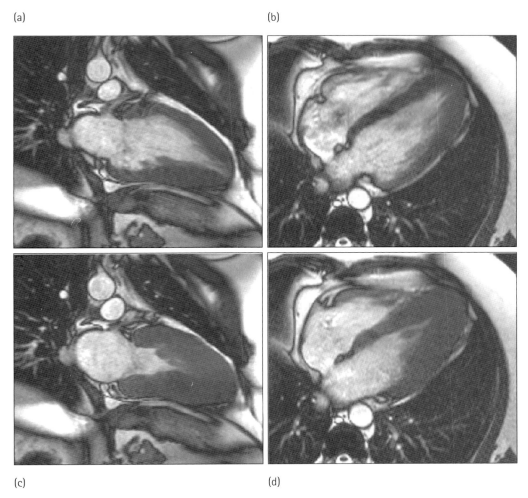

(c)   (d)

Figure 12.8
Apical hypertrophic cardiomyopathy. Apical HCM can be difficult to diagnose by echo, since the apical region is poorly visualized. CMR is not constrained by geometric planes or acoustic windows, and excellent views are obtainable to demonstrate apical hypertrophy in the vertical long axis (in diastole (a) and in systole (c)) and the four-chamber view (in diastole (b) and in systole (d)). In systole, there is cavity obliteration.

well documented,[45] and much interest has been focused on the role of tagging and better markers of diastolic dysfunction in the characterizing of these abnormalities. Variants of HCM such as Anderson–Fabry disease (which accounts for up to 4% of adult male HCM populations) can be distinguished from true HCM using the late enhancement pattern in lateral wall.[46] The reason for this specific finding is unknown.

Cardiomyopathy related to coronary disease

Clinical features

As a cause of LV dysfunction and congestive heart failure, CAD ranks as the leading cause of death in the Western world.[47] It is associated with an adverse prognosis. A

Table 12.4 Hypertrophic cardiomyopathy protocol

Morphology	*Transverse multislice T1-weighted spin-echo*
Function and mass	• Gradient-echo VLA and HLA • SA stack from mitral valve to apex • Tagging at basal, mid, and apical SA slices to assess regional wall motion
Outflow tract	• Gradient-echo cine of LVOT in two planes • Velocity flow map of LVOT undertaken in-plane and through-plane in LVOT and then above aortic valve
Fibrosis/scarring	• Late gadolinium-enhancement pattern using inversion recovery sequences

VLA, vertical long-axis; HLA, horizontal long-axis; SA, short-axis.

(a) (b)

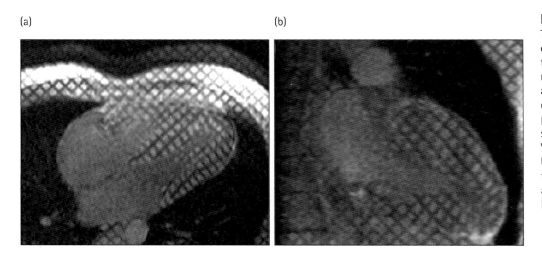

Figure 12.9
Tagging in hypertrophic cardiomyopathy. In addition to assessment of size and mass, MR has the ability to assess contractility through deformation of presaturation tag grids as shown in the HLA (a) and VLA (b) planes. This has been widely applied in HCM to determine regional abnormality in the hypertrophic regions.

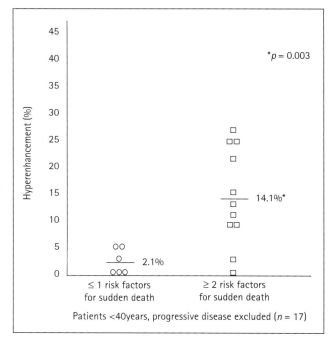

Figure 12.10
Hypertrophic cardiomyopathy and sudden death. In HCM patients, there is great hyperenhancement with gadolinium in those with risk factors for sudden death. This is particularly marked in patients aged under 40 years. (Reproduced from Moon et al. J Am Coll Cardiol 2003; 41:1561-7.[41])

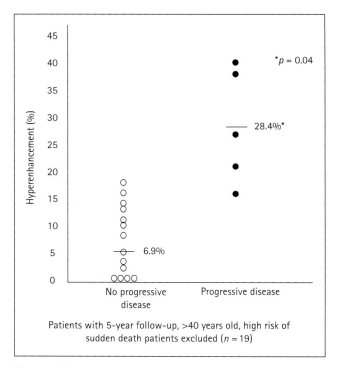

Figure 12.11
Hypertrophic cardiomyopathy and heart failure. In HCM patients, there is great hyperenhancement with gadolinium in those with progressive heart failure. This is particularly marked in patients aged over 40 years. (Reproduced from Moon et al. J Am Coll Cardiol 2003; 41:1561-7.[41])

unique feature of ischemic-related cardiomyopathy is hibernating myocardium, which is viable but with significantly impaired function that is recoverable with revascularization. It usually occurs in the presence of myocardial infarction, but this can be limited. In contrast, there is no functional improvement in scar tissue with revascularization. It is critical that any evaluation of function of this group of patients should determine the presence and extent of viable myocardium, since treatment is

believed to improve morbidity and prognosis.[48] Typically, dysfunction is chronic and associated with subendocardial infarction that affects <50% of the transmural wall.[49] Wall thickness is typically preserved. In contrast, nonviable myocardium shows dysfunction associated with near-transmural scarring and, particularly in the chronic stage, is thinned with fibrous replacement.

The evaluation of ventricular function and ischemic burden in patients with suspected or documented

(a)   (b)   (c)

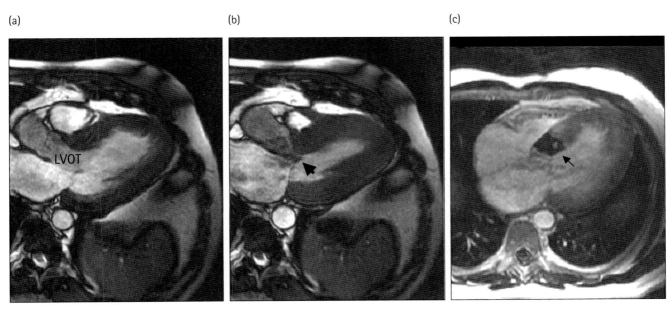

Figure 12.12
Septal ablation in a patient with hypertrophic cardiomyopathy. CMR of a 60-year-old patient with left-ventricular outflow tract (LVOT) obstruction who underwent alcohol septal ablation. CMR was performed 3 days post procedure. LVOT in diastole, and anterior motion of the mitral valve in systole (b: arrow). Following gadolinium, early enhancement images show decreased signal in a localized portion of the basal septum (c: arrow) suggestive of microvascular obstruction, and therefore correct localization of the infarct to relieve the obstruction.

ischemic heart disease can be made using various techniques, but all have their limitations. X-ray angiography has been considered the gold standard, but it has several limitations: it is invasive with a risk of morbidity and mortality, there is exposure to ionizing radiation, and it is well recognized that luminography provides little data on the myocardial substrate. Reflecting these factors is that in up to 60% of angiograms, subsequent management is by medical treatment rather than revascularization. Single-photon emission computed tomography (SPECT) is widely used to determine viability, and identifies reversible and fixed defects. SPECT also has limitations: the resolution is too limited to determine subendocardial changes, there is exposure to ionizing radiation, and artifacts significantly affect diagnostic accuracy. Positron emission tomography (PET) provides quantitative information on myocardial blood flow and glucose metabolism in hibernating myocardium and is not limited by attenuation artifacts, but resolution is still limited, and the technique comes with ionizing radiation, high cost, and lack of availability. Electron-beam computed tomography and multislice computed tomography are useful for identifying calcium deposition in coronary arteries with good resolution, but there is no significant published work on hibernation. Echocardiography is used clinically with a dobutamine stress protocol to identify recruitable contractile reserve in hibernation. It has good results when the acoustic access is satisfactory and it is widely available

and relatively cheap. However, subendocardial resolution is not available, and up to 15% of studies are non-diagnostic.

Role of CMR

Several CMR techniques are available to detect viable myocardium. Firstly, there is augmentation of contractility in response to inotropic agents such as dobutamine. Detecting improved contractile response after stress is suggestive of functional recovery after revascularization. Qualitative analysis consists of visualizing improvement in contractile response, whilst quantitative assessment compares end-diastolic wall thickness (EDWT) and systolic wall thickening (SWT). Criteria for viability include EDWT $\geq$5.5 mm and dobutamine-induced SWT $\geq$2 mm.[50] Myocardial tagging can also be used to detect any improvement with dobutamine.[51,52] Myocardial ischemia can also be detected, as a sign of both viability and adverse risk, through stress-induced wall motion abnormality,[53] which is better than that seen with dobutamine stress-echo.[54]

The second technique uses late gadolinium hyperenhancement (Figure 12.13). In the normal myocardium, >75% of tissue volume is intracellular leaving <25% of water space as the volume of distribution for contrast

(a)

(b)

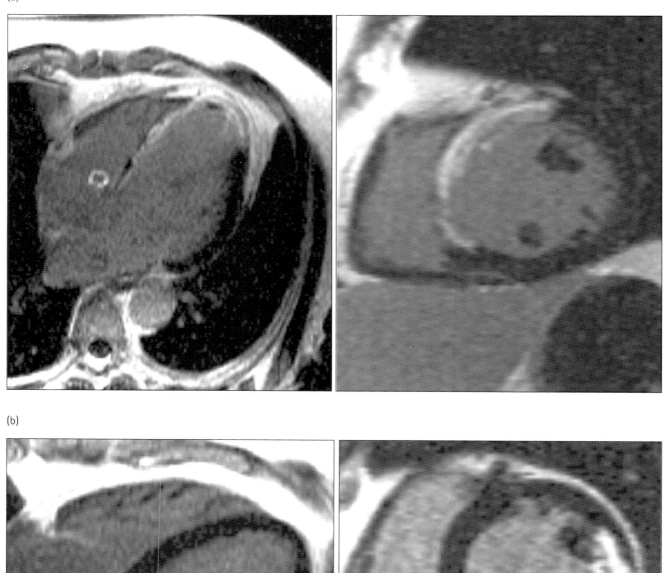

Figure 12.13

Cardiomyopathy due to ischemic heart disease. Extensive late enhancement in the anterior wall (arrows), seen in the four-chamber (a – upper left panel) and short-axis views (a – upper right panel) from a patient with a large anterior infarction. There is transmural and near transmural infarction. In contrast, in (b), there is subendocardial hyperenhancement seen in the lateral wall of the four-chamber (b – lower left panel) and short-axis views (b – lower right panel) in a patient with a lateral infarction (arrows). Substantial epicardial viable myocardium remains, and contractility in this region improved after revascularization.

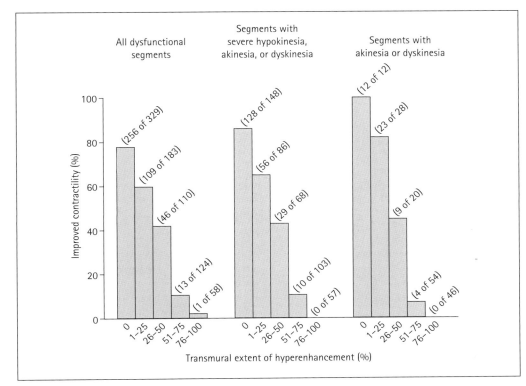

Figure 12.14
Transmural extent of gadolinium and functional recovery. There is a higher likelihood of functional recovery of dysfunctional segments affected by coronary disease when the gadolinium uptake is lower than when it is higher. This discrimination is particularly evident in the akinetic and dyskinetic segments. (Reproduced from Kim et al. N Engl J Med 2000; 343:1445–53.[49] © 2000 Massachusetts Medical Society.)

medium.[55] In infarcted tissue with nonviable myocytes, however, the tissue volume increases significantly. Animal and human studies show that following gadolinium, there is hyperenhancement of chronic infarct tissue in vivo.[56,57] The mechanism of such delayed enhancement is delayed washout and accumulation of contrast in necrotic, nonviable, myocardial tissue rich in collagen-filled fibrous scar with a larger interstitial compartment than in normal myocardium.[58] In a prospective study of 50 consecutive patients with ventricular dysfunction, cine and contrast CMR was performed before revascularization. The transmural extent of hyperenhancement correlated closely with the likelihood of increased contractility after revascularization (Figure 12.14).[49] Overall, 78% of segments with no hyperenhancement improved, compared with <2% of segments with >75% hyperenhancement. The high resolution and good predictive accuracy of CMR constitutes a significant advantage over other imaging modalities, whilst interpretation of stress responses and the use of ionizing radiation are not required. There is excellent correlation with PET data.[59]

Restrictive cardiomyopathy

Restrictive cardiomyopathy is a rare condition. The key common features are impaired diastolic function with restricted ventricular filling and reduction in diastolic volume. There are also dilated atria and inferior and supe-

rior vena cavae. Restrictive cardiomyopathy can be idiopathic or associated with systemic disorders, including hemochromatosis, sarcoid, and amyloidosis. The main diagnostic challenge is to differentiate this condition from constrictive pericarditis (Table 12.5). Using a combination of cines, T2-weighted spin-echo sequences, and postcontrast T1-weighted images, CMR has good diagnostic accuracy for assessment of restriction.[60] T2-weighted images are particularly helpful with this form of cardiomyopathy because of the edema associated with inflammatory and granulomatous lesions. It is important to bear in mind that conditions that may be classified as restrictive can also present with a dilated cardiomyopathy picture.

Myocardial siderosis

Iron deposition in the myocardium can be either primary or secondary. The primary form (hemochromatosis) is an autosomal recessive condition occurring mainly in Caucasians. The commonest secondary cause of siderosis is following frequent blood transfusions, notably in patients with thalassemia.

In primary myocardial siderosis, typical CMR findings include general functional abnormalities with initial impaired diastolic and systolic function. Ventricular dilatation also occurs. An important and unique role of CMR, however, is measurement of the iron overload, because iron decreases T1, T2*, and T2.[61] There is a

Table 12.5 Restriction versus constrictive pericarditis

	Restriction	Constrictive pericarditis
Pericardium	• Normal thickness	• Thickened (> 4 mm) • May be calcified
Atria	• Dilated	• Normal/dilated
Ventricle	• Small or normal-sized with preserved systolic function • Impaired diastolic function • Increased wall thickness and mass may be seen.	• Normal-sized ventricle. Normal wall size
Septum		• Contralateral bouncing of septum in diastole due to filling dysfunction
Late enhancement of myocardium	• Patchy myocardial uptake may suggest infiltrative process	• No late enhancement of myocardium reported, although myocardial fibrosis is known to occur in constriction • Pericardium may enhance with gadolinium if active inflammation is present
T1-weighted spin-echo	• May be patchy areas of increased signal intensity	• Thickened pericardium

correlation between the reduction in signal on T2-weighted spin-echo images and tissue iron content in animal models,[62] and this finding has been used to assess cardiac iron stores.[63] More recently, T2* imaging using gradient-echo images has proven a more robust technique to quantify tissue iron.[61]

Thalassemia is an inherited disorder in which there is an abnormality in one or more of the globin genes. It is

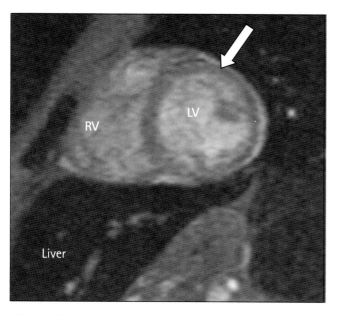
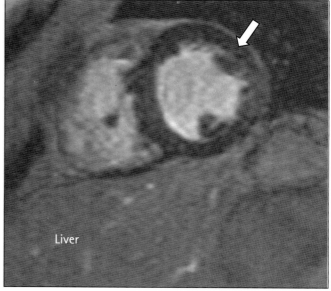

Figure 12.15
Myocardial siderosis. CMR is able to measure the T2* magnetic relaxation of the heart, which is significantly shortened by the tissue iron content. Thus, iron-loaded tissues are dark. In patient 1, there is considerable iron uptake in the liver but relatively little in the heart (large arrow). In contrast, in patients, there is marked iron overload (small arrow) with little hepatic uptake. Thus, liver iron levels are a poor guide to cardiac uptake.

the most common inherited condition worldwide, with 94 million heterozygotes affected, and 50 000 affected homozygote children born annually. Regular blood transfusions are required to treat the profound anemia and prevent death, but this results in the accumulation of iron in tissues, despite treatment with iron chelators such as desferrioxamine. Iron in the heart eventually leads to dilation and reduced function,[61] and heart failure causes up to 71% of all deaths in these patients,[64] with a 50% mortality rate by the age of 35 years.[65] The iron-induced cardiomyopathy is treatable and reversible with early and appropriate therapeutic intervention,[66] but mortality is high if treatment is delayed. LV dilatation and function as measured by echocardiography are insensitive as early markers of myocardial iron overload, but tissue Doppler has shown some encouraging results.[67] The key recent development has been the early detection of iron overload using T2*-weighted CMR sequences.[61,68] This allows direct quantification of myocardial iron, instead of the use of surrogate measures, which are later markers (Figure 12.15). The normal myocardial T2* >20 ms, and once iron accumulates to reduce T2* below this level, there is a clear relationship to adverse ventricular remodeling, including reduced ejection fraction and increased volumes (Figure 12.16).[61] This has allowed the evaluation for the first time of treatment responses to different iron-chelating drugs, and suggests that treatments specifically tailored to the heart can be developed, as deferiprone and desferrioxamine appear to have greater chelating ability in the heart and liver, respectively.[69]

Amyloidosis

Abnormal deposition of amyloid fibrils and associated fibrosis results in concentric hypertrophy of the ventricle and interatrial septal thickening. Frequently, the mitral and tricuspid valve leaflets are also thickened. The phenotypic manifestation can mimic hypertrophic cardiomyopathy but is distinguished by the concentric nature in the absence of hypertension, in conjunction with hypocontractility – notably loss of long-axis function – and reduced ejection fraction.[70] In addition, the atria are dilated and the T1 and T2 signal intensities reduced compared with normal. There is a loss of atrial function. Following gadolinium administration, there is a distinct endocardial pattern of uptake that also aids in the differentiation from other causes of hypertrophy.

Sarcoidosis

Sarcoidosis is a granulomatous condition associated with multisystem abnormalities. The incidence of cardiac involvement in systemic sarcoidosis is seen in 20–30% of cases at autopsy, although a smaller proportion are actually symptomatic.[71,72] The pathological features of cardiac sarcoidosis include patchy infiltration of the myocardium, with three successive histological stages: edema, granulomatous infiltration, and fibrosis leading to postinflammatory scarring.[73,74] Cardiac sarcoidosis is associated with an increased

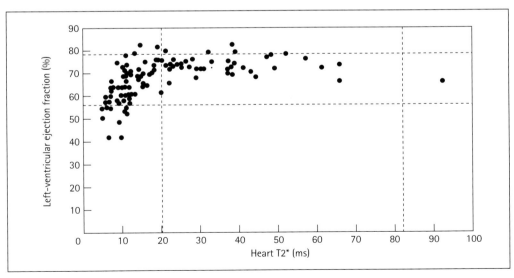

Figure 12.16
Relation between T2* of the myocardium and ejection fraction in thalassemia. The normal myocardial T2* >20 ms. In all patients with transfucsion dependent thalassemia, the ejection fraction was in the upper normal range, with T2* >20 ms. There was a linear decrease in ejection fraction, with T2* < 20 ms, clearly demonstrating the toxic iron effects on myocardial contractility and the value of measuring myocardial T2* in predicting the likelihood of deterioration in function. (Reproduced from Anderson et al. Eur Heart J 2001; 22:2171–9.[61])

risk of mortality,[75] including the risk of sudden death due to ventricular tachyarrhythmia or conduction block.[76] Typical symptoms suggestive of cardiac sarcoidosis are syncope, dyspnea, and, occasionally, acute cardiac failure.

Typical CMR findings are patchy regions of increased signal intensity on T2-weighted images and hyper-enhancement on T1-weighted images following gadolinium.[77–80] Increases in the thickness of the interventricular septum have also been noted.[81] A late feature of cardiac sarcoid involvement is ventricular dilatation associated with wall thinning and impaired function. Scarring is detected by gadolinium.[82] Occasionally, this can be difficult to distinguish from dilated cardiomyopathy, and attention should always be paid to the cardiac history. CMR is useful in sarcoid to guide biopsies, enhancing their otherwise low diagnostic success. In addition, it can be used both to initiate treatment and to monitor therapeutic response, particularly with corticosteroids.[74]

Arrhythmogenic right-ventricular cardiomyopathy

Arrythmogenic RV cardiomyopathy (ARVC) is characterized histologically by fibrofatty replacement primarily of the RV and clinically by life-threatening ventricular arrhythmias in apparently healthy young people.[83] When first described by Fontaine in 1977,[84] the original description related to six patients with sustained ventricular tachycardia who had no evidence of overt heart disease. Although initial descriptions have focused on localized RV involvement, it is now clear that ARVC can progress to diffuse RV and LV involvement and may culminate in biventricular failure.[85] ARVC is recognized as a cause of sudden death during athletic activity because of its association with ventricular arrhythmias provoked by exercise-induced catecholamine discharge. Diagnosis may be difficult because many of the electrocardiographic abnormalities mimic patterns seen in normal children, and the disease often involves only patchy areas of the RV. For this reason, international diagnostic criteria for ARVC were proposed by an expert consensus panel in 1994. Treatment is directed to preventing life-threatening cardiac arrhythmias with medications and the use of implantable defibrillators.

Histopathology

Characteristically, in ARVC, there is gradual replacement of myocytes by adipose and fibrous tissue. Morphological alterations usually begin in the subepicardium and progress to the endocardium with subsequent thinning of the wall.[86] The regions most frequently involved are the RV inflow area, the apex, and the infundibulum. These three areas form the so-called 'triangle of dysplasia'.[87] However, small amounts of fat are present in the epicardial layer and within the RV myocardium in normal subjects. In an autopsy study by Fontaine and Fontarilan[88] of hearts from individuals with no history of heart disorders, >50% of subjects had fat within their RV myocardial fibers, and the presence of intramyocardial fat increased with age. Consequently histological diagnosis of ARVC may be difficult in borderline cases. In a forensic autopsy of 20 patients with ARVC who died suddenly, the fatty replacement involved the outer half of RV free wall in 27%, the outer two-thirds in 28%, and the entire wall thickness in 45% of cases.[89] Curiously, the endocardial muscular trabeculae are generally spared, but may also be atrophied. The LV was involved in 40% of cases in this report, although other reports have identified LV involvement in up to 76% of individuals with ARVC at necropsy.[90] Typically, when the LV is involved, there is fibrofatty replacement of the subepicardial and midventricular wall, which is usually regional[91] although occasionally diffuse involvement can occur.[92] The pathological changes form the basis for ventricular arrhythmias, particularly in adolescents and young adults.

Etiology and epidemiology

A familial predilection has been identified with an autosomal dominant trait with variable penetrance and incomplete expression. The genetic basis involves chromosomes 10 and 14, but not all cases have been characterized. Problems have arisen due to incomplete penetrance and expression, polymorphic phenotype, age-related expression, and difficulties with accurate diagnosis of the disease. Recently, several additional theories have been proposed as the cause of or as environmental factors facilitating gene expression. These include inflammatory and degenerative changes, and apoptotic and myocyte transdifferentiation mechanisms.[93] The prevalence of the disease has been estimated at 1 in 5000 individuals.[94] This may reflect an under-representation, since diagnosis can be difficult. ARVC is an important cause of sudden death in individuals aged below 30 years, and in several studies is thought to account for up to 20% of the causes of sudden death in young people, particularly athletes.[95,96]

Clinical presentation

The typical presentation is in young adult men, with the diagnosis being made before the age of 40 years.[97] The mean age at diagnosis is 31 years.[98] ARVC should be considered in any young patients presenting with syncope, ventricular taehycardia (VT), or cardiac arrest, or in adult patients with congestive heart failure.[99] The mechanism of sudden death in ARVC is, in most cases, acceleration of VT with degeneration into ventricular fibrillation. The islands of fibrofatty tissue appear to generate macro re-entry electrical circuits and form the arrhythmogenic substrate for the onset of VT. Adrenergic stimulation such as physical exercise and catecholamine infusion appear to induce the arrhythmia. In a large follow-up review of 365 subjects, the mean age at death was 27 years. The annual mortality rate of ARVC has been estimated as 3% without treatment and as 1% with pharmacological medical treatment. This is significantly reduced by the use of implantable cardioverter–defibrillators (ICDs).

Diagnosis

The main diagnostic features of ARVC detected on CMR are quantitative measures of RV volumes, wall motion, and morphological abnormalities (Table 12.6).[100] When the LV

Table 12.6 CMR features of arrythmogenic right-ventricular cardiomyopathy

- Dilated or hypokinetic RV
- Increased RV end-systolic and end-diastolic volumes
- Localized aneurysms
- RV free-wall systolic bulging
- Increased signal intensity from fibrofatty myocardial replacement of RV
- Prominent trabeculations

is affected (15%), there is a mild decrease in LV function, although left-sided heart failure is unusual. Such dysfunction should be differentiated from biventricular myocarditis with fibrosis.[101] The definitive diagnosis of ARVC requires the histological finding of transmural fibrofatty replacement of RV myocardium at necropsy, surgery, or endomyocardial biopsy. The latter is problematic, since the usual area sampled is the intraventricular septum, which is rarely affected. For this reason, international diagnostic criteria for ARVC were proposed by an expert consensus panel in 1994. For the diagnosis of ARVC, a patient must

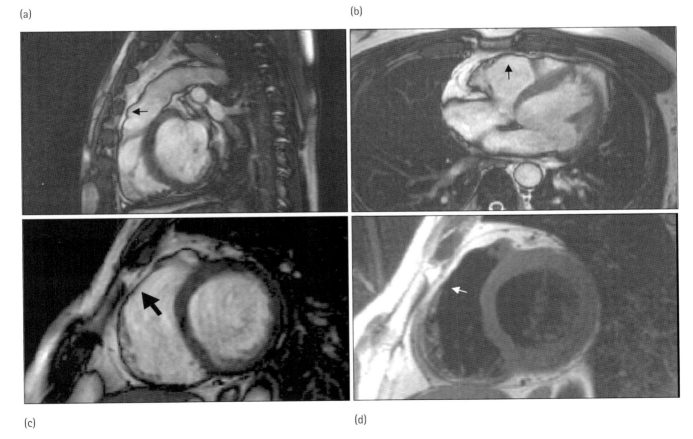

Figure 12.17
Arrythmogenic right-ventricular cardiomyopathy. (a) In this image of the RV outflow tract, there is bulging of the RV free wall (arrow). (b, c) RV dilatation with aneurysmal bulging of the RV free wall together with localized thinning. (d) Turbo spin-echo short-axis cut demonstrating fatty infiltration of the RV (arrow).

demonstrate either two major criteria, one major plus two minor criteria, or four minor criteria.[102]

CMR offers several advantages in the diagnosis of ARVC (Figure 12.17) and has helped to improve the diagnostic sensitivity and opportunity for early intervention; a protocol for acquisition and analysis is presented in Table 12.7. Cine CMR provides excellent contrast between the blood pool and the myocardial wall, and therefore can provide good quality information about regional RV wall motion and global RV function.[103] Impaired regional RV function is assessed in both the short-axis and transverse planes. Aneurysmal changes are also best appreciated with SSFP cines. Wall thinning and fibrofatty replacement of myocardium is best visualized by T1-weighted spin-echo, although frequent ventricular premature beats can make this difficult. Because significant fat infiltration of the RV has been described in a significant proportion of normal hearts in elderly patients, functional information is critical in establishing the diagnosis of ARVC.

Limitations of CMR

The RV free wall is thin (normal thickness 2.7 ± 0.4 mm), resulting in limited ability to adequately quantify the RV thickness, in addition to the normal presence of epicardial and pericardial fat, which can cause some difficulty in identifying intramyocardial fat.[104,105]

Management

Treatment options include pharmacological therapy such as beta-blockers and amiodarone. There is an increased trend towards the implantation of ICDs in patients at high risk for sudden cardiac death. These include patients who have been resuscitated from cardiac arrest, who have a history of syncope, or who have threatening arrhythmias that are not completely suppressed by antiarrhythmic therapy. From the CMR perspective, the practical implication is the contraindication to further scanning after ICD implantation.

Future considerations

Much interest is currently focusing on the role of myocardial velocity mapping, tagging and ventricular torsion to appraise systolic and diastolic function. It is likely that CMR will have an important role to play in the evaluation

---

Table 12.7 Protocol for evaluation of arrythrogenic right-ventricular cardiomyopathy.

A. Pharmacologic control of arrhythmia
B. 1.5 T MR scanner
C. Thoracic torso or cardiac coil (phase array receiver coil)
D. Sequences (preferred field of view 24–26 cm but <32 cm) Anterior surface coil may be used to reduce 'wraparound' artifact.
  1. Ventricular anatomy, wall thinning, fatty infiltration
    (a) ECG-gated spin-echo, transaxial plane, to cover from above the pulmonary valve to the diaphragm with suppression of blood pool signal (such as preparatory double inversion pulse) with either 3 mm multislice, 4 NEX, 5 mm gap, respiratory compensation or 5 mm single slices, 1 NEX, 3 mm gap with multiple acquisitions during breathholds. Fast spin-echo technique recommended only for breathhold images. In-plane pixel resolution should be $\leqslant$ 1.5 mm $\times$ 1.5 mm. Motion/artifact control techniques such as the use of a saturation band over the anterior chest wall are encouraged.
    (b) Same spin-echo sequence in the short-axis plane from base to apex of both ventricles.
  2. Ventricular function (regional and global):
    • Breathhold cine gradient echo sequences (steady-state free precession (SSFP) sequences preferred, such as TrueFISP, balanced fast field echo (FFE), Fiesta) encompassing the entire RV and LV in both transaxial and short-axis planes (planes to correspond with the spin-echo acquisitions above to allow direct comparison).
    • 10 mm gap between center of slices and optimal thickness according to local practice, but $\geqslant$ 5 mm.
  3. Other planes and sequences optional; for example fat-suppression double inversion recovery fast spin-echo images).
E. Analysis to include:
  1. Quantification of global RV and LV volumes, function, and mass.
  2. Examination for regional wall motion abnormalities on dynamic cines.
  3. Examination for RV anatomical abnormalities such as thinning, bulging, and abnormal trabeculation.
  4. Examination for possible fatty infiltration, excluding known sources of fat such as the RCA and LAD, atrial lipomatous hypertrophy, and obesity.
  5. Direct comparison of possible fatty infiltration sites with regional wall motion in corresponding areas on dynamic cines.
  6. Examination for LV involvement (clinically apparent in up to 15% of cases).

(Reproduced from Bluemke et al. Cardiology 2003; 99:153–62.[108])

of stem cell research. This is most obviously to assess functional response, but if tracker molecules can be generated, then it could also be used to guide and confirm the site of transplantation. In the assessment of cardiomyopathy it is now emerging that the same gene mutations can manifest in widely different ways, so that genotyping is not the panacea once expected – this highlights the importance of accurate phenotypic characterization.[106] As more patients with cardiomyopathy are genotyped, polymorphisms will be identified and there is the potential for pharmacogenomic-based therapy. Accurate phenotypic characterization will be integral to such therapeutic options,[107] and CMR is ideal in this role.

Conclusions

The diagnosis of cardiomyopathy can be comprehensively established in patients by a single CMR study. It is accurate and reproducible. Assessment can be made of function, mass, morphology, fibrotic/scarring changes, and infiltrative processes. Added to this armamentarium is the ability to assess remodeling, viability, and perfusion. Furthermore, CMR is extremely useful to monitor therapeutic response. An expanding role is in the early detection of phenotypic changes whilst screening family members for inherited cardiomyopathies. The future of CMR will be consolidated with greater phenotypic characterization of the cardiomyopathies, together with a better understanding of myocardial disease.

References

1. Ehlert FA. Comparison of dilated cardiomyopathy and coronary artery disease in patients with life-threatening ventricular arrhythmias: differences in presentation and outcome in the AVID registry. Am Heart J 2001; 142:816–22.

2. Richardson P, McKenna W, Bristow M, et al. Report of the 1995 World Health Organization/International Society and Federation of Cardiology Task Force on the Definition and Classification of cardiomyopathies. Circulation 1996; 93:841–2.

3. Schulz-Menger J, Friedrich MG. Magnetic resonance imaging in patients with cardiomyopathies: when and why. Herz 2000; 25:384–91.

4. Di Cesare E. MRI of the cardiomyopathies. Eur J Radiol 2001; 38:179–84.

5. Bellenger NG, Burgess MI, Ray SG, et al. Comparison of left ventricular ejection fraction and volumes in heart failure by echocardiography, radionuclide ventriculography and cardiovascular magnetic resonance: Are they interchangeable? Eur Heart J 2000; 21:1387–96.

6. Grothues F, Smith GC, Moon JC, et al. Comparison of interstudy reproducibility of cardiovascular magnetic resonance with two-dimensional echocardiography in normal subjects and in patients with heart failure or left ventricular hypertrophy. Am J Cardiol 2002; 90:29–34.

7. Redfield MM, Jacobsen SJ, Burnett JC Jr, et al. Burden of systolic and diastolic ventricular dysfunction in the community: appreciating the scope of the heart failure epidemic. JAMA 2003; 289:194–202.

8. van Kraaij DJ, van Pol PE, Ruiters AW, et al. Diagnosing diastolic heart failure. Eur J Heart Fail 2002; 4:419–30.

9. Varela-Roman A, Gonzalez-Juanatey JR, Basante P, et al. Clinical characteristics and prognosis of hospitalised inpatients with heart failure and preserved or reduced left ventricular ejection fraction. Heart 2002; 88:249–54.

10. Mandinov L, Eberli FR, Seiler C, Hess OM. Diastolic heart failure. Cardiovasc Res 2000; 45:813–25.

11. Bellenger NG, Davies LC, Francis JM, et al. Reduction in sample size for studies of remodeling in heart failure by the use of cardiovascular magnetic resonance. J Cardiovasc Magn Reson 2000; 2:271–8.

12. Takeda N. Cardiomyopathy: molecular and immunological aspects. Int J Mol Med 2003; 11:13–16.

13. Brown CA, O'Connell JB. Myocarditis and idiopathic dilated cardiomyopathy. Am J Med 1995; 99:309–16.

14. Dec GW, Fuster V. Medical progress: Idiopathic dilated cardiomyopathy. N Engl J Med 1994; 331:1564–70.

15. de Leeuw N Histopathologic findings in explanted heart tissue from patients with end-stage idiopathic dilated cardiomyopathy. Transplant Int 2001; 14: 299–306.

16. Moon JCC, Lorenz CH, Francis JM, et al. Breath-hold FLASH and FISP cardiovascular MR imaging: left ventricular volume differences and reproducibility. Radiology 2002; 223:789–97.

17. Pennell DJ. Ventricular volume and mass by CMR. J Cardiovasc Magn Reson 2002; 4:507–13.

18. Bellenger NG, Pennell DJ. Ventricular function. In: Magnetic Resonance Imaging in Clinical Cardiology (Manning WJ, Pennell DJ, eds). New York: Churchill Livingstone, 2002.

19. Rossi A, Cicoira M, Zanolla L, et al. Determinants and prognostic value of left atrial volume in patients with dilated cardiomyopathy. J Am Coll Cardiol 2002; 40:1425–30.

20. Myers J, Wagner D, Schertler T, et al. Effects of exercise training on left ventricular volumes and function in patients with nonischemic cardiomyopathy: application of magnetic resonance myocardial tagging. Am Heart J 2002; 144:719–25.

21. Friedrich MG, Strohm O, Schulz-Menger J, et al. Contrast media enhanced magnetic resonance imaging visualises myocardial changes in the course of viral myocarditis. Circulation 1998; 97:1802–9.

22. McCrohon JA, Moon JC, Prasad SK, et al. Differentiation of heart failure related to dilated cardiomyopathy and coronary artery disease using gadolinium enhanced cardiovascular magnetic resonance. Circulation 2003; 108:54–9.

23. Bellenger NG, Swinburn JM, Rajappan K, et al. Cardiac remodelling in the era of aggressive medical therapy: Does it still exist? Int J Cardiol 2002; 83:217–25.

24. Strohm O, Schulz-Menger J, Pilz B, et al. Measurement of left ventricular dimensions and function in patients with dilated cardiomyopathy. J Magn Reson Imaging 2001; 13:367–71.

25. Osterziel KJ, Strohm O, Schuler J, et al. Randomised, double-blind, placebo-controlled trial of human recombinant growth hormone in

patients with chronic heart failure due to dilated cardiomyopathy. Lancet 1998; 351:1233–7.

26. Doherty NE 3rd, Seelos KC, Suzuki J, et al. Application of cine nuclear magnetic resonance imaging for sequential evaluation of response to angiotensin-converting enzyme inhibitor therapy in dilated cardiomyopathy. J Am Coll Cardiol 1992; 19:1294–302.

27. Bellenger NG, Rajappan K, Lahiri A, et al. Effects of carvedilol on left ventricular remodelling in chronic stable heart failure demonstrated by cardiovascular magnetic resonance. Heart (in press).

28. Groenning BA, Nilsson JC, Sondergaard L, et al. Antiremodeling effects on the left ventricle during beta-blockade with metoprolol in the treatment of chronic heart failure. J Am Coll Cardiol 2000; 36:2072–80.

29. Prasad SK, Smith G, Dargie H, Cleland JCC, Pennell DJ. Enrasentan compared with enalapril in patients with asymptomatic left ventricular systolic dysfunction. Circulation 2002; 106:II-470.

30. Greatbatch W, Miller V, Shellock FG. Magnetic resonance safety testing of a newly-developed fiber-optic cardiac pacing lead. J Magn Reson Imaging 2002; 16:97–103.

31. Conway MA, Allis J, Ouwerkerk R, et al. Detection of low phosphocreatine to ATP ratio in failing hypertrophied human myocardium by P-31 magnetic resonance spectroscopy. Lancet 1991; 338:973–6.

32. Hardy CJ, Weiss RG, Bottomley PA, Gerstenblith G. Altered myocardial high-energy phosphate metabolites in patients with dilated cardiomyopathy. Am Heart J 1991; 122:795–80.

33. Neubauer S, Horn M, Cramer M et al. Myocardial phosphocreatine to ATP ratio is a predictor of mortality in patients with dilated cardiomyopathy. Circulation 1997; 96:2190–6.

34. Devlin AM. A comparison of MRI and echocardiography in hypertrophic cardiomyopathy. Br J Radiol 1999; 72:258–64.

35. Braunwald E, Seidman CE, Sigwart U. Contemporary evaluation and management of hypertrophic cardiomyopathy. Circulation 2002; 106:1312–16.

36. Pons-Llado G, Carreras F, Borras X, et al. Comparison of morphologic assessment of hypertrophic cardiomyopathy by magnetic resonance versus echocardiographic imaging. Am J Cardiol 1997; 79:1651–6.

37. Sipola P, Vanninen E, Aronen HJ. Cardiac adrenergic activity is associated with left ventricular hypertrophy in genetically homogeneous subjects with hypertrophic cardiomyopathy. J Nucl Med. 2003; 44:487–93.

38. Dong SJ, MacGregor JH, Crawley AP, et al. Left ventricular wall thickness and regional systolic function in patients with hypertrophic cardiomyopathy. A three-dimensional tagged magnetic resonance imaging study. Circulation 1994; 90:1200–9.

39. Dong SJ, Hees PS, Siu CO, et al. MRI assessment of LV relaxation by untwisting rate: a new isovolumic phase measure of tau. Am J Physiol Heart Circ Physiol 2001; 281:H2002–9.

40. Choudhury L, Mahrholdt H, Wagner A, et al. Myocardial scarring in asymptomatic or mildly symptomatic patients with hypertrophic cardiomyopathy. J Am Coll Cardiol 2002; 40:2156–64.

41. Moon JC, McKenna WJ, McCrohon JA, et al. Toward clinical risk assessment in hypertrophic cardiomyopathy with gadolinium cardiovascular magnetic resonance. J Am Coll Cardiol. 2003; 41:1561–7.

42. Kawada N, Sakuma H, Yamakado T, et al. Hypertrophic cardiomyopathy: MR measurement of coronary blood flow and vasodilator flow reserve in patients and healthy subjects. Radiology 1999; 211:129–35.

43. Sievers B, Moon JCC, Pennell DJ. Magnetic resonance contrast enhancement of iatrogenic septal myocardial infarction in hypertrophic cardiomyopathy. Circulation 2002; 105:1018.

44. Schulz-Menger J, Strohm O, Waigand J, et al. The value of magnetic resonance imaging of the left ventricular outflow tract in patients with hypertrophic obstructive cardiomyopathy after septal artery embolization. Circulation 2000; 101:1764–6.

45. Suzuki J, Shimamoto R, Nishikawa J, et al. Morphological onset and early diagnosis in apical hypertrophic cardiomyopathy: a long term analysis with nuclear magnetic resonance imaging. J Am Coll Cardiol 1999; 33:146–51.

46. Kampmann C, Wiethoff CM, Perrot A. The heart in Anderson Fabry disease. Z Kardiol. 2002; 91:786–95.

47. Poole-Wilson PA, Uretsky BF, Thygesen K, et al. Mode of death in heart failure: findings from the ATLAS trial. The Atlas Study Group. Assessment of treatment with lisinopril and survival. Heart 2003; 89:42–8.

48. Senior R, Kaul S, Lahiri A. Myocardial viability on echocardiography predicts long-term survival after revascularization in patients with ischemic congestive heart failure. J Am Coll Cardiol 1999; 33:1848–54.

49. Kim RJ, Wu E, Rafael A, et al. The use of contrast-enhanced magnetic resonance imaging to identify reversible myocardial dysfunction. N Engl J Med 2000; 343:1445–53.

50. Baer FM, Voth E, Schneider CA, et al. Comparison of low dose dobutamine gradient echo magnetic resonance imaging and positron emission tomography with fluorodeoxyglucose in patients with chronic coronary artery disease. A functional and morphological approach to the detection of residual myocardial viability. Circulation 1995; 91:1006–15.

51. Geskin G, Kramer CM, Rogers WJ, et al. Quantitative assessment of myocardial viability after infarction by dobutamine magnetic resonance tagging. Circulation 1998; 98:217–23.

52. Gotte MJ, van Rossum AC, Twisk JWR, et al. Quantification of regional contractile function after infarction: strain analysis superior to wall thickening analysis in discriminating infarct from remote myocardium. J Am Coll Cardiol 2001; 37:808–17.

53. Pennell DJ, Underwood SR, Manzara CC, et al. Magnetic resonance imaging during dobutamine stress in coronary artery disease. Am J Cardiol 1992; 70:34–40.

54. Nagel E, Lehmkuhl HB, Bocksch W, et al. Noninvasive diagnosis of ischemia-induced wall motion abnormalities with the use of high-dose dobutamine stress MRI: comparison with dobutamine stress echocardiography. Circulation 1999; 99:763–70.

55. Polimeni PI. Extracellular space and ionic distribution in rat ventricle. Am J Physiol 1974; 227:676–83.

56. Wu E, Judd RM, Vargas JD, et al. Visualisation of presence, location, and transmural extent of healed Q-wave and non-Q-wave myocardial infarction. Lancet 2001; 357:21–8.

57. Simonetti OP, Kim RJ, Fieno DS, et al. An improved MR imaging technique for the visualization of myocardial infarction. Radiology 2001; 218:215–23.

58. Rehwald WG, Kim RJ, Judd RM. Rapid cine MRI of the human heart using reconstruction by estimation of lines and inhibition of fold-in. Magn Reson Med 2002; 47:844–9.

59. Klein C, Nekolla SG, Bengel FM, et al. Assessment of myocardial viability with contrast-enhanced magnetic resonance imaging: comparison with positron emission tomography. Circulation. 2002; 105:162–7.

60. Masui T, Finck S, Higgins CB. Constrictive pericarditis and restrictive cardiomyopathy: evaluation with MR imaging. Radiology 1992; 182:369–73.

61. Anderson LJ, Holden S, Davies B, et al. Cardiovascular T2* magnetic resonance for the early diagnosis of myocardial iron overload. Eur Heart J 2001; 22:2171–9.

62. Liu P, Henkelman M, Joshi J, et al. Quantification of cardiac and tissue iron by nuclear magnetic resonance relaxometry in a novel murine thalassemia–cardiac iron overload model. Can J Cardiol 1996; 12:155–64.

63. Mavrogeni SI, Maris T, Gouliamos A, Vlahos L, Kremastinos DT. Myocardial iron deposition in beta-thalassemia studied by magnetic resonance imaging. Int J Card Imaging. 1998; 14:117–22.

64. Borgna-Pignatti C, Rugolotto S, De Stefano P, et al. Survival and disease complications in thalassemia major. Ann NY Acad Sci 1998; 850:227–31.

65. Kremastinos DT, Tsetsos GA, Tsiapras DP, et al. Heart failure in beta thalassemia: a 5-year follow-up study. Am J Med 2001; 111:349–54.

66. Anderson LJ, Holden S, Davis B, et al. Reversal of siderotic cardiomyopathy with myocardial iron elimination: a prospective CMR study. In review.

67. Vogel M, Anderson LJ, Holden S, et al. Tissue Doppler echocardiography in patients with thalassaemia detects early myocardial dysfunction related to myocardial iron overload. Eur Heart J 2003; 24:113–19.

68. Westwood M, Anderson LJ, Firmin DN, et al. A single breath-hold multiecho T2* cardiovascular magnetic resonance technique for diagnosis of myocardial iron overload. J Magn Reson Imaging 2003; 18:33–9.

69. Anderson LJ, Wonke B, Prescott E, et al. Comparison of effects of oral deferiprone and subcutaneous desferrioxamine on myocardial iron levels and ventricular function in beta thalassemia. Lancet 2002; 360:516–20.

70. Fattori R, Rocchi G, Celletti F, et al. Contribution of magnetic resonance imaging in the differential diagnosis of cardiac amyloidosis and symmetric hypertrophic cardiomyopathy. Am Heart J 1998; 136:824–30.

71. Flora GS, Sharma OP. Myocardial sarcoidosis: a review. Sarcoidosis 1989; 6:97–106.

72. Silverman KJ, Hutchins GM, Bulkley BH. Cardiac sarcoid: a clinicopathologic study of 84 unselected patients with systemic sarcoidosis. Circulation 1978; 58:1204–11.

73. Mana J. Magnetic resonance imaging and nuclear imaging in sarcoidosis. Curr Opin Pulm Med 2002; 8:457–63.

74. Vignaux O, Dhote R, Duboc D, et al. Clinical significance of myocardial magnetic resonance abnormalities in patients with sarcoidosis: a 1-year follow-up study. Chest 2002; 122:1895–901.

75. Shimada T. Diagnosis of cardiac sarcoidosis and evaluation of the effects of steroid therapy by gadolinium-DTPA-enhanced magnetic resonance imaging. Am J Med 2001; 110:520–7.

76. Valantine H, McKenna WJ, Nihoyannopoulos P, et al. Sarcoidosis: a pattern of clinical and morphological presentation. Br Heart J 1987; 57:256–63.

77. Chandra M, Silverman ME, Oshinski J, Pettigrew R. Diagnosis of cardiac sarcoidosis aided by MRI. Chest 1996; 110:562–5.

78. Doherty MJ, Kumar SK, Nicholson AA, McGivern DV. Cardiac sarcoidosis: the value of magnetic resonance imaging in diagnosis and assessment of response to treatment. Respir Med 1998; 92:697–9.

79. Statement on Sarcoidosis. Joint Statement of the American Thoracic Society (ATS), the European Respiratory Society (ERS) and the World Association of Sarcoidosis and Other Granulomatous Disorders (WASOG) adopted by the ATS Board of Directors and by the ERS Executive Committee, February 1999. Am J Respir Crit Care Med 1999; 160:736–55.

80. Riedy K, Fisher MR, Belic N, Koenigsberg DI. MR imaging of myocardial sarcoidosis. AJR 1988; 15:915–16.

81. Matsumori A, Hara M, Nagai S, et al. Hypertrophic cardiomyopathy as a manifestation of cardiac sarcoidosis. Jpn Circ J 2000; 64:679–83.

82. White ES. Sarcoidosis involving multiple systems: diagnostic and therapeutic challenges. Chest 2001; 119:1593–7.

83. Fontaine G, Fontaliran F, Hebert JL, et al. Arrhythmogenic right ventricular dysplasia. Annu Rev Med 1999; 50:17–35.

84. Fontaine G, Fontaliran F, Frank R, et al. Arrhythmogenic right ventricular dysplasia. A new clinical entity. Bull Acad Natl Med 1993; 177:501–12.

85. Corrado D, Basso C, Thiene G, et al. Spectrum of clinicopathologic manifestations of arrhythmogenic right ventricular cardiomyopathy/dysplasia: a multicenter study. J Am Coll Cardiol 1997; 30:1512–20.

86. Corrado D, Basso C, Thiene G. Arrhythmogenic right ventricular cardiomyopathy: diagnosis, prognosis, and treatment. Heart 2000; 83:588–95.

87. Gemayel C, Pelliccia A, Thompson PD. Arrhythmogenic right ventricular cardiomyopathy. J Am Coll Cardiol 2001; 38:1773–81.

88. Fontaine G, Fontaliran F. Arrhythmogenic right ventricular dysplasia masquerading as dilated cardiomyopathy. Am J Cardiol 1999; 84:1143.

89. Fornes P, Ratel S, Lecomte D. Pathology of arrhythmogenic right ventricular cardiomyopathy/dysplasia – an autopsy study of 20 forensic cases. J Forensic Sci 1998; 43:777–83.

90. Paul M, Schulze-Bahr E, Breithardt G, Wichter T. Genetics of arrhythmogenic right ventricular cardiomyopathy – status quo and future perspectives. Z Kardiol 2003; 92:128–36.

91. McCrohon JA, John AS, Lorenz CH, et al. Left ventricular involvement in arrhythmogenic right ventricular cardiomyopathy. Circulation 2002; 105:1394.

92. Corrado D, Basso C, Nava A, Thiene G. Arrhythmogenic right ventricular cardiomyopathy: current diagnostic and management strategies. Cardiol Rev 2001; 9:259–65.

93. Nava A, Bauce B, Basso C, et al. Clinical profile and long-term follow-up of 37 families with arrhythmogenic right ventricular cardiomyopathy. J Am Coll Cardiol 2000; 36:2226–33.

94. Corrado D, Buja G, Basso C, Thiene G. Clinical diagnosis and management strategies in arrhythmogenic right ventricular cardiomyopathy. J Electrocardiol 2000; 33 (Suppl):49–55.

95. Franz WM, Muller OJ, Katus HA. Cardiomyopathies: from genetics to the prospect of treatment. Lancet 2001; 358:1627–37.

96. Shen WK, Edwards WD, Hammill SC, et al. Sudden unexpected nontraumatic death in 54 young adults: a 30-year population-based study. Am J Cardiol 1995; 76:148–52.

97. Marcus FI, Fontaine GH, Guiraudon G, et al. Right ventricular dysplasia: a report of 24 adult cases. Circulation 1982; 65:384–98.

98. Folino AF, Buja G, Bauce B, et al. Heart rate variability in arrhythmogenic right ventricular cardiomyopathy correlation with clinical and prognostic features. Pacing Clin Electrophysiol. 2002; 25:1285–92.

99. Kullo IJ, Edwards WD, Seward JB. Right ventricular dysplasia: the Mayo Clinic experience. Mayo Clin Proc 1995; 70:541–8.

100. Blake LM, Scheinmann MM, Higgins CB. MR features of arrhythmogenic right ventricular dysplasia. AJR 1994; 162:809–12.

101. Pinamonti B, Sinagra G, Camerini F. Clinical relevance of right ventricular dysplasia/cardiomyopathy. Heart 2000; 83:9–11.

102. McKenna WJ, Thiene G, Nava A, et al. Diagnosis of arrhythmogenic right ventricular dysplasia/cardiomyopathy. Task Force of the Working Group Myocardial and Pericardial Disease of the European Society of Cardiology and of the Scientific Council on Cardiomyopathies of the International Society and Federation of Cardiology. Br Heart J 1994; 71:215–18.

103. Molinari G, Sardanelli F, Gaita F, et al. Right ventricular dysplasia as a generalized cardiomyopathy? Findings on magnetic resonance imaging. Eur Heart J 1995; 16:1619–24.

104. Burke AP, Farb A, Tashko G, Virmani R. Arrhythmogenic right ventricular cardiomyopathy and fatty replacement of the right ventricular myocardium: are they different diseases? Circulation 1998; 97:1571–80.

105. Fontaine G, Fontaliran F, Zenati O, et al. Fat in the heart. A feature unique to the human species? Observational reflections on an unsolved problem. Acta Cardiol 1999; 54:189–94.

106. Shaw T, Elliott P, McKenna WJ. Dilated cardiomyopathy: a genetically heterogeneous disease. Lancet 2002; 360:654–5.

107. Charron P, Komajda M. Genes and their polymorphisms in mono- and multifactorial cardiomyopathies: towards pharmacogenomics in heart failure. Pharmacogenomics 2002; 3:367–78.

108. Bluemke DA, Krupinski EA, Ovitt T, et al. MR Imaging of arrhythmogenic right ventricular cardiomyopathy: morphologic findings and interobserver reliability. Cardiology 2003; 99:153–62.

13

CMR of cardiac masses and thrombi

Christina M Bove, Christopher M Kramer

Introduction

Cardiac magnetic resonance (CMR) provides a noninvasive, comprehensive three-dimensional assessment of intra- and extracardiac structures. Although transthoracic echocardiography (TTE) has traditionally been the initial test of choice for evaluating cardiac and paracardiac masses, its limitations include a limited field of view and poor acoustic windows in some patients.[1] Additionally, TTE has difficulty evaluating apical, pericardial, and paracardiac masses, often making transesophageal echocardiography (TEE) necessary to provide complementary information. While TEE has higher resolution and better acoustic windows, which aids in the detection of paracardiac, apical, and left-atrial appendage masses, it has a limited field of view and is a semi-invasive test.

CMR is able to provide a detailed assessment of intra- and extracardiac masses, including their location, mobility, and relationship to other structures. The presence of pericardial and intramyocardial involvement and fine definition of tumor extent are easily evaluated. These features are important information for the clinician in order to guide therapeutic strategy. For example, extension into atrial walls generally precludes surgical removal of the entire tumor. In a study assessing the role of CMR for evaluating suspected cardiac and paracardiac masses involving the heart, CMR provided diagnostic information that affected clinical management or surgical planning in 53 of 61 patients, including showing lack of resectability or guiding the surgical approach.[2] The advantages of CMR include its large field of view, high spatial resolution, high contrast-to-noise ratio, and multiplanar imaging capabilities. Serial CMR has also become a common modality for monitoring tumor regression after surgical, pharmacologic, and radiologic therapies. CMR is also able to provide supplementary information, including tumor vascularity and tissue characterization for some tumors.

Tissue characterization and commonly used pulse sequences

Spin-echo imaging

Spin-echo CMR can often suggest the presence of a mass by demonstrating asymmetric thickening, cavity distortion, and intracavitary masses.[3] Using spin-echo, T1 and T2 relaxation times can be used to help differentiate tissue characteristics of different masses. While nonspecific for many primary cardiac tumors, tissue characterization by CMR can often be diagnostic for lipomas, myxomas, and lymphomas. Cysts and lipomas tend to have high signal intensity on T1-weighted (T1-W) spin-echo, similar to fat, whereas lipomas and lipomatous hypertrophy have reduced signal intensity using a T1-W fat-presaturation technique[4–6] (Figure 13.1). Conversely, tumors such as myxomas and lymphomas appear less intense on T1-W spin-echo.[2,7–9] Relaxation times can also be used to identify acute or subacute hematomas, which appear bright on T2-weighted (T2-W) spin-echo.[10]

Gradient-echo and steady-state free precession cine imaging

Cine CMR can be used to visualize valvular regurgitation or obstruction, which is important since intracavitary tumors may produce obstruction to flow into or within the heart. The dephasing of spins from turbulent blood flow provides excellent contrast in signal on gradient-echo cine imaging to help differentiate stationary from mobile objects. Cine imaging is also useful for depicting the site of attachment of tumors and prolapse of tumors through atrioventricular (AV) valves and can aid in the

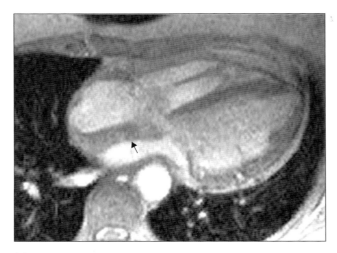

(a)

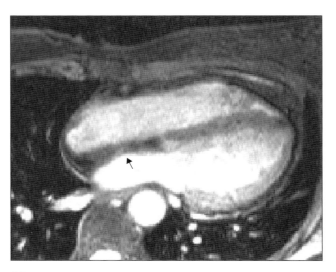

(b)

Figure 13.1
Lipomatous hypertrophy of the interatrial septum in a 55-year-old woman referred for CMR to evaluate an atrial mass. (a) Four-chamber end-diastolic T1-W gradient-echo cine MR image showing marked thickening of the interatrial septum (arrow). Note the homogeneous, isointense appearance of the interatrial septum in this sequence. (b) Corresponding T1-W Turbo-FLASH gradient echo image with fat presaturation showing large, nodular areas of low (reduced) signal intensity (arrow) within the interatrial septum, corresponding to fatty infiltration.

differentiation of certain tumors. With the exception of most atrial myxomas, tumors generally have higher signal intensities (greater than or equal to that of muscle) when compared with thrombi in the cardiac chambers.[11] Myocardial tissue tagging can be applied to gradient-echo cine or multi-phase T1-W spin-echo imaging to help differentiate tumor from myocardium.[12] Radiofrequency (RF) tags can be placed in any chosen angle to optimally

evaluate a particular tissue interface, thus visualizing relative motion of the myocardium and tumor and demonstrating potential planes of dissection to help plan surgical resection (Figure 13.2).

Use of contrast agents: first-pass and delayed imaging

The use of gadolinium-based contrast is helpful in many tumors and often shows differential contrast uptake with respect to normal myocardium[3] (Figures 13.3 and 13.4). On precontrast T1-W spin-echo images, cardiac tumors appear isointense in most cases and not clearly discernible from normal myocardium based upon signal intensity. Following administration of contrast, differential uptake of contrast within the tumor compared to normal myocardium is seen due to increased vascularity within the tumor.[3] This can better delineate tumor margins. Additionally, nonvascularized, necrotic, or cystic areas inside a tumor can be differentiated, since they do not accumulate contrast medium.[13] By delineating these areas within the tumor, contrast-enhanced CMR can help formulate differential diagnoses or assess efficacy of therapy on follow-up imaging studies. The administration of MR contrast agents can also help differentiate intracardiac thrombi, which generally do not take up contrast medium (see below) (Figures 13.5 and 13.6).

Cardiac tumors

Neoplasms of the heart may be either primary or secondary, and primary cardiac tumors may be either benign or malignant. Primary cardiac tumors are rare, with a prevalence of 0.001–0.3% in most autopsy series.[14,15] Secondary or metastatic neoplasms of the heart are much more frequent than primary neoplasms, being ~30–50 times more common.[16,17] Most primary cardiac tumors are benign, are most often myxomas, and are most commonly located in the left atrium. Benign cardiac tumors are typically well circumscribed. Malignant cardiac neoplasms are frequently invasive and may involve multiple structures. Only ~25% of primary cardiac tumors are malignant, and most of these are sarcomas. The primary malignant cardiac tumors typically involve the myocardium and the endocardial surface, while most secondary (metastatic) neoplasms to the heart involve the pericardium or epicardium and are often associated with pericardial and pleural effusions and may cause pericardial constriction.

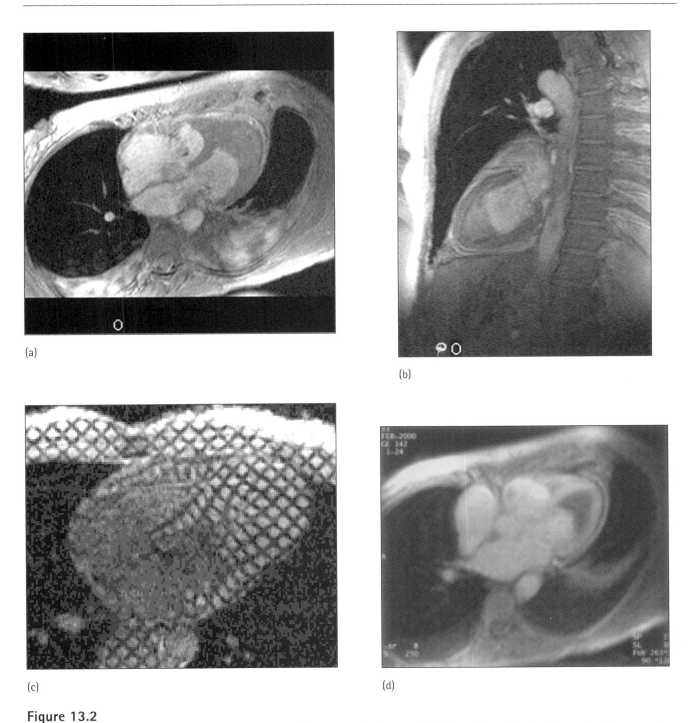

(a)

(b)

(c)

(d)

Figure 13.2

A 57-year-old woman with hypereosinophilic syndrome. (a) Four-chamber long-axis T1-W gradient-echo cine image showing masses in the apex of the right and left ventricles. (b) Two-chamber long-axis T1-W gradient-echo image showing differences in signal intensity between the apical mass and the myocardium. The mass exhibits lower signal intensity and there appears to be a distinct anatomic plane between the mass and myocardium. (c) T1-W gradient-echo end-systolic tagged cine image in the four-chamber long-axis plane demonstrating intramyocardial dysfunction in the apex (seen as lack of tag deformation), but normal tag deformation and myocardial function within the lateral wall and basal septum. (d) First-pass inversion recovery gradient-echo image following gadolinium contrast administration in the same four-chamber plane as (a) and (c). There is normal perfusion of the myocardium and no perfusion is seen in the apical masses, again defining a distinct plane. At the time of surgery, the masses were easily extracted and were shown to be thrombus and eosinophilic debris. (Adapted from Circulation 2001; 104: e3–4.)

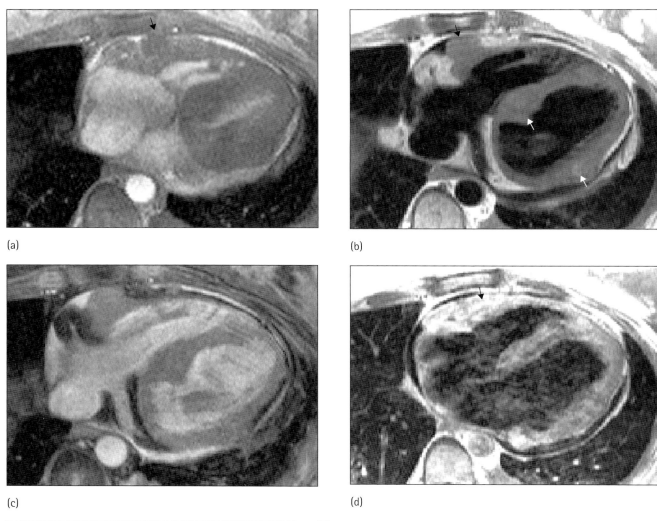

(a)

(b)

(c)

(d)

(e)

Figure 13.3

A 26-year-old woman with metastatic carcinoid. (a) Axial T1-W gradient-echo cine image showing several nodular densities within and adjacent to the right-ventricular (RV) wall within the pericardial space (see arrows), consistent with hematogenous spread. On gradient-echo imaging, the tumor infiltration appears slightly heterogeneous and isointense to the surrounding myocardium. (b) Axial T1-W fast spin-echo image showing tumor infiltration with heterogeneous signal within and adjacent to the RV wall (see black arrow), adjacent to an area of high signal consistent with fat within the right atrioventricular (AV) groove. There is also a nodular appearance to the basal left-ventricular (LV) septum and LV free wall (white arrows).
(c) Corresponding axial T1-W Turbo-FLASH image using fat presaturation, verifying isolated fat within the AV groove, but isointense appearance of tumor elsewhere within the myocardium. (d) Axial T1-W fast spin-echo image (same parameters as b) following administration of intravenous contrast showing increased signal within the tumor in the RV wall (see arrow). (e) Axial T1-W Turbo-FLASH inversion recovery image after contrast demonstrating low signal in the RV tumor (arrow) and regions of high signal surrounding low-signal areas in the LV septum and free wall (arrows).

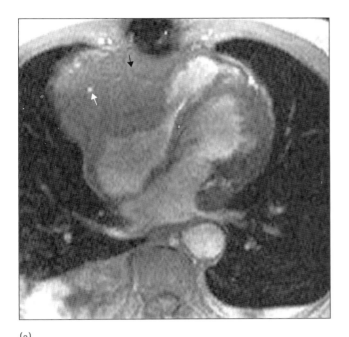

(a)

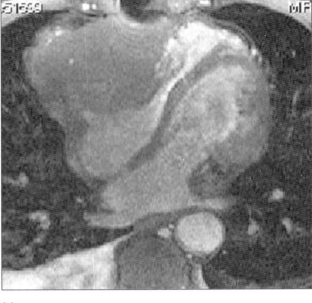

(b)

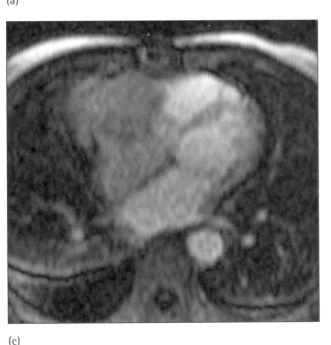

(c)

Figure 13.4

Large cell lymphoma in an elderly male with a history of coronary artery bypass grafting. (a) Axial gradient-echo cine MR end-diastolic image showing a large homogenous mass within the RV free wall and pericardial space (black arrow), consistent with tumor infiltration. This tumor appears isointense with myocardium on T1-W gradient-echo. Note compression of the RV in this end-diastolic image. In addition, the right coronary artery is completely surrounded by tumor (white arrow). Artifact from the sternal wire related to the patient's prior surgery is noted. (b) A T1-W gradient-echo FLASH image with fat presaturation in the same plane as (a) shows no change in signal intensity when compared with (a). (c) Axial T1-W inversion recovery gradient-echo MR image during the infusion of 0.1 mM/kg Gd-DTPA showing that, coincident with perfusion of the myocardium, the mass takes up contrast. This excludes thrombus or cyst and suggests mass vascularity.

Benign cardiac tumors

Myxomas

Myxomas are the most common primary cardiac tumors, accounting for ~25% of all cardiac masses and ~50% of all benign cardiac tumors.[14] They occur more often in women and middle-aged patients. The classic clinical presentation is the triad of obstructive symptoms, constitutional symptoms, and embolic phenomena. Obstructive cardiac symptoms are seen in over half of patients with cardiac myxomas, although 20% may be asymptomatic.[18] Myxomas are most often solitary, located in the left atrium (LA, 75%) or right atrium (RA, 23%) and attached by a narrow pedunculated (although sometimes broad) stalk to the interatrial septum at the region of the fossa ovalis.[14] On pathology, cardiac myxomas are heterogeneous, and may contain cysts and areas of hemorrhage, calcification, and necrosis. On CMR, they appear as spherical or ovoid lobular masses with heterogeneous signal intensity (Figures 13.7 and 13.8).

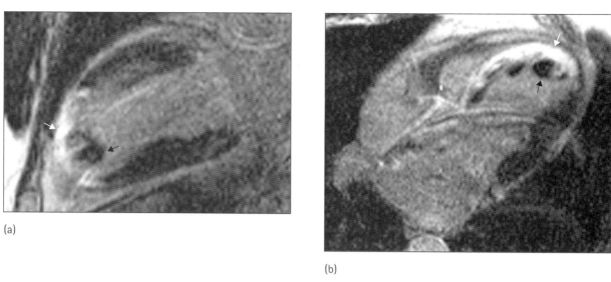

Figure 13.5

Apical left-ventricular infarction with associated thrombus. Two-chamber (a) and four-chamber (b) long-axis T1-W inversion recovery gradient-echo MR images performed 20 min following contrast injection. The infarct is visualized as the area of transmural hyperenhancement (white arrows), while the thrombus shows no contrast enhancement (black arrows).

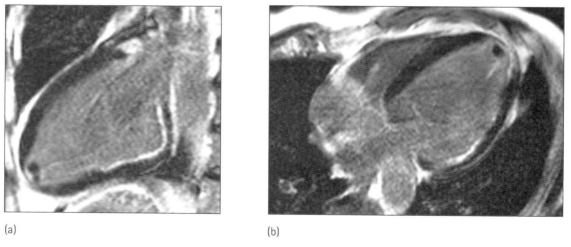

Figure 13.6

Apical thrombus in another patient with an ischemic cardiomyopathy demonstrated on T1-W inversion recovery gradient-echo MR images following contrast administration in two-chamber (a) and four-chamber (b) views.

Spin-echo imaging provides excellent anatomic visualization of myxomas, while cine imaging provides additional information regarding their movement relative to the cardiac chambers and the presence of valvular obstruction or regurgitation. Using cine imaging and multiple planes of view, the point of attachment to the endocardial surface can be accurately visualized (Figure 13.7). In one study, the point of attachment was correctly identified by CMR in 83% of cases.[19] Myxomas typically have an intermediate (isointense to myocardium), heterogeneous signal intensity on T1-W spin-echo imaging,[19]

with higher, generally heterogeneous signal intensity following contrast administration, due to areas of inflammation within the tumor (Figure 13.8c). There may be nonenhancing necrotic and cystic areas within the tumor as well.[3,20] Myxomas may exhibit markedly increased signal intensity on T2-W images, and typically demonstrate low signal intensity on gradient-echo images due to magnetic susceptibility artifact from their relatively high iron content[20–22] (Figure 13.7). On T1-W and T2-W images, calcification within the tumor is typically seen as regions of low signal intensity,[23] while subacute hemorrhage

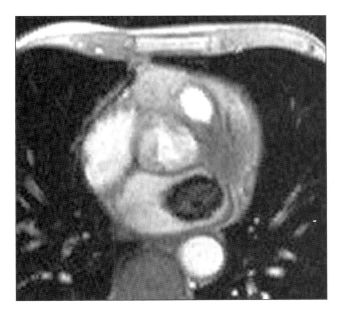

(a)

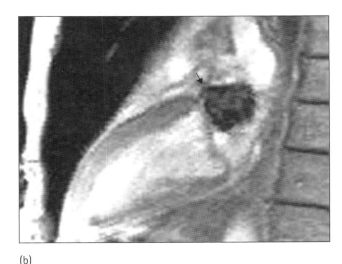

(b)

Figure 13.7

Left-atrial (LA) myxoma. (a) Axial image at the base of the heart showing typical heterogeneous and hypointense appearance of a cardiac myxoma on T1-W gradient-echo cine imaging. The attachment site (LA wall or mitral valve) is not clear from this image. (b) Parasagittal two-chamber T1-W gradient-echo cine image demonstrating that the attachment site is on the superior pole of the LA (see arrow). Cine imaging demonstrated the mass to hinge at that point and prolapse along the anterior leaflet of the mitral valve during diastole.

within the tumor shows high signal intensity. In contrast, fresh hemorrhage within the myxoma has intermediate to low signal intensity on T1-W and low signal intensity on T2-W images.[11,22]

Lipomas

Lipomas are benign tumors of mature adipose tissue; they are typically solitary, well-circumscribed, encapsulated lesions, and are most frequently subendocardial or subpericardial. Intramyocardial lipomas are usually small and encapsulated. Lipomas may also be located on valves. They arise most commonly in the RA or left ventricle (LV).[15] The ability of CMR to characterize fat makes it an ideal modality to diagnose cardiac lipomas, which generally appear as nodular masses with homogenous increased signal intensity on T1-W images, without any other distinguishing features. They do not exhibit any contrast enhancement. They also have low signal intensity when short inversion recovery fat-suppression techniques are used.[5,24]

Lipomatous hypertrophy

Lipomatous hypertrophy is a tumor-like condition characterized by non-encapsulated fatty infiltration within the myocardium. This occurs most commonly in the inter-atrial septum, which is usually contiguous with either the epicardial fat of the AV groove or transverse pericardial sinus, but spares the fossa ovalis.[25] Lipomatous hypertrophy commonly affects older, obese women, and is associated with cardiac arrhythmias. Because CMR can easily and accurately identify adipose tissue, it can help distinguish lipomatous hypertrophy of the interatrial septum from other interatrial septal masses, such as metastatic lesions, amyloidosis, and septal aneurysms. As with lipomas, lipomatous hypertrophy characteristically appears bright on T1-W spin-echo images, with high signal intensities similar to fat, and the signal is lowered with fat-suppression techniques[5,24] (Figure 13.1).

Papillary fibroelastomas

Papillary fibroelastomas (fibromas of the valves) are the third most common benign cardiac tumors[14] and have a high propensity to embolize.[26] On pathology, they appear as small (<1 cm), delicate, frond-like excrescences attached to the endocardium by a short pedicle.[14] There may be calcifications within the neoplasm. Over 90% of fibroelastomas are limited to the valves, and are thus the most common cardiac tumor occurring on valves. The aortic or mitral valves are typically involved, but fibroelastomas may also appear attached to the LV endocardium. They are usually visualized on echocardiography as small, pedunculated, mobile masses with a cystic appearance.

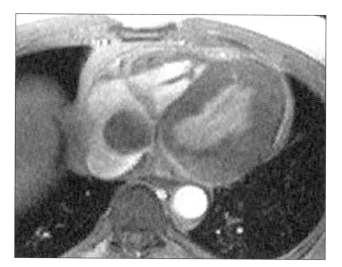

(a)

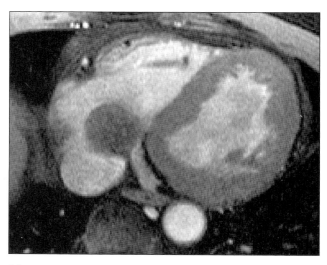

(b)

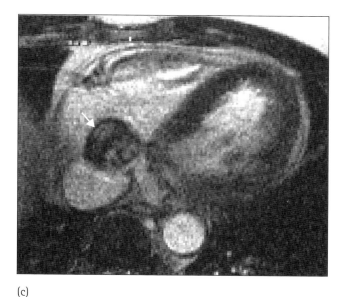

(c)

Figure 13.8

Right-atrial (RA) myxoma. (a) Axial T1-W gradient-echo cine image demonstrating a homogenous RA mass adjacent to the coronary sinus that, after resection, was proven to be a myxoma. (b) T1-W gradient-echo FLASH image with fat presaturation in the same plane showing the absence of fatty infiltration within the mass, demonstrated by the lack of signal change. (c) Corresponding axial contrast-enhanced T1-W inversion recovery Turbo-FLASH image revealing small areas of contrast uptake (arrows) within the myxoma, possibly due to inflammation or necrosis within the tumor.

They are generally not well visualized by CMR due to their small size and attachment to moving valves. When imaged by CMR, they appear as a small mass on either a valve leaflet or the endocardial surface of one of the cardiac chambers. Cine imaging may demonstrate turbulent blood flow associated with valvular papillary fibroelastomas.

Fibromas

Cardiac fibromas are rare and occur three times more frequently in children than adults. They are the second most common benign cardiac tumors in children and are frequently associated with lethal ventricular arrhythmias and heart failure, making early detection and excision important. Sudden death occurs in up to one-third of patients, due to conduction defects, arrhythmia, or obstruction of ventricular outflow. The tumor typically displaces, rather than invades and destroys, normal myocardium. They are typically solitary, 4–7 cm in diameter and located in the ventricular myocardium, most frequently in the anterior LV wall, septum, and right ventricle (RV), often extending into the ventricular cavity.[14,26] Unlike many other primary cardiac tumors, fibromas usually do not contain foci of hemorrhage, cystic changes, or necrosis.[14] On CMR, they appear as homogenous, well-demarcated, solitary intraventricular masses or as focal myocardial thickening. Because of their dense, fibrous consistency, they typically appear isointense or hyperintense relative to muscle on T1-W images and hypointense on T2-W images.[3,6] They usually demonstrate little or no contrast enhancement, although contrast-enhanced imaging may help delineate the borders of the tumor in some instances, and non-enhancing areas may correlate with poorly vascularized fibrous tissue.[3,27,28] CMR can help distinguish cardiac fibromas from other LV masses such as thrombi, malignant tumors (which are heterogeneous and typically enhance following contrast), eosinophilic cardiomyopathy, and endomyocardial fibrosis.

Rhabdomyomas

Primary cardiac tumors are rare in infants and young children, but rhabdomyoma is the most frequent cardiac tumor in this population, accounting for 90% of tumors, and typically presenting before 1 year of age.[14] They are benign myocardial hamartomas, and are associated with tuberous sclerosis in approximately one-third to one-half of patients. Most patients are asymptomatic, and the tumors are detected during prenatal screening ultrasonagraphy.[29] Clinical presentation is quite variable, ranging from no symptoms to severe heart failure and death. They typically appear in varying sizes and number within the myocardial wall of the LV or RV. They are generally well circumscribed but not encapsulated. They tend to have similar signal intensity to myocardium on CMR, making them difficult to detect. In fact, when the lesions are small and multiple, they are commonly seen as diffuse myocardial thickening on both ultrasound and CMR. CMR may allow more definitive definition of tumor margins and can prove to be extremely helpful when aggressive surgical resection is planned.[30] Rhabdomyomas typically appear isointense to surrounding myocardium on T1-W images and hyperintense to myocardium on T2-W images.[6]

Hemangiomas

Hemangiomas are typically single benign vascular tumors composed of proliferative endothelial cells that form blood channels. They account for 5–10% of benign cardiac tumors and are most often discovered incidentally in asymptomatic patients.[14] On CMR, they appear as solitary, poorly circumscribed, non-pedunculated, non-homogenous masses, and although they can occur in any chamber, they are most often located on the right side of the heart. They are often associated with a pericardial effusion, which may be hemorrhagic.[14] Like hemangiomas elsewhere in the body, they typically have intermediate signal intensity on T1-W images and hyperintense signal intensity on T2-W images[29,31,32] (Figure 13.9).

Paragangliomas

Paragangliomas are tumors arising from the paraganglia neuroendocrine cells (adrenal medulla, carotid, paraaortic, and sympathetic ganglia). They are extremely rare, with fewer than 50 cases reported, and typically occur in young adults, often presenting with hypertension or evidence of catecholamine overproduction.[33] These tumors are highly vascular and often involve the coronary arteries, making surgical resection difficult.[34] The tumors are usually large (3–8 cm) and may be encapsulated and contain hemorrhage. They typically occur in the location of cardiac paraganglia, and thus arise most often from the visceral paraganglia of the LA.[33] They typically have a broad base of attachment, and have markedly increased signal intensity on T2-W images and are iso- or hypo-intense compared with myocardium on T1-W images. Because of their increased vascularity, they demonstrate intense, heterogenous contrast enhancement, often with central non-enhancing areas due to tumor necrosis.[35,36]

Primary malignant cardiac tumors

Primary cardiac malignancies generally are not symptomatic until they grow large, at which point they present with nonspecific symptoms, making their diagnosis difficult and curative treatment infrequent. In one review of 40 years of experience, the mean time from onset of symptoms to diagnosis was 16 months.[37] With improvements in noninvasive imaging, the potential for earlier detection and even cure is possible. CMR features of malignant primary tumors can be nonspecific. However, primary cardiac malignancies may have differentiating features such as chamber of origin, presence of hemorrhage or calcification, and presence of pericardial or valvular involvement, making CMR a useful modality to help distinguish the type of malignant tumor when combined with the clinical presentation. CMR can also often distinguish malignant from benign cardiac neoplasms by evaluating size, location, and width of attachment, chamber involvement, infiltrative growth, and extracardiac extent.[38] Primary malignant cardiac tumors can involve any of the cardiac chambers, and often extend through anatomic planes into other chambers and the pericardium. Malignant primary cardiac tumors typically enhance following gadolinium contrast administration, are associated with pericardial effusions, and invade into the myocardium.[2,8] In patients with known or suspected primary malignant cardiac tumors, CMR is the test of choice for initial evaluation.[26]

Approximately 25% of primary cardiac tumors are malignant, with sarcomas accounting for 95% of these.[14] The most common cardiac sarcomas are angiosarcomas, undifferentiated sarcomas, malignant fibrous histiocytomas, leiomyosarcomas, and osteosarcomas.[14]

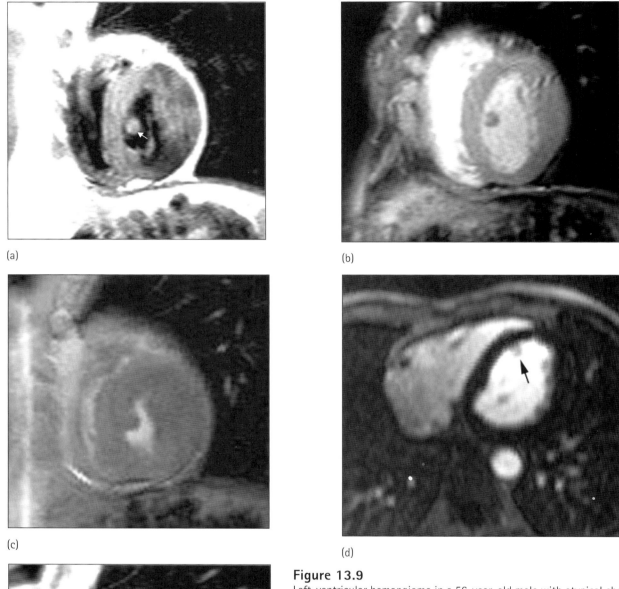

(a)

(b)

(c)

(d)

(e)

Figure 13.9

Left-ventricular hemangioma in a 56-year-old male with atypical chest pain. (a) Short-axis T1-W fast spin-echo image in the apical left ventricle at end-diastole demonstrating a well-circumscribed spherical mass attached to the septum. (b) Corresponding short-axis T1-W gradient-echo FLASH image with fat suppression demonstrating no suppression of the mass, and excluding a lipoma. (c) Short-axis T1-W gradient-echo cine image demonstrating attachment of the mass to the septum. The mass has heterogeneous, isointense signal intensity on this sequence. Myxomas generally demonstrate lower signal than myocardium on this sequence, making this less likely. (d) Long-axis T1-W inversion recovery gradient-echo image during the infusion of gadolinium contrast showing that, coincident with perfusion of the myocardium, the mass (arrow) takes up contrast. This excludes thrombus and suggests mass vascularity. (e) Short-axis T1-W spin-echo image with the same imaging parameters as (a), repeated 5 min after the contrast infusion. This figure shows marked enhancement of the mass, again confirming vascularity and excluding thrombus.

Angiosarcomas

Angiosarcomas are the most common sarcomas, accounting for >30% of sarcomas.[14] They are more common in males, and typically arise from the RA or epicardium. They have large vascular channels and are often associated with a precordial murmur due to the large amount of blood flowing through them. The CMR appearance is of irregular or nodular masses extending from the RA free wall, often with areas of central necrosis. Angiosarcomas may communicate with a cardiac chamber and invade into the myocardium, or present as diffusely infiltrative masses extending along the pericardium.[39] About 25% of angiosarcomas are at least partially intracavitary, and thus may be associated with obstruction to flow, right-sided heart failure, and pericardial tamponade due to hemorrhage.[40] Due to the associated hemorrhage, angiosarcomas often demonstrate focal or peripheral areas of increased signal intensity on T1-W sequences, with higher signal intensity on T2-W images. Due to their propensity for both hemorrhage and necrosis, angiosarcomas typically have heterogeneous signal intensity both prior to and following contrast administration.[41]

Osteosarcomas

Primary cardiac osteosarcomas account for 3–9% of cardiac sarcomas[14] and contain malignant, bone-producing cells. Primary osteosarcomas most often arise in the LA, and thus may be confused with LA myxomas on imaging. Osteosarcomas more typically have a broad base of attachment and an aggressive growth pattern that may involve the pulmonary veins, atrial septum, and epicardium[42], unlike LA myxomas, which present as discussed above.

Rare primary tumors

Rhabdomyosarcomas, liposarcomas, and leiomyosarcomas are very rare. Rhabdomyosarcomas are malignant tumors of striated muscle and account for ~4–7% of cardiac sarcomas. They are the most common primary malignancy in children and are the most likely primary malignancy to involve the valves.[43] They are often multiple, and while they may involve the pericardium, they always involve the myocardium, although no cardiac chamber in particular.[41] Because these tumors may have large areas of central necrosis, CMR may show a central defect that communicates with the pericardial space.[38] Signal intensity characteristics are typically quite variable but may be similar to myocardium, and contrast enhancement is generally seen.[38] Cardiac sarcomas tend to have a rapidly progressive clinical course, and are usually fatal.

Primary cardiac lymphomas and mesotheliomas are exceedingly rare, accounting for <5% of primary malignant tumors of the heart.[14] Primary cardiac lymphomas are typically non-Hodgkin lymphomas, are more common in immunocompromised patients, and are either diagnosed at autopsy or are rapidly progressive following diagnosis and fatal. CMR demonstrates poorly demarcated heterogeneous lesions that are isointense to slightly hypointense to myocardium on T1-W images and, unlike most other cardiac malignancies, isointense on T2-W and proton density images.[29] Contrast enhancement is usually heterogeneous. CMR is useful in early diagnosis and monitoring response to pharmacologic and radiation therapy.[44]

Secondary malignant cardiac tumors

Secondary malignant cardiac tumors are 30–50 times more frequent than primary tumors,[45] with an incidence of ~4% in autopsy studies, and up to 40% in patients with fatal malignancies.[26,46] Metastatic neoplasms most commonly affect the epicardium and may be single or multiple. Metastases from lung and breast carcinomas more often affect the pericardium and epicardium, suggesting regional lymphatic spread, whereas myocardial metastases are generally associated with lymphoma and melanoma, suggesting hematogenous spread.[47] Intramyocardial metastases may be single or multifocal and may affect all four chambers (Figure 13.3). Due to their direct contact with the pericardium and their relatively thin walls, the atria are more frequently affected by metastatic neoplasms than the ventricles.

These neoplasms commonly present with symptoms related to pericardial involvement, such as effusion, tamponade, or constriction, occur late in the disease process, and are associated with poor prognosis.[46] Intramyocardial metastases can produce obstruction to chamber inflow or outflow, and are often associated with systemic or peripheral embolization. Due to their high prevalence, lung and breast carcinomas are the most common neoplasms to metastasize to the heart. Percentage-wise, however, melanomas, lymphomas, and leukemias have the highest propensity of any malignancies to metastasize to the heart[48] (Figure 13.4). Mechanisms of metastasis include: (1) direct invasion, which is common in breast and bronchogenic carcinoma; (2) venous spread, which commonly occurs via the inferior vena cava from renal cell, hepatocellular, and adenocortical carcinomas, carcinoid, and Wilms' tumor; and (3) lymphatic spread, which occurs with lymphoma and leukemia.

On CMR, metastatic malignancies tend to have low signal intensity on T1-W images, appear brighter on

T2-W images, and enhance following contrast[3,49] (Figures 13.3b, d). One exception is cardiac metastases seen with melanoma. Unlike other metastases, they generally appear bright on T1-W images due to paramagnetic metals bound by melanin.[50,51] Metastatic carcinomas from the abdomen typically present as large masses extending from the inferior vena cava into the RA, and may also prolapse through the tricuspid valve. Carcinomas of the lung and breast most often invade the pericardium and lead to pericardial constriction or effusions. Metastatic lung cancers also often present as LA masses, since the pulmonary veins provide a direct conduit for spread. Hematogenous spread is the most common route of metastasis to the heart. Breast and lung carcinomas commonly pass through the lungs into the systemic circulation, entering cardiac structures through the coronary circulation.[26] Lymphomas and leukemias have a high propensity to metastasize to the heart, since mediastinal lymph nodes often fill with tumor and cause retrograde extension of the tumor.

Intracardiac thrombi

Thrombi are the most frequent intracardiac mass and are most commonly located in the LA when associated with atrial fibrillation or rheumatic heart disease, or in the LV when associated with myocardial infarction (Figure 13.5) or dilated cardiomyopathy (Figure 13.6). Detection is important due to the high risk of systemic embolization. Intracardiac thrombi often must be differentiated from tumors, trabeculations, and papillary muscles. CMR appearance is variable, depending on the age of the thrombus; fresh thrombi (acute and subacute) generally appear bright on the first-echo image, and even brighter on the second echo of a T2-W spin-echo study,[10] while older thrombi typically have lower signal intensity on T2-W images.[52] The high iron content in thrombi produces a magnetic susceptibility effect and thus low signal intensity on T2*-W imaging. In a study comparing T1-W spin-echo with gradient-echo cine imaging for differentiating tumor from nontumor thrombus, on gradient-echo imaging all 12 cases of blood clots were hypointense, with lower signal intensities, compared with skeletal muscle.[11] Additionally, cine imaging is very helpful in identifying ventricular thrombi, because of their association with segmental wall motion abnormalities.

Thrombi can be differentiated from most neoplastic masses by administration of MR contrast. Neoplasms typically enhance, while thrombi are nonvascular structures that do not enhance on T1-W spin-echo or T1-W inversion recovery gradient-echo images following contrast administration (Figures 13.5 and 13.6). Detection of ventricular thrombi has recently been evaluated with con-

trast-enhanced inversion recovery Turbo-FLASH CMR, balanced steady-state free precession (SSFP) cine CMR, and TEE in patients with acute and chronic myocardial infarction.[53] Contrast-enhanced CMR identified mural thrombus in 12 of 57 patients, which appeared as a dark, intracavitary mass clearly distinguishable from the contrast-enhanced blood pool. In this study, cine CMR only identified 6 and transthoracic echocardiography only identified 5 of the thrombi identified on contrast-enhanced CMR.

Differentiation between cardiac, paracardiac, and mediastinal masses

Numerous non-neoplastic conditions and extracardiac neoplasms are frequently mistaken for cardiac neoplasms. Thymomas, teratomas, lymphomas, hematomas, and cardiac sarcoid are abnormal structural findings that may be difficult to differentiate from cardiac neoplasms using other noninvasive imaging modalities. Similarly, extracardiac structures such as the descending aorta, pericardial cysts and epicardial fat pads, hiatal hernias, and the thymus are commonly mistaken for cardiac tumors, but can be clearly distinguished on CMR due to its high spatial resolution and soft tissue contrast.

Pericardial cysts are often discovered on routine chest radiographs, and appear as round, well demarcated masses along the right cardiac silhouette. They are most commonly located in the right costophrenic angle, but can also be present in the left costophrenic angle, and rarely in the anterior or posterior mediastinum. TTE typically provides limited information, while CMR can easily recognize and characterize pericardial cysts. They typically have low signal intensity on T1-W images and high intensity on T2-W images, although cysts that contain hemorrhage or increased protein levels have medium to high intensity on T1-W images.[28,54]

Pseudomasses

Pseudomasses or pseudotumors are intracardiac structures that appear as masses but are caused by normal cardiac structures such as the Chiari network and crista terminalis. These are well visualized by SSFP, gradient-echo cine, or spin-echo techniques, and often appear strandlike, attaching to the posterior wall of the RA. In one study evaluating CMR in 34 patients believed to have an intracardiac mass from 2D echocardiography, CMR demonstrated no intracardiac mass, but anatomic findings explaining the possible mass in 7 patients.[6] Other common pseudomasses seen on noninvasive modalities that are correctly identified on CMR due to greater spatial and contrast resolution include enlarged coronary sinuses, left superior vena cava, dilated proximal coronary arteries, anomalous pulmonary veins, prominent papillary muscles and trabeculae, asymmetric hypertrophy, moderator bands, atrial septal aneurysms, and lipomatosis.

References

1. Yang PC, Kerr AB, Liu AC, et al. New real-time interactive cardiac magnetic resonance imaging system complements echocardiography. J Am Coll Cardiol 1998; 32:2049–56.

2. Lund JT, Ehman RL, Julsrud PR, et al. Cardiac masses: assessment by MR imaging. AJR 1989; 152:469–73.

3. Funari M, Fujita N, Peck WW, Higgins CB. Cardiac tumors: assessment with Gd-DTPA enhanced MR imaging. J Comput Assist Tomogr 1991; 15:953–8.

4. Casolo F, Biasi S, Balzarii L, et al. MRI as an adjunct to echocardiography for the diagnostic imaging of cardiac masses. Eur J Radiol 1998; 88:226–30.

5. Dooms GC, Hricak H, Sollitto RA, et al. Lipomatous tumors and tumors with fatty component: MR imaging potential and comparison of MR and CT results. Radiology 1985; 157:479.

6. Winkler M, Higgins CB. Suspected intracardiac masses: evaluation with MR imaging. Radiology 1987; 165:117–22.

7. Pflugfelder PW, Wisenberg G, Boughner DR, et al. Detection of atrial myxoma by magnetic resonance imaging. Am J Cardiol 1985; 55:242.

8. Freedberg RS, Krozon I, Runnancik WN, et al. The contribution of magnetic resonance imaging to the evaution of intracardiac tumors diagnosed by echocardiography. Circulation 1988; 77:96–103.

9. Go R, O'Donnell JK, Underwood DA, et al. Comparison of gated cardiac MRI and 2D echocardiography of intracardiac neoplasms. AJR 1985; 145:21–5.

10. Dooms GC, Higgins CB. MR imaging of cardiac thrombi. J Comput Assist Tomogr 1986; 10:415–20.

11. Seelos KC, Caputo GR, Carrol CL, et al. Cine gradient refocused echo (GRE) imaging of intravascular masses: differentiation between tumor and nontumor thrombus. J Comput Assist Tomogr 1992; 16:169–75.

12. Bouton S, Yang A, McCrindle BW, et al. Differentiation of tumor from viable myocardium using cardiac tagging with MR imaging. J Comput Assist Tomogr 1991; 15:676–8.

13. Neuerburg JM, Bohndorf K, Sohn M, et al. Urinary bladder neoplasms: evaluation with contrast-enhanced MR imging. Radiology 1989; 172:739–43.

14. Burke A, Virmani R. Atlas of Tumor Pathology. Tumors of the Heart and Great Vessels. Washington, DC: Armed Forces Institute of Pathology, 1996.

15. Colucci W, Schoen F, Braunwald E. Primary tumors of the heart. In: Heart Disease: A Textbook of Cardiovascular Medicine (Braunwald E, ed). Philadelphia: WB Saunders, 1977:1464–77.

16. Lam KY, Dickens P, Chan ACL. Tumors of the heart. A 20-year experience with review of 12 485 consecutive autopsies. Arch Pathol Med 1993; 117:1027–31.

17. Reynan K. Frequency of primary tumors of the heart. Am J Cardiol 1996; 77:107.

18. Bjessmo S, Ivert T. Cardiac myxoma: 40 years' experience in 63 patients. Ann Thorac Surg 1997; 63:697–700.

19. Grebenc ML, Rosado-de-Christenson ML, Green CE, et al. From the archives of the AFIP: Cardiac myxoma: imaging features in 83 patients. RadioGraphics 2002; 22:673–89.

20. Matsuoka H, Hamada M, Honda T, et al. Morphologic and histologic characterization of cardiac myxomas by magnetic resonance imaging. Angiology 1996; 47:693–8.

21. Semelka RC, Tomei E, Wagner S, et al. Cardiac masses: signal intensity features on spin-echo, gradient-echo, gadolinium-enhanced spin-echo, and Turbo FLASH imaging. J Magn Reson Imaging 1992; 2:415–20.

22. Masui T, Takahashi M, Miura K, et al. Cardiac myxoma: identification of tumoral hemorrhage and calcification on MR images. AJR 1995; 164:850–2.

23. de Roos A, Weijers E, van Duinen S, van der Wall EE. Calcified right atrial myxoma demonstrated by magnetic resonance imaging. Chest 1989; 95:478–9.

24. Applegate PM, Tajik AJ, Ehman RL, et al. Two dimensional echocardiographic and MRI observations in massive lipomatous hypertrophy of the atrial septum. Am J Cardiol 1987; 59:489–91.

25. Levine RA, Weyman AE, Dinsmore RE, et al. Noninvasive tissue characterization: diagnosis of lipomatous hypertrophy of the atrial septum by nuclear magnetic resonance imaging. J Am Coll Cardiol 1983; 1:1352–7.

26. Salcedo EE. Cardiac tumors. In: Imaging in Cardiovascular Disease (Pohost GM, O'Rourke RA, Berman DS, Shah PM, eds). Philadelphia: Lippincott Williams & Wilkins, 2000:873–881.

27. Brown JJ, Barakos JA, Higgins CB. Magnetic resonance imaging of cardiac and paracardiac masses. J Thoracic Imaging 1989; 4:58–64.

28. Amparo EG, Higgins CB, Farmer D, et al. Gated MRI of cardiac and paracardiac masses: initial experience. AJR 1984; 143:1151–6.

29. Grebenc ML, Rosado-de-Christenson ML, Burke AP, et al. Primary cardiac and pericardial neoplasms: radiologic–pathologic correlation. RadioGraphics 2002; 20:1073–103.

30. Berkenblit R, Spindola-Franco H, Frater RW, et al. MRI in the evaluation and management of a newborn infant with cardiac rhabdomyoma. Ann Thorac Surg 1997; 63:1475–7.

31. Newell JC, Eckel C, Davis M, Tadros NB. MR appearance of an arteriovenous hemangioma of the interventricular septum. Cardiovasc Intervent Radiol 1988; 11:319–21.

32. Brizard C, Latremouille C, Jebara VA, et al. Cardiac hemangiomas. Ann Thorac Surg 1993; 56:390–4.

33. Araoz PA, Mulvagh HD, Tazelaar D, et al. CT and MR imaging of benign primary cardiac neoplasms with echocardiographic correlations. RadioGraphics 2000; 20:1303–19.

34. Jeevanandam V, Oz MC, Shapiro B, et al. Surgical management of cardiac pheochromocytoma: resection versus transplantation. Ann Surg 1995; 221:415–19.

35. Hamilton BH, Francis IR, Gross BH, et al. Intrapericardial paragangliomas (pheochromocytomas): imaging features. AJR 1997; 168:109–13.

36. Orr LA, Pettigrew RI, Churchwell AL, et al. Gadolinium utilization in the MR evaluation of cardiac paraganglioma. Clin Imaging 1997; 21:404–6.

37. Perchinsky MJ, Lichtenstein SV, Tyers GFO. Primary cardiac tumors: forty years' experience with 71 patients. Cancer 2002; 79:1809–15.

38. Siripornpitak S, Higgins CB. MRI of primary malignant cardiovascular tumors. J Comput Assist Tomogr 1997; 21:462–6.

39. Jannigan DT, Husain A, Robinson NA. Cardiac angiosarcomas: a review and a case report. Cancer 1986; 57:852–9.

40. Glancy DL, Morales JB Jr, Roberts WC. Angiosarcoma of the heart. Am J Cardiol 1968; 21:413–19.

41. Araoz PA, Eklund HE, Welch TJ, Breen JF. CT and MR imaging of primary cardiac malignancies. RadioGraphics 1999; 19:1421–34.

42. Reynard JS Jr, Gregoratos G, Gordon MJ, Bloor CM. Primary osteosarcoma of the heart. Am Heart J 1985; 109:598–600.

43. Wantanabe AT, Teitelbaum GP, Henderson RW, Bradley WG Jr. Magnetic resonance imaging of cardiac sarcomas. J Thorac Imaging 1989; 4:90–2.

44. Dorsay TA, Ho VB, Rovira MJ, et al. Primary cardiac lymphoma: CT and MR findings. J Comput Assist Tomogr 1993; 17:978–81.

45. Abraham DP, Reddy V, Gattusa P. Neoplasms metastatic to the heart: review of 3314 consecutive autopsies. Am J Cardiovasc Pathol 1990; 3:195–8.

46. Mukai K, Shinkai T, Tominaga K, Shomosato Y. The incidence of secondary tumors of the heart and pericardium: a 10 year study. Jpn J Clin Oncol 1988; 18:195–201.

47. Chiles C, Woodard PK, Gutierrez FR, Link KM. Metastatic involvement of the heart and pericardium: CT and MR imaging. RadioGraphics 2001; 21:439–49.

48. McAllister HA, Fenoglio JJ Jr. Atlas of Tumor Pathology. Tumors of the Cardiovascular System. Washington, DC: Armed Forces Institute of Pathology, 1978.

49. Fujita N, Caputo GR, Higgins CB. Diagnosis and characterization of intracardiac masses by magnetic resonance imaging. Am J Cardiac Imaging 1994; 8:69–80.

50. Enochs WS, Petherick P, Bogdanova A, et al. Paramagnetic metal scavenging by melanin: MR imaging. Radiology 1997; 204:417–23.

51. Mousseaux E, Meunier P, Azancott S, et al. Cardiac metastatic melanoma investigated by magnetic resonance imaging. Magn Reson Imaging 1998; 16:91–5.

52. Corti R, Osende JI, Fayad ZA, et al. In vivo noninvasive detection and age definition of arterial thrombus by MRI. J Am Coll Cardiol 2002; 39:1366–73.

53. Mollet NR, Dymarkowski S, Volders W, et al. Visualization of ventricular thrombi with contrast-enhanced magnetic resonance imaging in patients with ischemic heart disease. Circulation 2002; 106:2873–6.

54. Vinee P, Stover B, Sigmund G, et al. MR imaging of the pericardial cyst. J Magn Reson Imaging 1992; 2:593–6.

14

CMR of pericardial disease

David Bluemke, Gilberto Szarf

Introduction

The pericardium is a conical fibro-serous sac surrounding the heart and the roots of the great vessels. It is located within the mediastinal cavity behind the sternum and the cartilages of the third, fourth, fifth, sixth, and seventh ribs of the left side. Although the pericardium is usually described as a single sac, an examination of its structure shows that it consists essentially of two sacs intimately connected with one another, but totally different in structure. The outer sac, known as the fibrous pericardium, consists of fibrous tissue and has attachments to the diaphragm, sternum, and costal cartilage. The inner sac, or serous pericardium, is a delicate membrane that lines the walls of the fibrous pericardium. It is a thin mesothelial layer adjacent to the surface of the heart and is composed of a single layer of flattened cells resting on loose connective tissue.[1] The heart invaginates the wall of the serous sac from above and behind and practically obliterates its cavity, the space being merely a potential one.[2] This potential space between the heart and the pericardium normally contains a small amount of clear fluid, between 10 and 50 ml, an ultrafiltrate of plasma produced by the visceral pericardium. This fluid acts as a lubricant to minimize frictional forces between the heart and surrounding structures.[3] The pericardium limits cardiac displacement, protects the heart (reducing external friction, preventing inflammation from contiguous structures, and buttressing thinner portions of myocardium), and promotes cardiac efficiency, especially during hemodynamic overload.[4] The pericardium is susceptible to involvement by various kinds of diseases, and pericardial syndromes produce a range of clinical and physiologic abnormalities.

Imaging modalities

Two-dimensional echocardiography is the imaging modality initially applied in cases of suspected pericardial disease. However, this method is limited in its ability to image the entire pericardium because of restricted field of view, restricted acoustic windows, and the inherent difficulties in the evaluation of a structure surrounded by air-filled lungs.

Computed tomography (CT) or cardiac magnetic resonance imaging (CMR) best performs detailed anatomic display of the entire pericardium. These techniques provide a wide field of view of the entire chest. While CT has the advantage of detecting pericardial calcification better than the other methods, CMR has the advantage of not using ionizing radiation or iodinated contrast. In this chapter, we will focus on CMR of the pericardium.

Normal pericardium

CMR evaluation of the pericardium is performed using T1- and T2-weighted images in the transverse plane as well as steady-state, preprecession cine CMR in the short and long axes. If a mass is suspected, additional sequences should be performed incorporating contrast enhancement.

The normal pericardium is seen as a very thin linear structure surrounding the heart. It is represented by a dark line between the pericardial and epicardial fat layers. Visualization on CMR is improved when there is increased fat in these layers (Figure 14.1).[5]

Sechtem et al[6] found that the average pericardial width was 1.9 ± 0.6 mm in systole. This value, however, exceeds the thickness reported for pathologic measurements of pericardial thickness (0.4–1.0 mm). This discrepancy may be the result of the addition of fibrous tissue and nonlaminar motion of serous fluid when visualized on CMR.[6,7]

Sechtem et al[6] also found that although the pericardial line is visualized in all subjects on CMR, it is not seen with equal frequency in different regions of the heart. The contrast provided by the epicardial and pericardial fat better delineates the pericardium anteriorly to the right ventricle (RV) (sensitivity 100%). However, the pericardial region

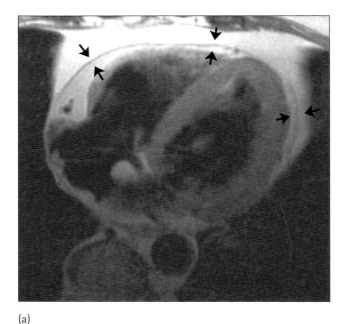

(a)

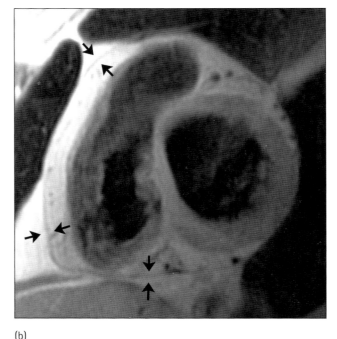

(b)

(c)

Figure 14.1

Normal pericardium. Axial (a), short-axis (b), and four-chamber (c) views of a normal pericardium.

located inferoposteriorly to the left ventricle (LV) is often less visible because of the proximity of the low-intensity lung (sensitivity 61%). In addition, pericardial visibility is improved on the caudal sections of the heart.[6]

Pericardial effusions

Accumulation of > 50 ml of fluid in the pericardial space is considered abnormal. Effusions develop as a response to injury of the pericardium. Excess fluid may develop in the pericardial space in all forms of pericardial disease. Most commonly, the fluid is exudative and reflects pericardial injury/inflammation.[5] When acute pericarditis is suspected clinically, CMR is able to identify the frequently associated effusion and also visualize inflammatory involvement of the pericardium and adjacent structures.[5] Serosanguinous effusions are typical of tuberculous and neoplastic disease, but may also be seen in uremic and viral/idiopathic disease or in response to mediastinal irradiation. Hemopericardium is most commonly seen with trauma, myocardial rupture following myocardial infarction, catheter-induced myocardial or epicardial coronary artery rupture, aortic dissection with rupture into the pericardial space, or primary hemorrhage in patients receiving anticoagulant therapy (often after cardiac valve surgery).[9,10] Chylopericardium is quite rare and results from leakage or injury to the thoracic duct.[3,11]

Although the presence of pericardial effusion is indicative of underlying pericardial disease, the clinical relevance of pericardial effusion is most closely associated with the rate of pericardial fluid collection, intrapericardial pressure, and subsequent development of tamponade.

Tuberculous pericarditis is the most common cause of chronic pericardial effusion. Hypothyroidism/myxedema is another common cause of very large pericardial effusions, especially in the elderly.[3,11]

Mulvagh et al[12] found that regional distribution of pericardial effusions was more clearly depicted by CMR than by echocardiography. Findings indicated that CMR detected small pericardial effusions that were not visualized by echocardiography. In addition, CMR was shown to be better at detecting fluid posteriorly at the LV apex, along the right atrial (RA) border and at the aortic–pericardial reflection site.

CMR is also sensitive for characterizing effusions. Transudates have low signal on T1-weighted spin-echo images and high signal on T2-weighted spin-echo images (Figure 14.2). Complex effusions/exudates exhibit greater signal intensity on T1-weighted images.[13] Hemorragic effusions can have variable signal, depending on the age of the blood, but frequently contain areas of medium and high intensity on T1-weighted images.[9,10] In exudative effusions, the pericardium and the pericardial adhesions may show greater signal intensities than normal pericardium. Also, pericardial inflammation may be recognized as thickened pericardium with higher signal intensity. Both adhesions and pericardial inflammation can be observed in association with uremia.[7]

Sechtem et al[8] observed that nonhemorragic effusions were mostly of low signal intensity throughout their extent. Patients with uremia, trauma, and tuberculosis (conditions known to be accompanied by effusions of high protein and cell content) had some regions of medium or high signal intensity within the pericardial sac. The regions of increased signal intensity are thought to represent inflammatory exudate with a high content of fibrinous material that is adherent to the pericardium.

Cine CMR images can depict right-sided chamber collapse during diastole, a useful signal in the diagnosis of cardiac tamponade. Cardiac tamponade is defined as hemodynamically significant cardiac compression by accumulating pericardial contents that evokes and defeats compensatory mechanisms. There is reduction of ventricular volume, producing rapidly rising diastolic pressures that resist ventricular filling with reduced stroke volume.[14] One of its main causes is myocardial rupture related to infarction.

Constrictive pericarditis

In constrictive pericarditis, there is impairment of mid and late ventricular filling from a thickened/noncompliant

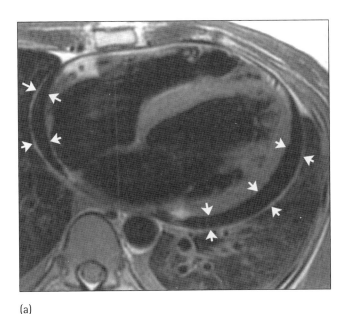

(a)

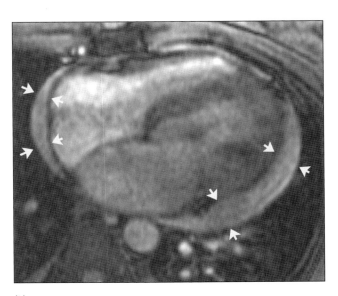

(b)

Figure 14.2
Pericardial effusion. Axial T1-weighted (a) and T2-weighted (b) images showing a moderate amount of fluid in the pericardial space.

pericardium. In the classic form, fibrous scarring and adhesions of both pericardial layers lead to obliteration of the pericardial cavity. Early ventricular filling is unimpeded, but diastolic filling is subsequently abruptly reduced as a result of the inability of the ventricles to fill because of physical constraints imposed by a rigid, thickened, and sometimes calcified pericardium. In less developed countries, tuberculosis remains the most common cause of chronic constrictive pericarditis, whereas in the USA, constriction may be associated with malignancy (lung cancer, breast cancer, or lymphoma), histoplasmosis, mediastinal irradiation, purulent or recurrent viral pericarditis, rheumatoid arthritis, uremia, chest trauma or hemopericardium, and cardiac surgery. Constriction may follow cardiac surgery by several weeks to months and may occur decades after chest wall irradiation. The cause may not be identified in many patients.[3]

On CMR, a pericardial thickness of > 4 mm is a key diagnostic feature. Other findings that confirm this diagnosis are dilatation of the inferior vena cava (IVC), hepatic veins and RA, whereas the RV shows normal or reduced volume (Figure 14.3).[7] Gradient-echo images demonstrate restricted diastolic filling of the RV and the RA. In chronic constriction, the thickened pericardium shows low-intensity signal on T1- and T2-weighted images. CMR is of limited value in the evaluation of patients with calcified pericarditis compared with CT when the calcifications are small (Figure 14.4).

The differential diagnosis is restrictive cardiomyopathy. It is important to distinguish those two entities, because constriction can be cured by surgical pericardiectomy whereas restrictive cardiomyopathy cannot be cured.

The ability to demonstrate a thickened pericardium in a patient within an appropriate clinical setting is used as a presumptive evidence of constrictive pericarditis.[15] Masui et al[16] demonstrated that CMR had sensitivity, specificity, and diagnostic accuracy rate of 88%, 100%, and 93%, respectively, in 29 patients who presented with the clinical purpose of establishing or excluding the diagnosis of constrictive pericarditis. They also found that localized, rather than generalized, thickening was common and the RV was the most common location to find thickened pericardium. A dilated atrium and IVC were identfied in 88% and 82%, respectively. None of the patients with restrictive cardiomyopathy had pericardial thickening, but 75% of them had dilatation of the RA and IVC. Sechtem et al[8] also found that CMR is able to exclude pericardial thickening in patients with restrictive cardiomyopathy.

Rienmuller et al[17] distinguished different forms of pericardial constriction as follows:

- *global* – bilateral thickening and/or calcification of the periepicardium along both ventricles and enlargement of both atria, superior vena cava (SVC) and IVC;
- *annular* – bilateral thickening and/or calcification of the periepicardium primarily in the atrioventricular (AV) grooves, with narrowing of both of them;

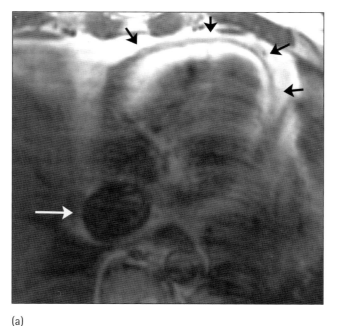

(a)

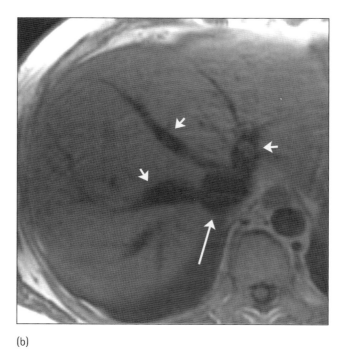

(b)

Figure 14.3
Constrictive pericarditis. Axial CMR showing (a) diffusely thickened pericardium (black arrows) with dilated inferior vena cava (white arrow) and (b) hepatic veins (short white arrows).

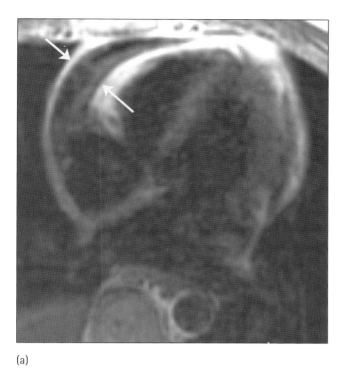

(a)

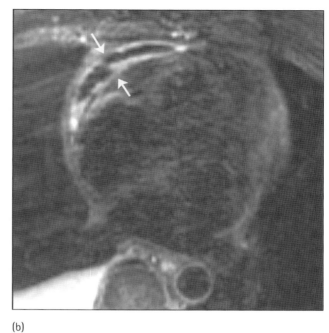

(b)

Figure 14.4

Pericardial thickening. Axial T1-weighted (a) and T2-weighted (b) images showing thickened pericardium over the right cardiac border, with areas of low signal corresponding to calcifications; note also right pleural effusion.

- *left-sided* – thickening or calcification of the periepicardium along the compressed LV with narrowing of the left AV groove;
- *right-sided* – thickening or calcification of the periepicardium in front of the compressed RV;
- *epicardial* – the global or focal form of constriction is predominantly caused by the involvement of the epicardial layer;
- *effusive* – the configuration of the epicardium does not change, regardless of the amount of pericardial fluid, but there is general epicardial constriction and pericardial effusion.

According to Rienmuller et al,[17] the description of the form of constriction is important in defining the surgical approach and the extent of pericardiectomy. Also they proposed that myocardial atrophy and fibrosis may be detected preoperatively by CMR and that patients with this condition are not candidates for pericardiectomy because of the higher perioperative mortality index in these subjects.

Neoplastic pericardial disease

Neoplastic pericardial disease usually occurs in the setting of relatively advanced neoplastic disease, often in patients in the terminal or near-terminal stage of cancer. However, a correct differential diagnosis is essential because of the frequent occurrence of pericardial disease due to other causes in patients who have cancer. Posner et al[18] showed in one series that 42% of patients with cancer who developed pericardial disease had no malignant involvement of the pericardium. CMR evaluation is advantageous because it provides a large field of view that allows evaluation of the disease throughout the thorax.

The diagnosis of malignant pericardial effusion can be confirmed by pericardiocentesis or open biopsy of the pericardium. Primary neoplasms of the pericardium are rare (Figure 14.5). Of those, mesothelioma and angiosarcomas should be remembered, both of them being highly malignant.[19] Pericardial mesothelioma is unrelated to asbestos exposure. In infants and children, intrapericardial teratomas may occur. Although usually benign tumors, teratomas can be life-threatening because of large pericardial effusions and cardiac compression.[20]

Most cases of neoplastic pericardial disease are the result of metastatic disease. Primary cancer of the lung is the most frequent source of pericardial neoplastic disease, and it may involve the heart by direct extension or by lymphatic/hematogeneous dissemination (Figure 14.6). Breast cancer is the second, and hematologic malignancies the third. Those three most frequent categories account for about three-quarters of cases of pericardial malignancies.[19]

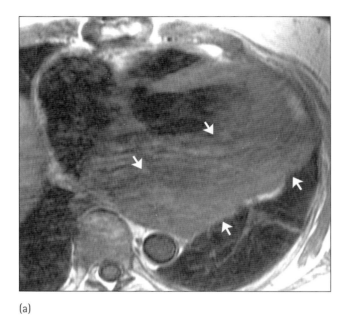

(a)

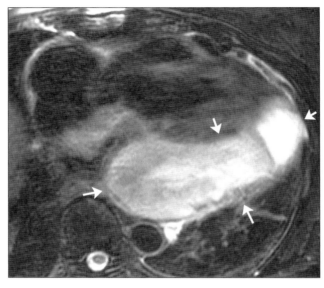

(b)

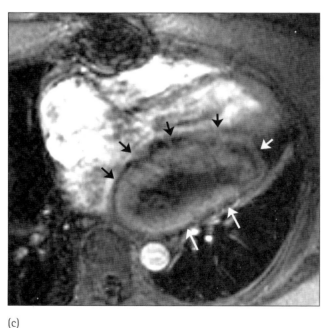

(c)

Figure 14.5
Hemangiopericytoma. Axial T1-weighted (a) and T2-weighted (b) images. (c) Note the enhancement in the peripheral region of the mass following intravenous injection of gadolinium.

Pericardial involvement is not usually the first clinical presentation of metastatic cancer. In most instances, the neoplastic disease has already been diagnosed and treated; the pericardial involvement occurs later as a manifestation of recurrent metastatic disease. Spread of cancer to the pericardium can occur through the bloodstream, through the lymphatic channels, or by direct grow from a nearby tumor. The predominant route is thought to be from lymph nodes in the mediastinum, with retrograde spread through lymphatic channels to the heart. Hematogenous metastasis to the pericardium are usually accompanied by evidence of hematogenous metastasis to other organs. Direct extension can occur in lung and esophageal carcinomas, among other tumors.

The symptoms and physical signs essentially reflect the severity of cardiac tamponade, but in rare instances neoplastic pericardial disease takes the form of encasement of the heart by solid tumor rather than pericardial effusion. The clinical picture in tumor encasement is one of constrictive pericarditis rather than tamponade.[19]

Any disease process that causes thickening or nodularity of the pericardium can mimic metastatic disease. This

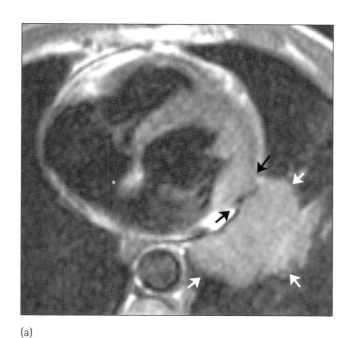

(a)

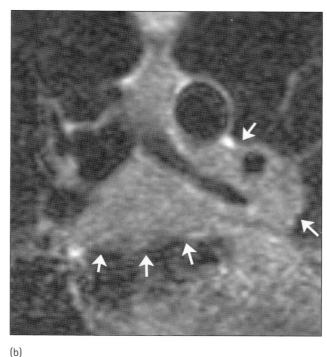

(b)

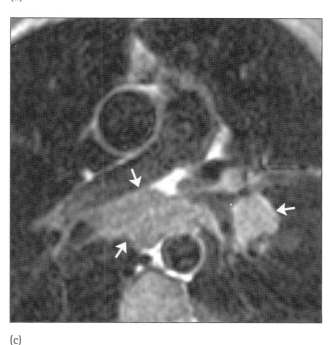

(c)

Figure 14.6
Bronchogenic carcinoma. (a) Axial CMR in a patient with bronchogenic carcinoma showing interruption of the pericardial line due to invasion. Coronal (b) and axial (c) CMR through the mediastinum showing extensive lymphadenopathy.

is especially true in a patient who has received radiation therapy, when the pericardium may appear thickened and nodular, mimicking metastatic disease. So, in a patient with a malignant tumor and pericardial effusion, the differential diagnosis includes malignant pericardial disease, drug-induced and/or radiation-induced pericarditis, infection, autoimmune disorders, and idiopathic pericardial disease.[21]

Congenital abnormalities of the pericardium

Pericardial cysts

Pericardial cysts represent a defect in the embryogenesis of the coelomic cavity. Their walls are composed of connective tissue and a single layer of mesothelial cells. They are usually filled with clear fluid. They are typically located in the right anterior cardiophrenic angle, but may be located anywhere within the pericardium (90% contact the diaphragm, 65% in the right cardiophrenic angle, 25% in the left cardiophrenic angle, and 10% are seen at higher levels).[22,23] Patients are generally asymptomatic, although rare complications have been reported.[24] The lesion is often discovered on a routine chest film and remains stable over time.[25]

Pericardial cysts appear as rounded or lobulated deformities of the cardiac silhouette, and their major clinical significance lies in the possibility of confusion with a tumor, ventricular aneurysm, or massive cardiomegaly. They show low signal intensity on T1-weighted spin-echo images and high signal intensity on T2-weighted spin-echo images; however, some pericardial cysts contain highly proteinaceous fluid that causes the signal to be high on T1-weighted spin-echo images.

Congenital absence of the pericardium

Congenital absence of the pericardium encompasses a range of congenital pericardial defects, ranging from a small foramen in the pericardium to a complete absence of the entire pericardium. This condition is rare and in most instances occurs on the left side.[26–28]

An explanation for the pericardial defects is that they result from incomplete development of either the transverse septum or of the pleuropericardial folds. This may be caused by deficient blood supply, and it has been hypothesized that the predominance of left-sided defects results from premature atrophy of the left duct of Cuvier or left common cardinal vein (the right duct of Cuvier normally persists as the SVC).[29]

Patients are most often asymptomatic, but can present with chest pain, which can be postural (precipitation by lying on the left side, relief by turning to the right).[30–32] Possible causes of pain are herniation of the left-atrial appendage through a foramen type of defect, torsion of the great vessels secondary to increased heart mobility, and constriction of the coronary arteries by fibrous bands on the lower edge of the absent pericardium, among others. Gatzoulis et al[31] suggested that the pain is most probably related to heart mobility, because they observed improvement or resolution of chest pain after surgical reconstruction of the pericardium (with immobilization of the heart) in all four patients who were submitted to surgery in their series.

On CMR, it is possible to confirm this diagnosis and determine the extent of the defect. The signs are nonvisualization/visualization of part of the pericardium, dis-placement of the heart into the left hemithorax, and lung parenchyma interposing between the main pulmonary artery and aorta, the later being the best marker of this condition.[31,33]

Conclusions

In conclusion, CMR represents the gold standard in imaging pericardial disease. CMR demonstrates excellent contrast resolution between normal and abnormal tissues, and functional images may be obtained for assessing the degree of both pericardial and myocardial involvement by inflammatory or malignant processes. Large fields of view and operator independence further improve the diagnostic capabilities of this method. Thus, while echocardiography is widely used for screening for pericardial disease, indeterminate cases should subsequently be evaluated by CMR.

References

1. Breen JF. Imaging of the pericardium. J Thorac Imag 2001; 16:47–54.

2. Gray H. Anatomy of the Human Body, 20th edn. Philadelphia: Lea & Febiger, 1918 (Bartleby.com, 2000. www.bartleby.com/107/): 524–6.

3. Goldman L, Bennett JC. Part VII, Cardiovascular Diseases. In: Cecil Textbook of Medicine, 21st edn. Philadelphia: WB Saunders, 2000: 348–53.

4. Spodick DH. Pericardial Anatomy and Physiology. In: Braunwald E. Heart Disease: A Textbook of Cardiovascular Medicine, 6th Ed. Philadelphia: WB Saunders, 2001, pp 1823–76.

5. Smith WHT, Beacock DJ, Goddard AJP, et al. Magnetic resonance evaluation of the pericardium. Br J Radiol 2001; 74:384–92.

6. Sechtem U, Tscholakoff D, Higgins CB. MRI of the normal pericardium. AJR 1986; 147:239–44.

7. Frank H, Globits S. Magnetic resonance imaging evaluation of myocardial and pericardial disease. J Magn Reson Imaging 1999; 10:617–26.

8. Sechtem U, Tscholakoff D, Higgins CB. MRI of the abnormal pericardium. AJR 1986; 147:245–52.

9. Vilacosta I, Gomez J, Dominguez J, et al. Massive pericardiac hematoma with severe constrictive pathophysiologic complications after insertion of an epicardial pacemaker. Am Heart J 1995; 130:1298–300.

10. Zellner C, Chou T, Higgins C, et al. Pericardial hematoma after primary angioplasty complicated by coronary rupture. Circulation 1998; 98:183.

11. Braunwald E. Pericardial disease. In: Harrison's Principles of Internal Medicine, 15th edn (Braunwald E, Fauci AS, Kasper DL, et al, eds). New York: McGraw-Hill, 2001: 1365–1372

12. Mulvagh SL,Rokey R, Vick GW, Johnston DL. Usefulness of nuclear magnetic resonance imaging for evaluation of pericardial effusions, and comparison with two-dimensional echocardiography, Am J Cardiol 1989; 64:1002–9.

13. White CS. MR evaluation of the pericardium. Top Magn Reson Imaging 1995; 7:258–66.

14. Spodick DH. The normal and diseased pericardium: current concepts of pericardial phisiology, diagnosis and treatment. J Am Coll Cardiol 1983; 1:240–51.

15. Vaitkus PT, Kussmaul WG. Constrictive pericarditis versus restrictive cardimyopathy: a reappraisal and update of diagnostic criteria. Am Heart J 1991; 122:1431–41.

16. Masui T, Finck S, Higgins CB. Constrictive pericarditis and restrictive cardimyopathy: evaluation with MR imaging. Radiology 1992; 182:369–73.

17. Rienmuller R, Gurgan M, Erdmann E, et al. CT and MR evaluation of pericardial constriction: a new diagnostic and therapeutic concept. J Thorac Imag 1993; 8:108–21.

18. Posner MR, Cohen GI, Skarin AT. Pericardial diseases in patients with cancer: the differentiation of malignant from idiopathic and radiation-induced pericarditis. Am J Med 1981; 71:407–13.

19. Hancock EW. Neoplastic pericardial disease. Cardiol Clin North Am 1990; 8:673–82.

20. Beghetti M, Prieditis M, Rebeyka IM, Mawson J. Intrapericardial teratoma. Circulation 1998; 97:1523–4.

21. Chiles C, Woodard PK, Gutierrez FR, Link KM. Metastatic involvement of the heart and pericardium: CT and MR imaging. RadioGraphics 2001; 21:439–49.

22. Pugatch RD, Braver JH, Robbins AH, Faling J. CT diagnosis of pericardial cysts. AJR 1978; 131:515–16.

23. Naidich DP, Muller NL, Zerhouni EA, et al. Computed Tomography and Magnetic Resonance of the Thorax 3rd edn. Philadelphia: Lippincott Williams & Wilkins, 1999: 128.

24. Ng AF, Olak J. Pericardial cyst causing right ventricular outflow tract obstruction. Ann Thorac Surg 1997; 63:1147–8.

25. Hoffmann U, Globits S, Frank H. Cardiac and paracardiac masses current opinion on diagnostic evaluation by magnetic resonance imaging. Eur Heart J 1998; 19:553–63.

26. Van Son JA, Danielson GK, Schaff HV, et al. Congenital partial and complete absence of the pericardium. Mayo Clin Proc 1993; 68:743–7.

27. Ellis K, Leeds NE, Himmelstein A. Congenital deficiencies in the parietal pericardium: a review with 2 new cases including successful diagnosis by plain roentgenography. AJR 1959; 82:125–37.

28. Ratib O, Perloff JK, Williams WG. Congenital complete absence of the pericardium. Circulation 103: 3154–5.

29. Perna G. Sopra un arresto di sviluppo della sierosa pericardica nell'uomo. Anat Anz 1909; 35:323–38.

30. Rusk RA, Kenny (??). Congenital pericardial defect presenting as chest pain. Heart 1999; 81:327–8.

31. Gatzoulis MA, Munk MD, Merchant N, et al. Isolated congenital absence of the pericardium: clinical presentation, diagnosis, and management. Ann Thorac Surg 2000; 69:1209–15.

32. Chapman JE, Rubin JW, Gross CM, Janssen ME. Congenital absence of pericardium: an unusual case of atypical angina. Ann Thorac Surg 1998; 45:91–3.

33. Raman SV, Daniels CJ, Katz SE, et al. Congenital absence of the pericardium. Circulation 104:1447–8.

15

Contrast-enhanced magnetic resonance angiography

Jeffrey H Maki, Michael V Knopp, Martin R Prince

Introduction

Rapid advances in the implementation and understanding of three-dimensional (3D) contrast-enhanced magnetic resonance angiography (CE-MRA) are making minimally-invasive vascular imaging safer and more accurate. For this reason, CE-MRA is increasingly utilized as the primary method of vascular imaging. This chapter describes the basic principles underlying 3D CE-MRA and demonstrates its applications throughout the body. Inherent advantages of 3D contrast MRA over 'conventional' MRA techniques such as time-of-flight and phase contrast will be discussed. Furthermore, we will explore techniques for improving spatial and temporal resolution, reducing respiratory motion artifacts, decreasing contrast dosing, and more accurately timing the contrast bolus. Finally, new contrast agents will be reviewed.

Conventional MRA

MR pulse sequences can exploit blood motion in order to directly visualize vascular structures without intravascular contrast material. One of the earliest MRA techniques, time-of-flight (TOF) angiography, is performed using a flow-compensated gradient refocused sequence. Data can be acquired as multiple 2D slices, or as a single 3D volume. In this technique, stationary tissues in the slice or volume of interest are 'saturated' and therefore have low signal intensity.[1–3] Blood upstream of the imaging volume, however, remains 'unsaturated'. When this blood flows into the imaging volume, it is bright compared with the stationary background tissues. This 'inflow' or 'time-of-flight' approach often works particularly well in relatively normal arteries and veins, including the inferior vena cava (IVC), iliac veins, carotid arteries, and cerebral vasculature.[4–12] It also has the benefit of allowing selective satura-

tion of blood adjacent to the imaging volume such that either arterial or venous signal can be suppressed. One major disadvantage of TOF angiography is in-plane saturation, which can be a problem with slowly flowing blood in tortuous arteries or when the long axis of the vessel coincides with the scan plane. A second limitation is turbulence-induced signal loss in and distal to a stenosis.[13,14] In addition, the relatively long echo times required for gradient moment nulling make TOF sensitive to susceptibility artifacts from metallic clips, metal implants, and bowel gas or other air–tissue interfaces. These artifacts have been implicated as a primary reason for inaccuracy in TOF MRA. As a further downside, TOF imaging times tend to be lengthy. This is due to the need to image perpendicular to the vessel axis in order to avoid in-plane saturation. Long acquisition times can lead to motion artifacts, including slice misregistration, particularly for those patients who have difficulty remaining still.

Phase contrast (PC) angiography makes use of phase shifts as blood flows in the presence of flow-encoding gradients.[1,15,16] Using phase difference images (created by subtracting two images created with opposite flow-encoding gradients), residual phase is proportional to velocity. Stationary background tissue, however, is suppressed because it has no phase shift on either image, and hence subtracts completely. The flow-encoding gradients can be applied in any or multiple directions, depending on the desired flow sensitivity. PC angiography can be implemented as a 2D or 3D gradient refocused sequence, and is substantially improved when performed after contrast administration.[17] It has proven useful for evaluation of the renal arteries, carotid arteries, and portal vein.[8,12,16–20] In normal vessels without stenoses or turbulence, the results are often spectacular.

Another strength of PC angiography is its ability to measure flow velocities. In combination with cine (synchronization with cardiac gating), a time-resolved velocity profile can be generated similar to an ultrasound Doppler waveform.[21,22] This provides physiologic flow data and allows the quantitative measurement of flow rates. Unfortunately, it is this same velocity sensitivity that limits PC angiography. Strong flow-encoding gradients make the sequence susceptible to degradation from bulk (cardiac, respiratory, and translational) motion. In addition, PC sequences only quantify a specified range of velocities.[19] In occlusive disease, turbulence causes a broad spectrum of rapidly varying velocities, which in turn causes intravoxel phase dispersion and signal loss. Thus artifactual loss of vessel visualization at a stenosis is common.[13] Interestingly, this apparent deficiency can be useful as an adjunct to 3D CE-MRA for characterizing the hemodynamic significance of a stenosis, since pressure gradients are known to occur in regions of high turbulence and jet flow.

Contrast-enhanced MRA: theory

Three-dimensional CE-MRA is performed in a manner analogous to conventional contrast angiography or helical computed tomography (CT). Rather than relying on blood motion to create intravascular signal, a contrast agent (traditionally a gadolinium chelate) is introduced to shorten the T1 (spin–lattice) relaxation time of blood such that it is significantly less than the surrounding tissues. Blood can then be directly imaged (using a T1-weighted sequence), irrespective of flow effects. This alleviates many of the problems inherent to TOF and PC angiography. In particular, sensitivity to turbulence is dramatically reduced, and in-plane saturation effects are eliminated.[13,14] The technique allows a small number of slices to be oriented in the plane of the target vessels to quickly image an extensive region of vascular anatomy (equal to the field of view) at high in-plane resolution. Thus, 3D CE-MRA is intrinsically fast, allowing high quality breath-hold MR angiograms.

Gadolinium chelates

At present, most CE-MRA examinations are conducted using gadolinium-based MR contrast agents. Gadolinium (Gd^{3+}) is a paramagnetic metal ion that decreases both the spin–lattice (T1) and spin–spin (T2) relaxation times.[23] Because the Gd^{3+} ion itself is biologically toxic, it is chelated with ligands such as DTPA (gadopentetate dimeglumine), HP-DO3A (gadoteridol), or DTPA-BMA (gadodiamide) to form low-molecular-weight contrast agents.[24] These 'extracellular' agents diffuse from the intravascular compartment into the interstitial space in a matter of minutes, meaning that selective imaging of the

vascular structures must be performed rapidly.[13,24] As compared with iodinated contrast agents, gadolinium chelates have a very low rate of adverse events and no nephrotoxicity, which is a significant advantage when evaluating patients with impaired renal function.[25–28]

Each gadolinium chelate decreases the T1 of blood according to the equation[14,29]

$$\frac{1}{T1} = \frac{1}{1200} + R_1[Gd], \qquad (1)$$

where R_1 is the field-dependent T1 relaxivity of the gadolinium chelate, [Gd] is the concentration of the gadolinium chelate, and 1200 ms is the T1 of blood without gadolinium (at 1.5 T). A similar equation applies for T2 (which is always <T1).

Pulse sequence

Dynamic CE-MRA exploits the transient shortening in blood T1 following intravenous administration of a contrast agent using a fast 3D spoiled gradient-echo (SPGR) sequence.[14,30,31] We use the term 'transient' because this technique exploits the 'first pass' of the contrast agent, since 80% of a typical gadolinium chelate leaks into the intravascular space within 5 min.[32] Typical repetition times (TR) for the 3D T1-weighted gradient-echo (SPGR, T1-FFE, FLASH) sequences used for CE-MRA are <5–6 ms, with echo times (TE) of 1–2 ms and total scan times in the 10–30 s range. This type of 3D sequence is ideally suited to MRA, as it has high spatial resolution and an intrinsically high signal-to-noise ratio (SNR). In addition, it is fast (it can be performed in a breathhold), and can be oriented and reformatted in any desired plane.[33–37] In addition, because intravascular signal is dependent on T1 relaxation rather than on inflow or phase accumulation, in-plane saturation and turbulence-induced signal loss are not a problem.[14]

The relative signal intensity (SI) for a 3D gradient-echo acquisition is given by[38]

$$SI = \frac{N(H)(1 - e^{-TR/T1})}{1 - e^{-TR/T1} \cos \alpha} \sin \alpha \ e^{-TE/T2^*}, \qquad (2)$$

where $N(H)$, TR, TE, and α are the proton density, repetition time, echo time, and flip angle, respectively. Examining Equation (2), SI is maximized when TR is long or T1 is short, since as TR/T1 becomes large, $e^{-TR/T1}$ approaches zero. Of these options, shortening T1 is the primary method for increasing intravascular signal intensity, since lengthening TR and thereby increasing scan time is not desirable. The Ernst angle α_E, which is important in understanding how to properly optimize parameters for a particular TR and expected T1, is defined as the

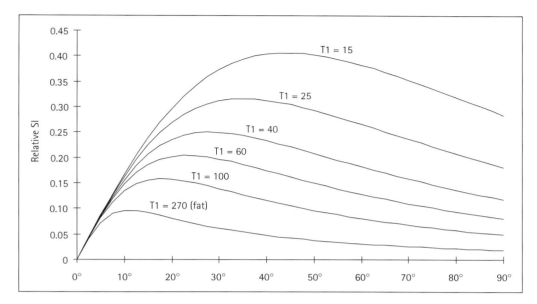

Figure 15.1
Relative signal intensity (SI) for different T1 values versus flip angle α for a spoiled gradient sequence. TR = 5 ms, TE <<T2*.

flip angle maximizing SI in Equation (2), and can be expressed as

$$\alpha_E = \cos^{-1}(e^{-TR/T1}). \qquad (3)$$

Figure 15.1 shows an example of relative signal intensity versus flip angle α for different values of T1 (assuming TR = 5 ms with TE<<T2*). Note the significant increase in signal intensity as T1 approaches zero.

Contrast dose and T1

In order for blood to appear bright with respect to background tissues during the arterial phase of dynamic 3D CE-MRA, sufficient contrast material must be administered to transiently reduce the arterial blood T1 to less than that of the brightest background tissue (i.e. fat), which has a T1 of ~270 ms. During the first-pass arterial phase, blood T1 is more related to infusion rate and contrast agent relaxivity than total contrast dose, since arterial phase imaging occurs well before intravascular contrast equilibration. This dynamic approach has the advantage of nearly eliminating steady-state background signal, but at the same time (considering non-blood-pool agents) is essentially a 'one shot' technique, meaning that once contrast is administered and dynamic imaging performed, the process cannot be repeated without a second contrast bolus. If a second bolus is adminstered, not only are there the issues of expense and total patient dose, but residual soft tissue enhancement can obscure vascular detail (as the biologic half-life of gadolinium chelates is ~90 min).[39] When using more than one injection, subtraction of a precontrast mask is desirable, and in some instances mandatory, for the second and third injections.[40]

Timing is extremely important in dynamic CE-MRA. In order to appreciate timing issues, the relationship between injection rate, blood T1, and resultant signal intensity must first be reviewed.

For times shorter than the recirculation time, contrast concentration of the bolus in blood can be approximated as[13,14,41]

$$[\text{contrast}] = \frac{\text{rate of contrast injection (mol/l)}}{\text{cardiac output in (l/s)}}. \qquad (4)$$

Although this simple equation ignores bolus dilution at leading and trailing edges, as well as extravasation of contrast in the lungs, a complex model originally developed for intravenous digital subtraction angiography arrives at the same value for maximum contrast concentration.[42] Combining Equations (1), (2), and (4), and assuming no recirculation, blood T1 can be calculated for a given cardiac output and injection rate. This is demonstrated in Figure 15.2 for cardiac outputs of 3, 5, and 7 l/min using a standard gadolinium chelate preparation with a concentration of 0.5 mol/l.

Note from Figure 15.2 that for a 'typical' cardiac output of 5 l/min, an injection rate of 1 cm³/s yields a blood T1 of 36 ms, while a 2 cm³/s injection gives a blood T1 of 18 ms. These T1 values are in fact much shorter than the T1 of fat, even though our own experience suggests that true T1 values are not quite this short, being instead nearer double this estimate. Such a rapid injection rate, however, can and need not necessarily be sustained over the entire acquisition time. For a typical 80 kg patient receiving a 'single dose' (0.1 mmol/kg) of gadolinium, this equates to 16 cm³ of a 0.5 mol/l gadolinium chelate preparation. Thus a 1 cm³/s injection can be sustained for 16 s, or a 2 cm³/s injection can be sustained for 8 s. Even though the acquisition time may be considerably greater than this, by

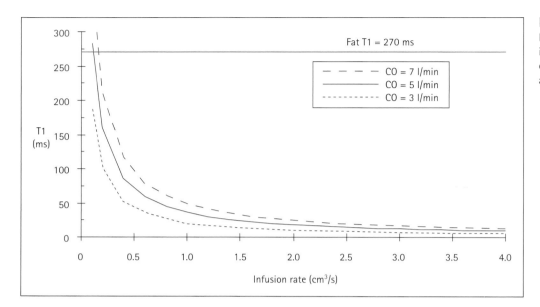

Figure 15.2
Blood T1 versus gadolinium infusion rate for changing cardiac output (CO), assuming no recirculation.

properly timing the bolus with respect to image acquisition, as well as by realizing that a contrast bolus lengthens as it propagates from the venous to the arterial circulation, full advantage of the dynamic blood T1 shortening can be obtained. This is largely due to the unique way in which MR data are acquired.

Fourier (k-space) considerations

MR imaging does not map spatial data linearly with respect to time as does conventional CT.[43] With 3D MR imaging, the entire 3D 'Fourier' or 'k-space' data set is collected before reconstructing individual slices. Because k-space maps spatial frequencies rather than spatial data, k-space data do not directly correspond to image space. Instead, different regions of k-space data determine different image features. For example, the center of k-space, or 'low' spatial frequencies, dominates image contrast, whereas the periphery of k-space, or 'high' spatial frequencies, contributes more to fine details such as edges.[44,45] This means that the state of the intravascular T1 in large vessels is essentially 'captured' at the instant corresponding to acquisition of central k-space.[44] If central k-space is collected when arterial contrast concentration is peaking but has not yet reached the venous structures (arterial phase), only the arteries will enhance. The fact that intravascular contrast concentration may not be uniform over the entire acquisition time may generate artifacts, but these have been shown to be relatively minor provided that the contrast is not rapidly changing over the critical central portion of k-space and at least some 'tail' of the contrast bolus is present during the collection of high-spatial-frequency data at the periphery of k-space.[41,44]

Thus, with proper timing, gadolinium injection duration need not be as long as the entire acquisition time, and in fact many protocols use injection durations much shorter than the acquisition time, with quite acceptable results.[46,47] For a given gadolinium dose, the injection strategy then becomes a tradeoff between a fast injection (shorter T1 – more intravascular signal) and long injection (more uniform T1 – fewer artifacts). We have a general rule of thumb that advocates injecting the total contrast dose over a duration of ~50–60% that of the acquisition for single-station examinations.

Another factor that must be considered is phase-encoding order. Traditionally, phase encoding is performed 'sequentially' such that central k-space is acquired at the midpoint of the scan. Alternatively, phase encoding can be performed in a 'centric' fashion such that central k-space is acquired at the beginning of the scan.[48,49] Although centric phase encoding order has been shown to be somewhat more prone to artifacts if the contrast concentration changes rapidly during acquisition of central k-space, it greatly simplifies bolus timing (discussed below) and is less susceptible to artifact from incomplete breathholds.[50,51]

Contrast material injection rate

Note from Figure 15.2 that for injection rates greater than ~2 cm³/s, there is diminishing return with respect to T1 shortening. But, based on Figure 15.1, even small decreases in T1 lead to tremendous increases in signal intensity. Combining Equations (1)–(4), signal intensity (for TR = 5, TE = 2) can be plotted verses injection rate for a fixed cardiac output (5 l/min) and flip angle (Ernst

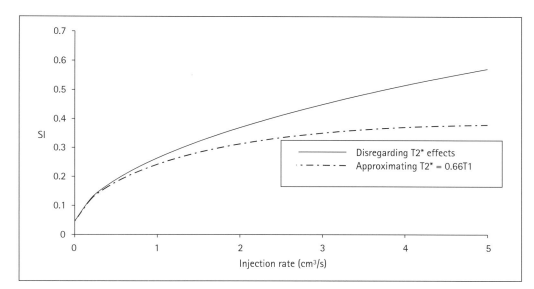

Figure 15.3
Relative signal intensity (SI) versus gadolinium injection rate for a spoiled gradient-echo sequence. Flip angle α = Ernst angle, cardiac output 5 l/min.

angle) as shown in Figure 15.3. This is done both disregarding T2* effects and using the approximation that T2* = 0.66 T1.[41] This graph demonstrates that signal intensity increases asymptotically as injection rate increases, particularly when taking into account T2* effects, with negligible increases seen beyond a rate of 4–5 cm³/s.[52,53]

Different authors have taken different approaches to optimizing injection rate. Before the advent of high-speed gradient systems that permitted total acquisition times of <1 min (in the realm of a breathhold), imaging times were ~3–5 min, and injections were typically performed so that a 'double dose' (0.2 mmol/kg) was administered at a uniform rate over the entire scan duration.[30,54] For a 4 min scan on a 70 kg patient, this amounted to an injection rate of just over 0.1 cm³/s. With the much shorter acquisition times currently possible, many investigators advocate a 'double dose' (0.2 mmol/kg, or alternatively a set volume of 20 or 30 cm³) of gadolinium chelate with injection rates of 1–2 cm³/s. Others use up to a 'quadruple dose' (0.4 mmol/kg) and rates of 4–5 cm³/s, while a new trend now advocates much smaller doses.[35,37,55–57] We feel, that using a single 20 cm³ vial of gadolinium chelate with an injection rate of 1.5–2.5 cm³/s is generally a good compromise between maximizing arterial signal and minimizing artifacts for breathhold scans.[58] Multistation exams, large aneurysms or dissections, and cases where venous evaluation is important are different, and will be discussed shortly.

Contrast-enhanced MRA: bolus timing considerations

As discussed above, the timing of the gadolinium bolus acquisition of central k-space is extremely important. The contrast travel time, defined as the time required for contrast to travel from the injection site to the vascular territory of interest, is highly variable, as is the degree to which the bolus 'broadens' as it transits the heart and pulmonary circulation. A mean transit time to the abdominal aorta of 23 ± 5 s, with a range of 13–37 s has been reported.[59] An example of time-resolved abdominal aortic SI (which is proportional to [Gd]) after intravenous injection of 9.5 cm³ gadolinium chelate at 2 cm³/s is shown in Figure 15.4.

Based on Figure 15.4, note first that arterial signal peaks relatively sharply. (If the bolus were of longer duration, i.e. larger total dose, the arterial peak would be somewhat lengthened.) This observation has important implications. Because it has been shown that intravascular signal intensity is determined by the gadolinium concentration at the time the center of k-space is collected,[44] whether central k-space is acquired at time t_1, t_2, or t_3 (Figure 15.4) has a dramatic influence over the resultant image. Perfect timing (t_2) yields maximum arterial signal with minimal venous signal, as shown in Figure 15.5a. If, however, central k-space data are acquired too early (t_1 – while arterial [Gd] is still rapidly increasing), 'ringing' or 'banding' artifacts of variable severity can be generated, as subtly demonstrated in the iliac arteries (Figure 15.5b).[44] These artifacts are also referred to as 'leading edge' artifacts since they result from imaging during the leading edge of bolus arrival. Acquiring central k-space data too late (t_3) leads to submaximal arterial signal intensity and associated venous enhancement. These two factors can be detrimental to evaluation of the arterial structures. A mild example of such delayed timing is shown in Figure 15.5c. Hence, if one knows or can predict or measure the time course of intravascular [Gd], the placement of central k-space can be tailored to achieve the desired image characteristics, be they maximum arterial signal, maximum portal venous signal, etc.

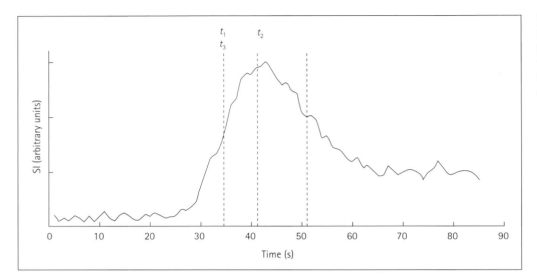

Figure 15.4
Relative signal intensity (SI) in the aorta versus time following a 9.5 cm³ injection of gadolinium chelate at a rate of 2 cm³/s.

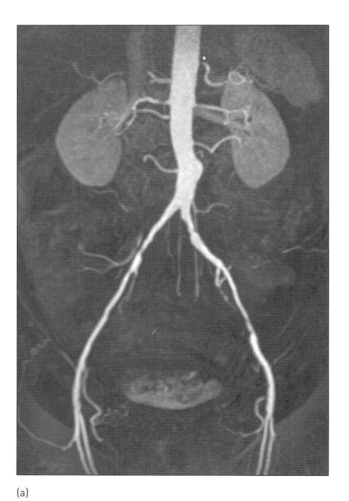

(a)

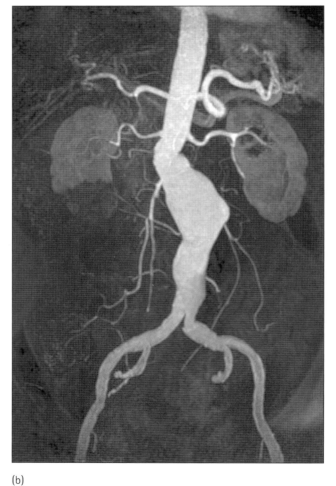

(b)

Figure 15.5
Maximum-intensity projection (MIP) images from different MRA studies demonstrating (a) good arterial phase timing in an abdominal aortic study, (b) slow flow through an abdominal aortic aneurysm with resultant leading edge artifact (mild ringing) and decreased SNR in the iliac arteries, and

(Figure 15.5c continues on the next page)

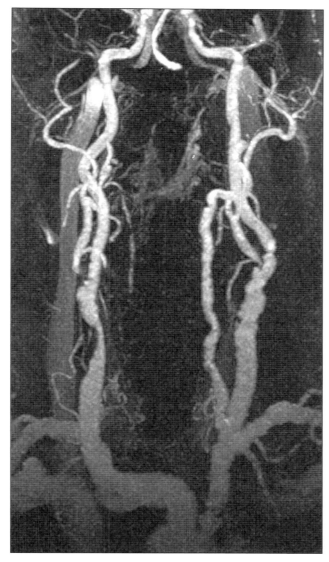

(c)

Figure 15.5 continued
(c) a carotid MRA with slightly delayed triggering leading to mild–moderate enhancement of the right jugular vein.

'Best guess' technique

Several solutions to proper bolus timing have been offered. Perhaps the simplest is to just make an educated 'best guess'. This involves estimating the contrast travel time from the site of injection to the vascular structure of interest. While this time is highly variable, an experienced MR angiographer can reliably achieve good results by taking factors such as injection site, age, cardiac output, and vascular anatomy into consideration. Sequential phase encoding is preferred when using 'best guess', since this encoding strategy is more tolerant of timing errors

(see the section below on logistical considerations).[44] Using this technique, timing can be calculated as follows:[35]

$$\text{imaging delay} = (\text{estimated contrast travel time})$$
$$+ (\text{injection time}/2) - (\text{imaging time}/2), \quad (5)$$

where the imaging delay is the delay between initiating the bolus and starting the scan (if negative, it refers to the delay between initiating the scan and starting the bolus). Equation (5) times the injection such that the midpoint of the bolus arrives at the desired vascular territory at the midpoint (center of k-space) of the scan. As an example, for a scan time of 18 s with an estimated contrast travel time of 20 s and a 20 cm^3 gadolinium bolus at 2 cm^3/s (10 s injection), the imaging delay would be 20 + 10/2 − 18/2 = 16 s (i.e. start the acquisition 16 s after initiating contrast injection). This timing is designed such that the midpoint of the bolus arrives as the center of k-space is collected, meaning that, depending on injection duration, there may already be venous enhancement by the time central k-space is collected. A potentially better timing strategy is as follows:

$$\text{imaging delay} = (\text{estimated contrast travel time})$$
$$- (\text{imaging time}/2 + \text{rise time}). \quad (6)$$

where the rise time is the expected time from arterial arrival to arterial peak, typically 3–5 s. This timing formula places the center of k-space at the approximate peak of contrast concentration.

The most difficult aspect of the 'best guess' technique is estimating the contrast travel time. As previously alluded to, it is better to image slightly late (increased venous phase) than slightly early (ringing/banding artifact: Figure 15.5b). With this in mind, as a general guideline for travel time from an antecubital vein to the abdominal aorta, we start with ~15 s for a young healthy patient. For a young hypertensive or athletic patient, it would be a few seconds less. For a healthy elderly patient it would be ~20–25 s. Patients with cardiac disease or an aortic aneurysm would have travel times in the 25–35 s range. In cases of severe cardiac failure in conjunction with aortic pathology, the travel time might be up to 40–50 s. We add 3–4 seconds if the injection is into the hand.

Test bolus technique

A better, and only slightly more time-consuming, way to estimate contrast travel time is through use of a 'test bolus'.[59–61] With this technique, 1–2 cm^3 of gadolinium (followed by 10–15 cm^3 saline flush) is injected at the same rate as planned for the actual injection. Multiple single-slice fast gradient-echo images of the appropriate vascular region are then obtained as rapidly as possible (at least every 1–2 s) for ~1 min. In order to minimize TOF effects and thereby maximize contrast conspicuity, the 2D test bolus image should either be oriented along the vessel of interest (i.e. sagittal or coronal for the aorta) or be relatively thick (>1 cm), with a superior saturation band or a blood-nulling inversion prepulse. The time of peak arterial enhancement (contrast travel time) is then determined visually or by using region of interest (ROI) analysis. Acquisition timing is then determined from Equation (6), keeping in mind that a longer bolus will take longer to peak than a test bolus, and therefore a 3–4 s rise time should be included. Alternatively, if centric encoding is desired (which is beneficial if the patient cannot breath-hold well),[50] the following equation should be used, again anticipating a rise time in the 3–4 s range:

$$\text{imaging delay} = \text{contrast travel time} + \text{rise time.} \quad (7)$$

Using the test bolus technique for abdominal aortic imaging, Earls et al[59] demonstrated a mean aortic SNR increase of 902% (15 patients) following a 1 cm³ bolus of gadopentetate dimeglumine.[59] By utilizing the resultant contrast travel time (24.0 ± 12.6 s), they were 100% successful in obtaining a 'pure' arterial phase study (as compared with 80% with 'best guess' timing), and saw significantly increased aortic SNR (29.8 versus 20.5).

There are three main drawbacks to the test bolus technique. First, setting up, performing, and analyzing the test bolus lengthens the overall examination time. In experienced hands, the average time penalty was reported as <5 min.[59] Second, the test bolus rapidly redistributes into the interstitial space, thereby increasing background signal. For such small test doses, however, these effects are negligible. Finally, there is no absolute guarantee that the imaging bolus will behave identically to the test bolus. This is because of moment-to-moment patient variables such as venous return and cardiac output, as well as the different total volume of injection. For example, a test bolus with the arm at the patient's side may not be accurate if the arms are above the head for the actual injection.

MR fluoroscopy

A third method of contrast bolus timing uses extremely rapid 'fluoroscopic' MR imaging.[45,62–64] With this technique, 2D sagittal gradient refocused images are rapidly (<1 s/image) obtained through the vascular structure of interest, ideally using complex subtraction to improve contrast-to-noise ratio and decrease artifacts. In this fashion, images are generated in near real time and updated at >1 image/s. The operator can watch the contrast bolus arrive, then switch over to the centric 3D MRA sequence when the desired enhancement is detected.

This technique has the advantage of allowing real-time operator-dependent decision making. This may be particularly advantageous in the evaluation of cases with unusual or asymmetric flow patterns such as unilateral stenoses and slow-filling aneurysms. As an example, an abdominal aortic aneurysm can be monitored such that triggering is somewhat delayed in order to allow for complete enhancement of the iliac vessels, which may fill slowly (see Figure 15.5b). The ability to assess the vasculature 'on the fly' under these circumstances is a great asset, as are the time and contrast savings associated with not performing a test injection.

A recent refinement is to electronically shift the MR fluoroscopic monitoring to a proximal region of vascular anatomy to get more advance warning of contrast arrival.[65] Using carotid CE-MRA as an example, MR fluoroscopic monitoring in the chest shows contrast arriving in the subclavian vein, then right heart, pulmonary arteries, left heart, arch, and finally proximal great vessels. Tracking the bolus over such a long period makes precise triggering easier. If the flow is very slow, the operator can compensate to allow for greater target vessel enhancement before triggering. This same work also demonstrates fluoroscopic triggering is improved by recessing the absolute center of k-space a few seconds from the beginning of the 3D acquisition, thus avoiding early triggering, which can cause the previously described 'leading edge' artifact.

Temporally resolved 3D contrast MRA

Because proper bolus timing is so difficult, and a timing mistake can ruin the study, some authors advocate 'temporally' resolved techniques whereby multiple 3D datasets are acquired (or synthesized) extremely rapidly (typically 2–8 s).[66–70] With such techniques, bolus timing is no longer a factor, since multiple vascular phases are obtained without any predetermined timing (i.e. inject and begin scanning simultaneously). The operator simply selects the desired image set, be it pure arterial, maximum venous, etc. This is particularly useful in the carotid and pulmonary arteries, where the venous phase is extremely rapid, and in the case of vessels such as in the calf, where variable rate filling may occur due to stenoses, occlusions, or rapid arteriovenous shunting due to soft tissue inflammatory disease.[66,70,71]

The most straightforward way to accelerate acquisition time is simply by scanning faster. This can be done using some combination of limiting the imaging volume, decreasing the resolution, decreasing TR, or using a parallel imaging technique such as SENSE.[72–75] Recent developments in gradient systems allow TRs of well under 2 ms on many systems, a threefold improvement compared with just a few years ago. In the pulmonary arteries, Goyen et al[73] achieved 4 s temporal resolution using partial k-space filling (TR = 1.6 ms), although slice thickness was relatively thick at 5.5 mm reconstructed to 2.75 mm. In another approach, taken by Finn et al,[74] the aorta is imaged in two alternating planes (oblique sagittal and coronal, TR = 1.6 ms) at ~1 s resolution per plane. This is in part possible due to a thick slab acquisition (~20 mm interpolated to 10 mm), meaning that the data are quasiprojectional. While off-plane reformats in this case are poor, in-plane Maximum-intensity projections (MIPs) (two planes) are of high resolution. Finn et al[76] have also used a 3D radial sampling scheme to further increase resolution. Once high-resolution temporal datasets are obtained, even if the temporal resolution is insufficient for isolating the desired vascular phase, postprocessing techniques such as correlation analysis can be used to synthesize images of a particular type, in this case pure pulmonary arterial versus pure pulmonary venous.[77]

Simultaneous high spatial resolution, high temporal-resolution, and increased volume coverage can be obtained using the 3D TRICKS (time-resolved imaging of contrast kinetics) technique and its variants.[67,71,78–80] In the most basic implementation of this technique, k-space is divided into multiple blocks. The central block of k-space (which contributes most to overall image contrast) is repeatedly collected every 2–8 s in an alternating fashion with the other blocks of more peripheral k-space. Images are then 'synthesized' at high temporal resolution by piecing together each unique central block of k-space with a linear interpolation of the remaining k-space blocks acquired in closest temporal proximity. This technique allows greater temporal and spatial resolution/volume coverage than with a streamlined conventional sequence. The technique lends itself to 'video' format, where passage of contrast material can be viewed directly. 3D TRICKS-type sequences are now finding their way into commercial packages. The biggest drawback, other than the tremendously large number of images generated, is the large amount of processing time required to perform the multiple reconstructions, although this is rapidly improving. Also, k-space discontinuities, in conjunction with varying intravascular gadolinium concentration, can potentially lead to artifacts. These artifacts, however, have been shown to be small provided the gadolinium bolus is not too compact.[78]

A recent refinement in this strategy is to traverse k-space using radial or spiral projections, which allow for sliding window reconstructions at very high temporal and spatial resolutions.[81] One variation, known as VIPR (vastly undersampled isotropic projection reconstruction), is particularly promising.[82]

Contrast-enhanced MRA: logistical considerations

The following logistical considerations apply to 3D CE-MRA in general, whether using 'best guess' timing, a test bolus, or triggering.

Artifacts: k-space-related

As previously discussed, the key to maximizing arterial enhancement is to image such that the center of k-space is collected when arterial contrast concentration is at a maximum. Acquiring central k-space data after arterial contrast has peaked leads to suboptimal arterial signal and increased venous signal (Figures 15.4 and 15.5c). Acquiring central k-space during the rapid upslope in arterial contrast arrival causes 'ringing'-type leading edge artifacts (Figure 15.5b). Even with optimal timing, similar artifacts can be generated with the use of very compact boluses such that contrast falls rapidly while still acquiring relatively central k-space.[78] If the bolus is too short, such that the contrast concentration tapers too rapidly toward the end of the acquisition (high k-space frequencies), blurring of the edges results.[44] These artifacts are not as severe if k-space is mapped in a sequential rather than a centric manner.[44]

Thus, when using 'best guess' timing, sequential phase encoding is more forgiving. Also, if using this technique, we suggest slightly overestimating the contrast travel time so that the (inevitable) timing errors are more likely to cause increased venous enhancement than 'ringing' artifacts. When using the test bolus technique such that contrast travel time is known, either centric or sequential phase encoding can be used. The advantage of centric is twofold: less degradation with an incomplete breathhold (see the discussion of respiratory artifacts below) and simplified operator logistics with respect to timing (no need to count backwards to the middle of the scan to figure out when to inject – just inject, wait the proper delay, initiate breathhold, and start imaging). For automated bolus detection, centric phase encoding is typically used. Because contrast rise times are not instantaneous, the delay from 'triggering' to initiation of data acquisition becomes crucial in order to avoid artifacts. Examining Figure 15.4, if the 3D MRA triggers at time t_1, the appropriate delay is $t_2 - t_1$. This delay, of course, varies by patient and vascular territory. A delay of 3–6 s typically works well for abdominal aortic imaging. In patients expected to have particularly slow flow (congestive heart failure or aneurysm), this time should be lengthened to 7–10 s. In the carotid arteries, however, which have a more rapid upslope and a very short arteriovenous window, shorter trigger delays of 2–3 s are more appropriate in order to avoid jugular venous enhancement.[63,83] Recessing the absolute center of k-space from the beginning of the scan improves consistency by providing high arterial phase contrast even if the trigger is premature.

Artifacts: respiratory

Respiratory motion causes ghosting, blurring, and signal loss.[84,85] In 3D imaging, blurring occurs in the direction of the motion, whereas ghosting is most pronounced in the slow phase-encoding direction. For elliptical centric phase-encoding order, the ghosting is spread out in both phase-encoding directions.[86] Before the advent of fast imaging systems, 3D CE-MRA acquisition times were ~3 min, making breathholding an impossibility. Thus early CE-MRA images suffered from significant image degradation, particularly when evaluating small vessels such as renal arteries.[14] Figures 15.6a,b illustrate the difference between good- and poor-quality breathholding.

There is no disagreement among researchers regarding the beneficial effects of breathholding on abdominal and thoracic 3D CE-MRA.[35–37,50,87] Holland et al[87] evaluated the same six patients using both breathhold and non-breathhold renal 3D CE-MRA. They found that the non-breathhold studies failed to identify three of four peripheral renal artery abnormalities, missed one of two accessory renal arteries, and were unable to visualize any of the renal artery bifurcations at the hilum. In contrast, breathhold 3D CE-MRA identified all abnormalities, all accessory renal arteries, and renal artery bifurcations at the hilum in all patients. In the carotid arteries, breathholding does not appear essential, although it does improve visualization of the arch vessels.[88]

Maki et al[50] looked at SNR loss and blur associated with incomplete breathholds. Their work demonstrated that for typical MRA acquisition matrices and scan times, breathholding during the acquisition of the central 50% of k-space was the most important for minimizing blur. This means that for centric phase encoding, the majority of the benefit from breathholding can be obtained even if the patient begins breathing at the midpoint of the scan. Data from Wilman et al[51] and Vasbinder et al[86] show that the more fully 'centric' the phase-encoding order is, the less the artifact from partial breathholds – and thus there is a preference for an elliptical versus a linear centric phase-encoding order. These data suggest that for centric phase-encoding orders, an optimistic assessment of a patient's breathhold ability is appropriate, since there is little to lose if they 'don't quite make it'. Recent data, however, have suggested that a large number of patients have a relatively large degree of diaphragmatic motion even during an apparently successful breathhold.[86] This causes blurring and ringing artifacts within the visceral arteries, obscuring small vessels and subtle abnormalities (such as occur with fibromuscular dysplasia) – in effect counteracting the spatial resolution inherent in the sequence. This argues toward shortening abdominal MRA acquisition times to well below potential breathhold times, making rapid-acquisition techniques such as SENSE and the ultrashort TR previously discussed above even more attractive. In anatomic regions that can remain

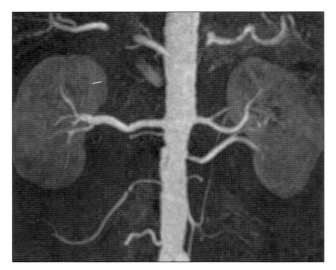

(a)

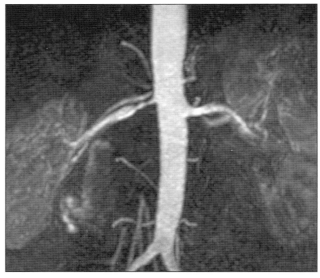

(b)

Figure 15.6
Coronal subvolume MIPs from renal MRA studies demonstrating (a) good breathholding and (b) poor breathholding.

truly motionless, such as the calves and feet, long acquisitions work well.[47]

We have found that patients are better able to breathhold if the procedure and expectations are described well in advance of the actual scan. The vast majority of ambulatory patients can breathhold for at least 20–30 s, while many have endurance well beyond this. While performing a test breathhold before the scan is always a good idea, watching a patient's respiratory pattern often gives you a clue to their breathhold potential. In our experience, patients who take slow deep breaths with relatively long expiratory pauses have no problem completing a 30–40 s breathhold. Patients who breath rapidly (>25 breaths/min) with no pause between expiration and subsequent inspiration often have trouble with a breathhold of this duration. Sick or postoperative inpatients often cannot or will not hold their breath at all, again making the high-temporal-resolution scanning more attractive.

We recommend the following breathing strategy. For 'best guess' or test dose bolus timing techniques, pre-breath the patient for three or four cycles ('deep breath in . . . and breath out . . .'), timed such that the last inspiration is held ('deep breath in and hold . . .') as the scan starts. Some authors advocate the use of supplemental oxygen during this prebreathing.[35,86] For fluoroscopic techniques, hyperventilating the patient for three or four cycles, then have them relax, start the fluoroscopic sequence, and wait for bolus arrival. Once the MRA sequence is triggered, use some prearranged signal such as squeezing the arm in addition to a loud verbal 'hold your breath' to initiate the breathhold. This needs to occur during the delay time, such that the patient is motionless once actual data collection starts and the critical center of k-space is collected.

Determining imaging time

The duration of a 3D CE-MRA acquisition (t_s) depends on several variables, and can be approximated as

$$t_s = TR \times y\text{-RES} \times z\text{-RES} \times \frac{\text{fractional } y\text{-FOV}}{SF}, \quad (8)$$

where TR is the repetition time, y-RES and z-RES are the number of phase-encoding steps in y and z, fractional y-FOV is the asymmetric y field-of-view fraction, and SF is the speedup factor due to parallel imaging techniques such as SENSE.[89] TR is itself a function of TE, echo type (i.e. full or fractional), and bandwidth. Spatial resolution is determined by voxel size, which is determined by

$$\text{voxel size} = \frac{y\text{-FOV}}{y\text{-RES}} \times \frac{z\text{-FOV}}{z\text{-RES}} \times \frac{x\text{-FOV}}{x\text{-RES}}, \quad (9)$$

where x-, y-, and z-FOV are the x, y, and z fields of view, and x-RES is the number of data points digitized during readout. Using fractional y-FOV decreases the number of y phase encodings, shortening scan time while maintaining resolution but collecting a smaller (or 'rectangular') FOV in the y-direction. This is particularly useful for large-FOV studies where structures at the periphery of the y-FOV are not important, and wraparound (aliasing) can be tolerated. Parallel imaging techniques, such as SENSE, require the use of multiple (phase array) coils. These techniques collect fewer phase encodings than are prescribed (phase and/or slice direction), effectively reducing the FOV(s), with resultant aliasing.[75,89,90] This can decrease scan time by up to a factor of the number of coils in the phased array, depending on geometry. SENSE has to date been most useful for cardiac imaging, although it appears to have great potential with MRA as well.[91,92] Using sensitivity data for each phased array coil obtained from a quick 'reference' scan, a mathematical algorithm can then 'unfold' the aliased dataset, restoring the original prescribed FOV with only a small geometry-related loss in SNR when coils are properly optimized. One important concept to remember when using SENSE is that the prescribed FOV must be such that there is no aliasing, or else the reconstruction algorithm breaks down and causes severe aliasing artifacts. Thus, SENSE is most advantageous when a full rectangular FOV is desired.

All of these parameters must be juggled to achieve the required volume coverage, spatial resolution, and SNR while keeping the scan time t_s within an acceptable range – hopefully as short as possible and certainly within the patient's anticipated breathhold duration t_b. Thus there are multiple tradeoffs. Increasing resolution (y-RES or z-RES with same overall slab thickness), increasing volume coverage (z-RES with same slice thickness), or increasing SNR (decreasing bandwidth or changing from fractional to full echo), all increase t_s. Decreasing the rectangular FOV or using a parallel imaging technique will decrease t_s. SNR must also be considered. In general, for all these techniques, SNR scales as the voxel size times the square root of t_s.[38,41] One interesting property unique to CE-MRA, however, is that, all other things being equal (e.g. without changing bandwidth), if the contrast injection rate is increased proportional to the decrease in scan duration (i.e. inject same total contrast dose faster), then the SNR is unchanged and the contrast-to-noise ratio increases. Maki et al[41] describe a mathematical analysis specific to breathhold Gd-MRA to optimize SNR by considering these variables.

A useful technique with no associated time penalty is to zero-fill k-space in multiple directions.[93] Most MR scanners have an option to zero-fill both frequency and phase to 256 or 512. In addition, a 2 × zero-fill in slice can be specified, yielding twice the number of slices. While the slice thickness is unchanged, the slices now overlap by one-half of a slice thickness. While zero-filling may not increase resolution, it permits smoother reformats by reducing partial-volume effects.

The art, then, of 3D breathhold CE-MRA boils down to a careful choice of the parameters in Equations (8) and (9), and is often an iterative process. As a general rule for non-time-resolved abdominal MRA, we start with a frequency resolution (x-RES) of ~400, with zero-filling to 512×512 in frequency and phase and times 2 in slice. We then consider the maximum estimated breathhold duration t_b and desired slice thickness. We increase z-RES to cover the required volume. If an asymmetric FOV can be used, we do so. Alternatively, we use SENSE with a SF of 2–3.[47,89] We then increase y-RES until t_b is reached. Always keep in mind the voxel dimension in z versus that in y. They should be roughly similar, since one fundamental purpose of a 3D data set is to generate relatively isotropic resolution so that multiplanar reformats (MPRs) maintain resolution in all planes.

If t_s cannot be made less than t_b after these manipulations, then sacrifices must be made. Partial Fourier techniques can be used (i.e. collect only a fraction of y phase encodes) at the cost of decreased SNR. Alternatively, bandwidth can be increased, again at the cost of decreased SNR, or slice thickness can be increased at the cost of decreased spatial resolution. Higher SENSE factors (>2.5–3.0) can be employed, although this also decreases SNR. Finally, incomplete breathholding can be anticipated at the cost of increased ghosting and blurring.

In cases where breathholding is not as important, such as in the extremities or carotids, there is more flexibility with regard to choosing imaging parameters. In these circumstances, the limiting factor becomes contrast bolus duration. As previously described, a 'compact' bolus (with respect to imaging duration) can cause artifacts such as ringing and blurring. So, assuming a double dose (0.2 mmol/kg) of a gadolinium chelate (0.5 mol/l) for a 80 kg patient administered at 2 cm³/s, the injection duration is only 16 s. Assuming that the bolus will broaden by several seconds before reaching the target vessels, this is still less than ~20–22 s. To avoid artifacts, this needs to be a substantial fraction of the scan time t_s, and scan times much greater than ~60 s are likely counterproductive. Nonetheless, this increase in imaging time allows for increased SNR and spatial resolution. When considering carotids or peripheral vessels with soft tissue disease, the rapidity of venous return must also be considered. This limits scan duration, since the longer the scan, the closer the proximity of phase encoding to central k-space when venous signal arrives. This leads to greater venous signal and 'leading edge' venous ringing artifact. With truly centric sequences, however, carotid scan times of up to 40 s and lower station peripheral scan times of well over 1 min have been shown to work extremely well, in part due to recirculation of contrast in the latter part of the scan.[47,63]

Patient preparation

The more relaxed and informed a patient is, the more easily they can remain still and perform a long breathhold. Therefore, reassurance and a brief description of the scan can really help. In patients who are particularly anxious, premedication with sedatives such as diazepam may be useful. This helps the patient to relax and lie still, and also decreases cardiac output.[14] This latter effect helps enhance image quality, since arterial phase [Gd] increases with decreasing cardiac output (Equation (4) and Figure 15.2).

Since most 3D CE-MRA is performed in the coronal plane, arm position is important to allow for a smaller FOV without aliasing, particularly if using SENSE. For carotid, large-FOV aortic, and peripheral studies, the arms can remain by the patient's side, since aliasing is not a factor. For pulmonary, small-FOV aortic, renal, and mesenteric studies, the arms must either be elevated out of the imaging plane using cushions or be extended over the head.[35] Both of these positions in which the arms are elevated have the added benefit of gravity-aided venous return from the intravenous (i.v.) injection site.

We recommend placing the i.v. before the patient is in the magnet. This alleviates anxiety and possible shifts in patient position that may occur if it is placed while in the magnet. If the MRA will be performed with the arms by the patient's side, placing the i.v. in the antecubital vein is adequate. If the arms will be over the head, it is preferable to place the i.v. below the antecubital fossa so it will not kink and obstruct should the patient's elbow bend. A 22-gauge catheter is usually adequate, although for smaller-diameter catheters (>22-gauge), warming the contrast to body temperature may decrease the viscosity enough to allow for adequate injection rates.

Contrast injection

As previously described, the total gadolinium dose and rate of delivery are tradeoffs between maximizing intravascular signal and minimizing artifacts. In the ideal situation, a large dose at a high rate would be optimal. This, however, must be weighed against safety, practicality, and cost. We feel that for breathhold CE-MRA with accurate bolus timing (test bolus or fluoroscopy), a single dose (0.1 mmol/kg) administered at a rate of ~1.5–2 cm³/s represents a good balance between these factors, depending on total scan time. In practice, however, once a bottle (typically 20 ml) of gadolinium is opened, it is best to inject the entire bottle, and hence we typically use 20 cm.³ For 'best guess' type techniques, we prefer closer to 0.2 mmol/kg (e.g. 40 cm³) at the same approximate rate. These recommendations can, under certain circumstances, be modified. For example, in a particularly small patient where the volume of a single dose is small, artifact from a compact bolus may be generated. To remedy this, either the injection rate can be decreased (thereby lengthening the bolus at the expense of intravascular signal) or the dose can be increased (at the expense of increased cost). If cost is an overwhelming concern, the dose and injection rate can be decreased at the expense of intravascular signal, or the dose alone can be decreased at the expense of compact bolus artifact.

In experienced hands, we find that manual injection works quite well. Since many smaller MR centers do not have a power injector, this is often the only choice. Manual injections are also simpler in some ways, since there is less 'plumbing' and less opportunity for mechanical difficulties. That said, a power injector offers a more constant and standardized bolus delivery. Either way, the contrast injection itself must be rapidly followed by adequate saline flush to complete delivery of the bolus and help flush the arm veins. Suggested flush volumes range from 15 to 50 cm[3], with most authors using 15–20 cm[3].[35,59] We suggest 25 cm[3] of saline flush at the same rate as the gadolinium bolus. For hand injections, a standardized tubing set that allows rapid switchover between gadolinium and saline injection works best (Smartset, TopSpins, Plymouth, MI).

Imaging different vascular phases

With most 3D CE-MRA studies, extensive efforts are made to optimally image the arterial phase, as has been extensively discussed. Once the arterial phase data set has been collected, however, the sequence can (and should) be repeated to obtain venous and equilibrium phases. Later phases are useful in evaluating unsuspected dissections, portal venous or venous structures, parenchymal enhancement patterns, and perhaps even renal glomerular function.[94,95] Temporal resolution is determined by a combination of scan time and the time required for the patient to prepare for another breathhold. Aside from techniques such as 3D TRICKS, the faster the scan, the better the potential temporal resolution.[67] In cases where high temporal resolution is desired (such as perhaps in the carotids or in cases of arteriovenous shunts), the previously described streamlined techniques can be used in a single breathhold, although SNR and spatial resolution decrease.[66] In more 'conventional' breathhold 3D CE-MRA, with a scan time of ~20–25 s, we advocate giving the patient ~8–10 s to 'catch their breath', then scanning again. In this manner, the second 'arteriovenous' phase occurs ~35 s after peak arterial phase. This is usually well timed for the portal venous phase, and often adequate for evaluating venous structures and parenchymal phases in the visceral organs. Sometimes a third phase may be

desired, usually to evaluate slow venous return or the renal collecting system.

Because these 'later' phase examinations occur more in the equilibrium phase of gadolinium distribution, intravascular T1 is increased, and therefore signal is reduced as compared with arterial phase (Figure 15.5c). In order to maximize signal in these later phases, the flip angle should, if possible, be reduced (see Figure 15.1). Whereas the optimum flip angle for the arterial phase may be 30°–40° at a TR of 4–6 ms, the optimal flip angle decreases to 15°–25° in later phases. To image gadolinium excreted into the collecting system and ureter, use a high flip angle (45°–60°) with the widest bandwidth and shortest possible TE.

Postproccessing and display

3D Gd-MRA produces a contiguous volume of image data. For a typical body MRA study, this volume is asymmetric, being perhaps $400 \times 300 \times 64$ mm^3. For a representative acquisition matrix size of $400 \times 150 \times 32$, this yields a true voxel size of $1.0 \times 2.0 \times 2.0$ mm^3. For diagnostic purposes, this dataset is best viewed interactively using a computer workstation allowing for thin multiplanar reformatting (MPR).[1,58] In this manner, thin (1.0–2.0 mm in this case) slices can be viewed in axial, sagittal, coronal, or oblique planes, thus eliminating overlapping structures and unfolding tortuous vessels. Because these reformatted slices remain thin and are not projections (see below), they not only provide the best achievable contrast, but also minimize the chance of diagnostic error (see Figure 15.8).[1,58,96]

Because thin reformations show only short vascular segments, it is advantageous to utilize the maximum-intensity projection (MIP) postprocessing technique.[97,98] Using this algorithm, the user first specifies the subvolume thickness and desired viewing plane. The algorithm then generates rays perpendicular to the viewing plane, takes the maximum value of any voxel encountered along that ray, and assigns that maximum value to the corresponding pixel in the output image. This technique is fast, and works extremely well with techniques such as Gd-MRA, since vascular signal is typically much greater than background signal. It provides projection images that are quite similar to conventional angiograms in appearance. The MIP algorithm is demonstrated in Figure 15.7, which shows a full-thickness coronal MIP of the thoracic aorta (Figure 15.7a), a thin slice axial reformation (MPR) through the aorta at the level of the pulmonary arteries (Figure 15.7b), and an oblique subvolume MIP taken from the axial reformat demonstrating the origins of the great vessels and a large Stanford B aortic dissection (Figure 15.7c). As can be seen, this technique is very

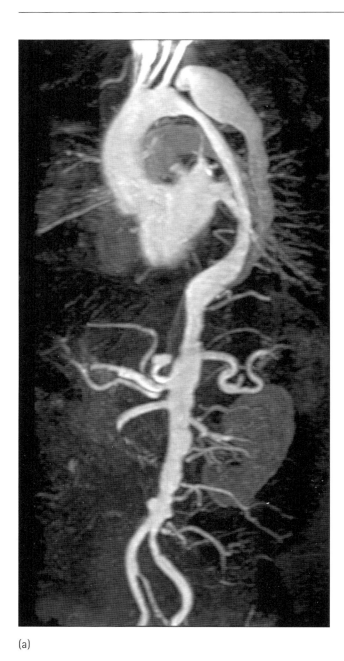

(a)

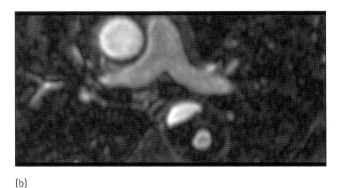

(b)

(c)

Figure 15.7
Stanford type-B aortic dissection. (a) Full-volume oblique sagittal MIP; note the bovine arch. (b) Subvolume MIP demonstrating the origin of the intimal flap. (c) Axial MPR showing the two lumens with mural thrombus in the false lumen.

helpful for displaying complex vascular anatomy, particularly when vessels are not oriented along a single plane.

Despite its usefulness, the MIP algorithm is subject to artifacts. Perhaps the most common artifact arises when stationary tissue has greater signal intensity than the vascular structures of interest, as can occur in the presence of other vessel segments, fat, hemorrhage, metallic susceptibility artifacts, or motion artifacts. This in turn leads to the mapping of nonvascular signal into the projection image and causes a discontinuity in vessel signal, potentially mimicking a stenosis or occlusion (Figure 15.8).[1] This type of artifact is best overcome by minimizing the thickness of the MIP subvolume, thereby excluding as much extraneous data as possible. Other artifacts inherent to the MIP technique have been described.[99] These mainly consist of underestimating vessel lumen, and are more of a problem with TOF or PC techniques. Because of these potential pitfalls, most authors agree that the MIP images should be used as a roadmap, utilizing the source images for definitive diagnosis.[1,58,99] New work suggests that volume rendering is more accurate than the MIP and similar to using the MPR, but should still not replace careful evaluation of the source images and MPRs.[100]

Subtraction techniques are also useful in image evaluation, particularly in vascular regions not subjected to significant respiratory motion. These areas include the

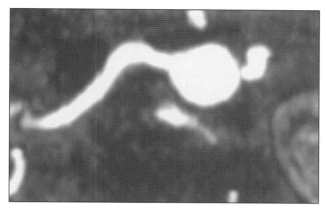

(a)

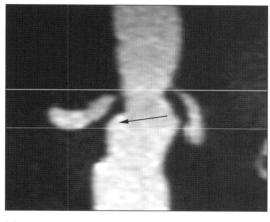

(b)

Figure 15.8
Demonstration of a potential MIP artifact. A subvolume axial MIP through the right renal artery (a) looks normal. Careful review of the source coronal images (b) demonstrates how the MIP volume (white lines) incorporates part of the ectatic aorta (black arrow), masking the high-grade right renal artery stenosis.

extremities, pelvis, and carotids. A 'digital subtraction' MRA can most easily be accomplished by subtracting pre- from postcontrast magnitude (reconstructed) images. Provided the patient maintains the same position on both studies, subtraction will eliminate background signal and improve vessel conspicuity. This technique has been used successfully in the extremities.[40,101] An improvement on this technique, particularly for thicker slice or 2D examinations, involves complex subtraction of the pre- and postcontrast 'raw' (k-space) datasets. This overcomes phase differences in voxels that contain both stationary and moving spins (i.e. very small vessels), allowing for increased vascular signal.[102,103]

Contrast-enhanced MRA: clinical applications

This section reviews techniques and imaging parameters for selective gadolinium-enhanced body MRA studies. The parameters provided here were largely derived from clinical experience with the Philips Intera 1.5 T system (Philips Medical Systems, Bothell, WA). The general techniques described here are easily applicable to other systems, although the parameters may need to be extrapolated as appropriate.

Based on the previous discussion, several general principles apply when performing Gd-MRA. First, TR and TE need to be as short as practical without excessively increasing the bandwidth. TE can and should be minimized using a partial (asymmetric) echo. For the Intera system using x-RES of 400 with a water–fat shift of ~0.8 (bandwidth ±36.8 kHz), minimum TR/TEs of ~4.0–5.0/ 1.2–2.0 ms are possible (somewhat dependent on choice of coil). Some systems are capable of even shorter TRs, although because SNR decreases as the square root of bandwidth, care should be taken not to increase bandwidth excessively to achieve minimal decreases in TR. Second, phase (y) and slice (z) resolution should be relatively balanced and ideally no greater than approximately one-third the smallest vessel of interest.[104,105] In general, most MRA practitioners tend to let the 2 resolution (slice thickness) drift somewhat lower than the phase (y) resolution. Note that the resolution in the frequency (x) direction is typically somewhat greater than in the phase and slice directions. For most abdominal applications, y- and z-resolutions of 1.8–2.4 mm are adequate, although for imaging large structures such as the portal vein or thoracic aorta, where fine detail is not of great concern, increasing resolution to 2.5–3.0 mm is often acceptable,[106] and for vessels such as peripheral below-the-knee vessels or carotids, isotropic resolutions of 1.0 mm are appropriate.[47,107] Third, to benefit from breathholding, which is essential in the abdomen, the number of slices and phase-encoding steps must be balanced between adequate volume coverage, adequate resolution, and estimated breathhold time. For a typical FOV of 400 × 300 mm², 192 phase encodings corresponds to a y-resolution of 2.1 mm. For 192 phase encodings and a TR of 5 ms, ~35 slices can be obtained in a 25 s breathhold. These imaging times can be further reduced using partial Fourier imaging (half-scan, 1/2 NEX) or SENSE. For example, a SENSE factor of 2.5 with an FOV of 400 × 400 and the same TR and y-RES, the same volume could be obtained in just over 13 s. Alternatively, 65 slices could be obtained instead of 35 in the same 25 s. Finally, for most arterial phase studies, it is best to use an automated bolus detection technique. This is particularly important for renal and carotid studies, where delayed timing causes artifacts due to adjacent venous opacification. If automated bolus detection is not available, a test bolus can be used. If neither of these techniques are feasible, educated 'best guess' timing can be used as a fallback.

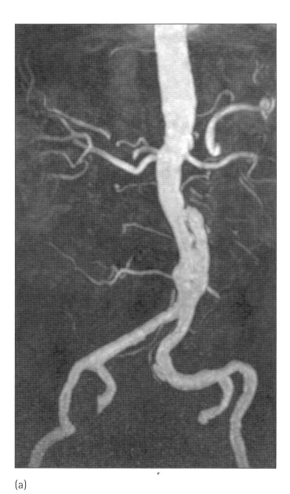

(a)

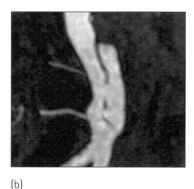

(b)

Figure 15.9

Coronal MIP from an abdominal aortic MRA demonstrating a focal infrarenal dissection.

Abdominal aorta/iliac arteries

3D CE-MRA of the abdominal aorta and iliac arteries is most often performed to evaluate aneurysmal disease (Figure 15.5a,b), dissection (Figure 15.9), or as part of a claudication workup. The acquisition is performed in the coronal plane to facilitate evaluation of the iliac and renal vessels, and a phased array body coil should be used whenever possible. The imaging volume can be prescribed from a breathhold sagittal 2D 'black-blood' gradient-echo or TrueFISP 'bright-blood' localizer, or alternatively from an MIP reformat of a fast low-resolution axial 2D TOF sequence. A breathhold localizer is preferred, since it captures the anatomy in the same position in which the CE-MRA will be performed, thus decreasing the chances of a vital structure (such as the anterior aspect of an aneurysm) falling outside the field of view. It also gives the patient a chance to practice a breathhold when the outcome is not crucial.

A 400×300 mm^2 FOV with a 400 matrix and a y-resolution of ~2 mm is a good starting point for CE-MRA of the abdominal aorta (~400×200 matrix). If the patient is large or has iliac/thoracic aortic disease, the FOV and slice thickness can be increased as needed. As previously described, slice thickness and number of slices are chosen based on desired resolution and breathholding capability. Ideally, the true slice thickness should be ≤2.4 mm. For very large aneurysms, however, it may be necessary to increase the slice thickness to 3 or 4 mm. Breathholding is important for aorto-iliac evaluation, particularly if good evaluation of the renal arteries is desired. Often, however, surprisingly good aortic and iliac image quality can be obtained even for patients who breathhold poorly.

Because large aneurysms have slow, swirling flow, extra time is required for the aneurysm to maximally opacify and allow filling of the iliac arteries (see Figure 15.5b). When using fluoroscopic bolus detection, we find it useful to trigger ~2–3 s beyond where we normally would (assuming a delay between fluoroscopy and 3D CE-MRA of 3–4 s). With a large aneurysm or known dissection, we typically use a full 40 cm^3 of gadolinium. Otherwise, 20 cm^3 works well. Obtaining a delayed phase immediately following the arterial phase is recommended, particularly for dissections or very slow-filling aneurysms.[70]

Thoracic aorta

As with the abdominal aorta, thoracic aortic MRA is most often performed for aneurysm or dissection (Figures 15.7 and 15.10). When evaluating the thoracic aorta, an oblique sagittal 3D volume oriented with the arch typically works best, minimizing the total number of slices. Obtaining two dynamic phases is extremely important, particularly with dissections, where slow-filling lumens may opacify much better on the venous phase (Figure 15.10a,b). We typically use 40 cm³ of gadolinium in the presence of a known dissection.

When targeting only the thoracic aorta, a phased array body coil and an FOV of ~380 × 266 mm² should be used,

since a moderate amount of aliasing can be tolerated. When evaluating the entire thoraco-abdominal aorta, the built-in body coil is typically used, since most phased array coils do not have sufficient cranio-caudal coverage. Using an FOV of ~440 × 290 mm², the entire aorta to the bifurcation can usually be covered, including the renal

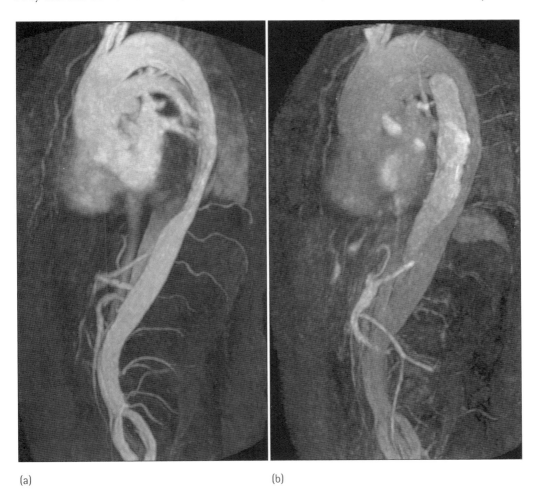

(a) (b)

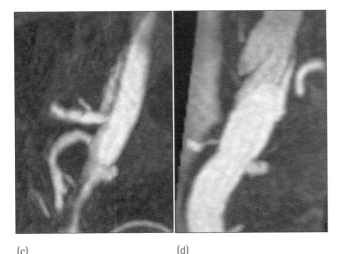

(c) (d)

Figure 15.10

Arterial (a) and immediate delayed phase (b) full-volume MIPs from a thoraco-abdominal MRA. The more posterior false lumen opacifies more rapidly and extends into the iliac arteries, with the delayed phase better demonstrating the more anterior true lumen. Sagittal (c) and coronal (d) arterial phase subvolume MIPs help define the extremely complicated anatomy in this case. A stenotic right renal artery and superior mesenteric artery originate from the true lumen, whereas the celiac axis and a proximally occluded left renal artery originate from the false lumen.

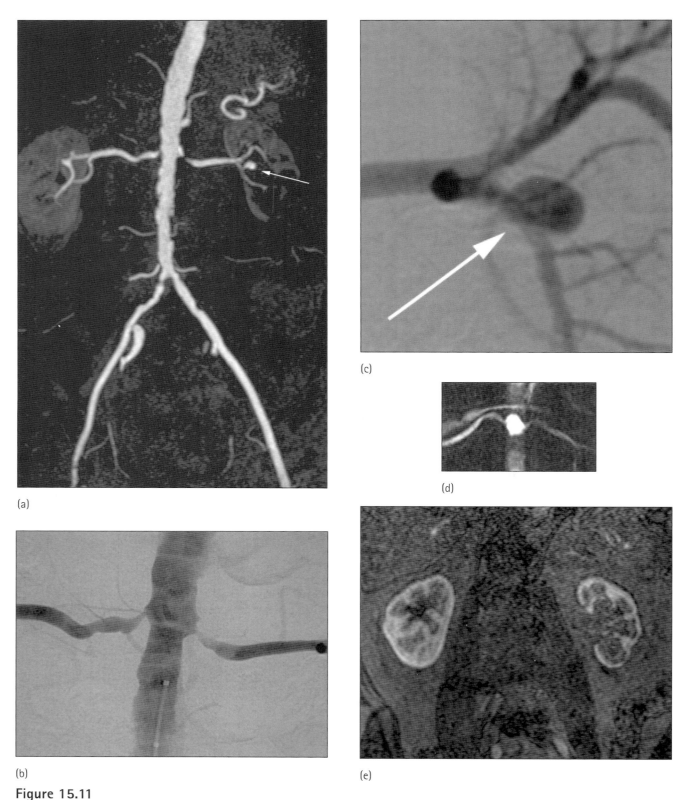

(a)

(b)

(c)

(d)

(e)

Figure 15.11
Full-volume MIP from a renal artery study (a) with angiographic correlation (b,c) demonstrating high-grade left and moderate- to high-grade right renal artery stenosis, as well as a small left renal artery aneurysm (arrows). An axial MIP from a phase contrast study (d) demonstrates no signal dropout on the right, with mild signal dropout on the left, indicating probable hemodynamic significance of the left renal artery stenosis. Examining the source images (e) can provide addition clues to the hemodynamic significance of a lesion, as in this case, where smooth left renal cortical thinning is seen.

artery origins (Figure 15.10d). In either case, the origins of the great vessels should be included in the imaging volume. True slice thickness can be as great as 3 mm, although if renal artery evaluation is important, thinner slices (~2.4 mm) are desirable. The total number of true slices depends on the size and tortuosity of the aorta, as well as the slice thickness, but is typically in the range of 30–40.

A complete evaluation of the thoracic aorta includes multiplanar cardiac-gated black-blood imaging of the aortic wall to detect intramural hematoma, an important prognostic indicator.[108] A complete description of this is beyond the scope of this review, but the reader is referred to the aforementioned reference.

Renal arteries

CE-MRA of the renal arteries is similar to an abdominal aortic study, with the exception that including the entire iliac vasculature is less important (although nice if possible). This allows for a thinner coronal slab, and therefore decreased slice thickness and/or acquisition time. Typically ~30 slices with a true slice thickness no greater than 2.2–2.4 mm, a matrix of 400 × 230, and an FOV of 400 × 300 mm^2 is sufficient. This allows for high resolution (1 × 1.7 × 2.2 mm^3) with relatively short scan times (<20–25 s). As discussed previously, breathholding is extremely critical, since distal branches and accessory renal arteries are difficult to evaluate in the presence of diaphragmatic motion.[86] This and other recent studies suggest that minimizing acquisition time (and thereby motion artifacts) is extremely beneficial. Techniques as simple as limiting the volume coverage or as advanced as SENSE are good choices for the renal arteries.[91]

Figure 15.11 demonstrates a mild–moderate right and a moderate–severe proximal left renal artery stenosis (Figure 15.11a), with angiographic correlation (Figure 15.11b,c). Note that 3D PC imaging (Figure 15.11d) can be a useful adjunct in the evaluation of renal artery stenosis. While the CE-MRA images demonstrate anatomy, the PC images show signal loss in regions of turbulence or extremely slow flow, suggesting which lesions are of hemodynamic significance.[109,110] In this example, there is no right-sided signal loss, but moderate signal dropout on the left, suggesting that the left-sided lesion is hemodynamically significant (confirmed by X-ray angiography; Figure 15.11b). Note also the left-sided cortical thinning (Figure 15.11e), a secondary sign of significant renal artery stenosis, as well as the incidentally noted small left renal artery aneurysm (a), nicely corroborated on a later phase X-ray angiogram (c). Figures 15.12(a) and (b) demonstrate an MIP and a volume-rendered image from a patient with proven fibromuscular dysplasia.

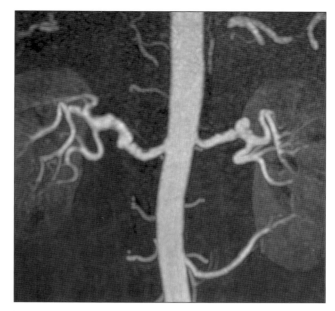

(a)

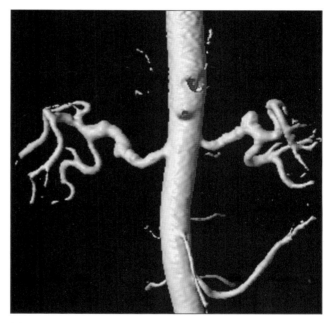

(b)

Figure 15.12
MIP (a) and volume-rendered image (b) from a renal MRA in a 49-year-old male with proven fibromuscular dysplasia.

Transplant renal arteries can be easily evaluated as well.[111,112] An example is shown in Figure 15.13, where the transplant artery has thrombosed with subsequent infarction of the renal graft. Since transplants are in the pelvis, respiratory motion is not as problematic, and breathholding is less critical. Nonetheless, it is best to have the patient breathhold if possible. While coronal imaging with

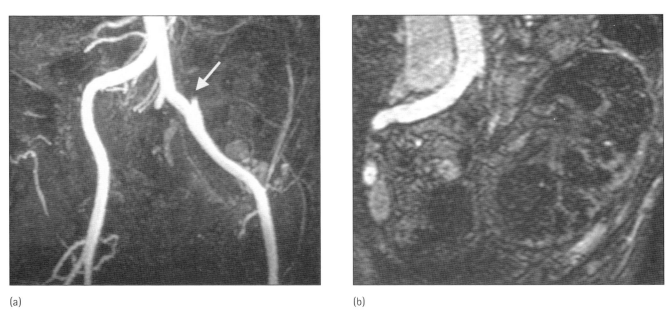

(a)   (b)

Figure 15.13
Oblique full-thickness MIP (a) from a renal artery MRA performed in a renal transplant patient with abdominal pain and rising creatinine 2 weeks following a motor vehicle accident. The arrow shows the occluded transplant renal artery. A delayed phase source image (b) shows near complete absence of renal blood flow. The graft could not be salvaged.

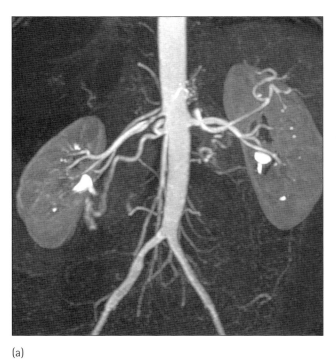

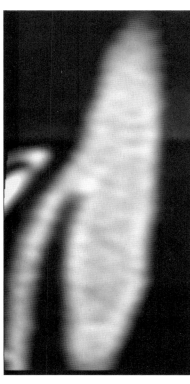

Figure 15.14
Full-thickness coronal MIP from an abdominal MRA (a). The sagittal subvolume MIP (b) demonstrates incidental complete occlusion of the proximal celiac axis. Note the long moderate main right renal artery stenosis with poststenotic dilatation.

(a)

(b)

a 320–360 mm FOV is usually adequate, oblique sagittal imaging can be performed with a smaller FOV. This gives higher resolution, but covers much less vascular territory. Transplant renal veins are easily seen on the venous phase of the study.

Mesenteric arteries

The proximal mesenteric vessels are included on renal or abdominal aortic CE-MRA studies, and are usually well visualized, even in the presence of respiratory motion (Figure 15.14). The inferior mesenteric artery is often seen as well.

Dedicated mesenteric artery studies, typically to evaluate for mesenteric ischemia or tumor encasement, are performed in either the coronal or sagittal plane, and are better suited to evaluating the more proximal vessels.[113,114] Slice thickness should be similar to that of a renal artery study (<2.4 mm), particularly when using the coronal plane, since the proximal mesenteric arteries travel primarily anteriorly. It should be kept in mind that the hepatic, gastroduodenal, and distal superior mesenteric arteries may be further anterior than usually included in a renal study, and

therefore volume coverage will need to be increased (or shifted anteriorly) in order to see these structures.

Portal/hepatic veins

Portal venous or hepatic vein studies are performed in a coronal plane with a phased array body coil (Figure 15.15).[115] Slice thickness can be increased to ~3 mm in order to adequately cover the relevant portal venous structures. Axial bright blood scout images, such as TrueFISP, are useful for determining the anterior and posterior extent of the portal/hepatic veins, and may even be diagnostic.

With portal venous/hepatic venous studies, timing is not as crucial as with arterial studies, since the portal venous phase is longer, and thus easier to isolate. After obtaining the arterial phase images, which allow for arterial evaluation, an ~10 s pause allows the patient to recover from the breathhold. Imaging is then repeated, followed by a second pause and a third scan. In this manner, the second set of images usually provides a nice portal venous and hepatic venous phase. The third set may show collaterals to better advantage.

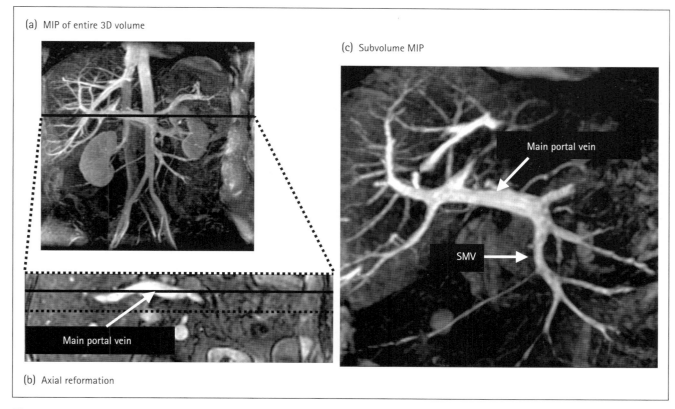

(a) MIP of entire 3D volume

(c) Subvolume MIP

Main portal vein

SMV

Main portal vein

(b) Axial reformation

Figure 15.15
Coronal 3D Gd-MRA of the portal vein using 40 cm³ gadolinium contrast. (a) Coronal MIP of the entire volume. (b) Axial reformation through the portal vein, with dotted lines indicating the optimal volume for performing MIP. (c) Subvolume MIP showing portal vein to better advantage by excluding more posterior structures.

This protocol has the added advantage of essentially being a dynamic liver study. Hence, if there is concern over a hepatic mass, this can be evaluated dynamically, provided it is included in the imaging volume.[116] Under these circumstances, further delayed phases should be obtained out to 5 or 10 min.

Pulmonary arteries

3D CE-MRA of the pulmonary arteries is gaining acceptance (Figure 15.16). A recent large-scale study comparing MRA with conventional DSA suggests that pulmonary MRA is similar in accuracy to helical CT, being sensitive and specific for emboli in segmental and larger vessels.[117] Creating high-quality pulmonary MR angiograms, however, requires considerable care. Good breathholding or extremely short acquisition times are extremely important, and unfortunately many patients requiring pulmonary angiography have significant respiratory compromise, and therefore cannot breathhold well. A phased array body coil should be used whenever possible.

The examination must be tailored to the individual patient. Two approaches can be used: single-acquisition coronal, and double-acquisition sagittal (separate injections and acquisitions for each lung).[117,118] Which approach to adopt is a matter of preference, breathhold capability, and machine speed. For the two-sagittal-acquisition approach, the volume coverage for each acquisition is smaller, and a high degree of rectangular FOV can be used. This reduces acquisition time, or alternatively allows for increased spatial resolution (as compared with a single coronal acquisition). In addition, the arms can remain by the patient's side, since the foldover direction is anterior–posterior. On the downside, two separate acquisitions requires more scanner and postprocessing time, and more contrast, and the pulmonary trunk and proximal pulmonary arteries may be excluded (although this is not usually clinically relevant).

For either approach, a total slab thickness of 100–150 mm is typical, with true slice thickness optimally

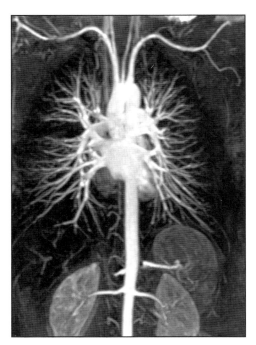

(a)

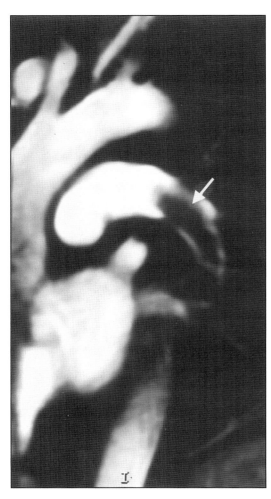

(b)

Figure 15.16
Pulmonary MRA of (a) a normal patient and (b) a patient with left descending pulmonary embolism (arrow). Data are acquired in the coronal plane with breathholding during infusion of 30 cm³ gadolinium contrast timed empirically with a 6 s delay between beginning the injection and beginning the scan; *k*-space is ordered sequentially.

<2.6 mm.[118] The frequency FOV is typically 300–360 mm, depending on patient size, with a higher degree of rectangular FOV possible for the sagittal approach (~45–70% versus ~65–70%). The matrix size should be on the order of 320 × 160, such that the overall resolution is <1.0 × 2.0 × 2.6 mm³. We always perform at least one practice run in order to evaluate the patient's breathholding capability, ensure the patient will comply with the breathing instructions, and check that any foldover is acceptable.

For a TR of 5 ms, acquisition times for coronal and sagittal acquisitions will be ~25 and 20 s, respectively. Shorter scan times are certainly desirable, especially given the difficulty these patients often have with breathholding and cardiac motion within the chest. We expect increased use of high-temporal-resolution techniques in the immediate future.[73,82] Correct bolus timing is important, but not as essential as for other vascular territories. It is difficult to isolate the pulmonary arterial phase from the pulmonary venous phase, although this is possible with extremely high temporal resolution or correlation analysis.[77] Fortunately, however, this is not a big problem, since pulmonary arteries and veins are easily distinguished on coronal images. The main pulmonary artery should be used for fluoroscopic triggering or calibrating a timing bolus. If these techniques are unavailable, transit time is typically 5–15 s. Gadolinium doses are approximately double dose for coronal imaging and single dose per side for sagittal imaging.

Extracranial carotid arteries

Carotid Gd-MRA is typically performed using a single contrast injection in the coronal plane (Figure 15.17). More so than in any other vascular territory, elliptical centric phase-encoding order and near-perfect timing are required to isolate the arterial phase, since jugular venous enhancement can severely degrade arterial evaluation.[63] This is due to the unique characteristics of the intracranial circulation, with its short arteriovenous window (4–6 s), and the blood–brain barrier, which prevents significant extraction of contrast (see Figure 15.5c). While one would expect shorter acquisition times (high temporal resolution) to increase the likelihood of isolating a pure arterial phase, excellent results have been achieved with long imaging times (40 s to >2 min) and high spatial resolution in combination with elliptical centric phase encoding.[63,79,83,119]

In order to accurately characterize a carotid stenosis according to NASCET criteria, particularly one with tortuous anatomy and high-speed turbulent jets, an accurate measurement of stenotic diameter is required. Given this, we suggest true 1 mm isotropic or better resolution, using as short a TE as practical to decrease signal dephasing in

the often very turbulent stenotic lumen. In order to maintain adequate SNR at these high resolutions, a birdcage or phased array coil is necessary. Unfortunately, depending on patient habitus, older neck coils suffer severe sensitivity dropoff near the arch, making evaluation of the important great vessel origins a problem (see Figure 15.5c). Recent coil advances (combination birdcage and anterior–posterior surface coils), however, make reliable evaluation of this important region possible as part of a routine carotid examination.[83]

A FOV of 360 × 180 mm² typically works well, allowing visualization down to the arch. The problem of arm aliasing into the chest is minimized due to inherent coil dropoff laterally, although this must be considered when using the built-in body coil (not suggested). A total slab thickness of 50–65 mm is usually adequate. 2D TOF or TrueFISP images can be used to evaluate the extent of the vertebral and carotid arteries for localization to ensure the CE-MRA volume is minimized. Typical scan parameters might be a 384 × 384 × 60 matrix with 1 mm slice thickness (reconstructed to 512 × 512 × 120), for a true resolution of 0.9 × 0.9 × 1.0 mm. For a TR of 5 ms, the acquisition time for such a sequence would be ~50 s. Carotid artery MRA is an exception to our general rule that injection time should be on the order of 50–60% of acquisition time, since rapid recirculation of contrast seems to support the longer acquisition times for the high-resolution sequences. We suggest 20–30 cm³ of gadolinium at 1.5–3.0 cm³/s. As stated previously, breathholding may help in evaluation of the arch vessels, but is not necessary for the carotid arteries.[88]

Peripheral MRA

The restricted FOV inherent to MR scanners has limited CE-MRA to analyzing only 400–500 mm chunks of vascular anatomy at one time. While this is acceptable for carotid, aortic, renal, pulmonary, and mesenteric studies, it has made peripheral CE-MRA studies challenging. While multiple injections and multiple acquisitions with intervening table movement can be performed,[120] a recent revolutionary advance has eliminated the FOV barrier. By moving the table while scanning, a single bolus of contrast can be imaged multiple times as it flows down the legs (Figure 15.18).[121–123] This 'moving table' or 'bolus-chase' approach allows arterial imaging from the abdominal aorta to the midfoot in just a few minutes, and is available in different varieties commercially. Even whole-body MRA using a single injection has been described.[124]

Once the FOV issue for peripheral MRA has been addressed, two further obstacles must be overcome. First, spatial resolution must be adequate for operative planning, since below-the-knee arteries are on the order of

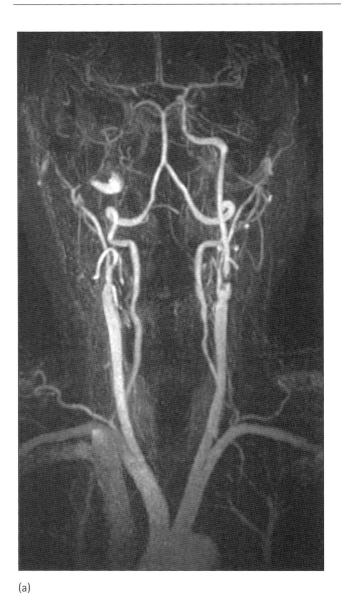

(a)

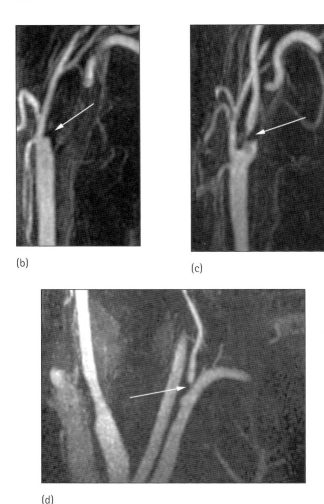

(b)

(c)

(d)

Figure 15.17
Carotid MRA. The full-thickness MIP (a) demonstrates the great vessels extending from the arch, although there is some signal dropoff due to the coil. Right (b) and left (c) sagittal subvolume MIPs demonstrate occlusion and high-grade stenosis of the internal carotid arteries, respectively. Note also the high-grade left vertebral artery 'tandem' stenoses in the coronal subvolume MIP (d).

2–3 mm, and grafting to an inadequate vessel can be a clinical disaster. In general, the upper (abdominal) and middle (thigh) station vessels are relatively large, and resolution requirements are not as strict as in the lower (calves/feet) station, where vessels may be only 2–3 mm. Thus spatial resolutions on the order of those previously discussed for the aorta and visceral arteries, with true 2.5–3.0 mm through-plane resolution, are likely adequate in the upper and middle stations. The lower station, however, requires spatial resolution more in keeping with a carotid examination, with true 1 mm isotropic resolution an attainable goal.[92] The cranio-caudal FOV for each station must be approximately 420–480 mm, with at least 30 mm of overlap between stations.

The second obstacle is that of venous enhancement, which must be absent or minimal, since the numerous paired veins in the leg can easily obscure and confuse the arterial anatomy. It seems surprising that numerous early works demonstrated the complete lack of venous enhancement in the majority of cases, even though acquisition in the lower station did not begin until ~60 s after initiating upper-station acquisition.[122,123,125] Several investigators have begun to explore this issue, which seems to be a complicated function of imaging delay, contrast injection rate, and patient specific parameters (particularly the presence/absence of claudication versus inflammatory conditions).[126,127] Of these, it is likely patient pathology that plays the largest role. In general, patients with claudication

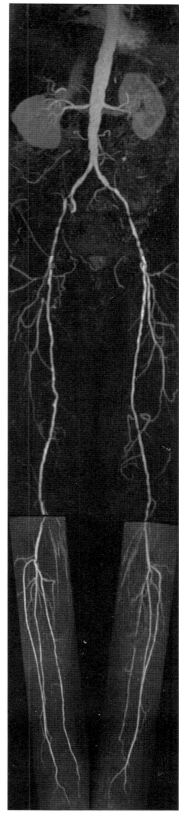

(a)

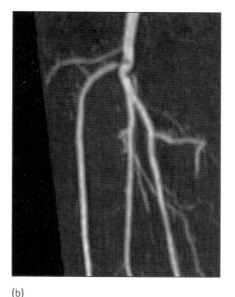

(b)

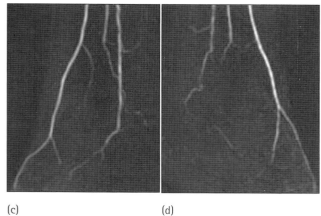

(c)   (d)

Figure 15.18

Composite coronal MIP from a three-station peripheral moving table MRA performed for bilateral calf claudication (a). The upper and middle stations were performed in a coronal plane, each requiring >12 s. The lower station was acquired as two sagittal slabs with true 1 mm isotropic resolution, and required 70 s. This allowed for inclusion of the pedal arteries. The upper and lower stations were performed using SENSE. Note the extensive disease throughout the arterial structures, with bilateral high-grade stenoses of the external iliac arteries. The 1 mm isotropic lower-station resolution provides excellent anatomic detail of the trifurcation (coronal subvolume MIP: b) and pedal arteries (right and left: c,d). These subvolume MIPs show that the dorsalis pedis arteries are widely patent bilaterally, but the left posterior tibial artery is occluded distally, with the right lateral plantar artery occluded at its origin.

do not demonstrate significant venous enhancement until quite late. Patients with rest pain or inflammatory conditions such as ulcers, cellulitis, or osteomyelitis tend to have early venous enhancement, likely secondary to arteriovenous shunting and increased perfusion. The trick then is to tailor the examination to the patient. We have begun using a 2-cm³ timing bolus in the calf to look for the presence of venous enhancement, and if present, to determine the length of the arterio-venous window.

We suggest the following protocol. If the patient has claudication or a timing study that indicates late venous enhancement, perform a moving table study with coronal upper and middle stations, and either a coronal or sagittal (two slabs – one for each calf/foot and easily includes the pedal vessels[128]) lower station. Every attempt should be made to image the upper and middle stations quickly (fast TR, SENSE, rapid table movement, etc.) so that acquisition of the lower station begins as soon as possible, decreasing the chances of venous enhancement.[47] Lower-station acquisition can and should be relatively lengthy, with spatial resolution at or near 1 mm isotropic and scan times >1 min very acceptable. [47,129] Phase-encoding orders should be reverse linear, linear, and elliptical centric respectively. This ensures adequate filling of the distal upper and middle stations (external iliac and proximal femoral arteries, popliteal arteries), and suppresses lower-station venous enhancement. We typically use 40 cm³ of gadolinium with a biphasic bolus and fluoroscopic triggering at the upper station (although a timing bolus will work equally well). Depending on acquisition time and table movement delay, an initial gadolinium infusion rate of 1.2–1.8 cm³/s (20 cm³) followed by 0.8–1.2 cm³/s (the remaining 20 cm³) works well. When determining bolus injection rates, consider that arterial flow down the diseased leg averages ~6 cm/s, such that travel time from aorta to foot is on the order of 15–20 s.[47,130] Also consider that the bolus broadens significantly, and, like the carotid, recirculation of contrast appears to be adequate for supporting high-resolution long acquisitions in the lower station.

If, on the other hand, the patient has distal rest pain, inflammatory disease, or demonstrates rapid venous enhancement on a lower-extremity test bolus, we suggest two separate injections. The first should target only the lower station, with parameters similar to those of a moving table examination, timing based on the test bolus (fluoroscopic triggering is difficult in the lower leg), and use of 15 cm³ of gadolinium at a rate of 0.8–1.0 cm³/s. A second injection of 25 cm³ (1.2–1.8 cm³/s) can then be performed to evaluate the upper and middle stations as a two-station moving table examination. Regardless of the technique used, subtraction is extremely important, particularly in the lower extremities, and a precontrast mask should always be obtained.[40] For the two-injection technique, subtraction becomes an absolute necessity following the second injection.

MR venograms

Gadolinium-enhanced MR venograms can be performed in a manner similar to a conventional contrast venogram.[131,132] By injecting a dilute gadolinium solution directly into the peripheral veins (arm or leg) during 3D image acquisition, structures such as the subclavian veins, SVC, and IVC can be evaluated (Figure 15.19). This provides much greater venous enhancement than the venous

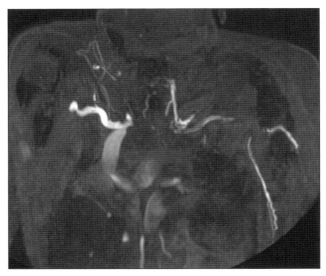

(a)

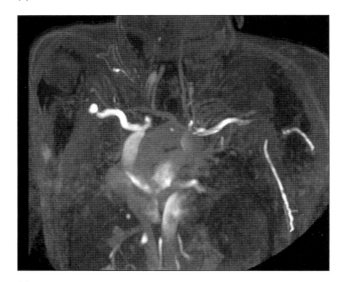

(b)

Figure 15.19
Early (a) and delayed (b) subvolume MIPs from a CE-MRV study where dilute (1 : 12.5) gadolinium was infused bilaterally into the antecubital veins. Note the complete occlusion of the left innominate vein, with high-grade stenosis at the confluence of the right innominate vein and SVC. The left subclavian vein signal void is secondary to slab positioning.

phase of an arterial study, since the gadolinium is delivered to the veins in a much higher concentration (less dilution of the bolus and no extravasation into extravascular structures). The arterial enhancement is also less than on the venous phase of a typical contrast MRA study, although such delayed phases can be effective as well.[133]

We find that diluting 1 bottle (20 cm^3) of gadolinium into a 250 cm^3 bag of saline (1 : 12.5) works well when injected into a peripheral vein at 2–3 cm^3/s. Multiple veins can be injected simultaneously, as in Figure 15.19. Imaging delay is not terribly important, since the dilute gadolinium solution can be delivered in large volumes. Volume coverage and slice thickness must be tailored to the individual case, and multiple phases should be obtained.

Future directions: contrast agents

First-pass gadolinium agents

Currently, the most widely used contrast agents in the USA, Europe and elsewhere for first-pass contrast-enhanced MRA are the 'conventional' gadolinium chelates (Table 15.1, column 1). These are available as 0.5 M formulations and possess T1 relaxivities (1.5 T) of between 4.3 and 5.0 s^{-1} mmol^{-1}.[134] The similar concentrations and relaxation properties of these agents generally translate into similar vascular imaging performance when injected at equal doses.

Recently, a number of gadolinium chelates have been developed that possess properties advantageous for first-pass CE-MRA.[135] These include conventional gadolinium agents formulated at 1.0 M rather than 0.5 M (e.g. gadobutrol), and agents with higher in vivo relaxivity due to a capacity for weak protein interaction (e.g. gadobenate dimeglumine). In the case of gadobutrol, studies have shown that the higher concentration of gadolinium combined with a more rapid bolus enables greater intravascular signal than is achievable with equivalent doses of traditional agents.[136–138] This may be useful for the improved visualization of smaller arteries in vascular regions in which the SNR is limited, such as in the calf and distal renal arteries. Improved visualization of smaller pelvic vessels has already been reported.[138]

Gadobenate dimeglumine (Table 15.1, column 2) also demonstrates increased intravascular signal as compared with conventional gadolinium chelates.[138–140] This agent differs from the other available gadolinium agents in that it possesses a higher in vivo T1 relaxivity (9.7 s^{-1} mmol^{-1}) due to weak and transient interactions between the Gd-BOPTA chelate and serum proteins, particularly albumin.[134,141] Clinical benefits of the increased relaxivity have been demonstrated for all vascular territories, including the peripheral vasculature.[142–144] Specifically, there is better visualization of lesions in larger vessels (Figure 15.20) as well as better depiction of smaller vessels themselves (Figure 15.21). Like the conventional non-protein-interacting gadolinium chelates, gadobenate dimeglumine demonstrates an excellent safety profile.[145]

Table 15.1. Classification scheme for 'vascular' MR contrast agents. The paramagnetic gadolinium chelates can be classified according to their degree of protein interaction. The ultrasmall iron oxide particles (USPIO) are 'blood pool agents', which demonstrate long intravascular enhancement.

Paramagnetic				Superparamagnetic
No protein interaction	*Weak protein interaction*	*Strong protein interaction*	*Macromolecular*	*USPIO*
Gadopentetate dimeglumine, Gd-DTPA (Magnevist) Gadoteridol, Gd-HP-DO3A (ProHance) Gadodiamide, Gd-DTPA-BMA (Omniscan) Gadoversetamide, Gd-DTPA-BMEA (Optimark) Gadoterate meglumine, Gd-DOTA (Dotarem) Gadobutrol, Gd-BT-DO3A (Gadovist)	Gadobenate dimeglumine, Gd-BOPTA (MultiHance)	MS-325: (Angiomark) B22956	P792 Gadomer-17	SHU 555A, (Resovist) AMI 227 NC100150 (Clariscan)

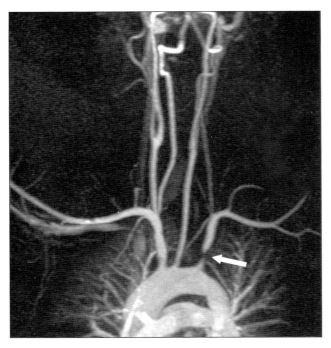

Figure 15.20
This full-thickness MIP (0.1 mmol/kg Gd-BOPTA) shows occlusion of the left subclavian artery (arrow) with collateralization from the left vertebral artery. The patient presented with typical clinical symptoms, and interventional therapy was performed. Due to the clear depiction of the size of the narrowed lumen, an interventional procedure could be accurately planned. Image courtesy of Günther Schneider (Department of Diagnostic Radiology, University Hospital, Homburg/Saar, Germany).

'Blood pool' gadolinium agents

Because of the rapid redistribution of the first-pass gadolinium chelates into the extracellular compartment, various attempts have been made to formulate intravascular 'blood pool' contrast agents for 3D CE-MRA. Currently, two main types of intravascular agent based on gadolinium are under development: agents that differ from the purely extracellular and weakly protein-interacting agents in having strong affinity for serum albumin (Table 15.1, column 3) and macromolecular agents whose size precludes their rapid extravasation (Table 15.1, column 4). Although no agents are yet approved for clinical use, two examples of agents with strong affinity for serum proteins are currently undergoing clinical trials: MS-325[146–148] (Figure 15.22) and B22956[149,150] (Figure 15.23). Both of these agents appear to he very promising, with excellent safety profiles and the capacity to perform conventional high-quality first-pass dynamic imaging in addition to delayed steady-state vascular imaging. This may be particularly useful for coronary studies.[149,151,152]

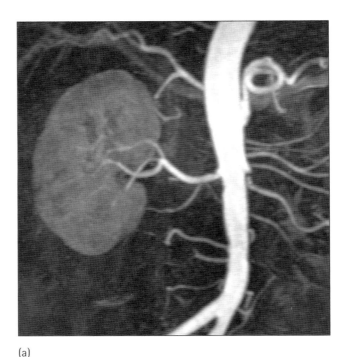

(a)

(b)

Figure 15.21
A 64-year-old patient post left-side nephrectomy with newly developed arterial hypertension. The full-thickness MIP image (a) reveals a proximal renal artery stenosis with slight poststenotic dilatation of the vessel. The corresponding DSA examination (b) performed during interventional therapy confirms the stenosis. Note the excellent depiction of smaller vessels on the MRA image and the good correlation with DSA. Images courtesy of Günther Schneider (Department of Diagnostic Radiology, University Hospital, Homburg/Saar, Germany).

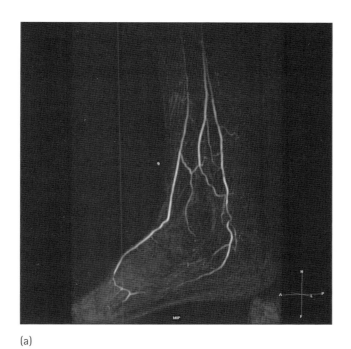
(a)

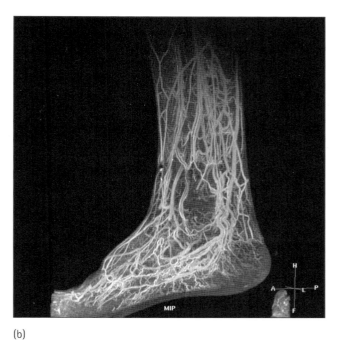
(b)

Figure 15.22

CE-MRA of the foot using the blood pool agent MS-325 in a patient with ischemic rest pain: arterial (a) and equilibrium (b) sagittal full-volume MIPs, with an MS-325 dose of 0.05 mmol/kg. The arterial study is subtracted, 46 s in duration, with true voxel size of $0.9 \times 0.9 \times 1.8$ mm^3. The equilibrium study is fat-suppressed at a delay of 5 min, 4:57 in duration, with a true voxel size of $0.9 \times 0.9 \times 0.8$ mm^3.

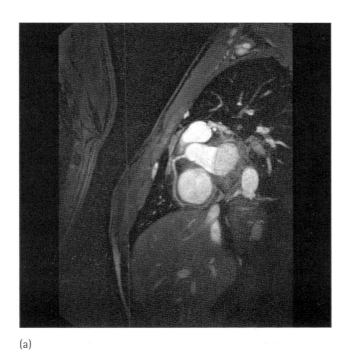
(a)

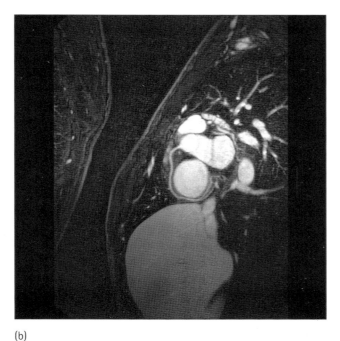
(b)

Figure 15.23

B22956 in imaging of healthy right coronary artery: (a) unenhanced (T2Prep acquisition) and (b) B22956-enhanced (0.075 mmol/kg) image acquired at 25 min postcontrast using 3D navigator-gated and corrected IR-FFE sequence. Images courtesy of Eckart Fleck and Ingo Paetsch (German Heart Institute, Berlin, Germany), Matthias Stuber (Beth Israel Deaconess Medical Center, Cardiovascular Division, Boston, MA, USA), and Friedrich Cavagna (Bracco Imaging SpA, Milano, Italy).

Examples of gadolinium-based blood pool agents with macromolecular structures are Gadomer-17[153] and P792.[154] Like MS–325 and B22956, preliminary results suggest these agents may prove beneficial for coronary MRA.[155,156]

Superparamagnetic iron oxide agents

The second major category of potential contrast agents for MRA consists of the superparamagnetic group, which is based on ultrasmall particles of iron oxide (USPIO) (Table 15.1, column 5). Currently, SHU 555A is the only clinically approved USPIO agent available for contrast-enhanced MRA, although few studies have been conducted in vascular territories other than the upper abdomen.[157] AMI 227 is another potentially useful repre-

sentative of this group, although again few studies have been conducted.[158]

Perhaps the most promising of the USPIO agents currently under development is the blood pool agent NC100150 (Figure 15.24).[159,160] As with the gadolinium blood pool agents, the potential advantages of this agent include a long intravascular half-life with minimal leakage into the interstitial space, thereby permitting steady-state vascular imaging. Preliminary studies on the use of this agent for coronary MRA have already been reported,[160] and work is ongoing to establish its potential for other applications, such as renal perfusion.[161]

As it stands today, the imaging quality achievable with first-pass agents has to some extent eliminated the initial target role for intravascular agents. It has become apparent that real benefits will most likely only be clinically achievable if the intravascular agents can be used both for first-pass and steady-state imaging. Nevertheless, it is doubtful whether this type of blood pool agent will ever have any advantage over the currently available gadolinium agents for dynamic arterial phase MRA. Conceivably, this type of agent may have benefits for ultrahigh-resolution imaging, for assessment of vasculature during intervention, and for real-time therapy monitoring. Other opportunities that may present themselves include perfusion applications combined with first-pass imaging.

While MRA using blood pool agents may ultimately prove beneficial, all current clinical work utilizes extracellular gadolinium chelates.

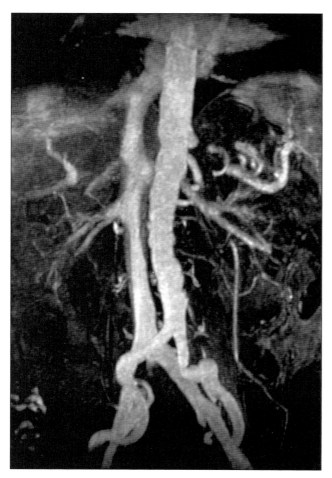

Figure 15.24
NC100150 (5.0 mg Fe/kg bodyweight, slow hand injection, third injection of an accumulating dose scheme) reveals occlusion of the left renal artery and a 60–70% stenosis of the right renal artery.

Future directions: hardware

Among the most important recent developments in MR hardware has been the introduction of whole-body 3.0 T scanners. The principal advantage of increasing the magnetic field strength is improved SNR, resulting in better resolution and conspicuity of vessels using similar acquisition times.[162] Although clinical experience with CE-MRA at 3.0 T is somewhat limited at present, early studies have indicated markedly improved performance of unenhanced TOF techniques, particularly in imaging of the intracranial and cervical vasculature.[162,163] Similarly, imaging at 3.0 T has been reported to improve the resolution and delineation of small venous vessels in the brain,[164] and appears advantageous for contrast-enhanced vascular and coronary imaging.[165–167] It remains to be seen just how the availability of 3.0 T machines will impact CE-MRA. Several challenges remain to be overcome, including developing new coils, overcoming SAR (RF power deposition) limitations, and optimizing protocols. This aside, however, it appears likely that the SNR-derived improvement in spatial and temporal resolution at 3.0 T will lead to significant improvements in CE-MRA image quality.

Summary

CE-MRA provides a safe, fast, and cost-efficient alternative to conventional diagnostic angiography throughout the vasculature. Numerous recent advances allow for high-resolution breathhold and multistation imaging with optimal arterial phase contrast bolus timing. As the technique is further refined, better coils, better contrast agents, and perhaps higher magnetic field strength will allow for greater spatial and temporal resolution, further increasing the effectiveness and utility of CE-MRA.

References

1. Saloner MRA: principles and display. In: Magnetic Resonance Imaging of the Body (Higgins C, Hricak H, Helms C, eds). Philadelphia: Lippincott-Raven, 1997:1345–68.

2. Gullberg G, Wherli F, Shimakawa A, Simmons M. MR vascular imaging with a fast gradient refocusing pulse sequence and reformatted images from transaxial sections. Radiology 1997; 165:241–6.

3. Doumolin C, Cline H, Souza S, et al. Three-dimensional time-of-flight magnetic resonance angiography using spin saturation. Magn Reson Imaging 1989; 11:35–46.

4. Owen R, Baum R, Carpenter J, et al. Symptomatic peripheral vascular disease: selection of imaging parameters and clinical evaluation with MR angiography. Radiology 1993; 187:627–35.

5. Cortell E, Kaufman J, Geller S, et al. MR angiography of the tibial runoff vessels: imaging with the head coil compared to conventional arteriography. AJR 1996; 167:147–51.

6. Glickerman D, Obregon G, Schmiedl U, et al. Cardiac-gated MR angiography of the entire lower extremity: a prospective comparison with conventional angiography. AJR 1996; 167:445–51.

7. Patel P, Kuntz K, Klufas R, et al. Carotid bifurcation. Can magnetic resonance angiography and duplex ultrasonography replace contrast arteriography? Stroke 1995; 26:1753–8.

8. Anderson C. MRA of the aortic arch and extracranial carotid arteries. In: Magnetic Resonance Imaging of the Body (Higgins C, Hricak H, Helms C, eds). Philadelphia: Lippincott-Raven, 1997:1369–81.

9. Blatter D, Parker D, Robinson R. Cerebral MR angiography with multiple overlapping thin slab acquisition. Radiology 1991; 179:805–11.

10. Kim D, Edelman R, Kent K, et al. Abdominal aorta and renal artery stenosis: evaluation with MR angiography. Radiology 1990; 174:727–31.

11. Yucel E, Kaufman J, Prince M, et al. Time-of-flight renal MR arteriography: utility in patients with renal insufficeincy. Magn Reson Imaging 1993; 11:925–30.

12. Loubeyre P, Cahan R, Grozel F, et al. Transplant renal artery stenosis. Evaluation of diagnosis with magnetic resonance angiography compared with color duplex sonography and arteriography. Transplantation 1996; 62:446–50.

13. Prince M. Body MR angiography with gadolinium contrast agents. MRI Clin North Am 1996; 4:11–24.

14. Prince M. Gadolinium-enhanced MR aortography. Radiology 1994; 191:155–64.

15. Bryant D, Payne J, Firmin D, Longmore D. Measurement of flow with NMR imaging using a gradient pulse and phase difference technique. Comput Assist Tomogr 1984; 8:588–93.

16. Gedroyc W. Magnetic resonance angiography of renal arteries. Urol Clin North Am 1994; 21:201–14.

17. Bass J, Prince M, Londy F, Chenevert T. Effect of gadolinium on phase-contrast MR angiography of the renal arteries. AJR 1997; 168:261–6.

18. Gedroyc W, Negus R, Al-Kutoubi A, et al. Magnetic resonance angiography of renal transplants. Lancet 1992; 339:789–91.

19. Yucel E. Magnetic resonance angiography of the lower extremity and renal arteries. Semir Ultrasound CT MRI 1992; 13:291–302.

20. Ngheim H, Winter R, Mountford M, et al. Evaluation of the portal venous system before liver transplantation: value of phase-contrast MR angiography. AJR 1995; 164:871–8.

21. Lundin B, Cooper T, Meyer R, Potchen E. Measurement of total and unilateral renal blood flow by oblique-angle velocity encoded 2D-CINE magnetic resonance angiography. Magn Reson Med 1992; 11:51–9.

22. Schoenberg S, Knopp M, Londy F, et al. Renal artery stenosis: stenosis grading by combined morphologic and functional MR imaging: results of a multicenter multireader analysis. J Am Soc Nephrol 2002; 13:158–69.

23. Weinman H, Brasch R, Press W, Wesbey G. Charcteristics of gadolinium-DTAP complex: a potential NMR contrast agent. AJR 1984; 142:619–24.

24. Schima W, Mukerjee A, Saini S. Contrast-enhanced MR imaging. Clin Radiol 1996; 51:235–44.

25. Goldstein H, Kashanian F, Blumetti R, et al. Safety assessment of gadopentetate dimeglumine in U.S. clinical trials. Radiology 1990; 174:17–23.

26. Niendorf H, Haustein J, Alhassan A, Clauss W. Safety of gadolinium-DTPA: extended clinical experience. In: Workshop on Contrast-Enhanced Magnetic Resonance (Brasch R, ed). Napa, CA: Society for Magnetic Resonance in Medicine, 1991:70–9.

27. Haustein J, Niendorf H, Krestin G, et al. Renal tolerance of gadolinium-DTAP/dimeglumine in patients with chronic renal failure. Invest Radiol 1992; 27:153–6.

28. Prince M, Arnoldus C, Frisoli J. Nephrotoxicity of high dose gadolinium compared to iodinated contrast. J Magn Reson Imaging 1996; 6:162–6.

29. Hohenschuh E, Watson A. Theory and mechanisms of contrast-enhancing agents. In: Magnetic Resonance Imaging of the Body (Higgins C, Hricak H, Helms C, eds). Philadelphia: Lippincott-Raven, 1997:1439–64.

30. Prince M, Yucel E, Kaufman J, et al. Dynamic gadolinium-enhanced three-dimensional abdominal MR arterography. J Magn Reson Imaging 1993; 3:877–81.

31. Runge V, Kirsch J, Lee C. Contrast-enhance MR angiography. J Magn Reson Imaging 1993; 3:233–9.

32. Ehman R, Revel D, Sievers R, Brasch R. Acute myocardial ischemia. Magnetic resonance contrast enhancement with gadolinium-DTPA. Radiology 1984; 153:157–63.

33. Moseley M, Sawyer A. Imgaing techniques: pulse sequences. In: Magnetic Resonance Imaging of the Body (Higgins C, Hricak H, Helms C, eds). Philadelphia: Lippincott-Raven, 1997:43–69.

34. Wehrli F. Principles of magnetic resonance. In: Magnetic Resonance Imaging (Stark D, Bradley W, eds). St Louis, Mo: Mosby-Year Book, 1992:3–20.

35. Prince M, Narasimham D, Stanley J, et al. Breath-hold gadolinium-enhanced MR angiography of the abdominal aorta and its major branches. Radiology 1995; 197:785–92.

36. Snidow J, Johnson S, Harris V, et al. Three-dimensional gadolinium-enhanced MR angiography for aortoiliac inflow assessment plus renal artery screening in a single breath hold. Radiology 1996; 198:725–32.

37. Leung D, McKinnon G, et al. Breath-hold, contrast-enhanced, three-dimensional MR angiography. Radiology 1996; 201:569–71.

38. Hendrick R, Roff U. Image Contrast and Noise. Chicago, IL: Mosby-Year Book, 1991.

39. Weinman H, Laniado M, Mutzel W. Pharmacokinetics of Gd-DTPA/dimeglumine after intravenous injection into healthy volunteers. Physiol Chem Phys Med NMR 1984; 16:167–72.

40. Lee V, Flyer M, Weinreb J, et al. Image subtraction in gadolinium-enhanced MR imaging. AJR 1996; 167:1427–32.

41. Maki J, Chenevert T, Prince M. Optimizing three-dimensional gadolinium-enhanced MR angiography. Invest Radiol 1998; 33:528–37.

42. Verhoeven L. Digital Subtraction Angiography: The Technique and an Analysis of the Physical Factors Influencing the Image Quality. Delft: Technische Hogeschule, 1985.

43. Barnes G, Lakshminarayann A. Conventional and spiral computed tomography. In: Computed Body Tomography with MRI Correlation (Lee J, Sagel S, Stanley R, Heiken J, eds). Philadelphia: Lippincott-Raven, 1998:1–20.

44. Maki J, Prince M, Londy F, Chenevert T. The effects of time varying intravascular signal intensity on three-dimensional MR angiography image quality. J Magn Reson Imaging 1996; 6:642–51.

45. Riederer S, Tasciyan T, Farzaneh F. MR fluoroscopy: technical feasibility. Magn Reson Med 1988; 8:1–15.

46. Fain S, Riederer S, Bernstein M, Huston J. Theoretical limits of spatial resolution in elliptical-centric contrast-enhanced 3d-MRA. Magn Reson Med 1999; 42:1106–16.

47. Maki J, Wilson G, Eubank W, Hoogeveen R. Utilizing SENSE to achieve lower station sub-millimeter isotropic resolution and minimal venous enhancement in peripheral MR angiography. J Magn Reson Imaging 2002; 15:484–91.

48. Bampton A, Riederer S, Korin H. Centric phase-encoding order in three-dimensional MP-RAGE sequences: application to abdominal imaging. J Magn Reson Imaging 1992; 2:327–34.

49. Wilman A, Riederer S. Improved centric phase encoding orders for three-dimensional magnetization-prepared MR angiography. Magn Reson Med 1996; 36:384–92.

50. Maki J, Chenevert T, Prince M. The effects of incomplete breath holding on 3D MR image quality. J Magn Reson Imaging 1997; 7:1132–9.

51. Wilman A, Riederer S, Breen J, Ehman R. Elliptical spiral phase-encoding order: an optimal, field-of-view-dependent ordering scheme for breath-hold contrast-enhanced 3D MR angiography. Radiology 1996; 201:328–9.

52. Hany T, Schmidt M, Hilfiker P, et al. Optimization of contrast dosage for gadolinium-enhanced 3D MRA of the pulmonary and renal arteries. Magn Reson Imaging 1998; 16:901–6.

53. Shetty A, Bis K, Kirsch M, et al. Contrast-enhanced breath-hold three-dimensional magnetic resonance angiography in the evaluation of renal arteries: optimization of technique and pitfalls. J Magn Reson Imaging 2000; 12:912–23.

54. Snidow J, Aisen A, Harris V, et al. Iliac artery MR angiography: comparison of three-dimensional gadolinium-enhanced and two-dimensional time-of-flight techniques. Radiology 1995; 196:371–8.

55. Steiner P, Debatin J, Romanowski B, et al. Optimization of breath-hold 3D MR pulmonary angiography. Radiology 1996; 201:201.

56. Hany T, Debatin J, Schmidt M, et al. Three-dimensional MR angiography of the renal arteries in a single breath-hold. Radiology 1996; 201:218.

57. Finn J, Baskaran V, Carr J, et al. Thorax: low-dose contrast-enhanced three-dimensional MR angiography with subsecond temporal resolution. initial results. Radiology 2002; 224:896–904.

58. Prince M, Grist T, Debatin J. 3D Contrast MR Angiography. Berlin: Springer-Verlag, 1997.

59. Earls J, Rofsky N, DeCorato D, et al. Breath-hold single-dose gadolinium-enhanced three-dimensional MR aortography: usefulness of a timing examination and MR power injector. Radiology 1996:705–10.

60. Krinsky G, Rofsky N, Flyer M, et al. Gadolinium-enhanced three-dimensional MR angiography of acquired arch vessel disease. AJR 1996; 167:981–7.

61. Kreitner K, Kunz R, Kalden P, et al. Contrast-enhanced three-dimensional MR angiography of the thoracic aorta: experiences after 118 examinations with a standard dose contrast administration and different injection protocols. Eur Radiol 2001; 11:1355–63.

62. Wilman A, Riederer S, King B, et al. Fluoroscopically-triggered contrast-enhanced three dimensional MR angiography with elliptical centric view order: application to the renal arteries. Radiology 1997; 205:137–46.

63. Huston J, Fain S, Riederer S, et al. Carotid arteries: maximizing arterial to venous contrast in fluoroscopically triggered contrast-enhanced MR angiography with elliptic centric view ordering. Radiology 1999; 211:265–73.

64. Fellner F, Fellner C, Wutke R, et al. Fluoroscopically triggered contrast-enhanced 3D MR DSA and 3D time-of-flight turbo MRA of the carotid arteries: first clinical experiences in correlation with ultrasound, x-ray angiography, and endarterectomy findings. Magn Reson Imaging 2000; 18:575–85.

65. Watts R, Wang Y, B R, et al. Recessed elliptical-centric view-ordering for contrast-enhanced 3D MR angiography of the carotid arteries. Magn Reson Med 2002; 48:419–24.

66. Levy R, Maki J. Three-dimensional contrast-enhanced MR angiography of the extracranial carotid arteries: two techniques. AJNR 1998; 19:688–90.

67. Korosec F, Grist T, Frayne R, Mistretta C. Time-resolved contrast-enhanced 3D MR angiography. Magn Reson Med 1996; 36:345–51.

68. Mistretta C, Grist T, Korosec F, Frayne R. 3D time-resolved contrast-enhanced MR DSA: advantages and tradeoffs. Magn Reson Med 1998; 40:571–81.

69. Schoenberg S, Bock M, Floemer F, et al. High-resolution pulmonary arterio- and venography using multiple-bolus multiphase 3D-Gd-mRA. J Magn Reson Imaging 1999; 10:339–46.

70. Schoenberg S, Essig M, Hallscheidt P, et al. Multiphase magnetic resonance angiography of the abdominal and pelvic arteries: results of a bicenter multireader analysis. Invest Radiol 2002; 37:20–8.

71. Stein B, DeMarco J, Zhou Y. 3D time-resolved MRA with elliptic centric view ordering. Initial clinical experience to evaluate tibo-peroneal arteries. In:XIIIth Annual International Workshop on MRA, Madison, WI, 2001:107.

72. Hennig J, Scheffler K, Laubenberger J, Strecker R. Time-resolved projection angiography after bolus injection of contrast agent. Magn Reson Med 1997; 37:341–5.

73. Goyen M, Laub G, Ladd M, et al. Dynamic 3D MR angiography of the pulmonary arteries in under four seconds. J Magn Reson Imaging 2001; 13:372–7.

74. Finn J, Carr J, Pereles S, et al. Time-resolved, contrast-enhanced MR angiography of the thorax. In:XIIIth Annual International Workshop on MRA, Madison, WI, 2001:25.

75. Pruessmann K, Weiger M, Scheidegger M, Boesiger P. SENSE: sensitivity encoding for fast MRI. Magn Reson Med 1999; 42:952–62.

76. Finn J, Larson A, Moore J, Simonetti O. Sub-second 3D contrast-enhanced MRA of the thorax with radial k-space sampling. In:Xth Scientific Meeting and Exhibition of the International Society for Magnetic Resonance in Medicine, Honolulu, HI, 2002:1793.

77. Bock M, Schoenberg S, Floemer F, Schad L. Separation of arteries and veins in 3D MR angiography using correlation analysis. Magn Reson Med 2000; 43:481–7.

78. Mistretta C, Grist T, Frayne R, Korosec F. Contrast and motion artifacts in 4D MR angiography. Radiology 1996; 201:238.

79. Turski P, Korosec F, Carroll T, et al. Contrast-Enhanced magnetic resonance angiography of the carotid bifurcation using the time-resolved imaging of contrast kinetics (TRICKS) technique. Top Magn Reson Imaging 2001; 12:175–81.

80. Mazaheri Y, Carroll T, Du J, et al. Combined time-resolved and high-spatial-resolution 3D MRA using an extended adaptive acquisition. J Magn Reson Imaging 2002; 15:291–301.

81. Peters D, Korosec F, Grist T, et al. Undersampled projection reconstruction applied to MR angiography. Magn Reson Med 200; 43:91–101.

82. Barger A, Block W, Toropov Y, et al. Time-resolved contrast-enhanced imaging with isotropic resolution and broad coverage using an undersampled 3D projection trajectory. Magn Reson Med 2002; 48:297–305.

83. Willinek W, Gieseke J, Von Falkenhousen V, et al. CD–3D MRA of the supraaoritc arteries at 512 and 1024 matrix: the use of randomly segmented central k-space ordering (CENTRA). In:Xth Scientific Meeting and Exhibition of the International Society for Magnetic Resonance in Medicine, Honolulu, HI, 2002:144.

84. Wood M, Runge V, Henkelman R. Overcoming motion in abdominal MR imaging. AJR 1988; 150:513–22.

85. Ehman R, Felmlee J. Adaptive technique for high-definition MR imaging of moving structure. Radiology 1989; 173:255–63.

86. Vasbinder G, Maki J, Nijenhuis R, et al. Motion of the distal renal artery during 3D contrast-enhanced breath-hold MRA. J Magn Reson Imaging 2002; 16:685–96.

87. Holland G, Dougherty L, Carpenter J, et al. Breath-hold ultrafast three-dimensional gadolinium-enhanced MR angiography of the aorta and the renal and other visceral abdominal arteries. AJR 1996; 166:971–81.

88. Carr J, Ma J, Desphande V, et al. High-resolution breath-hold contrast-enhanced MR angiography of the entire carotid circulation. AJR 2002; 178:543–9.

89. Weiger M, Pruessmann K, Kassner A, et al. Contrast-enhanced 3d MRA using SENSE. J Magn Reson Imaging 2000; 12:671–7.

90. Sodickson D, Manning W. Simultaneous acquisition of spatial harmonics (SMASH): fast imaging with radiofrequency coil arrays. Magn Reson Med 1997; 38:591–603.

91. Wilson G, Maki J, Evitts M, et al. A direct comparison study to evaluate the usefulness of sensitivity encoding (SENSE) in evaluating renal artery stenosis using MR angiography. In: XIII Annual International Workshop on MRA, Madison, WI, 2001:30–1.

92. Maki J, Wilson G, Hoogeveen R. 3D Gd enhanced moving table MR angiography of the aorta and outflow vessels using SENSE to achieve high resolution of the below knee vasculature. In: 7th Scientific Meeting of the International Society for Magnetic Resonance in Medicine, Glasgow, Scotland, 2001.

93. Du Y, Parker D, Davis W, Gao T. Reduction of partial-volume artifacts with zero-filled interpolation in three-dimensional MR angiography. J Magn Reson Imaging 1994; 4:733–41.

94. Ros P, Gauger J, Stoupis C, et al. Diagnosis of renal artery stenosis: feasibility of combining MR angiography, MR renography, and gadopentetate-based measurements of glomerular filtration rate. AJR 1995; 165:1447–51.

95. Schoenberg S, Bock M, Aumann S, et al. Quantitative recording of renal function with magnetic resonance tomography. Radiologie 2000; 40:925–37.

96. De Marco J, Nesbit G, Wesbey G, Richardson D. Prospective evaluation of extracranial carotid stenosis: MR angiography with maximum-intensity projections and multiplanar reformation compared with conventional angiography. AJR 1994; 163:1205–12.

97. Laub G. Displays for MR angiography. Magn Reson Med 1990; 14:222–9.

98. Rossnick S, Laub G, Braeckle R. Three dimensional display of blood vessels in MRI. In: Proceedings of the IEEE: Computers in Cardiology. New York: IEEE, 1986:193–95.

99. Anderson C, Saloner D, Tsuruda J, et al. Artifacts in maximum intensity projection display of MR angiograms. AJR 1990; 154:623–9.

100. Baskaran V, Pereles F, Nemcek AJ, et al. Gadolinium-enhanced 3D MR angiography of renal artery stenosis: a pilot comparison of maximum intensity projection, multiplanar reformatting, and 3D volume-rendering postprocessing algorithms. Acad Radiol 2002; 9:50–9.

101. Douek P, Revel D, Chazel S, et al. Fast MR angiography of the aortoiliac arteries and arteries of the lower extremity: value of bolus-enhanced, whole-volume subtraction technique. AJR 1995; 165:431–7.

102. Wang Y, Johnston D, Breen J, et al. Dynamic MR digital subtraction angiography using contrast enhancement, fast data acquisition, and complex subtraction. Magn Reson Med 1996; 36:551–6.

103. Wang Y, Winchester P, Khilnani N, et al. Contrast-enhanced peripheral MR angiography from the abdominal aorta to the pedal arteries: combined dynamic two-dimensional and bolus-chase three-dimensional acquisitions. Invest Radiol 2001; 36:170–7.

104. Hoogeveen R, Bakker C, Viergever M. Limits to the accuracy of vessel diameter measurement in MR angiography. J Magn Reson Imaging 1998; 8:1228–35.

105. Wilson G, Haynor D, Maki J. Resolution requirements for grading stenoses in 3D CE-MRA. In: 6th Scientific Meeting of the International Society for Magnetic Resonance in Medicine, Denver, CO, 2000:1787.

106. Stafford-Johnson D, Hamilton B, Dong Q, et al. Vascular complications of liver transplantation: evaluation with gadolinium-enhanced MR angiography. Radiology 1998; 207:153–60.

107. Wutke R, Lang W, Fellner C, et al. High-resolution, contrast-enhanced magnetic resonance angiography with elliptical centric *k*-space ordering of supra-aortic arteries compared with selective X-ray angiography. Stroke 2002; 33:1522–9.

108. Murray J, Manisali M, Flamm S, et al. Intramural hematoma of the thoracic aorta: MR image findings and their prognostic implications. Radiology 1997; 204:349–55.

109. Prince M, Schoenberg S, Ward J, et al. Hemodynamically significant atherosclerotic renal artery stenosis: MR angiographic features. Radiology 1997; 205:128–36.

110. Hood M, Ho V, Corse W. Three-dimensional phase-contrast magnetic resonance angiography: a useful clinical adjunct to gadolinium-enhanced three-dimensional renal magnetic resonance angiography? Mil Med 2002; 167:343–9.

111. Johnson D, Lerner C, Prince M, et al. Gadolinium-enhanced magnetic resonance angiography of renal transplants. Magn Reson Imaging 1997; 15:13–20.

112. Ferreiros J, Mendez R, Jorquera M, et al. Using gadolinium-enhanced three-dimensional MR angiography to assess arterial inflow stenosis after kidney transplantation. AJR 1999; 172:751–7.

113. Laissy J, Trillaud H, Douek P. MR angiography: noninvasive vascular imaging of the abdomen. Abdom Imaging 2002; 27:488–506.

114. Baden J, Racy D, Grist T. Contrast-enhanced three-dimensional magnetic resonance angiography of the mesenteric vasculature. J Magn Reson Imaging 1999; 10:369–75.

115. Stafford-Johnson D, Chenevert T, Cho K, Prince M. Portal venous magnetic resonance angiography. A review. Acad Radiol 1998; 5:289–305.

116. Rofsky N, Lee V, Laub G, et al. Abdominal MR imaging with a volumetric interpolated breath-hold examination. Radiology 1999; 212:876–84.

117. Oudkerk M, van Beek E, Wielopolski P, et al. Comparison of contrast-enhanced magnetic resonance angiography and conventional pulmonary angiography for the diagnosis of pulmonary embolism: a prospective study. Lancet 2002; 359:1643–7.

118. Meaney J, Johansson L, Ahlstrom H, Prince M. Pulmonary magnetic resonance angiography. J Magn Reson Imaging 1999; 10:326–38.

119. Wikstrom J, Johansson L, Rossitti S, et al. High resolution carotid artery MRA. Comparison with fast dynamic acquistion and duplex ultrasound scanning. Acta Radiol 2002; 43:256–61.

120. Sueyoshi E, Sakamoto I, Matsuoka Y, et al. Aortoiliac and lower extremity arteries: comparison of three-dimensional dynamic contrast-enhanced subtraction MR angiography and conventional angiography. Radiology 1999; 210:683–8.

121. Ho K, Leiner T, DeHaan M, et al. Peripheral vascular tree stenoses: evaluation with moving-bed infusion-tracking MR angiography. Radiology 1998; 206:683–92.

122. Meaney J, Ridgway J, Chakraverty S, et al. Stepping-table gadolinium-enhanced digital subtraction MR angiography of the aorta and lower extremity arteries: preliminary experience. Radiology 1999; 211:59–67.

123. Ho V, Choyke P, Foo T, et al. Automated bolus chase peripheral MR angiography: initial practical experiences and future directions of this work-in-progress. J Magn Reson Imaging 1999; 10:376–88.

124. Goyen M, Quick H, Debatin J, et al. Whole-body three-dimensional MR angiography with a rolling table platform: initial clinical experience. Radiology 2002; 224:270–7.

125. Ho K, de Haan M, Kessels A, et al. Peripheral vascular tree stenoses: detection with subtracted and nonsubtracted mr angiography. Radiology 1998; 206:673–81.

126. Ho K. MR Angiography of the Lower Extremities. Thesis, University of Maastricht, The Netherlands, 1999:93–108.

127. Ho K. First experiences with BPA for peripheral MRA. In:XI International Workshop on MRA, Lund, Sweden, 1999:43.

128. Maki J, Wilson G, Eubank W, et al. 3D Gd-enhanced moving table peripheral MR angiography using multi-station SENSE to include the pedal vasculature. In: 10th Scientific Meeting and Exhibition of the International Society for Magnetic Resonance in Medicine, Honolulu, HI, 2002:1743.

129. Leiner T, Kessels A, van Engelshoven J. Total runoff peripheral MRA in patients with critical ischemia and tissue loss can detect more patent arteries than IA-DSA. In:10th Scientific Meeting and Exhibition of the International Society for Magnetic Resonance in Medicine, Honolulu, HI, 2002:210.

130. Wang Y, Lee H, Avakian R, et al. Timing alogrithm for bolus chase MR digital subtraction angiography. Magn Reson Med 1998; 39:691–6.

131. Ruehm S, Zimny K, Debatin J. Direct contrast-enhanced 3D MR venography. Eur Radiol 2001; 11:102–12.

132. Li W, Kaplan D, Edelman R. Three-diensional low dose gadolinium-enhanced peripheral MR venography. J Magn Reson Imaging 1998; 8:630–3.

133. Thornton M, Ryan R, Varghese J, et al. A three-dimensional gadolinium-enhanced MR venography technique for imaging central veins. AJR 1999; 173:999–1003.

134. de Ha#aun C, Cabrini M, Akhnana L, et al. Gadobenate dimeglumine 0.5 M solution for injection (MultiHance) pharmaceutical formulation and physicochemical properties of a new magnetic resonance imaging contrast medium. J Comput Assist Tomogr 1999; 23 (Suppl 1):S161–8.

135. Knopp M, von Tengg-Kobligk H, Floemer F, Schoenberg S. Contrast agents for MRA: future directions. J Magn Reson Imaging 1999; 10:314–16.

136. Tombach B, Reimer P, Prumer B, et al. Does a higher concentration of gadolinium chelates improve first-pass cardiac signal changes? J Magn Reson Imaging 1999; 10:806–12.

137. Goyen M, Lauenstein T, Herborn C, et al. 0.5 M Gd chelate (Magnevist) versus 1.0 M Gd chelate (Gadovist): dose-independent effect on image quality of pelvic three-dimensional MR-angiography. J Magn Reson Imaging 2001; 14:602–7.

138. Herborn C, Lauenstein T, Ruehm S, et al. Intraindividual comparison of gadopentetate dimeglumine, gadobenate dimeglumine and gadobutrol for pelvic 3D magnetic resonance angiography. Invest Radiol 2003; 38:27–33.

139. Knopp M, Schoenberg S, Rehm C, et al. Assessment of gadobenate dimeglumine (Gd-BOPTA) for MR angiography: phase I studies. Invest Radiol 2002; 37:706–15.

140. Völk M, Strotzer M, Lenhart M, et al. Renal time-resolved MR angiography: quantitative comparison of gadobenate dimeglumine and gadopentetate dimeglumine with different doses. Radiology 2001; 220:484–8.

141. Cavagna F, Maggioni F, Castelli P, et al. Gadolinium chelates with weak binding to serum proteins. A new class of high-efficiency, general purpose contrast agents for magnetic resonance imaging. Invest Radiol 1997; 32:780–96.

142. Kroencke T, Wasser M, Pattynama P, et al. Gadobenate dimeglumine – enhanced magnetic resonance angiography of the abdominal aorta and renal arteries. AJR 2002; 179:1573–82.

143. Ruehm S, Goyen M, Barkhausen J, et al. Rapid magnetic resonance angiography for detection of atherosclerosis. Lancet 2001; 357:1086–91.

144. Goyen M, Herborn C, Lauenstein T, et al. Optimization of contrast dosage for gadobenate dimeglumine-enhanced high-resolution whole body 3D MR angiography. Invest Radiol 2002; 37:263–8.

145. Kirchin M, Pirovano G, Venetianer C, Spinazzi A. Safety assessment of gadobenate dimeglumine (MultiHance): extended clinical experience from phase I studies to post-marketing surveillance. J Magn Reson Imaging 2001; 14:281–94.

146. Grist T, Korosec F, Peters D, et al. Steady-state and dynamic MR angiography with MS-325: initial experience in humans. Radiology 1998; 207:539–44.

147. Lauffer R, Parmelee D, Dunham S, et al. MS–325: albumin-targeted contrast agent for MR angiography. Radiology 1998; 207:529–38.

148. Bluemke D, Stillman A, Bis K, et al. Carotid MR angiography: phase II study of safety and efficacy of MS-325. Radiology 2001; 219:114–22.

149. La Noce A, Stoelben S, Scheffler K, et al. B22956/1, a new intravascular contrast agent for MRI: first administration to humans – preliminary results. Acad Radiol 2002; 9(Suppl):S404–6.

150. Zheng J, Li D, Cavagna F, et al. Contrast-enhanced coronary MR angiography: relationship between coronary artery delineation and blood T1. J Magn Reson Imaging 2001; 14:348–54.

151. Stuber M, Botnar R, Danias P, et al. Contrast agent-enhanced, free-breathing, three-dimensional coronary magnetic resonance angiography. J Magn Reson Imaging 1999; 10:790–9.

152. Huber M, Paetsch I, Schnackenburg B, et al. Performance of a new gadolinium-based intravascular contrast agent in free-breathing inversion-recovery 3D coronary MRA. Magn Reson Med 2003; 49:115–21.

153. Dong Q, Hurst D, Weinmann H, Chenevert T, Londy F, Prince M. Magnetic resonance angiography with Gadomer-17. An animal study original investigation. Invest Radiol 1998; 33:699–708.

154. Gaillard S, Kubiak C, Stolz C, et al. Safety and pharmacokinetics of P792, a new blood-pool agent: results of clinical testing in non-patient volunteers. Invest Radiol 2002; 37:161–6.

155. Taupitz M, Schnorr J, Wagner S, et al. Coronary magnetic resonance angiography: experimental evaluation of the new rapid clearance blood pool contrast medium P792. Magn Reson Med 2001; 46:932–8.

156. Li D, Zheng J, Weinmann H. Contrast-enhanced MR imaging of coronary arteries: comparison of intra- and extravascular contrast agents in swine. Radiology 2001; 218:670–8.

157. Reimer P, Allkemper T, Matuszewski L, Balzer T. Contrast-enhanced 3D-MRA of the upper abdomen with a bolus-injectable SPIO (SHU 555A). J Magn Reson Imaging 1999; 10:65–71.

158. Mayo-Smith W, Saini S, Slater G, et al. MR contrast material for vascular enhancement: value of superparamagnetic iron oxide. AJR 1996; 166:73–7.

159. Weishaupt D, Ruhm S, Binkert C, et al. Equilibrium-phase MR angiography of the aortoiliac and renal arteries using a blood pool contrast agent. AJR 2000; 175:189–95.

160. Taylor A, Panting J, Keegan J, et al. Safety and preliminary findings with the intravascular contrast agent NC100150 injection for MR coronary angiography. J Magn Reson Imaging 1999; 9:220–7.

161. Bachmann R, Conrad R, Kreft B, et al. Evaluation of a new ultra-small superparamagnetic iron oxide contrast agent Clariscan, (NC100150) for MRI of renal perfusion: experimental study in an animal model. J Magn Reson Imaging 2002; 16:190–5.

162. Campeau N, Huston JR, Bernstein M, et al. Magnetic resonance angiography at 3.0 tesla: initial clinical experience. Top Magn Reson Imaging 2001; 12:183–204.

163. Al-Kwifi O, Emery D, Wilman A. Vessel contrast at three tesla in time-of-flight magnetic resonance angiography of the intracranial and carotid arteries. Magn Reson Imaging 2002; 20:181–7.

164. Reichenbach J, Barth M, Haacke E, et al. High-resolution MR venography at 3.0 tesla. J Comput Assist Tomogr 2000; 24:949–57.

165. Hugg J, Rofsky N, Stokar S, et al. Clinical whole body MRI at 3.0 T – initial experience. In: 10th Scientific Meeting and Exhibition of the International Society for Magnetic Resonance in Medicine. Honolulu, HI, 2002:569.

166. Leiner T, Vasbinder B, De Vries M, et al. Contrast-enhanced peripheral MRA at 3.0 T: initial results. In: 10th Scientific Meeting and Exhibition of the International Society for Magnetic Resonance in Medicine. Honolulu, HI, 2002:217.

167. Stuber M, Botnar R, Fischer S, et al. Preliminary report on in vivo coronary MRA at 3 tesla in humans. Magn Reson Med 2002; 48:425–9.

16

CMR of aortic disease

James C Carr, J Paul Finn

Introduction

Diseases of the thoracic and abdominal aorta are a significant cause of morbidity and mortality and have the potential to produce catastrophic consequences. Conventional digital subtraction angiography (DSA) has been the gold standard for imaging for many years. However, in addition to being time-consuming, costly, and providing only limited information about vessel morphology, DSA is relatively invasive and is associated with well-recognized side-effects.[1] DSA is now primarily used as a first-line investigation in the setting of trauma.[2] Computed tomography (CT) is now the most frequently utilized modality for evaluating the aorta and has high diagnostic accuracy for detection of aortic pathology, particularly with the advent of multidetector scanners.[3,4] CT has the advantage of being quick and readily available in most hospital settings; however, it employs ionizing radiation[5] and potentially nephrotoxic contrast agents. Transesophageal echocardiography (TEE) can be used to assess the thoracic aorta, particularly in the diagnosis of aortic dissection; however, it is invasive and provides limited coverage of the entire vessel.[6]

Cardiac magnetic resonance imaging (CMR) is increasingly becoming the first-line investigation for evaluating aortic diseases, particularly in the thoracic aorta.[7,8] CMR has the capacity for multiplanar imaging, does not involve ionizing radiation, and can be used with non-nephrotoxic contrast agents. With recent advances in gradient hardware, much shorter repetition times (TR) are now achievable, resulting in significant increases in acquisition speed. This has prompted the development of new pulse sequences and ultrafast magnetic resonance angiography (MRA) techniques. The principal challenge to universal implementation of CMR as a first-line imaging tool for the aorta remains its availability compared with CT.

MR imaging techniques

Most CMR strategies for assessing the aorta involve a technique to assess vessel morphology combined with contrast-enhanced (CE)-MRA. Recent improvements in gradient speed have seen a resurgence of steady-state free precession techniques (SSFP: TrueFISP, FIESTA, and Balanced FFE). In addition, shortened TRs and parallel acquisition allow ultrafast MRA to be implemented with near-real-time temporal resolution. These newer techniques can be used to supplement the older well-established strategies and in many cases stand poised to replace them.

Steady-state free precession

TrueFISP is a steady-state gradient-echo sequence originally described by Oppelt.[9] Because of its sensitivity to off-resonance artifacts, the clinical applications of TrueFISP were limited prior to the availability of high-performance gradients. With the advent of fast gradients, single-shot and segmented k-space versions of TrueFISP proved very powerful for cine imaging of the heart.[9–14] TrueFISP is a T2*-weighted pulse sequence, which produces high signal from blood without the need for a contrast agent. The contrast-to-noise ratio depends on T2/T1 differences, which, at short TR, are high for blood and soft tissues. In order to produce artifact-free images, TrueFISP must be implemented at short TR, and consequently can only be successfully used on scanners with high-performance gradients. The typical TR is 3.2 ms with an echo time (TE) of 1.6 ms. Signal intensity is maximal at a flip angle of 60°–70°. With a 256 imaging matrix, in-plane resolution with pixel sizes of approximately 2.0×1.5 mm^2 can be achieved.[12] TrueFISP can be implemented as either a single-shot or a cine technique for imaging both the thoracic and abdominal aorta.[15]

The single-shot strategy is an electrocardiographically (ECG)-controlled two-dimensional (2D) acquisition. A trigger delay (~200–400 ms) after the R-wave can be used to push the acquisition period further into diastole, depending on the R–R interval. The acquisition time per image is of the order of 450 ms, resulting in 1 image per heartbeat. Because of the acquisition speed, the technique is essentially independent of respiratory motion artifact. Consequently, imaging can be successfully carried out without breathholding, which is particularly advantageous in critically ill patients. The aorta is typically covered in an interleaved manner in axial, coronal, and sagittal orientations. Segmented k-space cine TrueFISP is a breathhold ECG-synchronized acquisition where multiple phases of the cardiac cycle are captured and may be reviewed in video format.[12,15] The image is acquired over several heartbeats, and selective line acquisition mode (SLAM)[16] may be utilized to decrease the acquisition duration, resulting in an imaging time of ~6–8 s/slice. Cine images are typically acquired at selected anatomic levels and orientations. A sagittal oblique 'candy-cane' image through the upper chest is particularly useful for demonstrating the aortic arch. In cases of type A aortic dissection, coronal and long-axis images through the aortic valve will exclude significant aortic insufficiency.

Real-time TrueFISP, which does not require breathholding or ECG triggering, is a useful alternative cine technique in patients who are poor breathholders or those with irregular cardiac rhythms.[17,18] An ultrashort TR of 2.8 ms and a reduced 128 matrix size is employed to minimize the acquisition time. This results in frame times of ~70–80 ms. Despite the lower spatial and temporal resolution with this technique, useful images of the thoracic aorta and aortic valve can usually be obtained.

'Black-blood' techniques

'Black-blood' techniques provide detailed imaging of the wall of the aorta and can be useful for evaluating abnormalities such as penetrating atherosclerotic ulcers and intramural hematomas. A number of different strategies are used.

ECG-triggered breathhold 'black-blood' turbo spin-echo (TSE)[19] utilizes a double inversion technique to null the blood signal. The first 180° inversion recovery pulse is non-slice-selective and occurs at the R-wave trigger. It inverts the magnetization in the entire tissue volume, including the blood signal. This is followed immediately by a slice-selective 'reversion' 180° pulse, which regenerates the magnetization in the slice to be imaged.[20] At a specific inversion time (TI), the blood signal is completely nulled. Blood flowing into the slice is nulled from the first 180° inversion pulse, resulting in a 'black-blood' appear-

ance. The image is acquired during diastole by incorporating a trigger delay after the R-wave. This has the effect of reducing cardiac motion artifact. Multiple lines of k-space are acquired in each R–R interval and the center of k-space is acquired at the TI. The entire image is produced over several heartbeats. T1-, T2-, or proton density-weighted images can be obtained, allowing improved characterization of tissues such as blood in an intramural hematoma or lipid in an atherosclerotic plaque.[21–24] ECG-triggered 'black-blood' HASTE (half Fourier acquisition single-shot turbo spin-echo) utilizes a 'black-blood' preparation to null signal from blood.[25] This is a single-shot technique, with the entire image being acquired in a single heartbeat. It is a useful alternative in patients who cannot hold their breath.

T1-weighted gradient-echo fat-saturated (GRE-FS) imaging

T1 GRE-FS imaging pre and post contrast injection is routinely used to evaluate pathology in the chest and abdomen. It provides an overview of the entire thoracic and abdominal aorta with adjacent structures.[26] It is particularly helpful in demonstrating intramural abnormalities, and may complement or replace 'black-blood' techniques in many situations. A 2D breathhold gradient-echo pulse sequence with fat saturation is used to cover the thorax or abdomen in an interleaved manner. A non-slice-selective preparatory pulse is employed to null the fat signal. Thirteen slices are acquired after each fat-saturation pulse, resulting in a total of 26 slices in a breathhold.[27] The thoracic or abdominal aorta is covered in axial, coronal, or sagittal orientations pre and post contrast injection. The postcontrast set of images is usually obtained following the MRA.

Contrast-enhanced magnetic resonance angiography (CE-MRA)

CE-MRA was originally developed in the early 1990s[28–30] and has rapidly overtaken time-of-flight (ToF) techniques as the method of choice for vascular imaging. CE-MRA is increasingly being used as a first-line investigation for evaluating disease in the carotid,[31–34] renal,[35–38] hepatic,[39] mesenteric, and lower-extremity arteries.[40–43] Likewise, it is ideally suited for assessment of aortic pathology.[30,41,44,45] Improvements in gradient subsystems and pulse sequence technology have expanded the abilities of CE-MRA, allowing unprecedented temporal and spatial information to be obtained in the same study. This has led to the development of newer CE-MRA techniques with near-real-time temporal resolution. (See also Chapter 15.)

Temporally resolved subsecond CE-MRA

Recent advances in gradient speed have made ultrashort TRs achievable for spoiled, 3D gradient-echo imaging. This has resulted in reduced acquisition times, permitting 3D CE-MRA to be implemented with near-real-time temporal resolution and small contrast doses.[46,47] This is particularly advantageous in the thoracic aorta, where high temporal resolution is useful for unwrapping overlying vascular structures and evaluating high-flow lesions such as shunts and dissections. Subsecond CE-MRA is also accurate in detecting other pathology in the thoracic aorta[48] and provides the same information as conventional CE-MRA in many situations. Subsecond CE-MRA is also useful in the abdomen, particularly for the diagnosis and characterization of arteriovenous fistulae. The basic pulse sequence is a 3D gradient-echo acquisition, similar to conventional CE-MRA. Asymmetric k-space scanning is utilized in all three axes, to further shorten the acquisition time. A TR <2 ms and a TE of 0.8 ms are used. The flip angle is typically 15°–25°. A 256 matrix size yields an in-plane resolution of 2.0 × 1.5 mm.[2] Six milliliters of gadolinium-based contrast is injected at 6 ml/s via an 18G cannula placed in an antecubital vein. The contrast injection and MR acquisition are started simultaneously, and patients are asked to breathhold in inspiration for the acquisition period or as long as is comfortable. Up to 50 3D volumes can be acquired in a single breathhold, the first 3D set serving as a mask for digital in-line subtraction from the remainder. Maximum-intensity projection (MIP) images can be automatically calculated, and the entire series can be viewed as a cine loop, with frame durations of 500–900 ms.

Although this represents true 3D acquisition, temporal resolution is purchased from through-plane resolution, while maintaining in-plane resolution. The result is quasi-projectional MRA with a limited number of partitions. This approach works well, because, in many circumstances, through-plane information is less helpful than temporal resolution. Furthermore, because of the rapid frame rates, image quality is usually diagnostic, even in patients who have trouble holding their breath. Moreover, because of the light contrast load, subsecond CE-MRA can be repeated and combined with conventional CE-MRA in order to provide a comprehensive assessment of vascular abnormalities.

Conventional CE-MRA

Conventional CE-MRA[29,30,44,49,50] provides detailed anatomic evaluation of the thoracic and abdominal aorta.

Although, in our experience, abnormalities in the thoracic aorta are already evident on the subsecond CE-MRA images, the near-isotropic spatial resolution of conventional CE-MRA is helpful in evaluating branch vessels and details of the vessel wall. The basic pulse sequence for conventional CE-MRA is a standard 3D, spoiled gradient-echo acquisition. The contrast transit time can be calculated from the subsecond CE-MRA or a separate bolus timing acquisition can be carried out. A 512 matrix size is used, yielding a typical voxel size of 1.5 × 0.8 × 1.5 mm.[3] We inject up to 40 ml of gadolinium at 2.5 ml/s via an 18G cannula placed in an antecubital vein. Images are acquired during breath holding. Subtracted 3D sets are calculated from the partition data, and these are subjected to MIP, volume-rendering (VR) or multiplanar reformatting (MPR) postprocessing algorithms.

Conventional CE-MRA is less useful for assessing the ascending thoracic aorta, which is commonly degraded by motion artifact from cardiac pulsation or obscured by overlapping vascular structures. This region is well evaluated by subsecond CE-MRA, which is essentially free from pulsation artifact.

Phase contrast MRA (PC-MRA)

PC-MRA may be used for calculating velocity and flow changes across a stenosis that has been detected on the CE-MRA.[51,52] PC-MRA utilizes velocity differences or phase shifts in moving spins to produce image contrast in vessels. Directional flow velocity is encoded in the phase of the MR signal by applying a directional bipolar gradient pulse. Relative to stationary tissues, spins flowing in the direction of the gradient pulse acquire a phase, the size of which is dependent on the size and duration of the gradient pulse. Phase can contain unique values only in the range $0–2\pi$ radians (0°–360°). Usually, half the available phase (π radians) is assigned to flow in the positive direction and the other half to flow in the negative direction. The velocity encoding (VENC) value determines the 'velocity bandwidth', or the maximum velocity that can be unambiguously encoded. The VENC is defined as the velocity that generates π radians (180°) of phase, or the maximum velocity that can be resolved. This is user-definable via the machine interface, and is typically in the range 150–200 cm/s in the aorta. If the VENC is too low, velocity aliasing or 'wraparound' will occur and may result in undesirable signal changes in the center of the lumen. If the VENC is set too high, then velocity contrast resolution is compromised, because only small phase increments separate spins flowing at different velocities. Choosing the correct VENC, therefore, requires some a priori information about the velocity ranges to be expected. PC-MRA results in two sets of data, namely

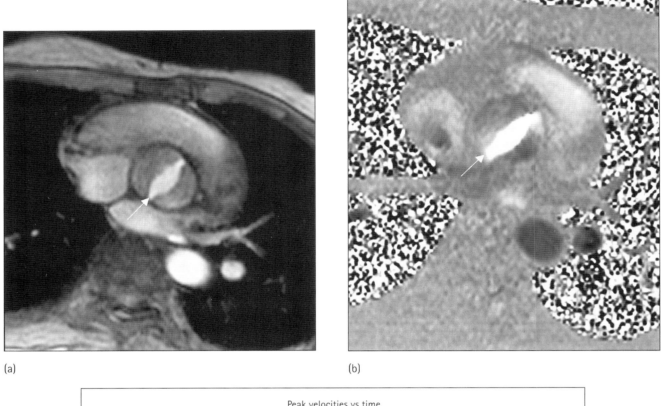

(a)

(b)

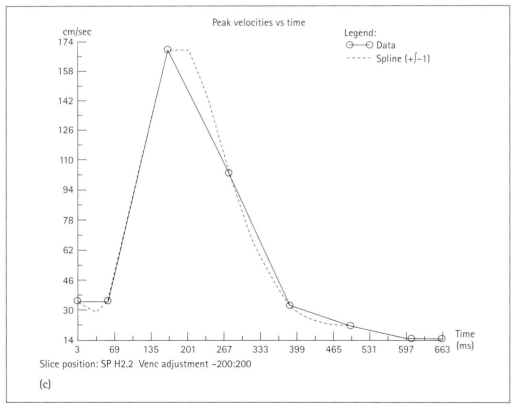

Peak velocities vs time

cm/sec

Legend:
⊖——⊖ Data
----- Spline (+∫−1)

Slice position: SP H2.2 Venc adjustment −200:200

(c)

Figure 16.1
Bicuspid aortic valve: (a) Magnitude and (b) phase images from flow quantification sequence showing bicuspid aortic valve.
(c) Time–velocity curves can be produced to evaluate the maximal velocity through the valve orifice.

phase images and magnitude images. The sequence can be either ECG-triggered or retrospectively gated. If through-plane velocity information is required, it is important that the 2D slice be orientated perpendicular to the vessel of interest and that the region of interest be positioned as close as reasonable to the center of the magnetic field to avoid additional sources of phase error.

Time–flow and time–velocity curves can be generated from the PC-MRA data, and peak flow and peak velocity values are calculated (Figure 16.1). Analysis of curve shape and slope may help decide whether stenoses are significant or not. These measurements can be useful for routine follow-up of stenoses.

Other techniques

The speed at which CE-MRA is carried out is primarily limited by the time it takes to acquire phase-encoding steps. This, in turn, is dependent on the performance of the gradient hardware. The limiting factor in gradient switching rates is ultimately physiological stimulation, as manifest in unwanted neuromuscular stimulation due to rapid gradient switching.

Recently, a number of parallel acquisition techniques have been described that attempt to improve temporal resolution by changing the way in which data are acquired and processed. With the SMASH (simultaneous acquisition of spatial harmonics)[53,54] and SENSE (sensitivity-encoding)[55,56] techniques, component coil signals in a radiofrequency (RF) coil array are used to partially encode spatial information by substituting for phase-encoding gradient steps that have been omitted. Each coil element encodes a small field-of-view (FOV) image with resultant overfolding due to k-space undersampling. The overfolding is unwrapped using the information present in the spatial sensitivity profiles of the individual coil elements. Either an initial calibration scan or some full-FOV k-space lines are acquired prior to the unfolding process. Parallel acquisition can in principle allow greatly enhanced imaging speed. The limiting factor at this point is diminished signal-to-noise ratio (SNR), which scales as the square root of the imaging time. At the time of writing, up to fourfold accelerations have been demonstrated in humans with reasonable SNR.

Techniques for CE-MRA have been described that allow more rapid acquisition of 3D data sets than with conventional imaging. Some of these employ a form of temporal interpolation or sliding window. With 3D TRICKS (time-resolved imaging of contrast kinetics),[57] the high spatial frequencies are sampled less frequently than the low spatial frequencies. As a result, high-contrast information is acquired more often than high-resolution information. By combination with 'nearest neighbor' high-spatial-frequency data, the full 3D data set is updated

at the rate determined by the low-spatial-frequency measurements.

Elements from all of the above approaches can be combined with conventional 3D CE-MRA pulse sequences and have the potential to produce unprecedented improvements in temporal resolution.

Aortic dissection

Aortic dissection results from a laceration of the aortic intima and inner layer of the aortic media, which allows blood to course freely along a false lumen in the outer third of the media.[58–60] There may be several entry and re-entry points between the true and false lumens, allowing the false lumen to enlarge over time and gradually compress the true lumen. The primary etiologic event in aortic dissection is somewhat controversial. Some authors propose that the intimal tear is the primary event, allowing the blood to spread through the outer two-thirds of the aortic media.[61] Others suggest that the etiology is related to spontaneous rupture of the aortic vasa vasorum, leading to subsequent intimal tear and aortic dissection.[62] Cystic medial necrosis is no longer regarded as the common structural disorder underlying aortic dissection.

Typically, the patient will present with tearing chest pain. Dissections are usually spontaneous events in middle-aged patients with poorly controlled hypertension and atherosclerosis. In younger patients, they may be associated with other entities such as aortic coarctation, Marfan syndrome, or Ehlers–Danlos syndrome. Dissection can also occur within aneurysmal aortic segments or as a result of iatrogenic injury to the vessel during catheter manipulations.

Complications of aortic dissection arise from either proximal or distal migration of the dissection to involve and occlude branch vessels of the aorta. Proximal migration of the dissection may cause occlusion of the coronary arteries or involvement of the aortic valve, causing aortic insufficiency. The dissection may cause aortic rupture into the pericardial and pleural spaces, which is commonly fatal. Distal migration of the dissection may cause occlusion or stenosis of the branches of the aorta. Involvement of the lumbar, mesenteric, and renal arteries may cause spinal cord infarction, bowel ischemia, or renal failure. The false lumen enlarges over time, and this may cause a functional blockage of branch vessels, such as the renal arteries.

Aortic dissections are classified as Stanford type A (i.e. involving the ascending thoracic aorta) or Stanford type B (i.e. without involvement of the ascending thoracic aorta). Type A dissections are surgical emergencies whereas type B dissections are treated medically. Dissections may also be divided further according to the

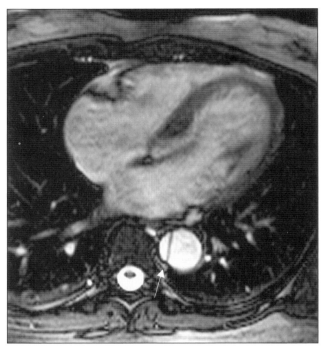

(a)

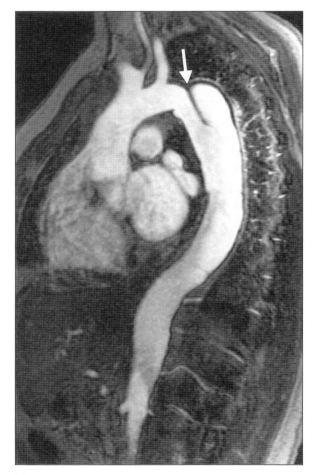

(b)

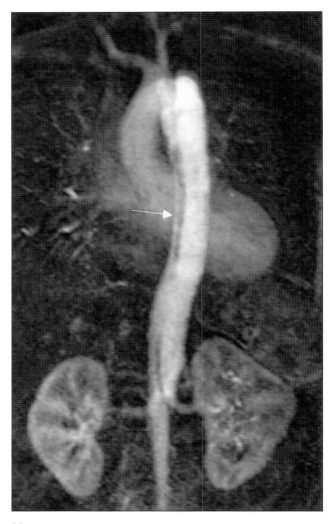

(c)

Figure 16.2

Type B aortic dissection: (a) axial TrueFISP image, (b) oblique
sagittal partition image from conventional MRA, and (c) coronal
MIP image from temporally resolved subsecond MRA showing
intimal flap (arrow) separating true lumen and false lumen.

DeBakey classification. Type 1 dissections involve the entire aorta. Type 2 dissections involve the ascending aorta only. Type 3 dissections involve the descending aorta only.

The main objective of imaging is not only to identify the presence of a dissection but also to distinguish type A from type B.

CMR has high sensitivity and specificity for the detection of dissection, and is now regarded as the gold standard for assessment of this abnormality[3,26,50] (Figure 16.2). In a study by Nienaber et al,[60] sensitivity and specificity for detection of aortic dissection were 93.8% and 87.1%, respectively, with conventional CT; 97.7% and 76.9%, respectively, with TEE; and 98.3% and 97.8%, respectively, with CMR. More recent studies have shown similar sensitivities and specificities for all three modalities.[26] CMR has the advantage of being able to assess the pericardial space, cardiac chambers, and aortic valve for complications arising from type A dissections. Because iodinated contrast is not used, it avoids the risk of renal failure, which is of particular importance in patients with extension of the dissection to involve the renal arteries. The primary disadvantage of CMR is the additional time it takes to carry out different pulse sequences, which is significant for critically ill patients with type A dissections.

There are a number of imaging features to assess during an evaluation for aortic dissection. The direct diagnostic signs are the presence of a double lumen and an intimal flap (Figure 16.2). The indirect signs include compression of the true lumen by the false lumen, thickening of the aortic wall, aortic insufficiency, branch vessel abnormality, ulcer-like projections from the aortic wall, pericardial effusion, and involvement of coronary artery ostia. The presence of extensive periluminal thrombus in the thoracic aorta should raise the suspicion of a thrombosed false lumen in an aortic dissection.

All of the above-mentioned techniques are well suited for diagnosis of aortic dissections. Single-shot TrueFISP has recently been shown to be highly accurate for diagnosis and classification of aortic dissection.[15] Because of the inherent high SNR from blood, both true and false lumen and dissection flap are clearly visible. In fact, the diagnosis is made on the TrueFISP localizers in many instances. Moreover, the technique can be implemented without breathholding in a total imaging time of <2 min. This is ideally suited to critically ill patients who cannot hold their breath. Breathhold cine TrueFISP can be used to evaluate aortic insufficiency and hemopericardium in type A dissections; however, these patients are rarely fit enough to suspend respirations. In these situations, non ECG-triggered real-time TrueFISP, although of lower spatial resolution, can be a useful alternative.[17,18] T1 GRE-FS imaging pre and post contrast is essential for detecting intramural hematoma or thrombosed false lumen associated with a dissection (Figure 16.3). Recent intramural hemorrhage will appear hyperintense on noncontrast

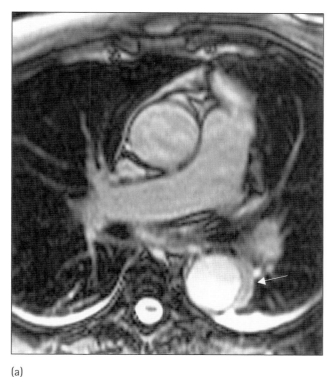
(a)

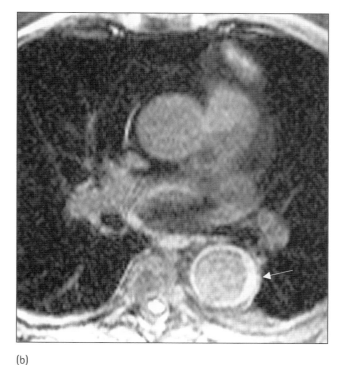
(b)

Figure 16.3
Thrombosed false lumen of type B aortic dissection: (a) Axial TrueFISP, (b) axial precontrast T1 GRE-FS, and   *(continued on next page)*

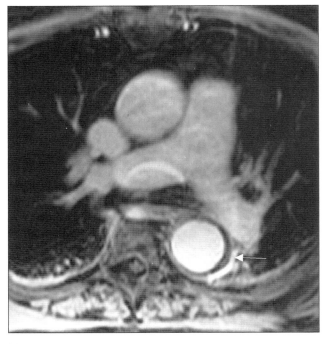

(c)

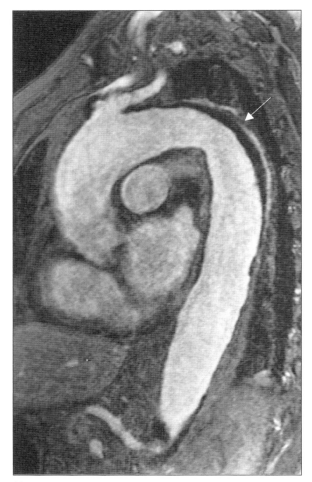

(e)

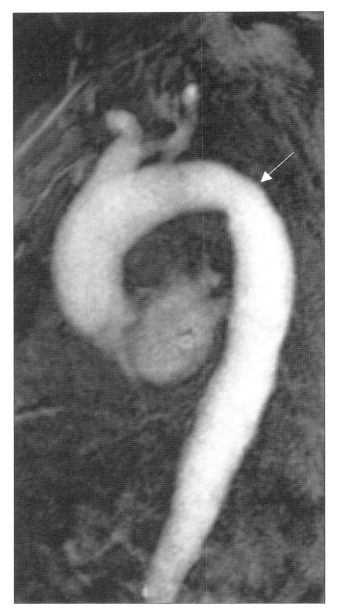

(d)

Figure 16.3 continued
(c) axial post-contrast T1 GRE-FS images showing eccentric periluminal thrombus in the descending thoracic aorta (arrow). The thrombus is hyperintense on the precontrast T1-weighted image, suggesting recent hemorrhage. (d) Sagittal oblique temporally resolved subsecond MRA showing apparent diffuse narrowing of the upper descending thoracic aorta (arrow). (e) Sagittal oblique MRA partition image showing a diffuse eccentric thrombus in the upper descending thoracic aorta (arrow). The shape and extent of the thrombus resembles a type B dissection, suggesting that this represents the thrombosed lumen of an aortic dissection.

T1-weighted images. It may also be very hard to distinguish intramural hematoma from a thrombosed false lumen of an aortic dissection. CE-MRA is also accurate in diagnosing aortic dissections; however, the diagnosis is usually made already on the TrueFISP images. CE-MRA is useful for assessing the proximal and distal extent of the dissection and its involvement of branch vessels. A separate CE-MRA study of the abdomen may be required to assess distal dissections extending into the abdominal aorta, particularly to evaluate involvement of the renal and mesenteric vasculature. Subsecond CE-MRA can demonstrate sequential filling of the true and false lumens, and may help identify the entry and exit points of the dissection. In addition, subsecond CE-MRA can clearly demonstrate pseudoaneurysms or intramural hematomas.

There are potential pitfalls of interpretation with CMR. A thrombosed false lumen of an aortic dissection may be mistaken for intramural clot (Figure 16.3). The shape and extent of the thrombus may be helpful in distinguishing between the two entities. Pulsation artifacts can occur in the ascending thoracic aorta on CE-MRA, and may be mistaken for an intimal flap. This usually clarified using other pulse sequences, such as SSFP or temporally resolved subsecond CE-MRA.

Intramural hematoma (IMH)

Intramural hematoma (IMH) and penetrating atherosclerotic ulcer (PAU; see below) were virtually unknown when aortic imaging was carried out using aortography. In the current era of 3D high-resolution imaging of the aorta with CT, CMR, and TEE, these two disorders have become increasingly recognized. The distinctions from classic aortic dissection have not always been clear.

Although classic aortic dissections begin with an intimal tear that allows blood to course rapidly along a plane in the outer third of an intrinsically diseased media, an IMH is thought to begin with rupture of the vasa vasorum of the aortic wall. This results in a circumferential blood-containing space within the media, without evidence of intimal discontinuity. IMH was originally described as a 'dissection without intimal tear'.[63] It may occur spontaneously in hypertensive patients or following blunt chest trauma. It has been speculated that IMH may also originate from ulceration in an atherosclerotic aorta. IMH usually occurs in the descending thoracic aorta. The incidence of IMH detected by CT and CMR is 13% in patients with acute aortic syndromes.[63] Patients are typically older and usually present with excruciating chest or back pain, similar to aortic dissection. The incidence of ischemic complications due to branch vessel occlusion is lower than aortic dissection; however, the frequency of aortic rupture is higher, occurring in up to one-third of cases.[64]

The diagnosis of IMH relies on visualization of intramural blood and evidence of localized increased wall thickness.[65] Both CT and TEE are useful for detecting IMH. This will appear as a high-attenuation, crescent-shaped abnormality within the wall of the aorta on non-contrast CT. TEE will also diagnose IMH, but may have difficulty differentiating it from severe atherosclerosis with wall thickening. CMR is probably the most useful modality because of its capability of multiplanar imaging and comprehensive characterization of the hematoma.

Intramural blood is best detected with T1-weighted GRE or TSE techniques. IMH appears as a curvilinear area of altered signal intensity within the vessel wall. The signal intensity varies depending on the age of the clot. Subacute IMH will appear hyperintense on T1-weighted images; however acute IMH may be isointense.[63,66] One potential pitfall for detection of IMH with CMR rests with CE-MRA. The MIP images will not demonstrate IMH, since they only depict a cast of the lumen and provide no information about mural abnormalities. IMH should be evident, however, on the unsubtracted partition images from the MRA.

Penetrating atherosclerotic ulcer (PAU)

PAUs ulcerate and disrupt the internal elastic lamina, burrowing deeply through the intima into the aortic media.[67,68] The plaque may precipitate a localized intramedial dissection associated with a variable amount of hematoma in the aortic wall, may break through into the adventitia forming a pseudoaneurysms, or may rupture completely into the right or left hemithorax. Ulceration of an atheroma occurs in patients with advanced atherosclerosis. The localized dissection is limited by areas of severe calcification associated with locally advanced atherosclerotic disease. The site of entry into the dissection is the ulcer itself.

The clinical presentation of patients with PAU is similar to aortic dissection and IMH. Patients typically have chest or back pain of excruciating intensity. The incidence of aortic rupture is slightly higher compared with dissection and IMH.[64]

The main imaging findings include an ulcer crater surrounded by varying degrees of intramural hemorrhage. PAU can be diagnosed with several imaging modalities, including aortography, CT, CMR, and TEE.

With CMR, PAUs are best depicted on postcontrast T1 GRE-FS images or the partition images from a conventional CE-MRA.[69] They appear as a contrast-filled outpouchings of the aorta in the absence of a false lumen or intimal flap and often in the presence of extensive aortic calcification (Figure 16.4).

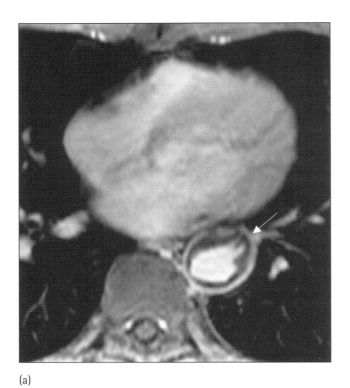

(a)

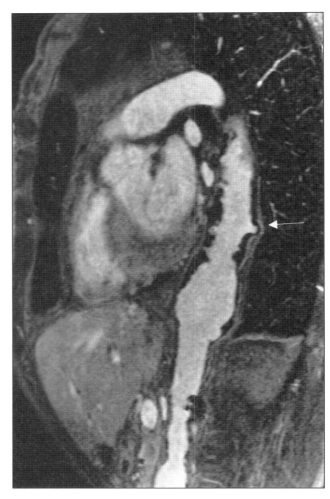

(b)

Figure 16.4
Penetrating atherosclerotic ulcer (PAU): (a) postcontrast axial T1 GRE-FS image and (b) oblique sagittal partition image showing PAU (arrow) in the wall of the descending thoracic aorta.

Aortic aneurysm

The normal values of aortic diameter have been reported and are related to age and body surface area. A diameter >4 cm in the ascending thoracic aorta is regarded as an aneurysm and a lower value is considered ectasia. A diameter >3 cm in the descending thoracic and abdominal aorta is considered aneurysmal. The aortic wall thickness should be <4 mm. The aortic diameter gradually increases over time. The normal expansion rate over 10 years is between 1 and 2 mm and is greater for patients with an aorta that is larger than normal.

Aneurysms of the aorta are relatively common and are important because of their potentially reversible lethal consequences.[70] Aneurysms can be classified as true or false. True aneurysms involve all layers of the aortic wall and result from degeneration of elastin fibers within the media. False aneurysms, or pseudoaneurysms, result from a contained perforation of the vessel wall where the actual wall is formed by the surrounding adventitia and perivascular tissues. Pseudoaneurysms commonly have a narrow 'neck' leading to the vessel lumen. Aneurysms can be further subdivided depending on their extent into localized or diffuse. They can also be subdivided into fusiform (i.e. with circumferential involvement of the vessel wall) or saccular (i.e. with involvement of a portion of wall).

Any disease that results in weakening of the aortic wall can result in dilatation. The commonest cause is atherosclerosis, where aneurysms most commonly affect the descending thoracic and abdominal aorta. They tend to be fusiform, involving long segments of the aorta. Atherosclerotic aneurysms are commonly true aneurysms, but may form pseudoaneurysms when a contained rupture occurs. Aneurysms caused by syphilis, Marfan syndrome, Ehlers–Danlos syndrome, and poststenotic dilatation from aortic stenosis are typically localized in the ascending aorta. The sinotubular junction is preserved in aortic stenosis but markedly dilated in the other entities. Traumatic aneurysms are pseudoaneurysms and typically result from an aortic transection. They are the second most common type of thoracic aneurysm and usually occur at the junction between the aortic arch and descending aorta. Mycotic aneurysms are rare and result from nonsyphilitic infection. Predisposing factors include intravenous drug abuse and immunocompromise. In addition to the aneurysm, features supporting an infectious source include periaortic gas and adjacent vertebral osteomyelitis.

The main complication of aortic aneurysms is rupture. The incidence of rupture of an abdominal aortic aneurysm (AAA) is related to size. Aneurysms with diameter <4 cm rupture in 10%, 4–5 cm in 23%, 5–7 cm in 25%, 7–10 cm in 46%, and >10 cm in 60%. AAAs usually rupture into the retroperitoneum, commonly on the left-hand side. Rarely, they can rupture directly into the gastrointestinal tract or inferior vena cava. AAAs may be a source of peripheral embolization or infection, and may cause spontaneous occlusion of the aorta. The 5-year survival rate for AAA without surgery is 17% while with surgery it is 50–60%. Thoracic aortic aneurysms usually rupture into the mediastinum, pericardium, pleural, or extrapleural space. Rarely, they cause an aortobronchopulmonary fistula. Untreated, the 5-year survival rate for thoracic aortic aneurysms is 19%.

The primary objectives of imaging in the assessment of aortic aneurysms are to define the size, extent, rate of growth, presence of thrombus or dissection, and involvement of adjacent structures, including the aortic valve.

CMR can consistently and comprehensively provide all this information. It has the ability to image in multiple planes, and can combine several pulse sequences to fully characterize the pathology.[7,71] Aortography may underestimate the size of an aneurysm if significant periluminal thrombus is present, and may fail to fully define saccular structures due to stagnant intra-aneurysmal flow. CT uses iodinated contrast and can only acquire axial images. TEE cannot image the entire aorta.

All of the previously mentioned CMR techniques are accurate in detecting aneurysms; however, CE-MRA is most useful for depicting location, extent and exact diameter (Figure 16.5). CMR is frequently utilized as a follow-up tool for monitoring the progression of disease, and, therefore, in order to produce consistent results, vessel dimensions should be measured at the same anatomic locations each time. It is important to remember that MIP images represent a cast of the lumen; therefore, measurements should be obtained from source images where the vessel wall is visible. Where aneurysms involve the ascending aorta or sinuses of Valsalva, concomitant aortic valve disease can be evaluated using cine imaging of the heart.

Aortic stenoses

Stenoses in the thoracic aorta are commonly caused by atherosclerosis, but are usually multifocal and rarely flow-limiting. Atherosclerotic narrowing may be more severe in the abdominal aorta, particularly in the infrarenal aorta, where it can cause Leriche syndrome. Coarctation of the aorta is an important cause of stenosis in the thoracic aorta, and is discussed in the next section. Pseudocoarctation resembles a true coarctation but is caused by aortic kinking just distal to the origin of the left subclavian artery. It is not hemodynamically flow-limiting and therefore is not associated with collaterals. Stenotic lesions can also occur at the site of surgical anastomoses following repair of aortic aneurysms. Less common causes of aortic stenosis include extrinsic compression from tumor or rare inflammatory conditions such as Takayasu's arteritis.

CE-MRA is the most useful technique for evaluating stenoses in both the thoracic and abdominal aorta. Image postprocessing on the 3D data set yields MIP, VR, and MPR images allowing the abnormality to be viewed in multiple orientations. Temporally resolved subsecond CE-MRA will accurately depict aortic stenoses, but is particularly useful in hemodynamically significant lesions such as coarctations, where it demonstrates gradual filling of chest wall collaterals. Multiplanar TrueFISP or T1 GRE-FS images are useful for evaluating an adjacent mass causing extrinsic compression. PC-MRA can be used to measure velocity and flow both proximal and distal to a stenosis, and helps assess the significance of a stenosis.[72] It may be more useful in monitoring disease progression over time; however, it is important to obtain measurements in similar anatomic locations in order to produce accurate and consistent results.

Congenital anomalies

Coarctation of the aorta

Coarctation of the aorta is a common congenital anomaly resulting from an abnormality of the media, and causes narrowing in the upper thoracic aorta.

There are two types of aortic coarctation. The first is localized coarctation, also known as adult or postductal type. In this, there is a short discrete narrowing at the junction of the aortic arch and descending aorta, close to the ligamentum arteriosum. It is usually asymptomatic and is detected as an incidental finding later in life. Coexistent cardiac anomalies are uncommon. The second type is diffuse coarctation, also known as infantile or preductal type. In this type, there is hypoplasia of a variable portion of the aortic arch between the innominate artery and the ductus arteriosus. Blood reaches the descending aorta via multiple collaterals. Intercostal arteries represent the most common collateral pathway, and may cause significant rib notching after ~10 years due to dilatation.

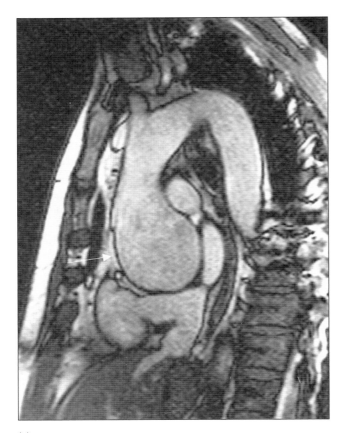

(a)

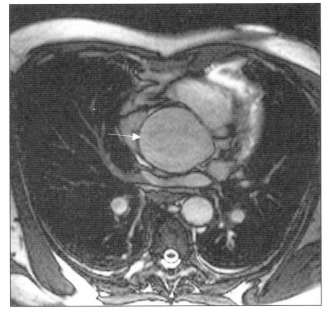

(b)

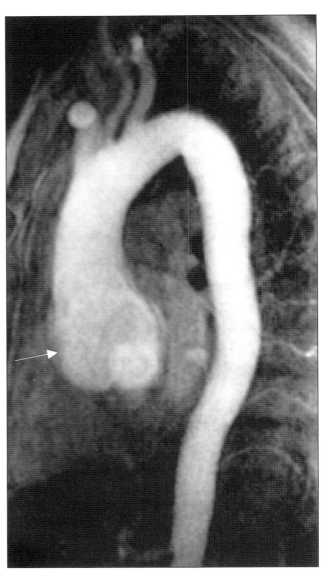

(c)

Figure 16.5

Thoracic aortic aneurysm: (a) oblique sagittal TrueFISP image, (b) axial TrueFISP, and (c) oblique sagittal MIP image from subsecond MRA showing an aneurysm of the ascending thoracic aorta (arrow) at the level of the sinuses of Valsalva.

This type presents shortly after birth and coexistent cardiac anomalies are common.

Coarctation of the aorta is associated with bicuspid aortic valve (25–50% cases), which may result in aortic stenosis later in life. It is also associated with intracardiac malformations such as patent ductus arteriosus (33% cases), atrial septal defect, and ventricular septal defects. Turner syndrome, cerebral berry aneurysms, and mycotic aneurysms may also occur with coarctation.

CE-MRA is the best technique for evaluating aortic coarctation. Image postprocessing of 3D sets allows the anomaly to be viewed from different angles. Temporally resolved CE-MRA provides better demonstration of collateral pathways, and can give an estimate of the hemodynamic severity of the coarctation. PC-MRA allows velocity and flow to be measured proximal and distal to the stenosis. These measurements may be useful for monitoring the abnormality over time. In addition, cine imaging of the heart can be carried out at the same time to look for coexistent cardiac abnormalities.

Aortic arch anomalies

There are a number of congenital abnormalities that affect the aortic arch, including left aortic arch with aberrant right subclavian artery, double aortic arch, and right-sided aortic arch. All of these anomalies result from a disruption of the hypothetical double aortic arch of Edwards.[73]

The commonest thoracic aortic arch anomaly, occurring in 0.5% of the population, is the left aortic arch with aberrant right subclavian artery. The right subclavian artery arises from the descending thoracic aorta distal to the origin of the left subclavian artery. It can originate directly from the aorta or can arise from an aortic diverticulum (diverticulum of Kommerell). The aberrant right subclavian courses posterior to the esophagus, but, because a vascular ring is not intact, it does not cause dyspnea or dysphagia. The right aortic arch passes to the right of the trachea and descends to the right or left of the thoracic spine. The right aortic arch with mirror-image branching is the second most common aortic arch anomaly and results from interruption of the embryonic left arch between left subclavian and descending aorta. In type 1, the left aortic arch is interrupted distal to the ductus arteriosus. There is no retroesophageal component and no vascular ring. It is nearly always associated with cyanotic congenital heart disease. In type 2, the interruption of the left aortic arch occurs proximal to the ductus arteriosus. This produces a true vascular ring and is rarely associated with congenital heart disease. The right aortic arch with isolated left subclavian artery results from interruption of the embryonic left arch between the left common carotid and left subclavian arteries and between the left ductus and descending aorta. There is a direct connection between the left subclavian and left pulmonary artery. The left common carotid arises as the first branch and the left subclavian connects to the left pulmonary artery through a patent ductus arteriosus. It is associated with tetralogy of Fallot and produces a congenital subclavian steal syndrome. The double aortic arch is a common cause of a vascular ring, but is usually asymptomatic. Two separate arches arise from a single ascending aorta, and each arch joins to form a single descending aorta.

All of these conditions are best assessed using CE-MRA.[74,75] In these situations, 3D postprocessing techniques can be used to great effect, allowing the abnormality to be viewed from different orientations. Cine imaging of the heart should always accompany an assessment for congenital abnormalities of the aorta in order to detect accompanying lesions in the heart.

Vascular shunts

Congenital vascular shunts can be intracardiac, such as atrial or ventricular septal defects, or extracardiac, such as a patent ductus arteriosus. Shunts can flow either left to right or right to left between systemic and pulmonary circulations. Eisenmenger syndrome occurs when pulmonary hypertension develops as a result of a longstanding left-to-right shunt and causes reversal of shunt direction from right to left.

Patent ductus arteriosus (PDA) is the main congenital shunt that affects the aorta (Figure 16.6). It results from persistence of the embryonic communication between the left pulmonary artery and the descending thoracic aorta. The ductus arteriosus is normally closed by 1 year in 99% cases. Most PDAs are usually asymptomatic, but may cause left-ventricular failure in neonates if the left-to-right shunt is large. A right-to-left shunt may occur across a PDA if Eisenmenger pulmonary hypertension develops.

Large shunts can be identified using morphologic imaging techniques such as TrueFISP. Temporally resolved subsecond CE-MRA is the most useful technique for detecting shunts and determining the direction of flow. Because only small doses of contrast are required each time, acquisitions can be repeated multiple times until the shunt has been accurately characterized. Furthermore, an estimate of shunt fraction can be obtained by generating time–intensity curves at different anatomic locations. A conventional CE-MRA is usually required to provided more detailed anatomic information about the shunt. PC-MRA can be utilized to calculate flow and velocity across the shunt.

Inflammatory diseases of the aorta

Aortitis results in weakening and thickening of the aortic wall, and this may progress to either focal dilatation or stenosis and occlusion of the aorta. There are many causes

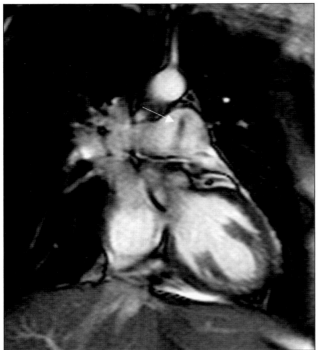

(a)

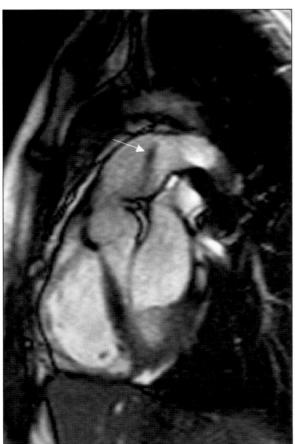

(b)

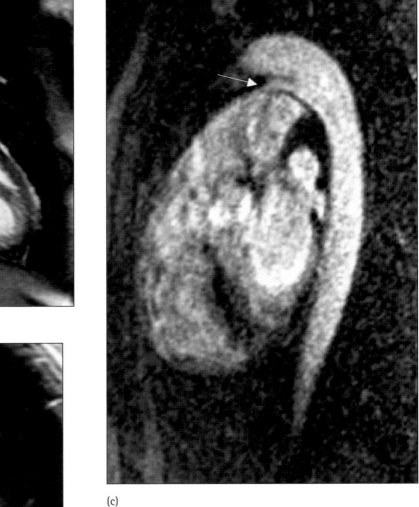

(c)

Figure 16.6

Patent ductus arteriosus: (a) coronal and (b) sagittal TrueFISP images showing a flow jet (arrow) from the descending aorta into the left main pulmonary artery, suggesting the presence of a patent ductus arteriosus. (c) Oblique sagittal partition image from MRA showing direct communication between pulmonary trunk and upper descending thoracic aorta (arrow) indicating the presence of a patent ductus arteriosus. (Images courtesy of FS Pereles MD, Northwestern University, Chicago, IL.)

of aortitis, including Takayasu's aortitis, giant cell arteritis, Behçet's disease, Cogan's disease, and aortitis with retroperitoneal fibrosis (Ormond's disease).

Takayasu's aortitis is a chronic inflammatory panarteritis of unknown pathogenesis affecting segments of the aorta, main aortic branches, and pulmonary arteries. It usually occurs in younger women, and produces diffuse wall thickening in the aorta with stenosis and occlusion of the aorta and branch vessels.

Asymmetric wall thickening in the aorta is best detected with T1 GRE-FS imaging and the partition images from CE-MRA.[76] CE-MRA is useful for demonstrating stenoses and occlusion of the aorta and branch vessels, and also outlines the extent of involvement of vascular structures.

Aortic trauma

Aortic transection is a relatively common complication of high-speed deceleration injury.[77] The site of injury is usually just distal to the origin of the left subclavian artery at the point of attachment of the ligamentum arteriosum (95% of cases). Tears also occur at the origins of the great vessels from the aortic arch, above the diaphragm, and in the descending aorta.[78] Transection of the aorta caused by motor vehicle accidents is fatal in 90% of cases. In survivors of aortic injury, the adventitia is intact and prevents exsanguination. If left untreated, 90% of survivors will die. Fifty percent rupture within the first 24 hours and most of the rest within the next few weeks. Only 2% of patients survive with a chronic pseudoaneurysm.[79]

Aortography remains the gold standard for evaluation of aortic trauma; however, it requires transport of the injured patient to the cath lab for a potentially lengthy procedure and has a 10% complication rate in that setting.[80,81] TEE can also evaluate the aorta rapidly in an injured patient, and has the advantage of being portable, allowing the examination to proceed at the bedside or in the operating room. However, the entire aorta may not be visualized with TEE, and branches are difficult to see well in a substantial proportion of patients. Spiral CT has become the investigation of choice in the setting of aortic trauma. A normal CT in the setting of trauma virtually excludes an aortic transection.[77] Reported sensitivities and specificities for detection of aortic injury are 100% and 83%, respectively, with CT and 92% and 99%, respectively, for conventional angiography.[82] Because aortic injuries usually occur following motor vehicle accidents, these patients usually have other life-threatening injuries that make CMR impractical. CMR is, however, appropriate in patients suspected of having chronic or missed aortic tears.

The imaging features of aortic injury include small intimal flap, hemorrhage localized to intima or media, pseudoaneurysm (Figure 16.7), mediastinal hemorrhage, abnormal contour of aortic lumen, or some combination of these.[78] Dissection of the media over more than a centimeter is rare in traumatic tears. The presence of a pericardial effusion is a bad prognostic sign in aortic injury.

The most useful sequences for detection of aortic injury include T1-weighted GRE-FS and CE-MRA. Intramural hemorrhage is visualized on T1-weighted imaging. Contour abnormalities and pseudoaneurysms are well seen with CE-MRA. Because of the excellent edge definition with TrueFISP, this technique may be useful for detecting localized intimal flaps or abnormal contours of the aortic wall.

Future developments

Whole-body 3 T systems are now becoming commercially available and have the potential to produce significant increases in SNR and contrast-to-noise ratio for most pulse sequences. This may substantially improve image quality with CE-MRA, allowing better definition of anatomic structures.

MR guidance, which was initially used for procedures such as biopsies, is now being investigated for endovascular intervention. Compared with other imaging modalities, CMR not only has the advantage of being able to depict vessel morphology but also can assess functional changes. This allows the efficacy of an endovascular intervention to be assessed directly at the time of the procedure. MR-guided angioplasty and stent placement has been successfully carried out in animal models, and has the potential to revolutionize endovascular treatment of disease in humans.[83–86]

Conclusions

There are numerous pulse sequences available now for evaluating the diverse pathology, which affects the thoracic aorta. Preliminary imaging using TrueFISP and pre- and postcontrast T1 GRE-FS is usually required to assess morphology of the aorta and adjacent structures. CE-MRA is the mainstay of the investigative approach. The addition of temporally resolved CE-MRA is particularly useful for assessing high-flow vascular lesions such as shunts, while at the same time not adding much to the overall contrast load. PC-MRA may help further characterize stenotic lesions, and can be useful for monitoring progression of disease.

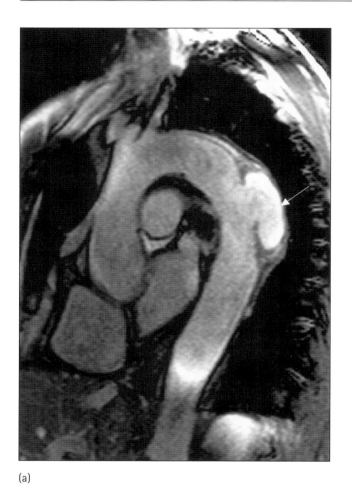

(a)

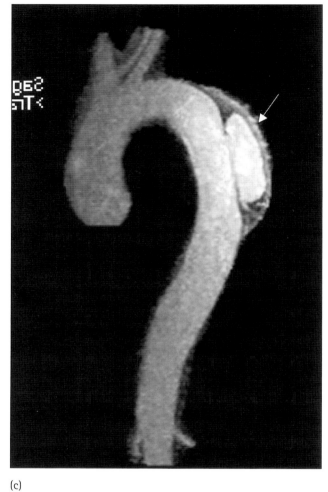

(c)

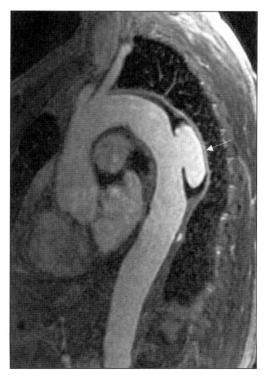

(b)

Figure 16.7

Chronic pseudoaneurysm: (a) oblique sagittal TrueFISP image, (b) oblique sagittal partition image, and (c) oblique sagittal MIP image from conventional MRA showing a pseudoaneurysm (arrow) arising from the posterior surface of the proximal descending thoracic aorta. The adventitia is intact and is the only structure preventing catastrophic hemorrhage.

References

1. Waugh JR, Sacharias N. Arteriographic complications in the DSA era. Radiology 1992; 182:243–6.

2. Mirvis S, Pais S, Gens D. Thoracic aortic rupture: advantages of intraarterial digital subtraction angiography. AJR 1986; 146:987–91.

3. Hartnell GG. Imaging of aortic aneurysms and dissections: CT and MRI. J Thorac Imaging 2001; 16:35–46.

4. Rubin GD. Helical CT angiography of the thoracic aorta. J Thorac Imaging 1997; 12:128–49.

5. Hidajat N, Maurer J, Schroder R, et al. Radiation exposure in spiral computed tomography – dose distribution and dose reduction. Invest Radiol 1999; 34:51–7.

6. Scott C, Keane M, Ferrari V. Echocardiographic evaluation of the thoracic aorta. Semin Roentgenol 2001; 36:325–33.

7. Roberts DA. Magnetic resonance imaging of thoracic aortic aneurysm and dissection. Semin Roentgenol 2001; 36:295–308.

8. Fattori R, Nienaber CA. MRI of acute and chronic aortic pathology: pre-operative and post-operative evaluation. J Magn Reson Imaging 1999; 10:741–50.

9. Oppelt A, Graumann R, Barfuss H. FISP – a new fast MRI sequence. Electromedica 1986; 54:15–18.

10. Fang W, Pereles FS, Bundy J, et al. Evaluating left ventricular function using real-time TrueFISP: a comparison with conventional techniques. In: Proceedings of the Annual Meeting of the International Society for Magnetic Resonance in Medicine, 2000:308.

11. Deimling M, Heid O. Magnetization prepared TrueFISP imaging. In: Proceedings of the Annual Meeting of the International Society for Magnetic Resonance in Medicine, 1994:495.

12. Carr J, Simonetti O, Bundy J, et al. Cine MR angiography of the heart with segmented true fast imaging with steady-state precession. Radiology 2001; 219:828–34.

13. Bundy J, Simonetti O, Laub G, Finn JP. Segmented TrueFISP imaging of the heart. Proceedings of the Annual Meeting of the International Society for Magnetic Resonance in Medicine, 1999:1282.

14. Barkhausen J, Ruehm S, Goyen M, et al. MR evaluation of ventricular function: true fast imaging with steady-state precession versus fast low-angle shot cine MR imaging: feasibility study. Radiology 2001; 219:264–9.

15. Pereles F, McCarthy R, Baskaran V, Carr J, et al. Thoracic aortic dissection and aneurysm: evaluation with non-enhanced TrueFISP MR angiography in less than 4 minutes. Radiology 2002; 223:270–4.

16. Rehwald W, Kim R, Simonetti O, et al. Theory of high-speed MR imaging of the human heart with the selective line acquisition mode. Radiology 2001; 220:540–7.

17. Barkhausen J, Goyen M, Ruhm SG, et al. Assessment of ventricular function with single breath-hold real-time steady-state free precession cine MR imaging. AJR 2002; 178:731–5.

18. Lee VS, Resnick D, Bundy JM, et al. Cardiac function: MR evaluation in one breath hold with real-time true fast imaging with steady state precession. Radiology 2002; 222:835–42.

19. Simonetti OP, Finn JP, White RD, et al. 'Black-blood' T2-weighted inversion-recovery MR imaging of the heart. Radiology 1996; 199:49–57.

20. Edelman R, Chien D, Kim D. Fast selective black blood MR imaging. Radiology 1991; 181:655–60.

21. Fayad ZA, Nahar T, Fallon J, et al. In vivo magnetic resonance evaluation of atherosclerotic plaques in human thoracic aorta: a comparison with transesophageal echocardiography. Circulation 2000; 101:2503–9.

22. Fayad Z, Fuster V, Fallon J, et al. Noninvasive in vivo human coronary artery lumen and wall imaging using black-blood magnetic resonance imaging. Circulation 2000; 102:506–10.

23. Fayad Z, Fuster V. Characterization of atherosclerotic plaques by magnetic resonance imaging. Ann NY Acad Sci 2000; 902:173–86.

24. Fayad Z, Fuster V. Clinical imaging of the high-risk or vulnerable atherosclerotic pla. Circ Res 2001; 89:305–16.

25. Stehling MK, Holzknecht NG, Laub G, et al. Single-shot T1 and T2 weighted magnetic resonance imaging of the heart with black blood: preliminary experience. Magma 1996; 4:231–40.

26. Summers RM, Sostman HD, Spritzer CE, et al. Fast spoiled gradient-recalled MR imaging of thoracic aortic dissection: preliminary clinical experience at 1.5 T. Magn Reson Imaging 1996; 14:1–9.

27. Finn J, Miller F, McCarthy R, Pereles F. Segmented fat-saturation for dynamic, multislice imaging of the pancreas. In: Proceedings of the Radiological Society of North America, 86th Annual Scientific Meeting, Chicago, 2000.

28. Prince MR, Yucel EK, Kaufman JA, et al. Dynamic gadolinium-enhanced three-dimensional abdominal MR arteriography. Magn Reson Imaging 1993; 3:877–81.

29. Prince M. Gadolinium-enhanced MR aortography. Radiology 1994; 191:155–64.

30. Prince MR, Narasimham DL, Stanley JC, et al. Breath-hold gadolinium-enhanced MR angiography of the abdominal aorta and its major branches. Radiology 1995; 197:785–92.

31. Carr JC, Ma J, Deshpande V, et al. High-resolution breath-hold contrast-enhanced MR angiography of the entire carotid circulation. AJR 2002; 178:543–9.

32. Carr JC, Shaibani A, Russell E, Finn JP. Contrast-enhanced magnetic resonance angiography of the carotid circulation. Top Magn Reson Imaging 2001; 12:349–57.

33. Scarabino T, Carriero A, Giannatempo GM, et al. Contrast-enhanced MR angiography (CE MRA) in the study of carotid stenosis: comparison with digital subtraction angiography (DSA). J Neuroradiol 1999; 25:87–91.

34. Scarabino T, Carriero A, Magarelli N, et al. MR angiography in carotid stenosis: a comparison of three techniques. Eur J Radiol 1998; 28:117–25.

35. Holland G, Dougherty L, Carpenter J, et al. Breath-hold ultrafast three-dimensional gadolinium-enhanced MR angiography of the aorta and the renal and other visceral arteries. AJR 1996; 166:971–81.

36. Debatin J, Spritzer C, Grist T, et al. Imaging of the renal arteries: value of MR angiography. AJR 1991; 157:981–90.

37. Grist T, Kennell T, Sproat I, et al. A prospective evaluation of renal MRA for detecting renal artery stenosis in 35 consecutive patients. In: Book of Abstracts, Society of Magnetic Resonance in Medicine, 12th Annual Meeting, 1993:187.

38. Kim D, Edelman R, Kent E, et al. Abdominal aorta and renal artery stenosis: evaluation with MR angiography. Radiology 1990; 174:727–31.

39. Carr J, Nemcek A, Abecassis M, et al. Pre-operative evaluation of the entire hepatic vasculature in living liver donors using contrast-enhanced MR angiography and TrueFISP. J Vasc Inter Radiol 2003; 14:441–9.

40. Koelemay MJ, Lijmer JG, Stoker J, et al. Magnetic resonance angiography for the evaluation of lower extremity arterial disease: a meta-analysis. JAMA 2001; 14:1338–45.

41. Grist TM. MRA of the abdominal aorta and lower extremities. J Magn Reson Imaging 2000; 11:32–43.

42. Adamis M, Li W, Wielopolski P, et al. Dynamic contrast-enhanced subtraction MR angiography of the lower extremities: initial evaluation with a multisection two-dimensional time-of-flight sequence. Radiology 1995; 196:689–95.

43. Morasch M, Collins J, Pereles F, et al. MR Angiography of the lower extremities. J Vasc Surg 2003; 37:62–71.

44. Krinsky GA, Reuss PM, Lee VS, et al. Thoracic aorta: comparison of single-dose breath-hold and double-dose non-breath-hold gadolinium-enhanced three-dimensional MR angiography. AJR 1999; 173:145–50.

45. Prince MR, Narasimham DL, Jacoby WT, et al. Three-dimensional gadolinium-enhanced MR angiography of the thoracic aorta. AJR 1996; 166:1387–97.

46. Carr J, McCarthy R, Laub G, et al. Subsecond, contrast-enhanced 3D MR angiography: a new technique for dynamic imaging of the vasculature. In: Proceedings of the Annual Meeting of the International Society for Magnetic Resonance in Medicine, 2001:302.

47. Finn JP, Baskaran V, Carr J, et al. Low-dose, contrast-enhanced 3D MR angiography of the thorax with sub-second temporal resolution. Radiology 2002; 224:896–904.

48. Carr J, Baskaran V, McCarthy R, et al. Accuracy and incremental value of TrueFISP, subsecond MRA and high resolution MRA in the evaluation of diseases of the thoracic aorta. In: Proceedings of the Radiological Society of North America, 87th Annual Scientific Meeting, Chicago, 2001:264.

49. Krinsky GA, Rofsky NM, DeCorato DR, et al. Thoracic aorta: comparison of gadolinium-enhanced three-dimensional MR angiography with conventional MR imaging. Radiology 1997; 202:183–93.

50. Prince MR, Narasimham DL, Jacoby WT, et al. Three-dimensional gadolinium-enhanced MR angiography of the thoracic aorta. AJR 1996; 166:1387–97.

51. Dumoulin CL, Yucel EK, Vock P, et al. Two and three dimensional phase contrast MR angiography of the abdomen. J Comput Assist Tomogr 1990; 14:779–84.

52. Lundin B, Cooper TG, Meyer RA, et al. Measurement of total and unilateral renal blood flow by oblique-angle velocity-encoded 2D cine magnetic resonance angiography. Magn Reson Imaging 1993; 11:51–9.

53. Sodickson DK, Manning WJ. Simultaneous acquisition of spatial harmonics (SMASH) – fast imaging with radiofrequency coil arrays. Magn Reson Med 1997; 38:591–603.

54. Sodickson D, McKenzie C, Li W, et al. Contrast-enhanced 3D MR angiography with simultaneous acquisition of spatial harmonics: a pilot study. Radiology 2000; 217:284–9.

55. Weiger M, Pruessmann K, Kassner K, et al. Contrast-enhanced 3D MRA using SENSE. J Magn Reson Imaging 2000; 12:671–7.

56. Weiger M, Pruessmann K, Boesiger P. Cardiac real-time imaging using SENSE. Magn Reson Med 2000; 43:177–84.

57. Korosec FR, Grist TM, Mistretta CA. Time-resolved contrast-enhanced 3D MR angiography. Magn Reson Med 1996; 36:345–51.

58. DeBakey M, Henly W, Cooley D, et al. Surgical management of dissecting aneurysms of the aorta. J Thoracic Cardiovasc Surg 1965; 49:130–48.

59. DeSanctis R, Doroghazi R, Austen W, et al. Aortic dissection. N Engl J Med 1987; 317:1060–7.

60. Nienaber C, Con Kodolitsch Y, Nicolas V, et al. The diagnosis of aortic dissection by non-invasive imaging procedures. N Engl J Med 1993; 328:1–9.

61. Murray C, Edwards J. Spontaneous laceration of the ascending aorta. Circulation 1973; 47:848–58.

62. Gore I. Pathogenesis of dissecting aneurysms of the aorta. Arch Pathol Lab Med 1952; 53:142–53.

63. Neinaber C, Von Kodolitsh Y, Peterson B, et al. Intramural hemorrhage of the aorta: diagnostic and therapeutic implications. Circulation 1995; 92:1465–72.

64. Coady M, Rizzo J, Elefteriades J. Pathologic variants of thoracic aortic dissections: penetrating atherosclerotic ulcers and intramural hematomas. Cardiol Clin North Am 1999; 17:637–57.

65. Woolf KA, Herold CJ, Tempany CM et al. Aortic dissection: atypical patterns seen at MR imaging. Radiology 1991; 181:489–95.

66. Von Kodolitsch Y, Nienaber C. Intramural hemorrhage of the thoracic aorta: natural history, diagnostic and prognostic profiles of 209 cases with in vivo diagnosis. Z Cardiol 1998; 87:797.

67. Shennan T. Dissecting aneurysms. Medical Research Council, Special Report Series 1934:193.

68. Stanson A, Kazmier F, Hollier L, et al. Penetrating atherosclerotic ulcers of the thoracic aorta: natural history and clinicopathological correlations. Ann Vasc Surg 1986; 1:15–23.

69. Mohiaddin RH, McCrohon J, Francis JM, et al. Contrast-enhanced magnetic resonance angiogram of penetrating aortic ulcer. Circulation 2001; 103:18–19.

70. Pitt MP, Bonser RS. The natural history of thoracic aortic aneurysm disease: an overview. J Card Surg 1997; 12:270–8.

71. Schmidta M, Theissen P, Klempt G, et al. Long-term follow-up of 82 patients with chronic disease of the thoracic aorta using spin echo and cine gradient magnetic resonance imaging. Magn Reson Imaging 2000; 18:795–806.

72. Mohiaddin RH, Kilner PJ, Rees S, et al. Magnetic resonance volume flow and jet velocity mapping in aortic coarctation. J Am Coll Cardiol 1993; 22:1515–21.

73. Stewart J, Kincaid O, Edwards J. An Atlas of Vascular Rings and Related Malformations of the Aortic Arch System. Springfield, IL: Charles C Thomas, 1964.

74. Roche KJ, Krinsky G, Lee VS, et al. Interrupted aortic arch: diagnosis with gadolinium-enhanced 3D MRA. J Comput Assist Tomogr 1999; 23:197–202.

75. Soler R, Rodriguez E, Requejo I, et al. Magnetic resonance imaging of congenital abnormalities of the thoracic aorta. Eur Radiol 1998; 8:540–6.

76. Yamada I, Nakagawa T, Himeno Y, et al. Takayasu arteritis: diagnosis with breath-hold contrast-enhanced three dimensional MR angiography. J Magn Reson Imaging 2000; 11:481.

77. Mirvis S, Shanmuganathan K, Miller B, et al. Traumatic aortic injury: diagnosis with contrast-enhanced thoracic CT – five

Table 17.1. Contrast at CMR imaging of main components of atherothrombotic plaque characterization is based on the signal intensity and morphology characteristics. Modified from Fayad et al[11]

	Signal intensity relative to adjacent muscle			
Sequence:	*T1W*	*PDW*	*T2W*	*TOF*
Recent thrombus	+ to +/−	− to +/−	− to +/−	+
Lipid	+	+	−	+/−
Fibrous	+/−	+	+/− to +	+/− to −
Calcium	−	−	−	−

+, hyperintense; +/−, isointense; −, hypointense.

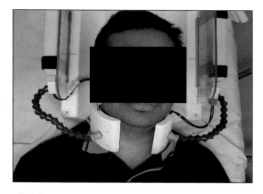

Figure 17.3
Photograph of the custom-built Mount Sinai Imaging Science Laboratories carotid phased array coil assembly. The assembly consists of a two-element bilateral phased array carotid coil. Each square element is 5.5 cm in length, and allows flexible positioning around the neck of the subject.

teins, their denaturation by oxidation, or the exchange between cholesteryl esters and water molecules (both from the fatty chain and from the cholesterol ring), with a further interchange between free and bound water.[27] Perivascular fat, composed mainly of triglycerides, has a distinct appearance on CMR as compared with atherosclerotic plaque lipids.[28] The plaque calcified regions consist primarily of calcium hydroxyapatite, and are associated with low signal intensities on the CMR images due to their low proton density and diffusion-mediated susceptibility effects.[29] Compared with black-blood sequences, bright-blood methods such as the TOF sequence create T2*-sensitive tissue signal that appears to improve the visualization of the intimal calfication and fibrous cap, which in general is a dense structured layer of collagen.[23] The CMR appearance and evolution of thrombus or hemorrhage have been investigated in the central nervous system,[30] pelvis,[31] and aorta.[32] These studies concluded that the different CMR signal intensities of hemorrhage depend on the structure of hemoglobin and its oxidation state.[30] Additional studies in the context of arterial thrombus and atherothrombosis are necessary.[33,34]

CMR has been used to study atherothrombotic plaques in human carotid, aortic, peripheral, and coronary arterial disease as described below.

In vivo CMR studies of human carotid artery plaques

In vivo CMR images of advanced lesions in the carotid arteries have been obtained from patients referred for endarterectomy.[35–37] The carotid arteries' superficial location and relative absence of motion present less of a technical challenge for imaging than the aorta or coronary arteries. Short-T2 components were quantified in vivo

before surgery and correlated with values obtained in vitro after surgery.[36] Some of the CMR studies of carotid arterial plaques include the imaging and characterization of atherosclerotic plaques,[38,39] the quantification of plaque size,[40] and the detection of fibrous cap 'integrity'.[17] Typically, the images are acquired with a resolution of $0.25 \times 0.25 \times 2$–$0.4 \times 0.4 \times 3$ mm^3 using a carotid phased array coil to improve signal-to-noise ratio (SNR) and image resolution (Figures 17.3 and 17.4).[41–43] Yuan et al[38] showed that in vivo multicontrast CMR of human carotid

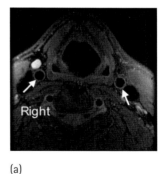
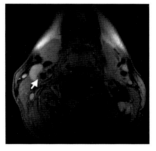

(a)   (b)

Figure 17.4
In vivo CMR carotid images of the common carotid arteries obtained with the phased array coil assembly demonstrated excellent high-resolution image quality of the vessel wall (arrows): T2-weighed ECG-gated fast spin-echo sequence black-blood imaging with double inversion recovery preparation pulses. Imaging parameters: repetition time 2 R–R intervals; echo time 45 ms; slice thickness 3 mm; acquisition matrix 256 × 256; number of signals averaged 2; echo train length 32; receiver bandwidth ±64 kHz; 512 zero-filling. A chemical shift suppression pulse is used to suppress the signal from perivascular fat. (A) 10 cm field of view (FOV) yielding an in-plane spatial resolution of ~390 × 390 μm^2; (B) 12 cm FOV yielding an in-plane spatial resolution of ~470 × 470 μm^2.

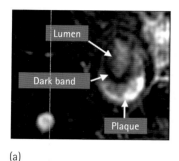

(a)

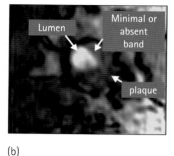

(b)

Figure 17.5

Time-of-flight (3D TOF) bright-blood CMR images of fibrous cap status. (A) CMR appearance of a plaque with intact, thick fibrous cap (>0.25 mm), in which there is a uniform dark band between bright lumen and gray plaque core. (B) CMR appearance of plaque with intact, thin fibrous cap (<0.25 mm), in which the dark band adjacent to lumen is absent. (Reproduced from Hatsukami et al. Circulation 2000; 102:959–64[17] with permission from Lippincott Williams & Wilkins.)

arteries had a sensitivity of 85% and a specificity of 92% for the identification of lipid core and acute intraplaque hemorrhage. Cai et al[39] demonstrated good agreement between the classification obtained by CMR and the American Heart Association (AHA) classification. The sensitivity and specificity, respectively, of CMR classification were as follows: type I–II lesions (near-normal wall thickness, no calcification) 67% and 100%; type III lesions (diffuse intimal thickening or small eccentric plaque with no calcification) 81% and 98%; type IV–Va lesions (plaque with a lipid or necrotic core surrounded by fibrous tissue with possible calcification) 84% and 90%; type Vb (calcified) lesions, 80% and 94%; type Vc lesions (fibrotic plaque without lipid core and with possible small calcifications) 56% and 100%; and type VI lesions (complex plaque with possible surface defect, hemorrhage, or thrombus) 82% and 91%. This study demonstrated that multicontrast CMR is capable of in vivo classification of human carotid atherosclerotic plaques

Using the 3D TOF bright-blood technique (Figure 17.5), Yuan et al[44] analyzed the integrity of fibrous caps of carotid atherosclerotic plaques in 53 patients scheduled for carotid endarterectomy. Results have shown that among symptomatic patients, 70% had ruptured caps, as opposed to 9% with thick caps. Furthermore, patients with ruptured plaques were 23 times more likely to have had an episode of transient ischemic attack (TIA) or stroke as compared with patients with intact-thick fibrous caps.

In vivo CMR studies of human aortic plaques

The principal challenges associated with CMR of the thoracic aorta are obtaining sufficient sensitivity for sub-millimeter imaging and exclusion of artifacts due to respiratory motion and blood flow. It has been shown by CMR that the wall thickness of the ascending aorta is increased in patients with homozygous familial hypercholesterolemia.[45] Fayad et al[46] assessed thoracic aortic plaque

composition and size using T1-, T2-, and proton density-weighted images. The acquired images had a resolution of $0.8 \times 0.8 \times 5$ mm^3 using a torso phased array coil.[41] Matched CMR and transesophageal echocardiography (TEE) cross-sectional aortic segments showed a strong correlation between plaque composition and mean maximum plaque thickness (Figure 17.6). Figure 17.7 shows a complicated plaque in the descending and aortic arch from another patient.

A study of asymptomatic subjects, the Framingham Heart Study (FHS), showed by CMR that aortic atherosclerosis prevalence and burden (i.e. plaque volume/aortic volume) increased significantly with age and was higher in the abdominal aorta than in the thoracic aorta.[47] It was also found that long-term measures such as risk factors

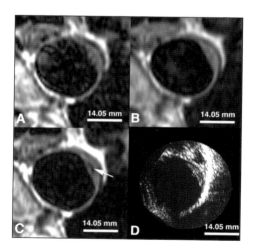

Figure 17.6

In vivo CMR images from a patient with 4.5 mm-thick plaque in the descending thoracic aorta: (A) T1-weighted; (B) proton-density-weighted; (C) T2-weighted; (D) corresponding TEE image. CMR images show an example of an AHA type IV/Va plaque with a dark area in the center, identified on the T2-weighted image (C, arrow) as a lipid-rich core. This lipid-rich core is separated from the lumen by a fibrous cap. Plaque characterization was based on information obtained from the T1-, proton density-, and T2-weighted CMR images. (Reproduced from Fayad et al. Circulation 2000; 22:849–54[46] with permission from Lippincott Williams & Wilkins.)

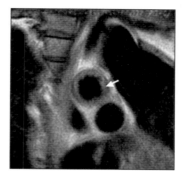

Figure 17.7
In vivo T2-weighted black-blood CMR image of a patient with a complicated, thrombus-rich, plaque in the aortic arch (white arrow). (Modified from Fayad et al. Neuroimaging Clin North Am 2002; 12:461–71.[22])

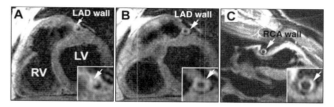

Figure 17.8
In vivo CMR black-blood cross-sectional images of human coronary arteries demonstrating a plaque, presumably with deposition of fat (A, arrow), a concentric fibrotic lesion (B) in the left anterior descending (LAD) artery, and an ectatic, but atherosclerotic, right coronary artery (RCA) (C). RV, right ventricle; LV, left ventricle. (Modified from Fayad et al. Circulation 2000; 102:506–10.[52])

and FHS coronary risk score are strongly associated with asymptomatic aortic atherosclerosis as detected by CMR.[47]

An alternative to surface coil aortic CMR was demonstrated by Shunk et al[48] using transesophageal CMR (TECMR) to improve visualization and quantitative assessment of the atherosclerotic plaque of the human thoracic aorta. This technique was tested in 22 subjects (8 normal subjects and 14 patients with atherosclerosis of the aorta) and in a human male cadaver with extensive aortic atherosclerosis, used for pathology correlation. The probe was introduced transnasally. When wall thickness and circumferencial extent of the plaque were compared, TEE and TECMR showed similar values. TECMR demonstrated a good SNR in the near field. The development of this technique may, in the future, be used as an alternative or complement to TEE and surface coil aortic CMR. TECMR is discussed in more detail in Chapter 18.

In vivo CMR studies of human peripheral arteries

High-resolution CMR of the popliteal artery and the response to balloon angioplasty has been reported.[49] In all patients, the extent of atherosclerotic plaque could be defined such that even in angiographically 'normal' segments of vessel, atherosclerotic lesions with cross-sectional areas ranging from 49% to 76% of the potential lumen area were identified. Following angioplasty, plaque fissuring and local dissection were easily identified, and serial changes in lumen diameter, blood flow, and lesion size were documented. This study showed that high-resolution CMR can define the extent of atherosclerotic plaque in the peripheral vasculature and can demonstrate the changes that occur with remodeling and restenosis following angioplasty.

In vivo CMR studies of coronary artery plaque

The ultimate goal is noninvasive imaging of plaque in the coronary arteries. Difficulties in CMR wall imaging of the coronary arteries are due to a combination of cardiac and respiratory motion artifacts,[50] the small size of the arteries (3–4 mm) as well as their tortuous course, and low contrast-to-noise ratio between the arteries and adjacent epicardial fat.[51] Attempts were made to overcome these problems, using breathhold[52] and navigator techniques[53] respectively for cardiac and respiratory synchronization, black-blood, fat-suppressed CMR sequences to improve lumen wall contrast-to-noise ratio, and tailored receiver coils to increase SNR.[54] High-resolution black-blood CMR images of atherosclerotic human coronary arteries are shown in Figure 17.8. Near-isotropic spatial resolution (0.7 × 0.7 × 1 mm³) black-blood imaging[55] may provide a quick way to image a long segment of the coronary artery wall, and may be useful for rapid coronary plaque burden measurements (Figure 17.9).[56]

Numerical simulations and phantom measurement of a vessel wall model showed that an in-plane spatial resolution of 330–500 μm could enable in vivo coronary plaque characterization.[57] We showed that, by using a new external receiver coil, in vivo high resolution (<0.5 mm in-plane resolution; 3–4 mm slice thickness) CMR imaging of the human coronary plaques could be obtained. Our new coil consists of an array (a four-elements phased array coil: two square coils 7.3 cm each, and two rectangular coils 6.4 × 9.7 cm² each) in which all of the coils are on the chest surface. Figure 17.10 shows the SNR plot as a function of depth for the two coil arrays. It is evident from the curves that the anterior array enjoys an SNR advantage for depths up to ~12 cm. We believe that this new approach can play an important role in applications such as high-resolution CMR wall characterization of atherosclerotic proximal coronary arteries (Figure 17.11).

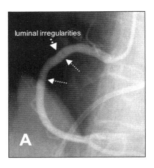
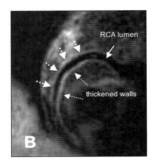

Figure 17.9

X-ray angiograph (A) from a 79-year-old patient with minor (~10% stenoses) luminal irregularities (white arrows) of the proximal RCA. The corresponding black-blood 3D CMR vessel wall image (B) demonstrates an irregularly thickened RCA wall (>2 mm) indicative of an increased atherosclerotic plaque burden. The inner and outer RCA walls are indicated by the white dotted arrows. (Modified from Kim et al. Circulation 2002; 106:296–9.[56] with permission from Lippincott Williams & Wilkins.)

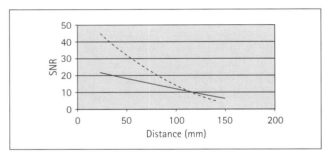

Figure 17.10

Signal-to-noise ratio (SNR) versus distance from the surface for the standard phased array whole-heart coil (solid line) and a newly designed four-elements anterior phased array chest coil (dashed line).

Further improvements in external coils and imaging acquisition, and the use of contrast agents that enhance the different vessel wall components, may lead to better in vivo noninvasive CMR characterization of high-risk plaque in the coronary arteries.

Plaque and thrombus characterization using CMR contrast agents

Plaque characterization

The characterization techniques described above utilize the inherent relaxation properties of different plaque components. Despite the use of multicontrast CMR (as

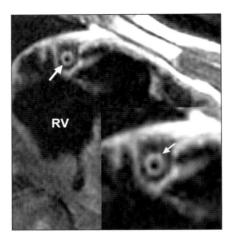

Figure 17.11

Very-high-resolution in vivo coronary wall CMR images of a patient with a plaque (arrows) in the right coronary artery. The images were obtained using a custom-built four-element anterior phased array chest coil. ECG-gated fast spin-echo sequence black-blood imaging with double inversion recovery preparation pulses (DIR) was used. Imaging parameters: repetition time 1 R–R interval; echo time 42 ms; slice thickness 4 mm; acquisition matrix 512 × 512; field-of-view 20 cm; number of signals averaged 2; echo train length 32; receiver bandwidth ±64 kHz. A chemical shift suppression pulse was used to suppress the signal from perivascular fat. The in-plane spatial resolution was ~390 × 390 μm². The insert represents a magnified view of the right coronary artery plaque. RV, right ventricle.

discussed earlier) or high-resolution (200 μm³) 3D imaging,[58] it is still not possible to uniquely identify plaque components. Overlap of signal intensities occurs, particularly between the lipid core and vessel media.[38,58] Moreover, approaches that are directed at the identification of the lipid core and fibrous cap are focused on relatively advanced lesions. More subtle distinctions within plaque and pre-atheromatous artery may be detectable by the introduction of conventional extracellular paramagnetic contrast agents, such as gadolinium.[21]

Paramagnetic metal cations such as chelated gadolinium are often used for enhancement of blood versus tissue contrast in magnetic resonance angiography (MRA). Gadolinium enhances T1 relaxivity and therefore increase contrast enhancement on T1-weighted pulse sequences with short TR and TE. Gadolinium contrast-enhanced CMR improves tissue differentiation. Free gadolinium is not appropriate for in vivo use because of its untoward effects. Chelation of gadolinium with, for example, free DTPA (diethylenetriaminepentaacetic acid) produces a highly stable metal chelate (Gd-DTPA) with low toxicity and excellent pharmacokinetics and systemic tolerance. Gd-DTPA does not penetrate phospholipid cellular membranes, because of its highly hydrophilic properties. It stays entirely confined in the extracellular space after intravenous administration, does not bind plasma proteins, and is eliminated unmetabolized by the kidneys.[59] Excellent renal tolerance was observed consistently in clinical studies, including those in patients with prior renal impairment.[60,61] Overall, the incidence of adverse effects was 1–2% after intravenous administration of the usual dose of 0.1–0.2 mmol Gd-DTPA/kg body weight.[59] Currently, Gd-DTPA is the CMR contrast agent most extensively used.

New microvessels form in atherosclerotic plaques, and this phenomenon may be associated with features of inflammation, such as upregulation of adhesion molecules and leukocyte infiltration.[62] The presence of new vessels has also been associated with carotid plaque instability.[63] These vessels may also be abnormally permeable, allowing the extravasation of plasma proteins, such as albumin and fibrinogen.[6,64] In some reports, contrast-enhanced CMR has utilized these and other features to aid plaque characterization.[65–67] On T1-weighted images of carotid arteries, a gadolinium-based contrast agent (namely Gd-DTPA) has been reported to enhance the signal intensities (SI) of three major plaque tissue types: fibrous tissue (SI increased by 80%), necrotic core (SI increased by 29%), and calcifications (SI increased by 47%).[67] In addition, contrast-enhanced CMR images showed increased SI (102%) in fibrotic areas irrigated by rich microvasculature within the plaque, allowing visualization and detection of the plaque at risk.[67] Wasserman et al[68] demonstrated enhanced contrast of fibrocellular tissue relative to lipid-rich components (Figure 17.12). Another recent application of dynamic contrast-enhanced CMR of atherosclerotic plaques has been the quantification of neovasculature.[69]

Using MS–325,[70] a gadolinium-based contrast agent that binds albumin, areas of high signal intensity, comparable to highly vascular tissue such as liver, have been observed in the aortic or iliac arterial wall. Maki et al speculated that this not only reflects increased plaque vascularity,[71] but a leakiness of these microvessels, which suggests active inflammation.[72] This is consistent with a report in which increased wall thickness, T2-weighted signal and/or gadolinium contrast enhancement in carotid arteries and aorta were associated with elevated serum levels of the inflammatory markers interleukin-6 (IL-6), C-reactive protein (CRP), intercellular adhesion molecule 1 (ICAM-1), and vascular cell adhesion molecule-1 (VCAM-1).[73]

Early inflammation of the arterial wall is known to be involved in the genesis of atherosclerotic plaques, and its response comprised of infiltration of monocyte-derived macrophages and T-lymphocytes.[74–76] In autopsy studies, a strong association was found between the presence and location of macrophages and the location of plaque rupture.[77] CMR imaging of the location and distribution of macrophages may be facilitated by the use of superparamagnetic nanoparticles of iron oxide (SPIO). These have unique magnetic properties and are avidly taken up by the macrophages.[78] In studies, injection of SPIO into hyperlipidemic rabbits was associated with accumulation in macrophages and, after 2 hours[79] to 5 days,[80] the appearance of signal voids studded on the luminal surface of the aorta. Similar appearances were incidentally observed in the aorta and intrapelvic arteries of humans who have received SPIO for oncological imaging (Figure 17.13).[81] This type of specific cellular targeting approach warrants further investigation.

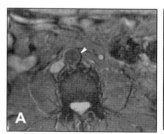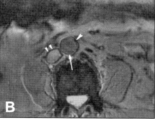

Figure 17.13
Axial T2* gradient-echo CMR precontrast (A) and postcontrast (ultrasmall superparamagnetic iron oxide (USPIO) particles (2.6 mg Fe/kg), 24–36 h) (B) aortic images. On the precontrast image (A), the aortic wall is homogeneously hyperintense (arrowhead). Following USPIO administration (B), pronounced signal loss of an area extending from the inner to the outer surface of the aortic wall can be seen (arrowhead). This vessel segment was considered positive. Note, however, that there is also a low-intensity ring at the interface between the aortic wall and lumen on the postcontrast image (B, long arrow). It is not possible to precisely determine whether the ring is truly confined to the aortic wall or to the lumen. This appearance is defined as a ring phenomenon, which is also seen in other vessels, such as the inferior vena cava (B, small arrowheads). (Reproduced from Schmitz et al. J Magn Reson Imaging 2001; 14: 355–61.[81])

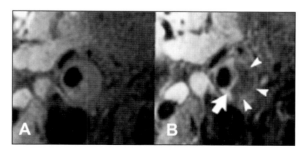

Figure 17.12
In vivo human common carotid artery CMR plaque precontrast (A) and postcontrast (Gd-DTPA; 0.1 mmol/kg) (B) images. A double inversion recovery, T1-weighted fast spin-echo sequence with fat saturation was used. The postcontrast image in (B) demonstrates heterogeneous enhancement (arrow enhancement along the margin of the lumen, while arrowheads indicate enhancement along the outer wall of the atheroma). Scale bars indicate 1 cm. (Modified from Wasserman et al. Radiology 2002; 223:566–73.[68])

Thrombus characterization

Plaque rupture or erosion exposes the prothrombotic core to circulating blood, which can lead to acute vessel occlusion and to myocardial infarction, unstable angina, or death.[82,83] Recent evidence suggests that layering and organization of thrombus may be responsible for plaque progression.[8] Early visualization of thrombus formation and rapid observation of its age may be clinically useful for the discrimination of treatment alternatives and secondary prevention of vascular events.

Time-related changes in the water diffusion properties of ex vivo thrombus in plaques have been identified using diffusion-weighted CMR methods.[84,85] In other studies, diffusion-weighted CMR was used for detection of cerebral venous thrombosis[86] and dural sinus thrombosis.[87,88] However, in vivo diffusion-weighted CMR for vivo atherosclerotic imaging is challenging due to its sensitivity to motion and limited available SNR.

CMR signal intensities of hemorrhage and 'altered blood' depend on the structure of hemoglobin and its oxidation state.[30] For example, the generation of methemoglobin within evolving thrombus is known to cause T1 shortening. This phenomenon has been exploited for the detection of fresh thrombus in the setting of deep vein thrombosis,[89,90] pulmonary embolus,[91] and acute carotid thrombus.[92] In these studies, direct imaging of thrombus against a suppressed background using 3D magnetization-prepared rapid gradient-echo (3D MPRAGE)[93] was found to be effective in the imaging of thrombus.

In vivo carotid images of recent intraplaque hemorrhages were identified by their multicontrast appearance (high signal on TOF, intermediate on T1-weighted, and variable intensity on proton density- and T2-weighted).[38] The results revealed that the CMR findings agreed well with the histological presence of a necrotic core or recent intraplaque hemorrhage, with a sensitivity of 85%, a specificity of 92%, and a calculated κ-value of 0.69.

The potential of CMR to detect arterial thrombotic obstruction and define thrombus age has recently been evaluated using black-blood T1- and T2-weighted imaging.[34] Carotid thrombi were induced in swine by arterial injury. Serial high-resolution in vivo CMR images were obtained at 6 hours, 1 day, and 1, 2, 3, 6, and 9 weeks. Thrombus appearance and relative signal intensity revealed characteristic temporal changes in the CMR images, reflecting histological changes in the composition. Age definition using visual appearance was highly accurate (Pearson's χ^2 with 4df in the range 96–132 and Cohen's κ in the range 0.81–0.94).

Using T2-weighted imaging, Johnstone et al[94] have identified the location and size of plaque-associated mural thrombus after pharmacological triggering of plaque disruption in vivo in an atherosclerotic rabbit model (Figure 17.14). Ultrasmall SPIO (USPIO)-enhanced T2*

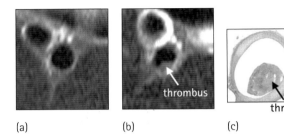

(a)   (b)   (c)

Figure 17.14
Cross-sectional CMR images of the abdominal aorta of a rabbit that develops a new thrombus. CMR images pre (A) and post (B) pharmacological triggering demonstrate the formation of the new thrombus. The corresponding histopathological section is shown in (C). (Modified from Johnstone et al. Arterioscler Thromb Vasc Biol 2001; 21:556–60.[94])

CMR imaging was used for the detection of thrombus induced in the jugular veins of rabbits.[95]

Contrast agents that characterize thrombus are under development: fibrin can be identified by lipid-encapsulated perfluorocarbon paramagnetic nanoparticles in vitro[96,97] and in vivo,[98] or by a paramagnetic dendrimeric contrast agent,[99] while activated platelets have been studied via the interaction of a USPIO–arginine–glycine–aspartic acid (RGD) peptide construct with the $\alpha_{IIb}\beta_3$ receptor.[100] A more detailed discussion of thrombus imaging and molecular of plaques with targeted contrast agents is given in Chapter 27.

Monitoring of therapy with CMR

CMR can be used to measure the effect of lipid-lowering therapy (statins) in asymptomatic untreated hypercholesterolemic patients with carotid and aortic atherosclerosis.[101,102] After 12 months of therapy, a regression of atherosclerotic lesions was observed in the aortic and carotid arterial wall. At 24 months, continued reduction of arterial wall area was observed, with a small increase in the arterial lumen (Figure 17.15 and Table 17.2).[101,102]

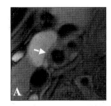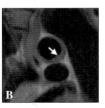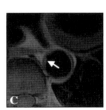

Figure 17.15
Complex carotid and aortic plaques (arrows) detected in a 71-year-old female patient using high-resolution in vivo CMR: (A) left carotid artery plaque; (B) aortic arch plaque; (C) descending aortic plaque.

Table 17.2. CMR-measured changes in plaque and lumen size after 24 months of lipid-lowering therapy.

	Aorta			Carotid artery		
	Baseline	24 months	p	Baseline	24 months	p
Lumen area	469.1 ± 28	495.2 ± 29	<0.01	32.6 ± 2	34.1 ± 2	0.01
VWA	288 ± 15	241.7 ± 12	<0.0001	46.5 ± 2	38.0 ± 2	<0.0001
Maximum VWT	4.91 ± 0.14	4.11 ± 0.12	<0.001	2.65 ± 0.9	2.14 ± 0.6	<0.001
Minimum VWT	1.73 ± 0.1	1.65 ± 0.1	NS	1.08 ± 0.5	1.04 ± 0.5	NS

VWA, vessel wall area; VWT, vessel wall thickness; NS, not statistically significant.
Values are given as mean ± SEM in mm^2 for area and mm for thickness.
(Modified from Corti et al. Circulation 2001; 102:249–52[102] with permission from Lippincott Williams & Wilkins.)

The results of prolonged intensive lipid-lowering therapy were demonstrated in a case–control study using in vivo CMR.[103] Patients with CAD receiving lipid-lowering therapy (niacin, lovastatin, and colestipol) for 10 years were selected from the Familial Atherosclerosis Treatment Study (FATS) group. Untreated patients with CAD were used as controls. A total of 32 carotid arteries were analyzed by CMR regarding calcium, fibrous tissue, and lipid content. CMR analysis showed a smaller lipid core area, a decreased lipid composition (estimated as a fraction of total plaque area), and an increased fibrous tissue composition in the treated group compared with the untreated group. There was a trend towards increased plaque calcium content in treated patients (Figure 17.16). The in vivo carotid CMR imaging application demonstrated in this study provides an alternative potential use of CMR therapy monitoring in secondary prevention.

Image analysis

As demonstrated above, a significant strength of CMR is the ability to noninvasively follow the progress of lesions in individual patients over a period of time. Comparisons of this nature will provide insights into the natural history

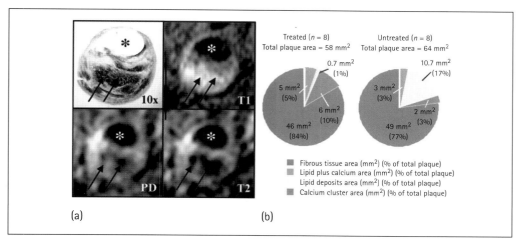

Figure 17.16

An eccentric and advanced plaque in the right common carotid artery from a patient who underwent carotid endarterectomy. (A) The matching in vivo CMR images were obtained before surgery. The histological specimen showed that this complex plaque with a large lipid core contains extracellular lipid, amorphous debris, cholesterol monohydrate crystals, calcifications, and hemorrhage (red). The matching CMR images showed that the area of hyperintense signal on T1 weighting and of hypointense signal on proton density and T2 weightings (see arrows) correlates well in size and appearance with the large lipid-rich region on the histological slide. * indicates the luminal area. (B) Comparisons of carotid plaque tissue components and composition. The treated plaques contained significantly less lipid than did the untreated plaques (p = 0.01). Quantities of fibrous tissue, calcium, and calcium plus lipid were not statistically different between the two groups. (Modified from Zhao et al. Arterioscler Thromb Vasc Biol 2001; 21:1623–9.[103])

of plaque and prospective information about plaques at risk of precipitating acute atherothrombotic events, and will also help determine response to treatment. However, changes in plaque size and composition within individuals may be small.[101–103] Reliable ways to ensure anatomical alignment of sections between successive scans and to measure small changes in measured parameters are required.

In one of the CMR studies of lipid-lowering in human aortic and carotid plaques,[101] the reproducibility of the vessel wall area measurement was assessed after repeated imaging. The error in vessel wall area measurement was found to be 2.6% for aortic and 3.5% for carotid plaques. Similar low measurement errors in plaque area and volume (4–6%) were reported by others, proving that plaque area and volume can be accurately assessed.[104,105]

To improve quantification, semiautomatic image processing techniques have been developed that improve the accuracy of vessel wall area measurements compared with manual morphometric analysis.[106,107] In one such model, a 'discrete dynamic contour' (DDC) is produced by image-derived edge characteristics moderated by elements to introduce contour tension and damping. Three-dimensional interpolation of DDCs obtained for inner and outer vessel wall has allowed the construction of vessel wall volume,[108] with the potential to quantify atherosclerotic plaque burden and distribution. Future work will concentrate on computer-aided segmentation and classification methods.[109]

Possible future improvements

More efficient imaging using a multislice black-blood sequence should shorten the total examination time.[110–113] Thinner slices such as those obtained with three-dimensional acquisition techniques could further improve artery wall imaging.[55,114] Additional CMR techniques, such as water diffusion weighting,[84] magnetization transfer weighting,[18] steady-state free precession (SSFP) sequences,[58] rapid *k*-space coverage methods such as spiral[55] and radial[115] imaging, parallel imaging,[116,117] contrast enhancement,[67] molecular imaging,[21] improved surface coils,[117] and higher-magnetic-field whole-body imaging (i.e. 3.0 T),[118] may provide complementary structural information and allow more detailed plaque characterization. New and improved blood-suppression methods[55] may be necessary for accurate plaque imaging, especially in the carotid artery bifurcation.

Using a combination of multidetector row computed tomography (CT) and CMR may enhance the clinical detection of atherothrombotic disease.[11] CT and CMR together identify flow-limiting coronary stenoses and calcified plaques, directly image the atherosclerotic

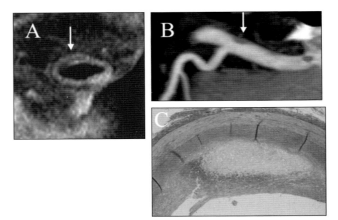

Figure 17.17
CMR and CT characterization of coronary artery calcified plaque: (A) cross-sectional ex vivo T2-weighted CMR image of a human left anterior descending (LAD) with a small calcified lesion (arrow) and vessel wall thickening; (B) multislice CT image of the same lesion (arrow), showing the typical blooming effect of calcified lesions in CT images; (C) corresponding histopathological section – calcium is washed out during the preparation process. (Reproduced from Fayad et al. Circulation 2002; 106:2026–34.[11])

lesions, measure atherosclerotic burden, and characterize the plaque components. Together, they may provide unique information that may predict cardiovascular risk, facilitate further study of the mechanisms of atherothrombosis progression and its response to therapy, and allow for assessment of subclinical disease. The advantage of CT is the complete assessment of the entire coronary artery tree within a very short scan time, while CMR offers excellent soft tissue contrast. CT may first be used to localize suspicious atherothrombotic lesions in the coronary and noncoronary arteries (Figure 17.17). The limited scan range of CMR can then take advantage of the knowledge of the problematic site in the coronary arteries and proceed with tissue characterization.

Invasive CMR approaches (see, e.g. reference 119) to plaque imaging and treatment monitoring are presented in Chapters 20 and 23.

Conclusions

In the future, the use of imaging methods to quantify the progression and regression of atherothrombosis could play a very strong role in the management of patients. High-resolution, noninvasive CMR imaging has the potential to provide three-dimensional anatomical information about the lumen and the vessel wall. Furthermore, CMR has the ability to characterize atherothrombotic plaque composition and micro-anatomy, and thus to

18

Transesophageal CMR of the aorta

Sandeep Gautam, William P Warren, Joao AC Lima

Introduction

In this chapter, we will discuss a novel technique of studying the thoracic aorta: transesophageal cardiovascular magnetic resonance imaging (TECMR). TECMR involves placement of a loopless MRI receiver coil into the esophagus to image the neighboring thoracic aorta in combination with MRI surface coils. The concept of TECMR is similar to the practice of transesophageal echocardiography (TEE), during which an ultrasound probe is inserted into the esophagus to image the heart and thoracic aorta with superior image quality compared with surface echocardiography. TECMR takes advantage of the higher signal-to-noise ratio (SNR) obtained by placing the receiver coil closer to the object of interest. TECMR has advantages for imaging the thoracic aorta compared with standard TEE or surface coil CMR alone.

Aortic atherosclerosis is an important marker of systemic atherosclerotic disease, including coronary artery and cerebrovascular disease.[1,2] This has been shown by various postmortem studies and observational studies utilizing TEE to study the aortic plaque.[3,4] Aortic wall and plaque characteristics and features such as aortic wall thickness, luminal irregularities, and plaque composition are strong predictors of future vascular events.[5,6]

Because the aorta is ten times larger in diameter than the average coronary artery, it is an ideal model for the in vivo study of human atherosclerosis using noninvasive imaging techniques.

Over the last several decades, accumulating evidence has shown that the process of atherosclerosis begins in the blood vessel wall as an extraluminal phenomenon.[7] Additionally, the atherosclerotic plaques that cause minor vessel stenoses may be lipid-rich and may be among the plaques most likely to rupture, causing clinical events such as stroke or myocardial infarction.[8,9] These realizations have sparked interest in plaque imaging methods that can quantify the extent of plaque, distinguish plaque components, and perhaps predict the likelihood of rupture. CMR

is one of the most promising of these noninvasive plaque-imaging modalities.

Imaging modalities

Current standard techniques for measuring the thoracic aorta include TEE, contrast aortography, intravascular ultrasound (IVUS), computed tomography (CT) and standard CMR.

TEE allows real-time imaging of the aorta, but suffers both from an inability to image clearly the quadrant of the aortic wall that is directly against the esophagus and from an inability to register images to a fixed frame of reference, making precise mapping of aortic lesions problematic. Kasprzak et al[10] used a technique to control movement of the TEE probe while imaging in multiple planes with subsequent offline three-dimensional (3D) image reconstruction. This system was complicated and not fully successful in obtaining adequate images. Montgomery et al[11] designed a semiquantitative atherosclerosis-grading scheme that uses orthogonal views to estimate the 3D characteristic of aortic lesions. The important concerns with TEE are limited imaging of the aortic arch and anterior wall of the descending aorta, in addition to the poor tissue characterization intrinsic to ultrasound imaging.

Contrast aortography was for a long time considered the 'gold standard' for aortic imaging. However, a more suitable term would be 'lumenography', since only lesions that protrude into the lumen can be seen as an absence of signal. Comparisons with an adjacent reference segment with normal vessel wall are used to conjecture inferences about the atherosclerotic involvement. This 'reference' normal segment is often unavailable.[12] This technique cannot make definite statements about the thickness and stiffness of the vessel wall at the site of a contrast-filling defect. Also, plaque characterization is not possible with this method. In clinical trials, statins cause a reduction in clinical events that is out of proportion to the degree of regression in angiographically defined coronary stenoses.[13]

IVUS, commonly used in the coronary arteries, is highly invasive and therefore unsuited as a method to follow the progression or regression of aortic atherosclerotic disease. Also, it provides poor contrast resolution between different intraplaque components.[14] Percutaneous transluminal angioscopic identification of plaque rupture and thrombus was independently associated with adverse outcome in patients with complex lesions after interventional procedures.[15] However, like IVUS, this technique is highly invasive. Newer invasive technologies for atherosclerotic plaque detection include thermography, optical coherence tomography, Raman spectroscopy, and near-infrared (NIR) spectroscopy.[16–20]

Standard CMR and CT allow complete visualization of the aortic wall, but presently lack adequate resolution for precise characterization of the aortic atheroma. Ultrafast computed tomography (UFCT) allows image acquisition at a faster rate than conventional CT. Fast imaging is essential to eliminate cardiac and respiratory motion artifacts. UFCT is able to image vessel wall calcification, which is found more frequently in advanced atherosclerotic lesions, but may occur in small amounts in early lesions.[21]

CMR is much superior to TEE at defining atheroma structure, and can help delineate the components of an atherosclerotic plaque.[22] The plaque fibrous tissues, consisting mainly of extracellular matrix elaborated by smooth muscle cells, are associated with a short T1. The plaque lipids consist primarily of unesterified cholesterol and cholesteryl esters, and are associated with a short T2. The plaque calcified regions consist primarily of calcium hydroxyapatite and are associated with low signal intensities on the MR images because of their low proton density and because of diffusion-mediated susceptibility effects.[23] The principal challenges associated with CMR of the thoracic aorta are obtaining sufficient sensitivity for submillimeter imaging and exclusion of artifacts caused by respiratory motion and blood flow.[22]

Intravascular CMR has overcome many of the limitations of CT and standard CMR, at the cost of invasiveness. Zimmerman et al,[24] in a study on heritable hyperlipidemic rabbits, concluded that intravascular CMR is feasible for detecting early atherosclerosis and characterizing more advanced plaque formations. In contrast to the externally placed surface coil in the study, the intravascular imaging device provided sufficient spatial resolution to accurately quantitate wall thickness as well as plaque area and differentiate various plaque. Rivas et al,[25] in their in vivo experiments, clearly showed real-time intravascular imaging of the rabbit aortic wall with minimal motion artifacts and effective blood signal suppression. By providing close proximity between the imaging coil and the vessel wall,

the CMR technique can achieve maximal spatial resolution.[26] In addition, positioning the coil next to the vascular wall allows the latter to fall within the area of maximal coil sensitivity. Thus, intravascular CMR provides much better SNR than standard CMR, at the cost of invasiveness. Martin et al[27] used this concept to study the aorta by placing an expandable radiofrequency (RF) receiver coil in the inferior vena cava. This approach to aortic wall imaging is certainly less invasive than intraaortic receiver coils, but still has the associated risks of a large-caliber central venous catheter placement.

Development of TECMR

Without invading a vascular space, we may obtain similar information by receiving the signal from an adjacent body structure. The concept of placing an RF receiver into a body cavity to image an adjacent structure was first described by Narayam et al,[28] who used an endorectal RF receiver coil to image the canine prostate, and by Schnall et al,[29] who used an expandable endorectal RF receiver coil to image the prostate in 15 humans with biopsy-proven prostate carcinoma and two normal volunteers. Siegelman et al[30] also used an endovaginal coil to image the vagina and adjacent structures.

An ideal technique, therefore, would be to find a minimally invasive method to place an MRI receiver coil in a structure adjacent to the aorta. The esophagus is an obvious candidate organ here, as demonstrated in the use of TEE to image the heart and in particular the left atrium and thoracic aorta. It should be possible to place an RF receiver coil in the esophagus and attempt to image the thoracic aortic wall. In pursue of this concept, a loopless RF receiver device designed for ease of placement into the esophagus was developed at the Johns Hopkins Hospital.[31] The device was a modification of an earlier intravascular catheter antenna used for intravascular imaging of rabbit aorta.[32]

TECMR probe device[31] (Figure 18.1)

The TECMR antenna consists of a flexible 1.2 mm-diameter loopless RF receiver constructed from 50 Ω coaxial cable ~$\lambda/4$ in length, with a 10 cm extension of the inner conductor at the distal end. The distal portion of the antenna is housed inside an 8 or 12 French Levin gastric tube. The proximal end of the antenna protrudes from the proximal end of the Levin tube, at which point the two are secured together to prevent the antenna from migrating out of the end of the Levin tube housing. The proximal end of the antenna is connected to an adjustable tuning and matching circuit, which is connected via coaxial cable to

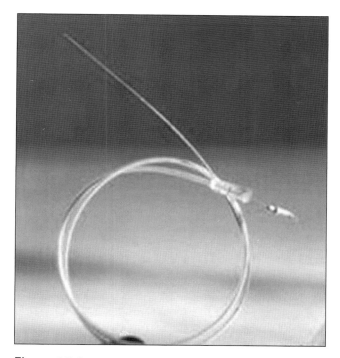

Figure 18.1
Transesophageal CMR (TECMR) coil.

the CMR scanner. The circuitry provides high-speed diode switching to decouple the antenna during external RF pulses and allows signal reception between pulses. A BALUN circuit is interposed to block the transmission of unbalanced currents. In theory, without the BALUN, if the CMR connector cable is inadvertently left in a loop configuration during scanning, induced currents might be transmitted to patient as heat.

Early TECMR studies

The TECMR probe was first tested in 1999 by Shunk et al[31] in an experiment on the miniswine and the New Zealand white rabbit. TECMR images of the thoracic aorta were obtained with tissue tagging and ECG gating. This animal experiment showed that the TECMR probe could be used safely to study the thoracic aorta. No evidence of esophageal injury was found in either animal after completion of the TECMR study. The presence of the TECMR probe in the esophagus did not interfere with standard CMR. The authors also found that the sensitivity of the TECMR antenna decreases with the longitudinal distance from its receptive center and linearly with the radial distance from the antenna, but is maintained at a reasonable level over a useful range. Therefore, it was not necessary to reposition the receiver to image the upper portion of the descending aorta or the aortic arch. The loopless receiver used in the experiment affords a theoretical and practical

advantage over a traditional coil receiver. The SNR for a receiver coil decreases as the inverse square of the distance from the coil, but the SNR for a loopless receiver decreases as the linear inverse of the distance. This means that beyond 1 cm from the probe, the loopless receiver provides a higher SNR. The linear inhomogeneity of signal from a loopless receiver is quite predictable across the field of view and can be corrected to homogeneity after image acquisition with an appropriate algorithm.[32] An expandable coil can extend the region over which a coil design outperforms a loopless receiver by increasing the diameter of the coil.[27] However, this would add further to the complexity of device design and placement, since coil receivers require additional capacitor components near the distal end of the device. Thus, for imaging the human aorta, which is normally 2–3 cm in diameter, a loopless receiver may be ideal through a TECMR probe, since the esophagus is immediately adjacent to the aorta.

TECMR versus TEE

The first in vivo human TECMR study was performed by Shunk et al[33] in 2001 in a comparison of TECMR with TEE in a cohort of 14 patients referred for TEE to rule out a cardiac or aortic source of thromboemboli. Eight normal controls and a formalin-fixed human male cadaver were also studied by TECMR. The studies demonstrated the feasibility of performing TECMR in humans. No sedation was required for TECMR and the probe maintained its SNR along much of its length, allowing TECMR at multiple locations over ~20 cm without repositioning the device. Figure 18.2 shows a cross-sectional TECMR image of the descending aorta in a 33-year-old

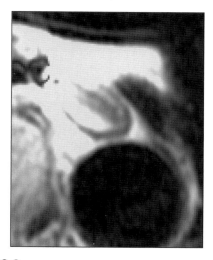

Figure 18.2
TECMR view of the descending aorta in a 33-year-old healthy male.

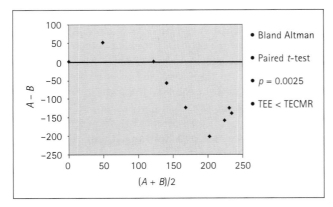

Figure 18.3
Bland Altman paired *t*-test comparison of circumferential plaque extent by TECMR (*A*) versus TEE (*B*), showing underestimation by TEE at the higher range of plaque values.

healthy male control. Although there was good correlation between TECMR and TEE for measurement of circumferential plaque extent, relative underestimation of the disease was found by TEE, particularly at the higher range of values, as shown in Figure 18.3.

Figure 18.4 shows corresponding TECMR and TEE images of the distal aortic arch in a 77-year-old male patient with remote stroke, depicting heterogeneous atherosclerotic thickening, and this illustrates the differences in circumferential plaque extent according to the two methods. Comparison of TECMR and TEE studies in the cadaver showed that TECMR allows for evaluation of the aorta over its entire circumference, whereas TEE aortic imaging is hampered by near-field limitations inherent to the ultrasound method (Figure 18.5). This highlights an important limitation of TEE in the quantification of aortic atherosclerosis.

TECMR versus surface coil CMR

Warren et al[34] compared the image acquisition using combined TECMR and surface coils versus standard surface coil CMR in a group of patients enrolled in a cholesterol-lowering study to assess changes in thoracic aortic atherosclerotic plaque size over a 6-month follow-up period. Data from each receiver coil (anterior chest, posterior

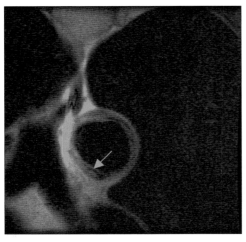

(a)

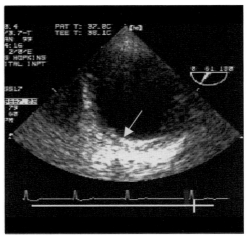

(b)

Figure 18.4
Aortic plaque by TECMR (a) versus TEE (b) in a 77-year-old with remote stroke. The TECMR picture shows a heterogenous plaque consistent with intraplaque calcification or hemorrhage.

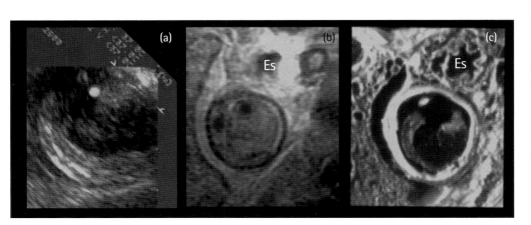

Figure 18.5
Descending thoracic aorta in a male cadaver with diffuse aortic atherosclerosis. TEE fails to image the entire aortic cross-section. (a) TEE; (b) TECMR; (c) histopathology. Es, esophagus.

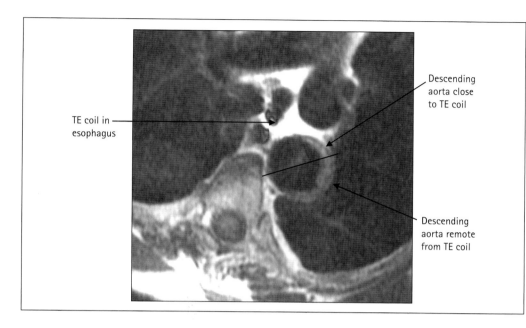

Figure 18.6
Schematic division of descending aorta into 'close to' and 'remote from' transesophageal (TE) coil for signal-to-noise ratio (SNR) measurement.

Labels on figure:
TE coil in esophagus
Descending aorta close to TE coil
Descending aorta remote from TE coil

chest, and transesophageal) were obtained individually, along with a composite image of all coils combined. Scion image 4.02 software was used to measure the signal for aortic atherosclerotic plaques close to and remote from the esophagus (Figure 18.6). Signal as well as the background image noise were measured for each coil individually and for both proton density-weighted (PDW) and T2-weighted (T2W) images using a region-of-interest (ROI) tool. The combined image SNR, the surface coil SNR (anterior plus posterior coils), and the transesophageal coil SNR were calculated using established methodology.[35] The percentage contribution of the transesophageal coil to the total image SNR was calculated using the following formula:

$$\frac{(\text{TE coil SNR})^2}{(\text{combined image SNR})^2}.$$

The percentage contribution of the surface coils to the total image SNR was calculated as follows:

$$\frac{(\text{surface coil 1})^2 + (\text{surface coil 2})^2 + (\text{surface coil 3})^2}{(\text{combined image SNR})^2}.$$

The SNR of the combined approach was superior to the SNR of any coil alone 93% of the time. In the descending aorta closest to the transesophageal coil (180° arc), the transesophageal coil SNR was 72% of the combined SNR for PDW images and 68% for T2W images. In the descending aorta remote from the transesophageal coil, the transesophageal coil SNR was 43% of combined SNR for PDW and 37% for T2W. Using only a small area of the descending aorta adjacent to the esophagus for image analysis, the transesophageal coil accounted for 80% of total image SNR for PDW and 79% for T2W images. In

the aortic arch, the transesophageal coil SNR was 66% of the combined SNR for PDW and 63% for T2W images for the segment of aorta nearest the esophagus. Fpr the aortic arch remote from the esophagus, the transesophageal coil SNR was 41% of combined image SNR for PDW images and 40% for T2W images (Figure 18.7).

In the ascending aorta, the transesophageal coil contributed <25% to the combined SNR. Inter-observer agreement ($r = 0.94$ for T2W and $r = 0.90$ for PDW images) and intra-observer agreement ($r = 0.90$ for both T2W and PDW) were high. This study found that the combined transesophageal and surface CMR approach provides improved SNR as compared with surface coil or TECMR techniques alone. Especially for the aortic arch and descending thoracic aorta, the transesophageal coil adds significantly to the combined image SNR. The value of the transesophageal coil in aortic plaque imaging is particularly apparent in the portion of the aorta closest to the esophagus. However, the transesophageal coil had little role in imaging the ascending aorta. The SNR of the combined coil image was superior to that of any single coil alone.[36]

In 10 patients imaged by TECMR, a second CMR study was obtained within 1 week of the index CMR examination for reproducibility of plaque size measurements (Figure 18.8).[37] Plaque thickness (mm) and plaque area (cm²) were measured for each image and the 3D plaque volume (cm³) was calculated for the composite of all images using Simpson's rule:[38]

$$\left[\tfrac{1}{3}A_1 + A_5 + 4(A_2 + A_4) + 2A_3\right] + \tfrac{1}{2}(A_5 + A_6),$$

where A_n ($n = 1, \ldots, 6$) is the area of image n. Table 18.1 shows the results of the reproducibility analysis. The

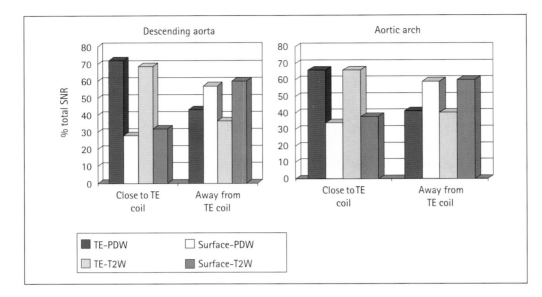

Figure 18.7
SNR analysis for TECMR versus CMR using only surface coils, 'close to' and 'remote from' the TE coil, for T2-weighted (T2W) and proton density-weighted (PDW) images.

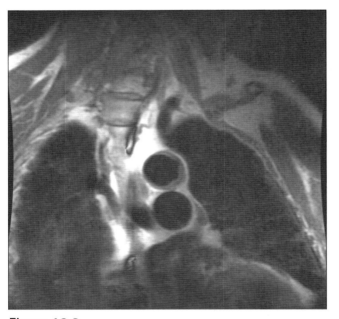 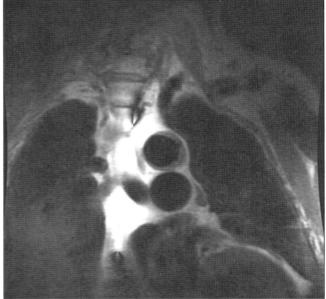

Figure 18.8
The same patient imaged twice with TECMR at a gap of 1 week.

Table 18.1. Reproducibility analysis for TECMR-measured aortic plaque thickness, area, and volume

Reproducibility measurement	Thickness		Area		Volume	
	PDW	T2W	PDW	T2W	PDW	T2W
Intraclass correlation coefficient R	0.82	0.84	0.90	0.91	0.95	0.97
Coefficient of variation (%)	18.9	18.2	21.3	23.9	5.7	4.8

Inter-observer reliability was high between two independent observers, $r = 0.97$. PDW, proton density-weighted; T2W, T2-weighted.

inter-observer reliability for plaque volume was high, $r = 0.96$. The reproducibility analysis showed significant variability of 1D and 2D measurements of plaque. This variability was improved by measuring a 3D volume of atherosclerosis in the entire imaged segment of aorta. The authors also computed the percentage change in plaque volume for each patient (difference in plaque volume from study 1 to study 2/study 1 plaque volume* 100%). From this, they calculated that the background standard error using this technique of TECMR is 2.24–2.65% for measurement of aortic plaque volume.[37]

TECMR technique

In this section, we will describe the process of acquisition of a TECMR study. The TECMR receiver probe (Intercept Esophageal MR Coil, Surgi-Vision, Gaithersburg, MD) has been described above. This is placed through the nose into the esophagus via a Levin tube, using topical benzocaine spray only when needed. Proper positioning is confirmed by aspiration and auscultation, and adjusted once after scout images if necessary. The distal portion of the receiver is placed at the gastroesophageal junction (Figure 18.9).

The TECMR device is arrayed with a standard cardiac phase array surface coil using a specially designed CMR interface connector. The indicated location of the TECMR probe is recognized in each image by the characteristic appearance of a small dark region reflecting the actual silver and copper coaxial RF receiver within the brightest

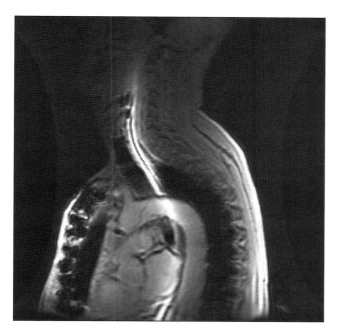

Figure 18.9
Proper positioning of the TECMR probe in the distal esophagus confirmed by CMR.

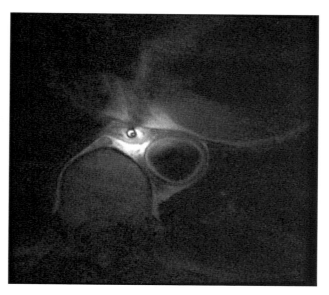

Figure 18.10
Appearance of the transesophageal coil in a cross-sectional view.

region of the image. The metallic conductor can be seen in the center (dark), surrounded by gastric fluid (light), surrounded in turn by plastic (dark) from the Levin tube probe housing, all within the brightest region of the image (Figure 18.10).

Guided by scout images, oblique slices of the thoracic aorta perpendicular to blood flow are prescribed. The present protocol includes the acquisition of six images of the thoracic aorta with a 4 mm slice thickness and no gap encompassing the area with the thickest plaque seen on sagittal image planes. One or two segments of the thoracic aorta are targeted, depending on patient compliance and scan time. Imaging is done with both T2W and PDW techniques during breathholds, with an ECG-gated fast spin-echo imaging pulse sequence and inversion recovery RF pulses to produce black-blood images. Additional imaging parameters are 16–24 cm field of view, 4 mm slice thickness, no gap, repetition time (TR) = 2R–R intervals, echo delay time (TE) = 20 ms (PDW) and 65 ms (T2W), image matrix 256 × 160, echo train length (ETL) = 16–24, 1 NEX (number of excitations), and no phase wrap. After the completion of the study, the Levin tube and TECMR receiver are removed.

Aortic atherosclerosis research using TECMR

At the Department of Cardiology, Johns Hopkins University School of Medicine, we are using TECMR as a measurement tool for studying the effect of lipid-lowering agents on atherosclerotic plaque in the thoracic aorta.[37]

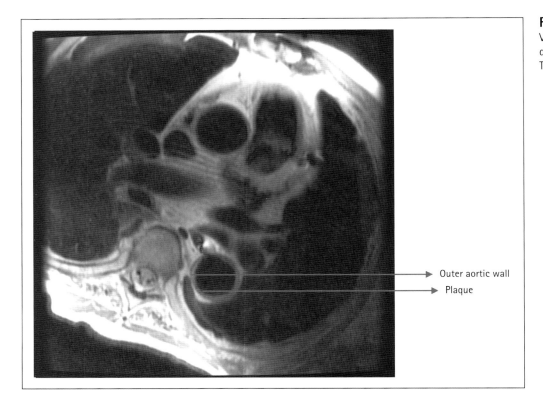

Figure 18.11
Visualization of plaque in descending aorta using TECMR.

Outer aortic wall
Plaque

Eligible participants are patients with documented atherosclerosis in at least one vascular territory, such as aortic disease seen by TEE for stroke evaluation or in the cardiac operating room during bypass or valve surgery, multivessel coronary disease seen at cardiac catheterization, or aortic or peripheral vascular disease necessitating vascular surgery. Patients are then randomly assigned to a high- or low-dose statin (simvastatin 80 mg or 20 mg) and followed with serial lipid panels every 3 months and serial TECMRs every 6 months.

In 37 patients, we have measured the baseline plaque thickness, plaque area and the 3D volume of thoracic aortic plaque using combined surface CMR and TECMR. Figure 18.11 shows atherosclerotic plaque in the descending aorta in one of these patients. The average plaque thickness per patient was 3.7 ± 1.1 mm (mean $\pm$ SD).

The average plaque area was 140 ± 69.5 mm^2. The plaque volume averaged 2.9 ± 1.4 cm^3. Fourteen patients have been followed for 6 months after randomization. In these patients, the mean atherosclerotic plaque volume by TECMR decreased by 13% from 3.5 ± 0.3 cm^3 to 3.0 ± 0.3 cm^3 ($p < 0.02$) at 6 months. The change in aortic plaque volume was well above the upper limit of 5.3% attributable to error (double the calculated standard error). The role of CMR in the longitudinal follow-up of aortic atherosclerotic plaque has been also recognized in other studies.[39–41]

Advantages of TECMR

1. Close proximity to the thoracic aorta affords higher SNR and image resolution. This aspect of TECMR is important for characterization of the aortic atherosclerotic plaque (Figure 18.9).
2. When combined with surface coils, TECMR provides more accurate quantification of plaque burden. Plaque volume measurement is much more reproducible than presently used measures of plaque size, i.e. plaque thickness and plaque area.[37]
3. As opposed to TEE, there are no near-field limitations and artifacts, and the entire aortic wall circumference can be imaged.
4. The probe is introduced transnasally in nonsedated patients, with minimal risk of complications. Also, there is no need for highly trained conscious-sedation personnel during imaging.
5. Once positioned in the esophagus, the probe provides multiple views without further manipulation.

Limitations of TECMR

1. As opposed to TEE, this technique is not portable to the bedside and does not allow for true real-time imaging.

2. Compared with surface-coil CMR, TECMR is slightly invasive and therefore carries more potential risk. However, this risk is minimized by the small caliber of the nasogastric tube housing for the probe.

3. In terms of safety, the potential for heating of the device is the primary concern. Intrinsic to MRI technology is a feature that detects a change in the bias current used to decouple the antenna. If a change in this bias current is detected, the system will alarm and shut down the pulse sequence. While this safety feature has been triggered during deliberate attempts to operate the device in a phantom with the decoupling disabled, it has not triggered during any studies in which the decoupling feature of the tuning, matching, and decoupling circuit (TMD box) was enabled.[31]

Potential uses of TECMR

1. *Quantitative and qualitative studies of aortic atherosclerosis, including therapeutic trials of change in plaque size and vulnerability.* TECMR combined with surface CMR may well be the ideal method of measurement of plaque burden and plaque characterization.[37] Plaque thickness or area measured in the most stenosed slice or as the average of all slices are subject to significant variation caused by minimal errors of prescription. Global plaque measurements such as total plaque volume would be more representative of plaque burden.[37,42] TECMR measured plaque volume is a highly reproducible index.

2. *Study of adjacent cardiac structures, particularly the left atrium.* The higher SNR by TECMR for left-atrial studies merits clinical trials comparing with TEE for the diagnosis of left-atrial thrombi and masses.

3. *Study of coronary arteries.* Recent studies have highlighted the use of CMR to visualize plaque in coronary vasculature.[43] TECMR would be more useful, considering the closer proximity to coronary anatomy. We know that human coronary arteries enlarge in relation to plaque area (Glagov phenomenon), and this compensatory enlargement may delay the recognition of significant atherosclerotic disease by traditional coronary angiography.[7] Animal experiments using TECMR to study coronary vessels are ongoing.

4. *Electrophysiological studies and therapeutic procedures.* Ongoing trials at the Johns Hopkins Hospital are using CMR to guide cardiac RF ablation therapy.[44]

Conclusions

In conclusion, the TECMR technique is a promising tool for quantification of atherosclerotic plaque extent in the aortic arch and the descending thoracic aorta. Because the entire circumference of the aorta can be visualized at any level and orientation, the relationship of individual plaques to structural landmarks is straightforward, making the technique ideal for serial studies. This is particularly important in serial studies of qualitative and quantitative response of aortic plaque to treatment modalities such as lipid-lowering therapies. Emerging data are showing that lipid-lowering therapy causes significant changes in plaque composition and burden.[45] The minimally invasive nature of TECMR and the lack of a requirement for sedation are additional advantages. The potential for detailed assessment of plaque composition and characterization makes TECMR an important addition to cardiovascular medicine and clinical investigation.[46]

References

1. Kallikazaros IE, Tsioufis CP, Stefanadis CI, et al. Closed relation between carotid and ascending aortic atherosclerosis in cardiac patients. Circulation 2000; 102(19 Suppl 3):III263–8.

2. Fayad ZA, Nahar T, Fallon JT, et al. In vivo magnetic resonance evaluation of atherosclerotic plaques in the human thoracic aorta: a comparison with transesophageal echocardiography. Circulation 2000; 101:2503–9.

3. Solberg LA, Strong JP. Risk factors and atherosclerotic lesions: a review of autopsy studies. Arteriosclerosis 1983; 3:187–98.

4. Tunick PA, Kronzon I. Atheromas of the thoracic aorta: clinical and therapeutic update. J Am Coll Cardiol 2000; 35:545–54.

5. Fazio GP, Redberg RF, Winslow T, et al. Transesophageal echocardiographically detected atherosclerotic aortic plaque is a marker for coronary artery disease. J Am Coll Cardiol 1993; 21:144–50.

6. Cohen A, Tzourio C, Bertrand B, et al. Aortic plaque morphology and vascular events: a follow-up study in patients with ischemic stroke. FAPS Investigators. French Study of Aortic Plaques in Stroke. Circulation 1997; 96:3838–41.

7. Glagov S, Weisenberg E, Zarins CK, et al. Compensatory enlargement of human atherosclerotic coronary arteries. N Engl J Med 1987; 316:1371–5.

8. Little WC. Angiographic assessment of the culprit coronary artery lesion before acute myocardial infarction. Am J Cardiol 1990; 66:44G–7G.

9. Libby P. Current concepts of the pathogenesis of the acute coronary syndromes. Circulation 2001; 104:365–72.

10. Kasprzak JD, Salustri A, Taams M, et al. Three-dimensional echocardiography of the thoracic aorta. Eur Heart J 1996; 17:1584–92.

11. Montgomery DH, Ververis JJ, McGgorisk G, et al. Natural history of severe atheromatous disease of the thoracic aorta: a transesophageal echocardiographic study. J Am Coll Cardiol 1996; 27:95–101.

12. Thomas AC, Davies MJ, Dilly S, et al. Potential errors in the estimation of coronary arterial stenosis from clinical arteriography with reference to the shape of the caronary artery lumen. Br Heart J 1993; 55:144–50.

13. Brown G, Albers JJ, Fisher LD, et al. Regression of coronary artery disease as a result of intensive lipid-lowering therapy in men with high levels of apolipoprotein B. N Engl J Med 1990; 323:1289–98.

14. Mintz GS, Nissen SE, Anderson WE, et al. American College of Cardiology Clinical Expert Consensus Document on Standards for Acquisition, Measurement and Reporting of Intravascular Ultrasound Studies (IVUS). A report of the American College of Cardiology Task Force on Clinical Expert Consensus Documents. J Am Coll Cardiol 2001; 37:1478–92.

15. Feld S, Ganim M, Carell ES, et al. Comparison of angioscopy, intravascular ultrasound imaging and quantitative coronary angiography in predicting clinical outcome after coronary intervention in high risk patients. J Am Coll Cardiol 1996; 28:97–105.

16. Casscells W, Hathorn B, David M, et al. Thermal detection of cellular infiltrates in living atherosclerotic plaques: possible implications for plaque rupture and thrombosis. Lancet 1996; 347:1447–51.

17. Stefanadis C, Diamantopoulos L, Vlachopoulos C, et al. Thermal heterogeneity within human atherosclerotic coronary arteries detected in vivo: a new method of detection by application of a special thermography catheter. Circulation 1999; 99:1965–71.

18. Tearney GJ, Brezinski ME, Bouma BE, et al. In vivo endoscopic optical biopsy with optical coherence tomography. Science 1997; 276:2037–9.

19. Romer TJ, Brennan JF 3rd, Puppels GJ, et al. Intravascular ultrasound combined with Raman spectroscopy to localize and quantify cholesterol and calcium salts in atherosclerotic coronary arteries. Arterioscler Thromb Vasc Biol 2000; 20:478–83.

20. Charash WE, Lodder RA, Moreno PR, et al. Detection of simulated vulnerable plaque using a novel infrared spectroscopy catheter. J Am Coll Cardiol 2000; 35:38A(abst).

21. Wexler L, Brundage B, Crouse J, et al. Coronary artery calcification: pathophysiology, epidemiology, imaging methods, and clinical implications. A statement for health professionals from the American Heart Association Writing Group. Circulation 1996; 94:1175–92.

22. Fayad ZA, Fuster V. Review. Clinical Imaging of the high-risk or vulnerable atherosclerotic plaque. Circ Res 2001; 89:305.

23. Toussaint JF, LaMuraglia GM, Southern JF, et al. Magnetic resonance images of lipid, fibrous, calcified, hemorrhagic, and thrombotic components of human atherosclerosis in vivo. Circulation 1996; 94:932–8.

24. Zimmermann-Paul GG, Quick HH, Vogt P, et al. High-resolution intravascular magnetic resonance imaging. Monitoring of plaque formation in heritable hyperlipidemic rabbits. Circulation 1999; 99:1054–61.

25. Rivas PA, Nayak KS, Scott GC, et al. In vivo real-time intravascular MRI. J Cardiovasc Magn Reson 2002; 4:223–32.

26. Correia LC, Atalar E, Kelemen MD, et al. Intravascular magnetic resonance imaging of aortic atherosclerotic plaque composition. Arterioscler Thromb Vasc Biol 1997; 17:3626–32.

27. Martin AJ, McLoughlin RL, Chu KC, et al. An expandable intravenous RF coil for arterial wall imaging. J Magn Reson Imaging 1998; 8:226–34.

28. Narayan P, Vigneron DB, Jajodid P, et al. Transrectal probe for ^{1}H and ^{31}P MR spectroscopy of the prostate gland. Magn Reson Med 1989; 11:209–20.

29. Schnall MD, Lenkinski R, Pollack HM, et al. Prostate: MR imaging with an endorectal surface coil. Radiology 1989; 172:570–4.

30. Siegelman ES, Outwater EK, Banner MP, et al. High resolution MR imaging of the vagina. Radiographics 1997; 17:1183–203.

31. Shunk KA, Lima JAC, Heldman AW, et al. Transesophageal magnetic resonance imaging. Magn Reson Med 1999; 41:722–6.

32. Ocali O, Atalar E. Intravascular magnetic resonance imaging using a loopless catheter antenna. Magn Reson Med 1997; 37:112–18.

33. Shunk KA, Garot J, Atalar E, et al. Transesophageal magnetic resonance imaging of the aortic arch and descending thoracic aorta in patients with aortic atherosclerosis. J Am Coll Cardiol 2001; 37:2031–5.

34. Warren WP, Gautam S, Lima JAC. E-selectin and P-selectin are markers of aortic plaque burden as measured by transesophageal MRI. J Am Coll Cardiol 2003; 41(Suppl A):259A.

35. Constantinides CD, Atalar E, McVeigh ER. Signal-to-noise measurements in magnitude images from NMR phased arrays. Magn Reson Med 1997; 38:852–7.

36. Warren WP, Gautam S, Steen H, Lima JAC. Combined transesophageal and surface MRI provides optimal imaging of aortic atherosclerosis. J Am Coll Cardiol 2003; 41(Suppl A):458A.

37. Warren WP, Gautam S, Lima JAC. Effect of statin therapy on aortic atherosclerotic plaque volume measured by transesophageal MRI. Circulation 2002; 106:II-524.

38. Jeffreys, H, Jeffreys BS. Methods of Mathematical Physics, 3rd edn. Cambridge: Cambridge University Press, 1956:286.

39. Corti R, Fayad ZA, Fuster V, et al. Effects of lipid-lowering by simvastatin on human atherosclerotic lesions: a longitudinal study by high-resolution, noninvasive magnetic resonance imaging. Circulation 2001; 104:249–52.

40. Worthley SG, Helft G, Fuster V, et al. Serial in vivo MRI documents arterial remodeling in experimental atherosclerosis. Circulation 2000; 101:586–9.

41. Helft G, Worthley SG, Fuster V, et al. Progression and regression of atherosclerotic lesions. Monitoring with serial noninvasive magnetic resonance imaging. Circulation 2002; 105:993.

42. Morrisett JD, Insull W Jr. Evaluating atherosclerotic lesions by magnetic resonance imaging. From dimensional to compositional quantitation. Arterioscler Thromb Vasc Biol 2001; 21:1563–4.

43. Kim WY, Danias PG, Stuber M, et al. Coronary magnetic resonance angiography for the detection of coronary stenoses. N Engl J Med 2001; 345:1863–9.

44. Lardo AC, McVeigh ER, Jumrussirikul P, et al. Visualization and temporal/spatial characterization of cardiac radiofrequency ablation lesions using magnetic resonance imaging. Circulation 2000; 102:698–705.

45. Zhao XQ, Yuan C, Hatsukami TS, et al. Effects of prolonged intensive lipid-lowering therapy on the characteristics of carotid atherosclerotic plaques in vivo by MRI: a case–control study. Arterioscler Thromb Vasc Biol 21:1623–9.

46. Shunk KA, Atalar E, Lima JA. Possibilities of transesophageal MRI for assessment of aortic disease: a review. Int J Cardiovasc Imaging 2001; 17:179–85.

19

CMR in the assessment of pulmonary hypertension

Howard V Dinh, Jeffrey P Goldman, Michael Poon

Introduction

In the past two decades, magnetic resonance imaging (MRI) has been transformed from a research tool of organic chemists and physicists for deciphering molecular structures of chemical compounds to a robust and user-friendly imaging modality for clinicians and clinical scientists. Because of recent advances in hardware and software technology as well as in contrast agent, current MR images may be obtained rapidly and with exquisite morphologic detail in a noninvasive manner.[1–4] These images may be viewed from various tomographic orientations both in stilled frames and in dynamic cine format. The use of MRI in the assessment of cardiovascular diseases (i.e. cardiovascular MRI: CMR) is a rapidly growing field. One potential clinical application has been the assessment of pulmonary hypertensive diseases and right-ventricular (RV) dysfunction. RV dilatation and hypertrophy are adaptive changes in response to worsening pulmonary hypertension. These changes are analogous to that of left-ventricular (LV) hypertrophy and dilatation in response to chronic essential hypertension. The irregular shape of the RV and the unpredictable alterations in the dimension of this chamber in response to high pulmonary artery pressures pose a major challenge for many conventional cardiac imaging modalities. Compared with ultrasound-, radionuclide-, and X-ray-based imaging methods, CMR offers significant advantages in the evaluation of RV function and morphology. In this chapter, we explore current and potential applications of CMR in the diagnostic workup and subsequent follow-up of patients with pulmonary hypertension.

Pulmonary hypertension

Classification

Pulmonary hypertension (PH) is a devastating disease characterized by the progressive elevation of pulmonary artery (PA) pressure leading to RV failure and eventual death. However, it is not a single disease entity, but a common clinical endpoint for a host of diseases that are still being actively investigated. Traditionally, PH was classified into primary pulmonary hypertension (PPH) and secondary pulmonary hypertension (SPH). The major difference between these two groups of patients is that patients with SPH have a clear etiology or associated underlying disorder, which directly leads to elevated pulmonary artery pressure, while those with PPH are seemingly without a clear underlying cause. A newer, clinically more useful, treatment-based classification of pulmonary hypertension was proposed by a team of experts at the World Health Organization (WHO) meeting on the diagnostic classification of PH in 1998.[5] Five categories of PH were recognized: pulmonary arterial hypertension (PAH), pulmonary venous hypertension, pulmonary hypertension associated with disorders of the respiratory system and/or hypoxemia, pulmonary hypertension due to chronic thrombotic and/or embolic diseases, and pulmonary hypertension due to disorders directly affecting the pulmonary vasculature. PAH is perhaps the most intriguing group of all and has been an active area of research in the past two decades. PAH is further divided into PPH and pulmonary hypertension related to a variety of diseases (Table 19.1). The pathobiology of pulmonary

Table 19.1. The 1998 World Health Organization diagnostic classification of pulmonary hypertension

Diagnostic classification	Clinical entities	Pathobiology
1. Pulmonary arterial hypertension (PAH)	• Primary pulmonary hypertension (PPH) • Collagen vascular disease • Congenital systemic-to-pulmonary shunts • Portal hypertension • HIV infection • Anorexigen use • Persistent pulmonary hypertension of the newborn	Unclear etiology of increased pulmonary arterial pressures. Potential mechanisms include imbalance of vasoconstrictors versus vasodilators, increased prothrombotic or proinflammatory factors, reduced vasoreactivity, microvascular thrombosis, and uncontrolled proliferation of endothelial and vascular smooth muscle cells.
2. Pulmonary venous hypertension	• Left-sided atrial or ventricular heart disease • Left-sided valvular heart disease • Extrinsic compression of central pulmonary veins • Pulmonary veno-occlusive disease	Increased pulmonary artery pressure is thought to be a direct result of prolonged increased pulmonary venous pressure.
3. Pulmonary hypertension related to hypoxemia or respiratory diseases	• Chronic obstructive pulmonary disease • Interstitial lung disease • Sleep disordered breathing • Alveolar hypoventilation disorders • Chronic exposure to high altitude • Neonatal lung disease • Alveolar–capillary dysplasia	Chronic hypoxia may lead to increased vasoconstriction and/or vascular remodeling, which reduces pulmonary vascular compliance.
4. Pulmonary hypertension secondary to chronic thromboembolic disease	• Thromboembolic obstruction of proximal pulmonary arteries • Obstruction of distal pulmonary arteries (in situ thrombosis, sickle cell disease, or pulmonary embolism)	Vascular thrombotic/embolic obstruction leading to hypoxia, shunting, and vasoconstriction may be the initial process. Other mechanisms as for PAH may apply.
5. Pulmonary hypertension secondary to disorders directly affecting the pulmonary vasculature	• Inflammation-inducing disorders (sarcoidosis, schistosomiasis) • Pulmonary capillary hemangiomatosis	Increased inflammation leading to upregulated expression of cytokines and vasoconstrictors may be the underlying process.

Modified from World Symposium on Primary Pulmonary Hypertension, www.who.int/ncd/cvd/pph.html.[5]

hypertension has been reviewed recently, and includes endothelial and smooth muscle cell dysfunction, abnormal activation and release of vasoactive mediators, vascular remodeling, microvascular thrombosis, increased proinflammatory cytokines, and abnormal ion channels.[6–10]

Clinical evaluation

The main goal of clinical evaluation remains the detection of secondary and potentially reversible causes of PH. Patients with PH often present with symptoms of dyspnea at rest or with exertion. Other commonly reported symptoms include fatigue, angina, and, in severe cases, syncope. Because these symptoms are nonspecific, all patients suspected of having PH should have a minimal screening

evaluation that includes a detailed history and physical examination, electrocardiogram (ECG), chest radiography, and transthoracic echocardiogram (Table 19.2a). This initial cardiopulmonary evaluation can aid the clinician in assessing for potential risk factors, defining the severity of the PH, and ruling out common secondary causes such as pulmonary parenchymal diseases and congenital/structural heart diseases, including valvular and other cardiac diseases of the LV.

Once PH is suggested by the initial evaluation, additional testing should be done to confirm its presence and to further characterize the severity of the disease (Table 19.2b). Pulmonary function testing should be performed to rule out chronic obstructive or restrictive pulmonary disease. Nuclear medicine ventilation and perfusion scans are often performed to identify thromboembolic process as a contributing cause in those with high clinical suspicion of chronic thromboembolism. A positive six-minute

Table 19.2. Clinical evaluation of a patient suspected of having pulmonary hypertension (PH)

(a) Minimal evaluation/screening
1. *History and physical examination*, to define:
- The severity of symptoms and functional status
- The presence of underlying diseases, which may be causative and/or reversible
- The use of certain anorexigens strongly associated with pulmonary hypertension, such as aminorex, fenfluramine, and dexfenfluramine
- Family history of PPH

2. *Electrocardiogram*, to identify:
- Right-atrial enlargement
- Right-ventricular hypertrophy
- Right-bundle branch block
- Right-axis deviation
- S1,Q3,T3 suggesting pulmonary embolism as an underlying cause
- Left-ventricular hypertrophy, suggesting left-sided failure as cause of PH

3. *Chest X-ray* to evaluate:
- The lung parenchyma for underlying pulmonary diseases
- Prominence of the pulmonary artery and hilar vessels with pruning of peripheral vessels
- RV hypertrophy as suggested by diminished retrocardiac space on the lateral chest X-ray
- Cardiomegaly or congestive heart failure, suggesting left-sided failure
- Hyperinflation and flattening of the diaphragm, suggesting chronic obstructive pulmonary disease

4. *Echocardiogram (transthoracic)*, to assess:
- Pulmonary artery pressure (estimate)
- Congenital heart disease such as septal defects, pulmonary valve stenosis, patent ductus arteriosus, etc.
- Valvular defects, such as tricuspid regurgitation or mitral stenosis/regurgitation
- Left- and right-ventricular function
- Peak right-ventricular pressure
- Atrial hypertrophy

(b) Additional testing once PH has been highly suspected by above testing
1. *Pulmonary function testing*, to identify:
- Evidence of obstructive pulmonary disease

2. *Ventilation–perfusion scan,*[a] to rule out:
- Pulmonary embolism

3. *Chest CT or MRI*, to evaluate:
- Lung parenchyma and perfusion
- Valvular heart disease
- Ventricular and atrial morphology
- Ventricular function

4. *Six-minute walk test*, to assess:
- Functional capacity and symptoms during exercise
- Response to medical therapy (if appropriate)

5. *Right- and left-heart catheterization*, to assess:
- Pulmonary artery diastolic and systolic pressure
- Right-atrial pressure
- Pulmonary capillary wedge pressure
- Pulmonary vascular resistance index
- Cardiac output/index
- Pulmonary and systemic arterial saturation
- Underlying coronary artery disease (if indicated)
- Pulmonary vascular reactivity to various vasodilators (e.g. adenosine, nitroglycerin, epoprostenol, nitric oxide, calcium channel blockers)

Table 19.2. *Continued*

(c) **Specialized testing when diagnosis of PH is uncertain**
 1. *Laboratory tests*, to detect:
    - Underlying hypercoagulable states (e.g. PT, PTT, factor V Leiden mutation, prothrombin gene mutation, lupus anticoagulant, antiphospholipid antibodies, homocysteine, protein C and S, antithrombin III, lipoprotein a)
    - Underlying rheumatologic disorders such as systemic lupus (ANA, anti-dsDNA, anti-smRNP), Sjögren syndrome (anti-SSA, anti-SSB), scleroderma (anti-centromere, Scl-70, U3-RNP), mixed connective tissue diseases (anti-U1-RNP), and rheumatoid arthritis (rheumatoid factor)
    - Underlying proinflammatory states (CRP, ESR)
    - Underlying infectious diseases (HIV, hepatitis B, hepatitis C, schistosomiasis)
 2. *Lung biopsy*, to identify:
    - Vasculitis

---

[a] For patients with abnormal chest-X-ray or a low-intermediate probability V-Q scan, a CT-angiogram or definitive pulmonary angiogram should be performed

---

walk test, in which the walk and rest distances, reported symptoms at the end of the test, and the changes in oxygen saturation are used to assess exercise tolerance, has been shown to correlate strongly with mortality.[11]

The gold standard for diagnosing PH is right-heart catheterization. Measurements of cardiac chamber pressures and pulmonary oxygenation are helpful in identifying the presence of PH and the degree of RV failure. Patients diagnosed with PH (i.e. mean pulmonary artery pressure > 25 mmHg at rest or > 30 mmHg with exercise) but without evidence of left-sided heart failure (i.e. mean pulmonary wedge pressure <18 mmHg) should undergo vasodilator challenge. A diagnosis of PPH can only be made after other secondary and associated disorders have been excluded. Initial workup includes extensive blood work in search of underlying disorders caused by various rheumatologic diseases, proinflammatory conditions, hypercoagulable states, and infectious etiologies (Table 19.2c). Open lung biopsy is rarely needed except for the very unusual cases where the diagnosis of PPH, in situ thrombosis, or vasculitis cannot be delineated with conventional diagnostic modalities.

CMR in the evaluation of pulmonary hypertension

The clinical workup of PH can be enormously costly and time-consuming. Echocardiography, due to its relatively low cost and wide availability among practicing cardiologists, is often used as an initial cardiac screening technique for patients with a possible diagnosis of PH. Estimation of PA pressures can be made with echocardiography by measuring the velocities of regurgitant jets through either the tricuspid valve or the pulmonic valve. There is a wide variation in the literature in the reported accuracy of this method, ranging from 53% to 97%.[12,13] Echocardiography also has limitations in the assessment of cardiac function, especially that of the RV (Table 19.3). Problems with geo-

---

Table 19.3. **Comparison of echocardiography versus CMR in the evaluation of pulmonary hypertension**

	Advantages	*Disadvantages*
Echocardiography	• Low equipment cost • Portable	• Low spatial resolution (~2 mm) • Acoustic window difficulties • Inaccurate assessment of RV function • Operator variability
CMR	• High spatial resolution (~0.5 mm) • Accurate assessment of all chamber sizes and functions • Ability to assess intramyocardial and pericardial abnormalities • Does not depend on body habitus • Wide spectrum of clinical utilities (MRA, perfusion, 3D imaging, etc.)	• Image quality depends very strongly on good cardiac and respiratory gating/breathholding • High equipment cost • Not portable

metric assumptions and subsequent magnification of imaging errors, operator variability, and difficult acoustic windows have made echocardiography less than optimal for use in this group of patients.[14]

CMR is particularly useful in the evaluation of patients with severe PH. RV morphology and function may be imaged with high resolution using CMR. Quantitative changes in chamber size, the presence of cardiac mass, pericardial or pleural effusion, and septal deformity can be identified and may explain the cause and severity of PH and RV failure. CMR is also an important diagnostic modality in ruling out secondary causes of PH. For example, valvular heart diseases, coexisting pulmonary parenchymal disorders, pericardial and infiltrative myocardial diseases, cardiac tumors or extracardiac masses, and various congenital and structural heart diseases may be adequately evaluated in the same setting. Finally, contrast-enhanced MR angiography (MRA) is extremely valuable in the functional assessment of pulmonary vascular abnormalities and cardiac shunts, which are also important causes of PH.

Evaluation of right heart failure

Right-ventricular function and mass

The RV shares an intimate relationship with the pulmonary vasculature. Normally, it pumps desaturated blood into the low-resistance pulmonary vascular bed. Compared with the LV, which acts against a higher afterload, the RV wall is about half as thick.[15] Pulmonary hypertensive diseases alter the geometry and pathology of the RV by causing a compensatory hypertrophy and remodeling of the RV chamber in an attempt to maintain cardiac output in the setting of increased afterload. These responses are adequate until a critical mass or 'strain' has been reached, after which RV failure ensues. The ability to detect RV failure early, accurately, and noninvasively is clinically important, for these changes are a harbinger of poor prognosis for patients with PAH.[16,17]

Accurate assessment of RV morphology can be obtained with ECG-gated spin-echo sequences and ECG-gated, breathhold gradient-echo sequences. These sequences are available with most CMR scanners.[18] A series of gradient-echo scout images is obtained, from which the MR operator may prescribe the various axes through the cardiac chambers to produce the standard cardiac views for analysis. Typically, cine images are obtained in the short and transverse axes to obtain views analogous to the conventional views obtained by echocardiography (Figure 19.1a–c). One of the main advantages

of CMR is the freedom to view the heart from any angle, including those that have been traditionally difficult or impossible to be obtained using echocardiography (Figure 19.1d). From these views, an overview of the cardiac chambers, valves, pericardium, and outflow tracts can be assessed qualitatively for abnormalities. Quantitative analysis of RV function is performed from dynamic cine images in the short-axis views and is based on Simpson's rule, whereby the operator applies contours to the endo- and epicardial borders on various slices through the RV in both diastole and systole. From this, automatic computer-generated calculations of RV ejection fraction, stroke volume, cardiac output, diastolic and systolic volumes, and cardiac mass may be obtained. Normal values for the above CMR parameters have been assessed in comparison with autopsy, echocardiography, X-ray angiography and computed tomography (CT).[15]

Quantitative CMR parameters such as RV mass and stroke volume in patients with PH have been studied in small populations, and have shown good correlation with the severity of PA pressure. Using ECG-gated, spin-echo MR, Katz et al[19] showed that CMR was able to quantify the mass of excised calf RV with a high degree of accuracy as compared with direct weighing (a correlation coefficient $r = 0.97$). Patients with PH ($n = 13$) have a mean RV mass more than twice that of normal subjects ($p < 0.01$); furthermore, these mass measurements correlate positively with mean PA pressures ($r = 0.75$, $p < 0.01$) as measured by right-heart catheterization. Marcus et al[20] used cardiac-triggered cine CMR and found that in 8 patients with PH secondary to chronic obstructive pulmonary disease (COPD), the mean RV mass was 17% greater ($p < 0.005$) than that of age-matched normal controls.[20] Furthermore, there were statistically significant increases in RV wall thickness and decreases in RV stroke volume indicative of the physiologic burden on RV function exerted by elevated PA pressures.

Chronic PH leads to RV hypertrophy. While elevated RV mass is a useful indicator of this progression, it may not be useful once the PH exceeds the contractile reserve of the RV. This was illustrated by Hoeper et al,[21] who compared CMR- and catheterization-derived hemodynamics of 16 patients with severe PH (mean PA pressure >45 mmHg) and found that there was no statistically significant correlation between RV mass and mean PA pressure. These findings may be explained in part by the selection of patients with extremely high PA pressure and significant tricuspid regurgitation. In this population, the RV hypertrophy is offset by a dilatory response due to volume overload caused by the regurgitant flow. Nevertheless, RV mass remains a highly useful parameter that signifies significant chronic PH. The differences in the CMR volumetric parameters between normal and PH patients are summarized in Table 19.4.

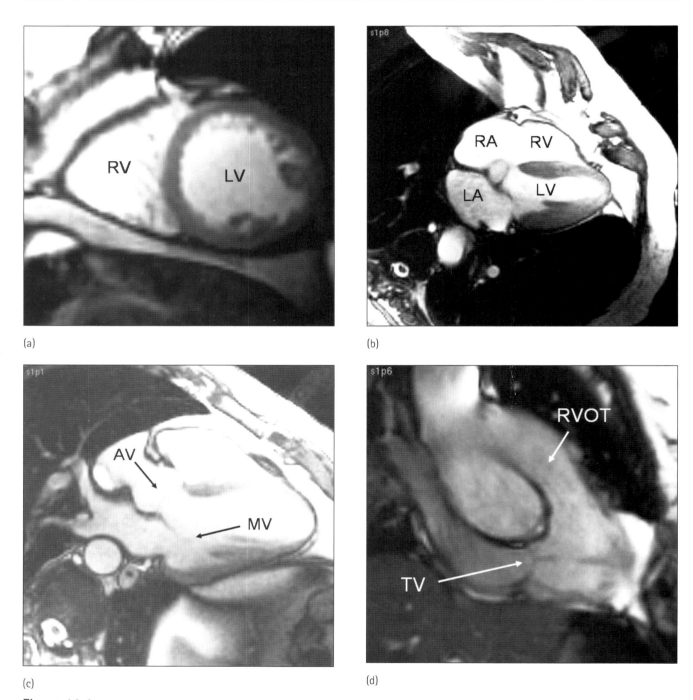

(a)

(b)

(c)

(d)

Figure 19.1
CMR views of the heart. (a) Short-axis view showing normal right and left ventricles (RV and LV). (b) Long-axis view (four-chamber view) showing normal right and left atria (A) and ventricles (V). (c) Left-ventricular outflow tract view showing normal mitral and aortic valves (MV and AV). (d) Right-ventricular outflow tract view showing tricupid valve (TV) and right-ventricular outflow tract (RVOT).

Septal deviation

The ventricular septum may be visualized on CMR with great spatial resolution. The position of the ventricular septum at end-diastole is an important marker of ventricular function and biventricular interplay.[22] Normally, the end-diastolic septal position is proportional to the difference between the RV and LV end-diastolic pressures (RVEDP and LVEDP). Because this value is ~3 mmHg (i.e. LVEDP>RVEDP) at end-diastole, the septum is slightly convex (or 'bowed') toward the RV (Figure 19.2a). Using 2D echocardiography, Dong et al[23] showed that in

Table 19.4. CMR characteristics suggestive of severe pulmonary hypertension

	Normal[15]	*Severe pulmonary hypertension*[19–21]
Volumetric parameters		
• Mean RV ejection fraction	61% ± 7%	34% ± 10%
• Mean RV mass	46 ± 11 g	109.6 ± 27 g
Anatomic parameters		
• RV wall thickness	Normal	Hypertrophied
• End-diastolic septal bowing	Towards the RV	Towards the LV
• Pulmonary Artery (PA)	Normal	Dilated main PA; pruning of the peripheral pulmonary vessels
Functional parameters		
• MR angiography	Normal	In situ PA thrombus or peripheral perfusion defect

animals with RV pressure overload secondary to PA constrictions, the end-diastolic septum progressively straightens out and deviates toward the LV as the transeptal pressure decreases and becomes negative (i.e. when RVEDP>LVEDP). This so-called leftward ventricular septal bowing (LVSB) (Figure 19.2b) was assessed in patients with PH. Using breathhold cine CMR, Marcus et al[24] noted statistically significant differences in the end-diastolic LVSB between normal control and 12 patients with PH (septal curvature of 0.30 ± 0.05 versus –0.14 ± 0.07; p <0.0001). This study confirmed previous animal models of RV overload, and suggests that the LVSB index may be an important marker of PH. Investigation led by

Sulica et al[25] have also assessed the degree of septal bowing by measuring the septal eccentricity index (EI). EI, defined as the ratio of the distance between the septal–lateral wall and the anterior–posterior wall measured in the short-axis view of breathhold CMR, was measured in both systole and diastole (SEI and DEI, respectively) in 16 controls and 21 patients with significant PH. Both SEI and DEI were significantly lower in PH patients compared with normal controls, and were highly correlated with worsening hemodynamic parameters. Abnormal septal deformity is a noninvasive parameter that may be an important surrogate marker of severe PH and may prove useful in following patients' response to various treatments.

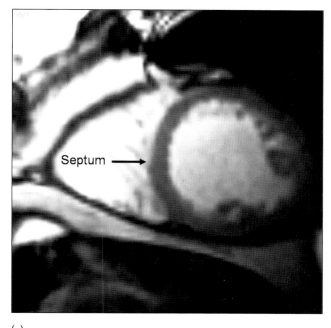

(a)

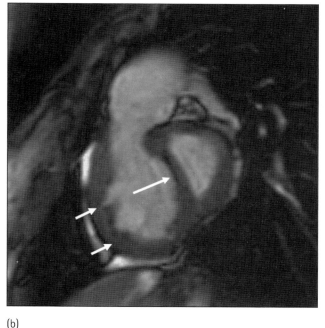

(b)

Figure 19.2
Abnormal septal movement in pulmonary hypertension. (a) Short-axis view of a normal heart. Note that the end-diastolic septal position (arrow) is bowed toward the right ventricle. (b) Short-axis view of the heart of a patient with severe pulmonary hypertension and right-ventricular hypertrophy (white short arrows). Note the 'D-shaped' deformity of the septal wall during diastole (long arrow).

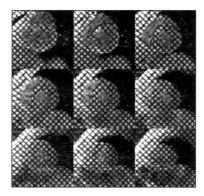

Figure 19.3
Myocardial tagging in pulmonary hypertension. Note the embedded saturation effects in the myocardial tissue, which deform with contraction of the myocardium.

Myocardial tagging

CMR has enabled the assessment of not only the function of the ventricular chamber (i.e. ejection fraction, volume, etc.), but also strain on the myocardium itself. This distinction is important, since it has long been understood that myocardial function may be compromised even when the ventricular pumping action is preserved secondary to reactive ventricular hypertrophy. Myocardial tagging can be used to measure myocardial strain. This method has been reviewed by Reichek.[3] In brief, the saturation effects by tagging techniques are embedded in the tissue and deform with the contraction of myocardial tissue, thus permitting the detailed characterization of myocardial fiber strain and shortening in normal and stressed ventricles (Figure 19.3).

Myocardial tagging has been applied to the study of the LV and RV function. The percentage segmental shortening (%S) is derived from analysis of designated-tagged regions of myocardium during diastole and systole. Using one-dimensional spatial modulation of magnetization (SPAMM) tags and a breathhold gradient-echo segmented *k*-space imaging technique, Fayad et al[26] compared the %S of various regions of the RV in 7 patients with chronic PH and 10 healthy normal volunteers. The results showed that in both short- and long-axis views, there were statistically significant depressions in the %S of all regions tested in the RV free wall in patients with PH as compared with controls. In addition, PH patients also showed depressions in %S in all regions of the septum (except for the midventricular septum as seen in the long-axis view). These results reconfirm the suspicion that prolonged elevation of pulmonary pressure cause RV strain even in patients who showed no overt RV pump failure. Although these preliminary data need to be confirmed and intra- and inter-observer variability needs to be reduced, this study is one of the few to apply this new CMR method to non-invasively assess RV strain patterns. Another potential application of this technology is its use in assessing medical therapeutics that potentially may improve patient symptoms via direct or indirect effects on the RV myocardium itself.

Currently, myocardial tagging software packages are available for use in most CMR scanners. Its clinical application is not widespread and still falls mainly in the purview of clinical investigation secondary to the lack of easy-to-use analysis packages. However, its use in the assessment of RV strain has important potential.

Evaluation of cardiac function under stress

The development of RV dysfunction in patients with severe PH is an ominous sign. Although the etiology of this phenomenon is unclear, myocardial ischemia secondary to abnormalities in the microcirculation has been hypothesized.[27,28] Gomez et al[29] have provided data to suggest that PH patients who develop evidence of RV failure based on echocardiographic or hemodynamic data might indeed have RV ischemia. In a prospective study, 23 PH patients underwent evaluation with echocardiography, right-heart catheterization, and exercise-stress single-photon emission computed tomography (SPECT). The right-atrial (RA) pressure, RV end-diastolic pressure, and mixed venous oxygenation in the 9 patients who had evidence of RV ischemia on SPECT were significantly higher than in the remaining PH patients who did not have ischemia ($p = 0.07$, 0.001, and 0.0001, respectively). All patients had normal coronary angiographies, and thus RV ischemia was not secondary to major epicardial artery disease, but perhaps as a result of increased metabolic demand and poor coronary blood flow.

Microvascular ischemia of the RV may be an important contributor to decompensating PH patients. However, which PH patients are prone to this and why some patients are better at compensating for high PA pressures needs further study. RV contractile reserve – the ability of the RV to augment its function upon demand may have prognostic value. Using a low-dose dobutamine stress CMR protocol, preliminary data from Goldman et al[30] demonstrated that PAH patients who had no significant augmentation or a decrease in RV ejection fraction in response to the dobutamine challenge were associated with poorer functional status and worse clinical symptoms (Figure 19.4). This study suggests that those with less severe disease (or RV dysfunction) may have better RV contractile reserve that is only apparent during pharmacologic stress testing. This finding may have important clinical implications in aiding the selec-

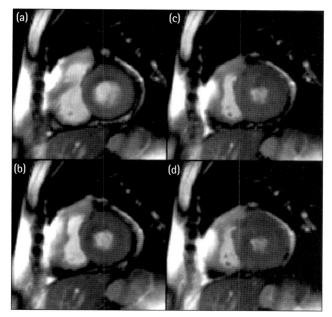

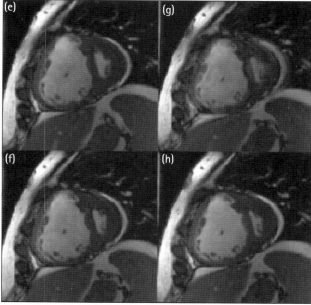

Figure 19.4
Dobutamine stress function of the right ventricle in normal and severe pulmonary hypertension. Right-ventricular ejection fraction:
(a) 66% (baseline); (b) 69% (dobutamine at 10 μg/kg/min); (c) 71% (dobutamine at 20 μg/kg/min); (d) 77% (dobutamine at
40 μg/kg/min); (e) 24% (baseline); (f) 22% (dobutamine at 5 μg/kg/min); (g) 15% (dobutamine at 10 μg/kg/min); (h) 16% (dobutamine at
20 μg/kg/min).

tion of patients who should receive early aggressive pharmacologic treatment.

Interstitial and chronic obstructive lung diseases are an important cause of secondary pulmonary hypertension. At present, the imaging of the lung parenchyma is performed

Evaluation of the pulmonary circulation

Pulmonary anatomy and morphology

Patients with chronic PH show pathologic changes in the pulmonary vasculature, most commonly central PA dilatation and peripheral PA pruning (Figure 19.5). Early studies in small cohorts of patients with PPH evaluated various CMR characteristics of the pulmonary vasculature in patients with elevated PA pressures and pulmonary vascular resistance. Using single-breathhold gradient-recalled acquisition in a steady-state technique, Gefter et al[31] compared the CMR of 8 patients with PH with 12 normal controls. Patients with PH showed dilatation and pruning of PA not noted in normal subjects. Attenuation of the peripheral branches of the PA was more prominent in PH. Furthermore, there was significant dampening in the percentage increase of PA diameter during systole in patients with PH as compared with healthy controls.

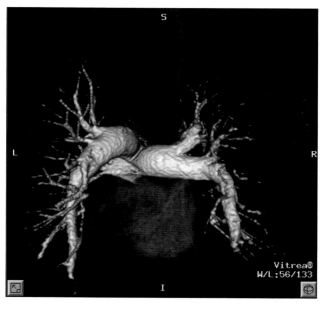

Figure 19.5
MRA of the pulmonary artery in pulmonary hypertension. Volume-rendered MR angiogram of a PH patient whose main pulmonary arteries are dilated and where there is evidence of pruning of the peripheral pulmonary arterial vessels.

using conventional X-ray-based modalities (chest roentgenograms and computed tomography). A few CMR centers have been exploring the use of inhaled or aerosolized contrast agents such as oxygen, gadolinium chelates, sulfur hexaflouride, perfluorcarbons, helium-3, and xenon-129 to demonstrate lung morphology, gas exchange, and ventilation abnormalities.[32] This technology has advanced tremendously, and a potential role for it in the clinical diagnosis of ventilation defects is anticipated.

Pulmonary perfusion and angiography

While worsening PH with elevated pulmonary vascular resistance may itself lead to in situ thrombus formation, chronic pulmonary embolism in patients with hypercoagulable states is a well-known risk factor for PH.[7,33] Anticoagulation of PH patients, even those where there are no objective findings of pulmonary embolus, has been proven to improve survival, indicating either that PH predisposes a patient to a hypercoagulable state, or that thromboembolic events occur but are underdiagnosed with current imaging studies. There is evidence to support both theories.[5,33–35]

Pulmonary embolism, a major cause of mortality and morbidity in the USA, may be diagnosed via various techniques. The current gold standard is X-ray angiography, but other techniques may also be utilized. These include ventilation–perfusion scanning, CT angiography, and, more recently, contrast-enhanced MRA. The use of these various techniques in the detection of pulmonary embolus is an area of active clinical research and has been recently reviewed.[36–38]

MR characteristics of pulmonary embolus include intravascular filling defects, 'trailing-embolus' and 'vessel cutoff'[2] (Figure 19.6). MR sequences, such as time-of-flight (TOF) and phase contrast (PC) MRA, are able to produce adequate contrast between laminar flowing blood and allow for imaging of vascular perfusion without the addition of a contrast agent. TOF methods involve the use of multiple radiofrequency pulses with short repeat times to suppress MR signals emanating from the nonmobile perivascular tissue but allow bright signals to be produced from the fresh incoming flowing blood. PC methods exploit the magnetic spin phase shifts acquired by blood moving in the direction of the magnetic field as opposed to the minimal or lack of phase shifts of the surrounding stationary tissue. The differences in phase shifts are manipulated to produce imaging contrast, and information regarding blood flow and velocity may also be generated. Patients with PH or with pulmonary embolism have abnormalities in the pulmonary vasculature, and disturbance to laminar flow may give rise to image artifacts.[39]

Contrast-enhanced MRA is a technique pioneered by Prince in the early 1990s that overcomes many artifacts inherent in TOF imaging. Small prospective studies have

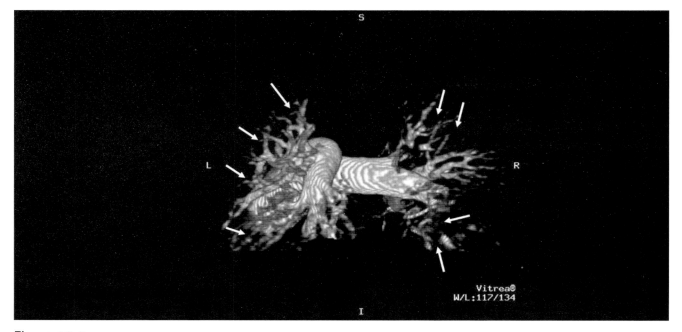

Figure 19.6
MRA of pulmonary embolism. Multiple pulmonary perfusion defects (white arrows) are detected on this volume-rendered MRA image of a patient with pulmonary hypertension and pulmonary thromboembolisms.

Table 19.5. Comparison of MR angiography (MRA) with CT angiography (CTA) in the diagnosis of pulmonary thromboembolic disease

	MRA[40–42]	CTA[43–52]
Sensitivity (%)	68–100	63–100
Specificity (%)	62–97	78–100
Imaging technology	Magnetic resonance of tissue protons	Tissue density detection via X-ray
In-plane spatial resolution (through-plane) (mm)	2–3 (3–4)	1 (1–3)
Ionizing radiation	No	Yes
Concomitant ventilation–perfusion assessment	Yes	No
Multiplanar image acquisition	Yes	No
Concomitant venography to detect deep venous thrombosis	Yes	No

shown that contrast-enhanced MRA, as compared with the current gold standard pulmonary angiograms, has a sensitivity between 68% and 100% and a specificity between 62% and 100%, depending on the levels of branching that are analyzed.[32,40–42] In comparison, pulmonary CT angiography (CTA), which has enjoyed greater acceptance in the clinical setting, has been assessed extensively in small to moderate sized studies. The sensitivities and specificities of pulmonary CTA are comparable to that of pulmonary MRA (63–100% and 78–100%, respectively) (Table 19.5).[43–52] Advantages of contrast-enhanced MRA over CTA include the much lower incidence of anaphylactic reaction, lack of exposure to ionizing radiation, lack of contrast-induced nephrotoxicity, and ease of postprocessing and viewing.[39] Current advantages of CTA over MRA in assessing pulmonary embolism include higher spatial resolution and wider availability, technical ease of performing the study, and less dependence on time-intensive postprocessing. The major advantage of contrast-enhanced MRA is the ability to acquire pulmonary perfusion information. This is currently undergoing research evaluation.

Encouraging results from a small study of PH patients and chronic thromboembolic pulmonary hypertension (CTEPH) showed that 2D gradient-recalled MRA was able to distinguish PH from CTEPH in 92% of cases (in comparison with ventilation–perfusion scans).[53] In another study, MRA had a sensitivity of 89% and a specificity of 100% compared with transthoracic echocardiography in the detection of PH and has a sensitivity of 100% in the detection of PE in this group of patients.[54] These studies were limited by the relatively small patient numbers and were not randomized. Furthermore, not all patients were uniformly assessed with the gold-standard diagnostic modality, namely pulmonary angiography. At present, the use of MRA to detect PE remains within specialized medical centers highly familiar with this technology.

Traditional obstacles to the widespread use of MRI in angiography studies include blurring artifacts and respiratory/cardiac pulsation interference. New faster MRI techniques are allowing the acquisition of pulmonary MR angiograms in several seconds, which is important in patients who have difficulty holding their breadth. The use of gadolinium-enhanced MRA requires meticulous attention to the time of image acquisition. A test bolus is instrumental in determining the time of maximal contrast enhancement of the region of interest (i.e. the pulmonary arterial vasculature). Because the contrast agent will extravasate out of the capillary network, uptake of the contrast into surrounding tissue and passage into the pulmonary venous system will render the MR images useless. Therefore, the operator must time the acquisition of images when the signal intensity in the pulmonary artery is brightest. We have had good success in visualizing the pulmonary vasculature using time-resolved contrast-enhanced MRA with digital subtraction images in the detection of pulmonary perfusion defects (Figure 19.7a).[55] This method is independent of contrast transit times, and allows for simultaneous acquisition of the images and injection of contrast. The 3D data sets that are acquired during this time include multiple phases of contrast enhancement, including the arterial, tissue, and venous phases. The cine format allows for functional assessment of major perfusion defect and vascular bed right-to-left shunts (Figure 19.7b).

Evaluation of adult congenital heart disease

Congenital systemic-to-pulmonary shunts are an important cause of pulmonary hypertension (Table 19.1). With improved medical and surgical advances in the past

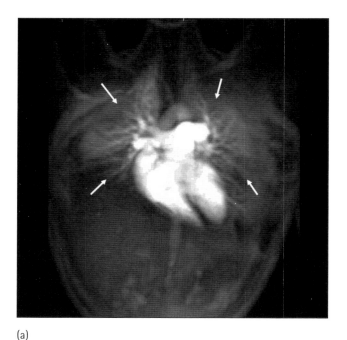

(a)

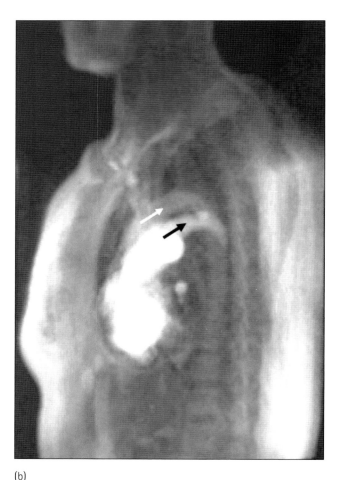

(b)

Figure 19.7
Time-resolved gadolinium-enhanced MRA of the lungs. (a) Coronal pulmonary MRA of an individual with a history of chronic pulmonary embolism. Note the multiple pulmonary perfusion defects (white arrows) in both lower lung fields. (b) Left anterior oblique view showing simultaneous contrast flow into both the aorta (white arrow) and the left main pulmonary artery (black arrow) demonstrating pulmonary-to-systemic shunting (Eisenmenger syndrome) in an individual with an unrestricted ventricular septal defect.

decade, it has been estimated that >90% of patients with congenital heart disease live for more than 10 years after surgical repair.[56] Although CMR may be used initially as a diagnostic procedure when such conditions are suspected during the clinical examination in childhood, its usefulness in the adult population lies in postoperative follow-up and assessment of potential long-term complications of the corrective procedures.[57] A combination of spin-echo and gradient-echo pulse sequences together with contrast-enhanced MRA allows for detailed morphologic assessment of the precise location of the anatomic abnormalities, surgically altered anatomy, cardiac shunts, associated valvular abnormalities, vascular flow, and physiologic impact of such abnormalities.[57,58] Common congenital conditions that lead to elevated PA pressures and RV failure include atrial septal defect (ASD), ventricular septal defect (VSD), patent ductus arteriosus, valvular heart disease, transposition of the great vessels, and tetralogy of Fallot (see Chapter 11 for a detailed discussion on the application of CMR in the evaluation of these congenital heart defects).

Septal defects and patent ductus arteriosus

In conditions such as patent ductus arteriosus, ASD and VSD, chronic systemic-to-pulmonary shunting leads to increased blood flow in the pulmonary arterial system. This volume and/or pressure overload results in the development of increased PA resistance and RV hypertrophy. The increased pulmonary vascular resistance eventually leads to reversal of blood flow from the pulmonary to the systemic circulation, resulting in cyanosis (also known as Eisenmenger syndrome). CMR may be useful in the non-invasive assessment of these patients in a number of ways. Firstly, the anatomic abnormality may be visualized and the area of the defect quantified (Figure 19.8). If a surgical correction is contemplated, visualization of surrounding structures such as the great vessels, outflow tracts, and coexisting valvular abnormalities may be assessed. Secondly, the clinical impact of the congenital abnormality may be calculated (via measurement of volumetric

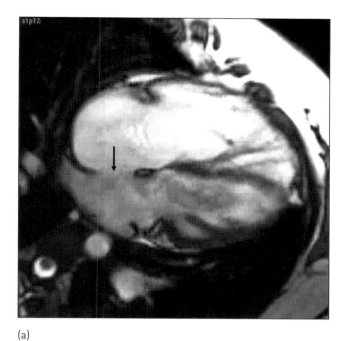

(a)

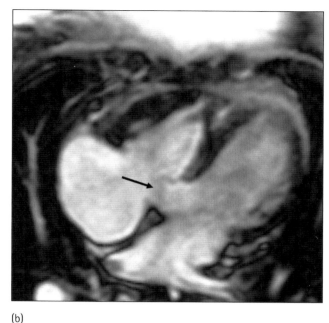

(b)

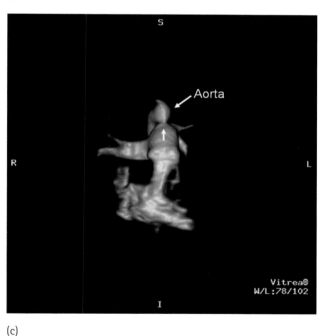

(c)

Figure 19.8
Congenital communications of the heart. (a) Four-chamber view of the heart in an individual with an atrial (secundum) septal defect (arrow). (b) Four-chamber view of the heart in an individual with a membranous ventricular septal defect (arrow). (c) Volume-rendered MRA of an individual with a patent ductus arteriosus (arrow) – a communication between the main pulmonary artery and the aorta.

parameters such as ejection fraction, stroke volume, and diastolic and systolic volumes, as well as ventricular mass). Abnormalities in these parameters may precede the onset of symptoms and thus may signal the need for further hemodynamic investigation or early intervention. Thirdly, by using flow-mapping CMR, measurement of flow across a septal defect allows for the quantification of the shunt direction, shunt volume, and Q_p/Q_s ratio.[59]

Transposition of the great vessels

Transposition of the great vessels accounts for 4.5% of all congenital cardiac malformations[60] (Figure 19.9). Uncorrected, this condition may be fatal. The transposition is corrected by redirecting systemic venous blood return directly to the morphologic LV and pulmonary venous blood return to the morphologic RV (Mustard or

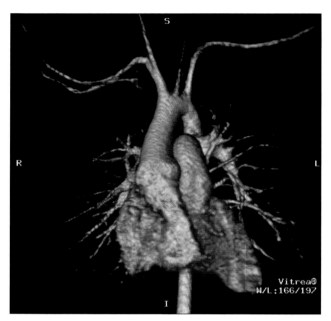

Figure 19.9
Transposition of the great vessels. Volume-rendered MRA of an individual with transposition. Note that the morphologic right ventricle is connected to the systemic outflow tract while the morphologic left ventricle communicates with the pulmonary outflow tract.

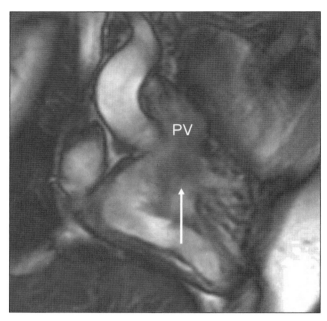

Figure 19.10
Surgically corrected tetralogy of Fallot. Right-ventricular outflow tract view of an individual at follow-up. Note the pulmonary valve (PV) regurgitant jet (arrow).

Senning techniques). Currently, the Jatene (or arterial switch) procedure is the surgery of choice. Long-term postoperative complications are seen with both techniques. With the arterial switch procedure, pulmonary stenosis is a serious complication and has been estimated to occur at an incidence of up to 1% per year.[61] Complications seen after the Senning or Mustard procedures include severe RV hypertrophy and failure, the incidence of which may be as high as 10% of patients. Other sequelae include baffle leaks and venous pathway obstructions. CMR is ideal in following these patients. RV function and mass as well as assessment of baffle patency and leakage may be obtained without the need for an invasive procedure. Valvular stenosis or insufficiency may be qualitatively assessed with gradient-echo CMR. The regurgitant blood volume and maximum velocity of blood flow in valvular stenosis may be quantitatively assessed by flow mapping and reconstruction of flow curves.[62]

Tetralogy of fallot

Tetralogy of Fallot is another congenital heart condition that affects the PA and RV. Tetralogy accounts for about 5.5% of all congenital heart conditions and consists of VSD, overriding aorta, RV outflow tract obstruction, and RV hypertrophy.[60] Surgical treatment of this syndrome

involves correction of the VSD and transannular patch placement to relieve the RV outflow tract obstruction. Postoperative complications in these patients consist of pulmonary valve insufficiency (Figure 19.10), pulmonary valve stenosis, and persisting or recurrent VSD. Pulmonary valve regurgitation may lead to RV dilatation due to chronic volume overload, whereas pulmonary stenosis may further increase RV hypertrophy. The consequences of a clinically significant VSD, as discussed above, include stress to the RV and pulmonary arterial system as well as cardiac shunting. Using standard gradient-echo CMR as well as phase-contrast CMR, anatomic and functional assessment of biventricular function and valvular defects may be obtained.

Indications and contraindications for the use of CMR

CMR is a state-of-the-art imaging modality with a wide spectrum of clinical utilities. It is currently considered to be the gold standard for the quantitative assessment of overall cardiac mass and function.[63–65] Currently, the use of CMR in the assessment of patients with pulmonary hypertensive diseases is restricted to centers with sophisticated CMR machines and experts dedicated and experi-

Table 19.6. Indications for CMR/MRA assessment of pulmonary hypertensive patients

Indications	Specific assessment	Typical patient
Pulmonary hypertension	• Evaluate right- and left-ventricular function • Identify valvular heart disease • Identify congenital heart disease • Identify presence of thromboembolic disease • Follow-up assessment of therapeutic intervention • Identify intracardiac shunting • Detect the presence of pericardial effusion/tamponade	• Complex patients with unclear etiology for pulmonary hypertension • Patients who cannot undergo or refuse cardiac catheterization • Patients with poor acoustic window (e.g. secondary to body habitus) and who refuse transesophageal echocardiography • Patients with renal disease who have relative contraindications to dye load
Congenital heart disease	• Similar to above • Assess anatomic anomalies • Evaluate abnormal or complex vascular flow • Identify surgically altered anatomy/conduits	• Patients with suspected pulmonary hypertension *and* a history of suspected congenital heart defects • Adults with congenital heart defects and surgically altered anatomy who now present with symptoms
Acute or chronic thromboembolic disease	• Similar to above • Identify presence of pulmonary embolus • Assess for venous thrombosis in pelvis and extremities for thromboembolic source	• Patients with pulmonary hypertension with risk factors for hypercoagulable states

enced with the use and interpretation of this technology. As more clinicians become familiar with the clinical usage of CMR and receive specialty training in this area, CMR will become widely available for the general practising clinicians. The current indications for the use of CMR/MRA in the assessment of pulmonary hypertensive patients are listed in Table 19.6.

Absolute contraindications to CMR include the presence of brain aneurysm clips, artificial pacemakers and automatic implantable cardiac defibrillators, retained metallic pacer wires, cochlear implants, ocular chips or fragments, and a hemodynamically unstable patient (Table 19.7). Because CMR is highly sensitive to movement artifact, patients who cannot remain relatively still or have claustrophobia are relatively contraindicated.

Conclusions

Pulmonary arterial hypertension, a disease with a poor prognosis, is often missed or misdiagnosed. Because the clinical presentation of this disease is often nonspecific, the differential diagnosis is considerable. Accurate diagnosis

Table 19.7. Contraindications to the use of CMR

Absolute contraindications
• Central nervous system aneurysm clips
• Implantable electronic devices (automatic implantable cardioverter defibrillators and artificial pacemakers)
• Pacer wires
• Metallic inner ear implants
• Ocular metallic fragments/chips
• Metallic insulin pumps
• Metal shrapnel or bullets
• Hemodynamically unstable patients

Relative contraindications
• Claustrophobia
• Pregnancy
• Patients requiring cumbersome life-support equipment (depends on institution and accommodation of CMR suite)
• Patients unable to cooperate or with excessive movement disorders (and who cannot be sedated)

and proper surveillance of disease progression is important in the clinical management of these patients. CMR/MRA has emerged as an important imaging modality that may facilitate the initial evaluation of PH and allows for an accurate assessment of the disease progression. It is noninvasive and devoid of radiation, and its contrast agent is non-nephrotoxic. New MR pulse sequences allow the test to be done quickly with short periods of breathholding or free breathing. CMR may be used to assess the pulmonary vasculature for signs of high PA pressure, the pulmonary parenchyma for associated lung abnormalities, the RV for signs of chronic and worsening disease, the left heart for secondary causes of pulmonary hypertension, and the vascular flow for coexisting thromboembolic or congenital cardiac anomalies. Current CMR technology provides clinicians with a useful modality to streamline the diagnostic evaluation of patients suspected of having elevated PA pressure. Advances are being made to further expand the clinical utility of CMR, which may become the true 'one-stop shop' examination for patients suffering from PH.

References

1. Saeed M, Wendland MF, Higgins CB. Blood pool MR contrast agents for cardiovascular imaging. J Magn Reson Imaging 2000; 12:890–8.

2. Meaney JF, Johansson LO, Ahlstrom H, Prince MR. Pulmonary magnetic resonance angiography. J Magn Reson Imaging 1999; 10:326–38.

3. Reichek N. MRI myocardial tagging. J Magn Reson Imaging 1999; 10:609–16.

4. Pettigrew RI, Oshinski JN, Chatzimavroudis G, Dixon WT. MRI techniques for cardiovascular imaging. J Magn Reson Imaging 1999; 10:590–601.

5. Rich S. Executive Summary: World Symposium on Primary Pulmonary Hypertension. WHO Publication on Internet 1998:www.who.int/ncd/cvd/pph.html.

6. Archer S, Rich S. Primary pulmonary hypertension: a vascular biology and translational research 'Work in Progress'. Circulation 2000; 102:2781–91.

7. Farber HW, Loscalzo J. Prothrombotic mechanisms in primary pulmonary hypertension. J Lab Clin Med 1999; 134:561–6.

8. Loscalzo J. Genetic clues to the cause of primary pulmonary hypertension. N Engl J Med 2001; 345:367–71.

9. Bando K, Vijayaraghavan P, Turrentine MW, et al. Dynamic changes of endothelin-1, nitric oxide, and cyclic GMP in patients with congenital heart disease. Circulation 1997; 96(9 Suppl):II-346–51.

10. Fartoukh M, Emilie D, Le Gall C, et al. Chemokine macrophage inflammatory protein-1α mRNA expression in lung biopsy specimens of primary pulmonary hypertension. Chest 1998; 114(1 Suppl):50S–1S.

11. Miyamoto S, Nagaya N, Satoh T, et al. Clinical correlates and prognostic significance of six-minute walk test in patients with primary pulmonary hypertension. Comparison with cardiopulmonary exercise testing. Am J Respir Crit Care Med 2000; 161:487–92.

12. Abramson SV, Burke JB, Pauletto FJ, Kelly JJ Jr. Use of multiple views in the echocardiographic assessment of pulmonary artery systolic pressure. J Am Soc Echocardiogr 1995; 8:55–60.

13. Borgeson DD, Seward JB, Miller FA Jr, et al. Frequency of Doppler measurable pulmonary artery pressures. J Am Soc Echocardiogr 1996; 9:832–7.

14. Nicholas G. Bellenger DJP. Assessment of cardiac function. In: Cardiovascular Magnetic Resonance (Warren J Manning, Dudley J Pennell, eds). Philadelphia: Churchill Livingstone, 2002:99–111.

15. Lorenz CH, Walker ES, Morgan VL, et al. Normal human right and left ventricular mass, systolic function, and gender differences by cine magnetic resonance imaging. J Cardiovasc Magn Reson 1999; 1:7–21.

16. Poon M, Goldman JP, Fayad ZA, Fuster V. Right ventricular dilatation as determined by MRI correlates closely with clinical deterioration of functional class in patients with primary pulmonary hypertension. In: Proceedings of the Annual Meeting of the International Society for Magnetic Resonance in Medicine, 2001.

17. Eysmann SB, Palevsky HI, Reichek N, et al. Two-dimensional and Doppler-echocardiographic and cardiac catheterization correlates of survival in primary pulmonary hypertension. Circulation 1989; 80:353–60.

18. Sodickson DK. Clinical cardiovascular magnetic resonance imaging techniques. In: Cardiovascular Magnetic Resonance (Warren J Manning, Dudley J Pennell, eds). Philadelphia: Churchill Livingstone, 2002:18–30.

19. Katz J, Whang J, Boxt LM, Barst RJ. Estimation of right ventricular mass in normal subjects and in patients with primary pulmonary hypertension by nuclear magnetic resonance imaging. J Am Coll Cardiol 1993; 21:1475–81.

20. Marcus JT, Vonk Noordegraaf A, De Vries PM, et al. MRI evaluation of right ventricular pressure overload in chronic obstructive pulmonary disease. J Magn Reson Imaging 1998; 8:999–1005.

21. Hoeper MM, Tongers J, Leppert A, et al. Evaluation of right ventricular performance with a right ventricular ejection fraction thermodilution catheter and MRI in patients with pulmonary hypertension. Chest 2001; 120:502–7.

22. Nelson GS, Sayed-Ahmed EY, Kroeker CA, et al. Compression of interventricular septum during right ventricular pressure loading. Am J Physiol Heart Circ Physiol 2001; 280:H2639–48.

23. Dong SJ, Smith ER, Tyberg JV. Changes in the radius of curvature of the ventricular septum at end diastole during pulmonary arterial and aortic constrictions in the dog. Circulation 1992; 86:1280–90.

24. Marcus JT, Vonk Noordegraaf A, Roeleveld RJ, et al. Impaired left ventricular filling due to right ventricular pressure overload in primary pulmonary hypertension: noninvasive monitoring using MRI. Chest 2001; 119:1761–5.

25. Sulica R, Boxt L, De Palo L et al. A novel MRI-index of pulmonary hypertension. Am J Resp Crit Care Med 2002; 165:A336.

26. Fayad ZA, Ferrari VA, Kraitchman DL, et al. Right ventricular regional function using MR tagging: normals versus chronic pulmonary hypertension. Magn Reson Med 1998; 39:116–23.

27. Murray PA, Vatner SF. Reduction of maximal coronary vasodilator capacity in conscious dogs with severe right ventricular hypertrophy. Circ Res 1981; 48:25–33.

28. Bache RJ. Effects of hypertrophy on the coronary circulation. Prog Cardiovasc Dis 1988; 30:403–40.

29. Gomez A, Bialostozky D, Zajarias A, et al. Right ventricular ischemia in patients with primary pulmonary hypertension. J Am Coll Cardiol 2001; 38:1137–42.

30. Goldman JP, Gentile J., Poon M. Dobutamine challenge: a novel technique for the noninvasive MR assessment of right ventricular reserve in pulmonary arterial hypertension. In: Proceedings of the Annual Meeting of the International Society for Magnetic Resonance in Medicine, 2002: Abst 1652.

31. Gefter WB, Hatabu H, Dinsmore BJ, et al. Pulmonary vascular cine MR imaging: a noninvasive approach to dynamic imaging of the pulmonary circulation. Radiology 1990; 176:761–70.

32. Kauczor HU, Kreitner KF. Contrast-enhanced MRI of the lung. Eur J Radiol 2000; 34:196–207.

33. Fuster V, Steele PM, Edwards WD, et al. Primary pulmonary hypertension: natural history and the importance of thrombosis. Circulation 1984; 70:580–7.

34. Rubin LJ. Primary pulmonary hypertension. N Engl J Med 1997; 336:111–17.

35. Rich S, Kaufmann E, Levy PS. The effect of high doses of calcium-channel blockers on survival in primary pulmonary hypertension. N Engl J Med 1992; 327:76–81.

36. Kauczor HU, Heussel CP, Thelen M. Update on diagnostic strategies of pulmonary embolism. Eur Radiol 1999; 9:262–75.

37. Bloomgarden DC, Rosen MP. Newer diagnostic modalities for pulmonary embolism. Pulmonary angiography using CT and MR imaging compared with conventional angiography. Emerg Med Clin North Am 2001; 19:975–94.

38. Woodard PK, Yusen RD. Diagnosis of pulmonary embolism with spiral computed tomography and magnetic resonance angiography. Curr Opin Cardiol 1999; 14:442–7.

39. Agnes E. Holland JWG, Edelman RR. Magnetic resonance angiography – aorta and peripheral vessels. In: Cardiovascular Magnetic Resonance (Warren J Manning, Dudley J Pennell, eds). Philadelphia: Churchill Livingstone, 2002:364–84.

40. Erdman WA, Peshock RM, Redman HC, et al. Pulmonary embolism: comparison of MR images with radionuclide and angiographic studies. Radiology 1994; 190:499–508.

41. Gupta A, Frazer CK, Ferguson JM, et al. Acute pulmonary embolism: diagnosis with MR angiography. Radiology 1999; 210:353–9.

42. Meaney JF, Weg JG, Chenevert TL, et al. Diagnosis of pulmonary embolism with magnetic resonance angiography. N Engl J Med 1997; 336:1422–7.

43. Remy-Jardin M, Remy J, Wattinne L, Giraud F. Central pulmonary thromboembolism: diagnosis with spiral volumetric CT with the single-breath-hold technique – comparison with pulmonary angiography. Radiology 1992; 185:381–7.

44. Teigen CL, Maus TP, Sheedy PF 2nd, et al. Pulmonary embolism: diagnosis with contrast-enhanced electron-beam CT and comparison with pulmonary angiography. Radiology 1995; 194:313–19.

45. Goodman LR, Curtin JJ, Mewissen MW, et al. Detection of pulmonary embolism in patients with unresolved clinical and scinti-graphic diagnosis: helical CT versus angiography. AJR 1995; 164:1369–74.

46. Bergin CJ, Rios G, King MA, et al. Accuracy of high-resolution CT in identifying chronic pulmonary thromboembolic disease. AJR 1996; 166:1371–7.

47. van Rossum AB, Pattynama PM, Ton ER, et al. Pulmonary embolism: validation of spiral CT angiography in 149 patients. Radiology 1996; 201:467–70.

48. Remy-Jardin M, Remy J, Deschildre F, et al. Diagnosis of pulmonary embolism with spiral CT: comparison with pulmonary angiography and scintigraphy. Radiology 1996; 200:699–706.

49. Mayo JR, Remy-Jardin M, Muller NL, et al. Pulmonary embolism: prospective comparison of spiral CT with ventilation-perfusion scintigraphy. Radiology 1997; 205:447–52.

50. Garg K, Welsh CH, Feyerabend AJ, et al. Pulmonary embolism: diagnosis with spiral CT and ventilation-perfusion scanning – correlation with pulmonary angiographic results or clinical outcome. Radiology 1998; 208:201–8.

51. Kim KI, Muller NL, Mayo JR. Clinically suspected pulmonary embolism: utility of spiral CT. Radiology 1999; 210:693–7.

52. Blachere H, Latrabe V, Montaudon M, et al. Pulmonary embolism revealed on helical CT angiography: comparison with ventilation–perfusion radionuclide lung scanning. AJR 2000; 174:1041–7.

53. Bergin CJ, Hauschildt J, Rios G, et al. Accuracy of MR angiography compared with radionuclide scanning in identifying the cause of pulmonary arterial hypertension. AJR 1997; 168:1549–55.

54. Kruger S, Haage P, Hoffmann R, et al. Diagnosis of pulmonary arterial hypertension and pulmonary embolism with magnetic resonance angiography. Chest 2001; 120:1556–61.

55. Goldman JP, Lai W, Golinko R, Poon M. Time resolved contrast enhanced MRA in the evaluation of adult congenital heart disease. In: Proceedings of the Annual Meeting of the Society for Magnetic Resonance in Medicine, 2002: Abst 1774.

56. Joyce L. Mended hearts grow up. Stanford Med 1994; 11:18–25.

57. Perloff JK, Warnes CA. Challenges posed by adults with repaired congenital heart disease. Circulation 2001; 103:2637–43.

58. Wimpfheimer O, Boxt LM. MR imaging of adult patients with congenital heart disease. Radiol Clin North Am 1999; 37:421–38, vii.

59. Roest AA, Helbing WA, van der Wall EE, de Roos A. Postoperative evaluation of congenital heart disease by magnetic resonance imaging. J Magn Reson Imaging 1999; 10:656–66.

60. Hoffman JI. Incidence of congenital heart disease: I. Postnatal incidence. Pediatr Cardiol 1995; 16:103–13.

61. Rolf Wyttenbach JB, Higgins CB. Cardiovascular magnetic resonance of complex congenital heart disease in the adult. In: Cardiovascular Magnetic Resonance (Warren J Manning, Dudley J Pennell, eds). Philadelphia: Churchill Livingstone, 2002:311–23.

62. Roest AAW, Groenink M, Helbing WA, et al. Cardiovascular magnetic resonance of simple congenital cardiovascular defects. In: Cardiovascular Magnetic Resonance (Warren J Manning, Dudley J Pennell, eds). Philadelphia: Churchill Livingstone, 2002:295–310.

63. Holman ER, Buller VG, de Roos A, et al. Detection and quantification of dysfunctional myocardium by magnetic resonance imaging. A new three-dimensional method for quantitative wall-thickening analysis. Circulation 1997; 95:924–31.

64. Semelka RC, Tomei E, Wagner S, et al. Interstudy reproducibility of dimensional and functional measurements between cine magnetic resonance studies in the morphologically abnormal left ventricle. Am Heart J 1990; 119:1367–73.

65. Shapiro EP, Rogers WJ, Beyar R, et al. Determination of left ventricular mass by magnetic resonance imaging in hearts deformed by acute infarction. Circulation 1989; 79:706–11.

20

Internal coils in CMR

Ergin Atalar

The use of internal coils in magnetic resonance imaging (MRI) is under investigation. The purpose of this chapter is to provide an overview of the state-of-the-art technology and describe briefly its possible uses in cardiovascular MRI (CMR).

In MRI, the body emits a radiofrequency (RF) signal in the form of an echo in response to an excitation RF signal.[1] This echo is a very weak signal and is usually picked up by specialized receiver coils. This weak RF signal is then amplified using ultralow-noise amplifiers and later used in image reconstruction.

One of the main criteria in the design of the receiver coil is its signal-to-noise ratio (SNR) performance. For optimum performance, the shape, size, and position of the receiver coil is critically important in MRI. Although we might be interested in imaging a small region, if we receive the MR signal with a coil that is sensitive to a large area, the noise level increases. On the other hand, if the sensitivity of the receiver coil does not cover the region of interest, the signal becomes low. Therefore, there is a need for a critical match between coverage and image quality. Ideally, a good receiver coil needs to be small and placed very close to the point of interest. If one is interested in regions of interest that are deep in the body, such as the aorta or the heart, the optimum size of a coil placed outside the body becomes relatively large and therefore the resulting image will have limited SNR. One possible solution to this problem is to place the probe inside the body.

In 1984, Kantor et al[2] placed a coil inside the left ventricle of a dog for the purpose of increasing the SNR in the heart image. Later, this idea formed the basis for the first MRI coils that were placed inside blood vessels to increase the SNR in the imaging of atherosclerotic plaques. In 1992, Martin et al[3] and Hurst et al[4] in two independent studies, utilized opposed-solenoid coils in vessels to image the vessel wall at ultrahigh resolution. The main challenges of these designs were miniaturization without loss of performance, the flexibility of the probes, and the lack of proper imaging sequences. Our group and many others worked to solve these problems.[5] Currently, there are internal probes[6] that have US Food and Drug Administration (FDA) approval for use in clinical practice, and initial tests on human patients have been promising.[7] However, for the widespread use of such probes in medicine, specific applications that may benefit patients must be identified and the devices and imaging methods must be further optimized for these applications.

With regard to the technical details of these devices, the basics of the design principles will be explained in this chapter with a view toward an audience of radiologists and cardiologists who may not have a technical background in coil design. For those who are interested in details, references are given extensively in the text. We will begin with the definition of the SNR and how one can measure it on an MR image.

Signal-to-noise ratio of MRI

If one applies a very high magnetic field to an object, the object can become magnetized. Although the amount of magnetization is very small, it can be detected using nuclear magnetic resonance techniques. The magnetized object, if exposed to an additional RF pulse, generates an echo at its resonance frequency and an RF signal originating from the object can be detected by specialized antennas.[1]

As can be seen in Figure 20.1, the transmission of the RF pulse and the reception of the MR signal can be done by two separate antennas. In some designs, these two functions are performed by a single antenna. Internal coils, which are the subject of this chapter, are usually designed to work as receive-only antennas, and therefore we will discuss only their signal reception properties.

The received signal in MRI is mixed with noise generated by various sources. A significant amount of noise cannot be separated from the signal, and this appears on the reconstructed images as a factor that degrades image quality. The absolute values of the signal and noise levels

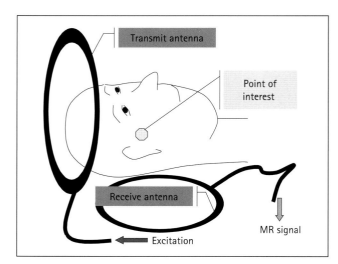

Figure 20.1
An object in an MRI scanner. A radiofrequency (RF) signal is applied to the transmit antenna to deliver RF energy to the object. The echo generated by the magnetic resonance phenomenon in the object is received by a specialized receiver coil and converted to a very weak electrical signal. This signal is later amplified and used in image reconstruction.

have no significant meaning in MRI; instead, the ratio of the signal to noise, the SNR, is used to measure the signal reception quality. The value of the SNR on the reconstructed image is usually taken as one of the primary measures of image quality in MRI.

There are multiple sources of noise.[8] In a well-designed MRI scanner, the main noise source is that originating from thermal radiation from the body. The other sources of noise originate from the scanner's receiver system, and usually can be decreased below the body noise level by proper instrument design.

Although the body noise level cannot be eliminated, the amount of received body noise can be decreased by proper antenna design. Understanding the relation between the SNR and the design of the antenna requires knowledge of advanced electromagnetic theory. While leaving these details to the other textbooks,[9] here we will briefly explain the components necessary to understand the operating principles of the design.

In the analysis of the design, reciprocity principles are utilized,[10] i.e., in order to understand reception performance, we analyze transmit performance. The magnetic field B, generated by an antenna at a point of interest is proportional to the signal received from an object at that location. In addition, the total power P delivered to the antenna to generate the field is proportional to the noise level, and therefore the SNR satisfies the following relation:

$$\text{SNR} \propto \frac{B}{\sqrt{P}}.$$

Therefore, with the optimum antenna design, when we have a high magnetic field at the point of interest, we deposit a minimum amount of power in the body.

Limits of external coils

The performance of an external MRI coil depends on multiple parameters including the shape and position of the coil, the electromagnetic properties of the body (namely its electrical conductivity, permittivity, and permeability), the magnetic resonance frequency, and the shape of the object.[11,12]

The upper limit of the SNR in MRI has been formulated.[13] The calculated limit is independent of the shape and position of the coil in use. It is interesting to note that the maximum SNR that one can get using an external coil is a function of the position of the point of interest (Figure 20.2: note that the scale of the figure is logarithmic). While for a point of interest deep inside the body, the SNR limitation is severe, for a point of interest close to the surface of the body, very high SNR may be achieved.

The simple circular loop coil is very close to the optimum design for objects close to the surface of the body. Studies on circular antennas showed that both signals and noise levels are monotonic functions of radius and that they increase as the radius of the antenna increases. The more important parameter, SNR, however, has a peak value at a certain radius.[14] As a rule of thumb, the optimum coil diameter is equal to the depth of the point of interest. Note that this rule is only valid if the distance between the point of interest and the surface of the body is much less than the wavelength in the body. For example, 5 cm is considered to be small enough for a 1.5 T MRI scanner. Another requirement for this rule to be valid is that the object must be considerably larger than the coil; in other words, the point of interest must be close to the surface. For points of interest that are deep in the body, circular loop coils are not optimum; the shape of the optimum coil for such cases is not known and is under investigation, but the maximum SNR that one can get with such a coil is known (Figure 20.2 and reference 13).

This upper bound on the SNR in an MRI experiment causes limitations in the diagnostic quality of MR images. This is especially important when imaging small structures such as atherosclerotic plaques.[15–17] As discussed extensively elsewhere in this book, atherosclerotic plaques are complex in nature, and detecting morphological changes in the arterial wall requires very high-resolution images.[18] It is known that the SNR of an image is proportional to voxel size.[1] Therefore, the limitations associated with the SNR cause limits in the resolution of MRI images. Since the maximum SNR that one can get depends on the distance from the point of interest to the

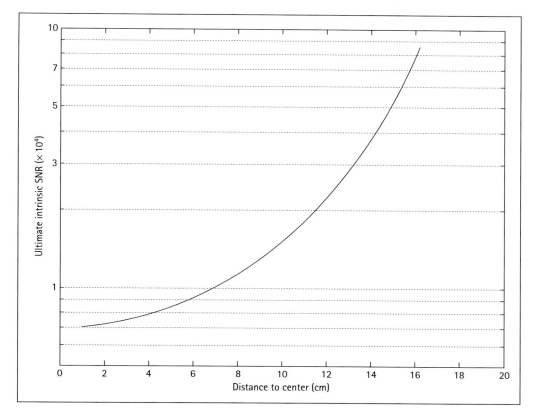

Figure 20.2
The ultimate intrinsic SNR as a function of the position of interest in a cylindrical phantom with a radius of 20 cm. Note that > 10-fold variation in SNR is observed between 20 mm and 150 mm deep points of interest.

surface, the resolution that one can get in MRI also depends on the distance to the surface. High-resolution MR images of carotid arteries can be obtained using external coils, mainly because of their proximity to the surface of the body;[19] however, for points deep in the body, such as the aorta or renal arteries, images of plaques with similar image quality cannot be obtained.

Internal coils

Internal MRI coils are defined as coils that can be placed inside the body through various body openings in order to increase the SNR and therefore the resolution of the images.

It should be noted that, just like external coils, internal coils also have an upper bound on their SNR performance.[20] In Figure 20.3, the ultimate SNR for a cylindrical object with a cylindrical hole for placement of internal coils is calculated. The inner and outer radiui are assumed to be 3 mm and 200 mm, respectively. As can be seen, internal coils significantly increase the upper bound, especially in regions deep inside the body. An important rule to remember is that as the internal coil gets closer to the point of interest, the performance increases.

Multiple versions of internal MRI coils have been designed to overcome SNR limitations. Each coil comes in different sizes and shapes and with its own limitations. In order to give some insight into their design, we will describe some of the basic designs that are being investigated.

Loopless antenna design[13]

This design is essentially a coaxial cable with an extended inner conductor, as shown in Figure 20.4. The antenna has a cylindrical sensitivity profile with a fall in signal as the distance from the antenna increases, and characterized approximately by $1/r$ where r is the distance from the point of interest to the antenna. The length of the extended inner conductor (whip) is adjusted for optimum performance. The signal level is low at the tip of the whip, and maximum where the whip joins the coaxial cable. Signal reception on the coaxial cable is possible, and generally decreases with increased distance from the junction point.

It should be pointed out that in this design there is no need for placement of the tuning/matching and decoupling circuit in the body since the antenna impedance is very close to the coaxial cable impedance.

The loopless design structurally resembles a guidewire. The mechanical properties of guidewires, such as their ability to be twisted and pulled, which enable easy maneuvering inside blood vessels, are very critical. To convert

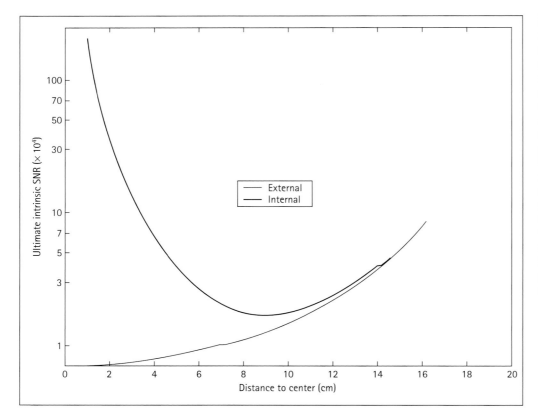

Figure 20.3
Ultimate intrinsic SNR that can be obtained using external coils compared with internal coils. In this analysis, internal coils are assumed to be used in conjunction with external coils; therefore, internal coil performance is always better than that of an external coil. The two curves are similar when the point of interest is close to the external surface. At around 100 mm from the surface, the performance of the internal coil is significantly higher than that of an external coil.

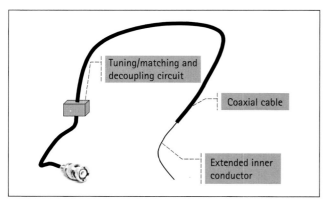

Figure 20.4
Loopless antenna. This design is essentially a coaxial cable with an extended inner conductor. The tuning/matching and decoupling circuit is located away from the sensitive part of the antenna.

the loopless design into a guidewire, mechanical design criteria that are commonly used in standard guidewire and catheter designs are applied directly to this design. Unfortunately, the most commonly used material in guidewires, steel, is not MRI-compatible. The second most commonly used material, NiTi, is suitable for this purpose, although its electrical conductivity is not high enough. The electrical conductivity can, however, be improved by plating NiTi with gold, silver, and/or copper.

Because of the simple structure of the loopless antenna, miniaturization to 0.75 mm diameter can be achieved without a significant reduction in either mechanical or electrical performance. Even smaller diameters have been designed (0.35 mm), but a loss in SNR was observed because of difficulties in balancing the mechanical stability of the design and it electrical performance. Designs that enable even smaller diameter guidewires are under investigation.

In a modified version of the loopless antenna design, the intravascular extended sensitivity (IVES) antenna design,[21] the whip is coiled in a solenoidal form and insulation is applied (Figure 20.5). This increases the overall longitudinal coverage. In the design example given in reference,[21] the coverage reaches 25 cm.

The loopless design has been tested on animals with atherosclerotic diseases (Figure 20.6). The small size of these antennas enables their insertion into the femoral artery of the rabbits. This design has also been tested on patients. One of the first human patient images obtained using a loopless design is shown in Figure 20.7.

Elongated loop design[22]

Another important class of internal coil design is the elongated loop (Figure 20.8). The active part of the design is

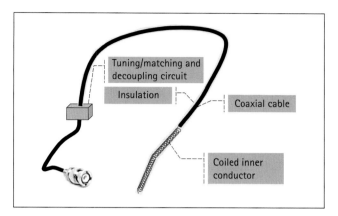

Figure 20.5
IVES (intravascular extended sensitivity) antenna. This is an extension of the loopless design and extends the useful range of the antenna while increasing its mechanical stability.

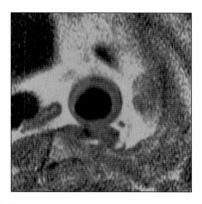

Figure 20.6
Aortic plaque imaging using a loopless antenna design. The abdominal aortic plaque in a Watanabe rabbit was imaged using a loopless antenna in a 1.5 T GE clinical MRI scanner. For the data acquisition, blood-suppression pulses were used in a T2-weighted fast spin-echo pulse sequence.

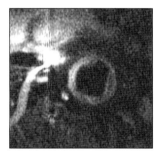

Figure 20.7
MR image of a human patient aorta obtained using a loopless antenna inserted into the vena cava. The T1-weighted image was obtained after contrast (Gd-DTPA) injection. The imaging parameters are fast spin-echo, TR/TE=820/7.2 ms, FOV=9.2 cm, slice thickness 3 mm, ETL=20, and matrix 256 × 256. The loopless antenna in the vena cava creates a bright spot around it. Aortic plaques are visible. (Courtesy of Dr Lawrence Hofmann, Johns Hopkins University.)

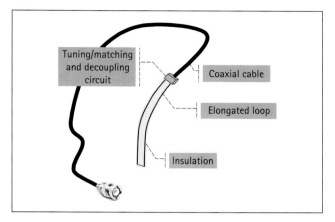

Figure 20.8
Elongated loop design. The active part of the design consists of two parallel wires that are short-circuited at one end and connected to the coaxial cable after a tuning/matching circuit. The wires are insulated.

fashioned from two parallel wires that are short-circuited at one end and connected to a coaxial cable after a tuning/matching circuit. The whole assembly, including the wires, is insulated for the best performance. Since the tuning of the design depends on the length of the wires as well as the separation between them, the wires can be flexed (together) without a significant change in their impedance, and therefore fixed tuning elements can be used. The presence of this electronic circuit in the vicinity of the sensitive part of the design imposes a lower bound on the size of this design. In addition, the separation between the wires has a significant effect on the performance of the wires (SNR is approximately proportional to wire separation). Therefore, there are limits on the miniaturization of this design but it has been shown that a 3 mm diameter design is feasible. Because of its relatively large size and its mechanical properties, this type of coil is placed in the body with the aid of a catheter.

The parallel wires can be made flexible without significant SNR degradation because the inductance of the elongated loop depends primarily on the length of the wire and its separation. As long as the structure of the design allows flexing without causing an alteration in the wire separation, the overall design can be made flexible.

For improved performance, a balun circuit can be placed on the coaxial cable. However, a balun circuit was not used in the published designs, mostly because of the miniaturization problem. In addition, the unbalanced currents on the wire allow some signal reception on the coaxial cable, thus facilitating the placement of the probe inside the body.

The signal of this design is more concentrated around the antenna compared with the loopless design. The signal drops faster with radial distance ($1/r^2$, compared with $1/r$ with the loopless design, where r is the radial distance to

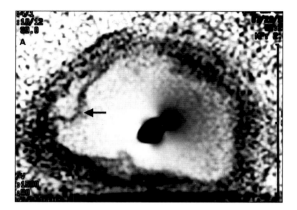

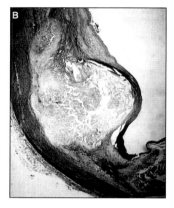

Figure 20.9
Intravascular MR image of a human aorta specimen (A) and the corresponding histological section (B). The arrow on the MR image indicates where the plaque is. The signal void at the center of the image represents the position of the intravascular MRI coil. The design is an elongated coil. (Reproduced from Correia et al. Arterioscler Thromb Vasc Biol 1997; 17:3626–32.[23])

compared with the loopless design. To date, this design has been tested only in animals and in vitro (Figure 20.9).

Expandable loop design[24,25]

An extension of the elongated loop design, the expandable loop design was proposed to eliminate size limitations. In this design, the antenna is collapsed into a catheter for ease of delivery (Figure 20.10). The separation between the wires is increased when the antenna is on the target location. After the imaging has been completed, the loop is collapsed back in order to ease pullback.

For optimum performance, as in all loop designs, the tuning/matching and decoupling circuits need to be close to the coil and therefore inside the body. However, miniaturizing the circuits and making them flexible is a serious design challenge. In the original design proposed by Quick et al,[24] these circuit elements are placed outside the body, far from the loop. Although this decreases the maximum possible SNR obtainable from this design, its implementation is much easier. Alternatively, only a small portion of the circuit can be placed inside the body for optimum performance.[25] In the design by Quick et al,[24] the coil was not insulated. For high performance, insulation is important, but manufacturing an insulated and expandable loop may be difficult. With the possibility of to increasing the separation of the wires, this design shows future promise.

Sample images have been published in the literature using this design.

the antenna). The longitudinal coverage is limited by the length of the parallel wires, which is usually <10 cm.

In large vessels, this design can be used in a relatively straightforward way and has significant SNR advantages

Opposed solenoid coil design[3,4]

One of the common shortcomings of the designs that we have discussed so far is the rapid variation in their sensi-

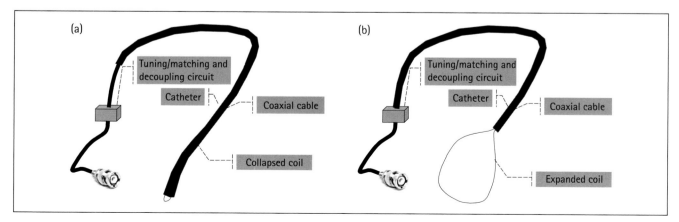

Figure 20.10
Expandable loop design. (A) The loop is collapsed inside a catheter. (B) The loop is expanded by pulling the catheter back. The tuning/matching and decoupling circuit is remote.

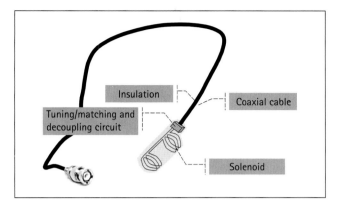

Figure 20.11
Opposed solenoid coil design. Two opposing solenoids with a small separation are used, with a tuning/matching and decoupling circuit in the catheter.

tivity. This results in a very bright signal around the antenna and in difficulties adjusting the contrast and brightness of the image for its proper visualization. Although this problem may be solved using signal intensity correction algorithms, this high sensitivity around the antenna sometimes causes image artifacts.[26] To alleviate this problem, the opposed solenoid design is a good alternative.

In this design, two solenoid coils are used, with a small separation and opposed winding directions (Figure 20.11). This design is known as the inside-out design, and was used in 1980 in nuclear magnetic resonance (NMR) in the oil-drilling industry in order to detect the NMR signal of the ground at a drilled point.[27] The main purpose was to generate a useful region where the field inhomogeneity was tolerable. The intravascular version of this

design was implemented by Hurst et al[3] and Martin et al[4] in two independent studies. They show that with this design, high-resolution images of large vessels can be obtained.

As in the loop designs, the tuning/matching and decoupling circuit needs to be placed close to the coils, and therefore causes some size limitations. In this design, remote tuning may not be a solution to the size limitation, because the windings of the coils are also difficult to miniaturize. Since the imaging volume is limited to the small region between two opposing solenoids, this design is not very effective for surveys of arteries in search of plaques. It is, however, excellent if the portion of the vessel to be imaged is predetermined using other coils. With low field inhomogeneity, this design may have significant applications for the imaging of large vessels.

These devices may be delivered using a catheter. To date, placement of these probes inside the blood vessels through femoral access has not been shown. However, testing on animals and tissue specimens (Figure 20.12) has shown very encouraging results.

Alternative tuning mechanisms

All the designs discussed so far have standard tuning mechanisms. Alternative tuning methods have also been proposed.

When the coil flexes or expands as in the expandable coil design, its tuning changes. Since the amount of expansion or flexion may not be known beforehand, the tuning of the coil may need to be modified just before scanning. This is not possible with fixed circuit elements.

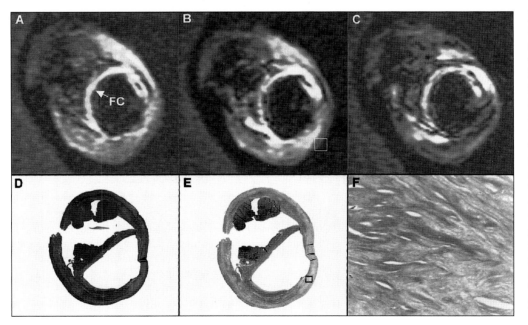

Figure 20.12
Carotid specimen containing a dense fibrous cap (FC) well visualized on intravascular MRI: (A) proton density; (B) inversion recovery; (C) gradient-echo. The region of loose connective tissue and edema (box) on trichrome (E) is seen as a region with reduced signal on the inversion recovery image (box, B). Neither trichrome (E) nor hematoxylin–eosin (D) showed evidence of lipids beneath the cap. (Reproduced from Rogers et al. Arterioscler Thromb Vasc Biol 2000; 20:1824–30.[26])

If the antenna is not tuned properly, its performance degrades and therefore the SNR of the resultant image decreases. In order to solve this problem, an autotuning mechanism was proposed.[28] The main circuit element for this purpose is called a varactor and is commonly used in radio receivers. The main problem with using varactors in tuning circuits is that they add additional noise to and thereby degrade the image. A balance between the loss in SNR due to a varactor and the loss due to a change in tuning because of the change in antenna geometry is necessary.

An old but very effective alternative method of tuning antennas is to use pieces of coaxial cables.[29] Open-ended long coaxial cables can act as capacitor and can replace the capacitors used in the circuits. This design strategy was proposed as an alternative to existing designs as a solution for the miniaturization problem.

Pulse sequences and artifacts related to the use of internal coils

Researchers are continually developing new pulse sequences to improve image quality. For example, imaging techniques that use steady-state free precession (SSFP) sequences have recently become very popular and have improved cardiac imaging capabilities significantly. Although the performances of most of these new sequences have been demonstrated with external coils, most of them can be used directly with internal coils. The use of internal coils with these sequences will increase the image SNR and therefore enable shorter data acquisition times (which is especially important for real-time catheter tracking) and higher image resolution (which is important for detailed analysis of structures such as atherosclerotic plaques).

The use of internal coils not only increases signal but also increases image artifacts. Special care must be taken in order to minimize these artifacts. Most problems arise from the fact that the signal is not uniform, and small artifacts around the catheter are multiplied by the sensitivity of the antenna. These artifacts may appear in the form of 'ghosts' in the region of low sensitivity[30]

The fundamental causes of the motion artifacts remain unchanged with the use of internal coils. The common motion artifact reduction techniques such as ECG gating, breathholding, and flow compensation are very effective in reducing motion artifact problems. However, pulse sequence-dependent artifacts are rather difficult to address. For example, the RF spoiling technique used in spoiled gradient-echo sequences causes artifacts to appear on a stationary phantom.[30]

Safety of internal coils

The safety of internal coils is a serious concern if proper care is not taken. An MRI scanner can be compared to a microwave oven with regard to safety. The amount of power delivered to the body is controlled by system software and hardware in order to minimize the role of excessive heating to the body.[31] The FDA regulates the calibration of MRI scanners to limit the total RF power output.[32] In the calibration of MRI scanners, however, the presence of metallic objects, such as internal RF coils, is not considered. Depending on the shape and size of the internal coil, and the performance of the electronic decoupling circuit, the RF power may be concentrated around the RF coil and its wires, and may cause excessive heating and burns. In order to avoid this undesired heating problem, a complete understanding of the heating process is necessary.

The RF power applied to the transmitter causes a distribution of power in the body, and this distribution is measured by the specific absorption rate (SAR), usually in units of watts per kilogram. Applied heat causes an increase in body temperature, but the distributions of heat and temperature do not necessarily match. Using thermodynamics, a bioheat equation can be formulated to determine the relationship between heat distribution and temperature distribution, and this is a function of perfusion, heat conduction, and body shape.[33]

If there are metallic objects implanted in the body, a local SAR increase around these objects may be observed during an MRI examination, and hence alter the temperature distribution in the body.[34]

The relationship between metallic objects and temperature rise can be formulated in terms of a measure called the safety index.[34] The expected peak temperature rise can be calculated by multiplying the local SAR value in the absence of the metallic object by this index (see Figure 20.13). For example, in a 1.5 T scanner, a piece

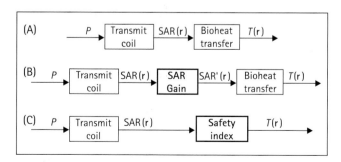

Figure 20.13
(A) Flow-chart model of RF heating in MRI. (B) Addition of an implanted wire causes an amplification of the local SAR, modeled by the SAR gain. (C) The safety index combines SAR gain and bioheat transfer to provide a relevant measure of the temperature change that can occur when using the wire in vivo for each unit of applied SAR.

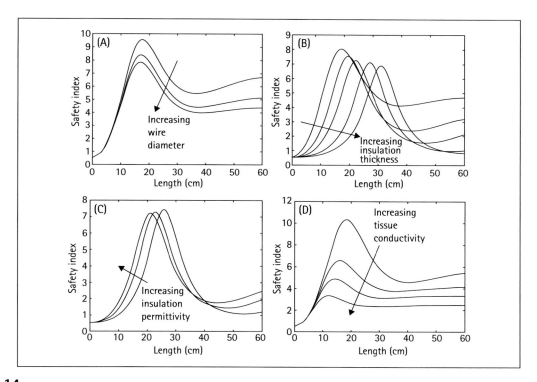

Figure 20.14
Theoretically predicted safety index when each of the following parameters are varied: (A) wire diameter (bare wire: 0.2, 0.4, and 0.8 mm); (B) insulation thickness (bare: 12, 25, 50, and 75 μm); (C) relative permittivity of insulation (25 μm-thick insulation: ϵ_r = 2, 3, and 4); (D) electrical conductivity of tissue (bare wire: σ = 0.4, 0.6, 0.8, and 1.2 S/m). The safety index (in °C/(W/kg)) incorporates the effects of both raw SAR gain due to the presence of wire and convolution with the Green's function of the bioheat equation. There is a stronger dependence on conductivity and insulation thickness than on wire diameter or insulation permittivity. The following standard parameters were used unless that parameter was the variable: wire diameter 0.5 mm (24 AWG); tissue thermal conductivity 0.4 W/m °C; resting muscle perfusion 2.7 ml/min/100 g; relative permittivity of insulation 3.3; tissue electrical conductivity 0.5 S/m.

of 18 cm-long bare wire has a safety index of 8°C kg/W, and if 1 W/kg of SAR is applied to a body while this bare wire is placed inside the body, a maximum temperature of 8°C could be observed. This excessive heat can easily be avoided by imposing limitations on the applied RF power. In this example with an 18 cm-long wire, the temperature rise cannot exceed 2°C if the applied heat never exceeds 0.25 W/kg.

Note that the safety index is a function of the device characteristics only. Once this number is known, the amount of power applied to the body can be formulated and the amount of power applied by the scanner can be controlled to remain within the safety limits. With this method, safety can be achieved with any arbitrary device once the safety index is known.[34]

There are methods that reduce heating concentration around the implant. These methods can be translated as methods of reducing the safety index and therefore allowing more power to be delivered to the body without causing significant heating. One very simple and effective method is insulation. For example, the

18 cm-wire that was given as an example earlier can have a safety index as low as 1.2 with only 75 μm of insulation. Other safety index reduction methods include using decoupling circuits, balun circuits,[35] and safe coaxial cable designs.[36]

If internal MRI coils are used to transmit the RF power as well as receive it, the SAR distribution in the body can be calculated in a rather straightforward manner, and therefore the limit on the amount of power that can be applied to the coil can be determined.[37]

In conclusion, internal MRI coils can be used safely in the body if the associated safety index is known and scanners are calibrated to limit the amount of power accordingly.

Applications

Although internal coils are not being used in current clinical practice in CMR these coils hold very strong promise in two main areas: characterization of atherosclerotic plaques and cardiovascular interventions.

Atherosclerosis and internal CMR probes

It is not necessary to discuss how important it is to develop imaging tools to fight atherosclerosis, the number one killer of humankind in developed countries. However, it is important to emphasize that current non-CMR-based imaging methods have either poor or no capabilities to characterize atherosclerotic plaques. CMR of the plaques is an emerging technology and shows great promise. Extensive studies using surface coils in MRI show that high image resolution provides a significant amount of information about plaque composition.[15] In addition, in recent years, researchers have found that small (1–2 mm thick) plaques are at least as risky as occlusive large plaques. It is still not known how much image resolution is necessary in order to image the plaques that are at risk for rupture. In studies of carotid arteries, MR images acquired with 200 μm of in-plane resolution provided useful information;[16,19] however, there are significant problems in imaging of vessels that are deep within the body, such as the renal arteries.[18]

To alleviate this problem, the use of internal coils has been proposed.[3,4] By placing the antenna inside the blood vessel of interest, one can get much higher image resolution[23,38,39] Although using catheters in the arteries for diagnostic purposes only is a common practice (X-ray angiography), the preferred method would be not to use any invasive device inside the artery. Two alternative solutions have been proposed. The use of an antenna inside a vein[25] (Figure 20.7) that is close to the artery, is one option. Another proposal is the use of an antenna inside the esophagus for imaging the aorta and especially the aortic arch[40] (Figure 20.15). Because safety is less of a

concern for these approaches, studies on patients have already begun and are showing very promising results (see Chapter 23 for extensive discussions on this topic).[41]

Role of internal coils in cardiovascular interventions

Up to now, we have discussed the role of RF coils in diagnostic procedures. There is a strong interest, however, in the use of MRI to guide cardiovascular interventions.

Most cardiac intervention procedures would benefit from the high soft tissue contrast of MRI and its ability to monitor therapy. Some of these applications are discussed elsewhere in this book. Common to all of them is a need to determine the position of interventional devices in real-time in the MRI scanner. This need motivated researchers to develop devices such as catheters or guidewires that can be tracked by MRI.[42]

An alternative method for vascular device visualization is to incorporate an MRI coil into the device. The intravascular RF coils described above can be modified to make them suitable for this purpose.[43] Alternative designs have been proposed solely for device visualization. For example, in one study, a twisted pair of wires was used to visualize the significant portion of the antenna.[44] In another study, a very small solenoid coil was used to determine the position of the tip of an intravascular device.[45] In the simplest of all of these designs, a single wire was connected to the scanner preamplifier for direct visualization.[46–48]

For rapid device localization, the slice-selection capability of the MRI scanner can be turned off and the scanner can then be operated in the projection mode, similar to that used in X-ray. Since these internal coils produce signal in a very limited region, large field-of-view imaging is not necessary, and this enables a high frame rate and complete visualization of catheters.[49,50]

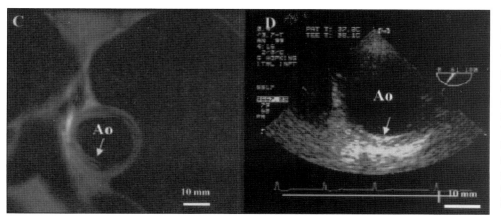

Figure 20.15
(A) Transesophageal CMR (TEMRI) of the distal aortic arch of a 77-year-old man with remote stroke, showing heterogeneous atherosclerotic thickening consistent with intraplaque calcification or hemorrhage; TR/TE = 1690/15 ms. (B) Corresponding transesophageal echocardiography (TEE). Ao, aorta. (Reproduced from Shunk et al. J Am Coll Cardiol 2001; 37:2031–5.[41])

Multifunctional internal coils in CMR

As discussed above, internal MRI coils may have a very simple structure and therefore can easily be incorporated into almost all intravascular devices. These multifunctional internal MRI coil designs include guidewires, guiding catheters, stents, balloon angioplasty catheters, electrophysiology catheters, and injection catheters.

Guidewires

As discussed above, for example, the loopless design was modified to conform to the mechanical properties of a guidewire[43,51] It is important to remember that a guidewire is used in vascular interventions to help in the placement of other vascular devices in target locations. In a typical vascular intervention, a guidewire and guiding catheter combination is used to reach the target location. Once the location has been reached, the guiding catheter

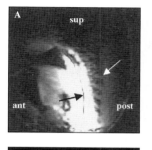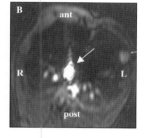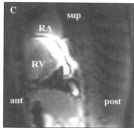
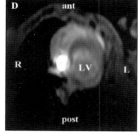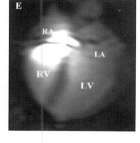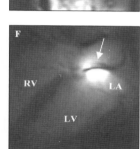

Figure 20.16

Guidewire tracking with a loopless miniature antenna wire in the closure of an atrial septal defect (ASD). With the conventional external phased array coils turned off, the short-range receiver profile makes the vicinity of the wire visible (white arrow, spine). In the initial frames (A, sagittal; B, coronal) the antenna wire (black arrow) is advanced in the vena cava using real-time MR fluoroscopy. It is then advanced into the right atrium (C, sagittal; D, coronal), and crosses the atrial septum (E) through the ASD. In the final frame (F), the wire (white arrow) is in the left atrium. ant, anterior; post, posterior; sup, superior; L, left; R, right. (Reproduced from Rickers et al. Circulation 2003; 107:132–8[54] with permission from Lippincott Williams & Wilkins.)

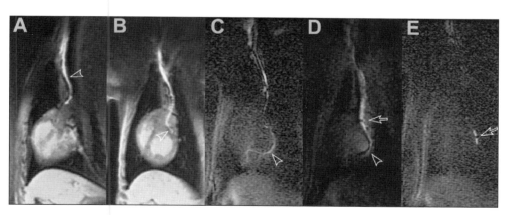

Figure 20.17

Complete MRI-guided intervention in a circumflex artery. (A) Placement of the MRI guiding catheter (arrowhead) in the ascending aorta using the oblique sagittal view. (B) Catheterization with the MRI guiding catheter (arrowhead) of the left main coronary artery and circumflex artery using the oblique coronal view. (C) Real-time projection angiography of the circumflex artery (arrowhead) on an oblique coronal view after injection of diluted gadolinium (31 mM) in the MRI guiding catheter. (D) Placement of the MR imaging-guidewire (MRIG, arrowhead) in the circumflex artery in the oblique coronal view. The balloon angioplasty catheter can be localized and advanced on the MRIG by using a black artifact created by a platinum ring localized in the center of the balloon angioplasty catheter (long arrow). (E) Injection of diluted Gd-DTPA (31 mM) in the balloon enhances the balloon on the real-time projection angiography images (long arrow); oblique coronal view. Sequences: fast spoiled gradient-echo, TR/TE = 4.4/1.3 ms, FOV = 32 mm × 16 mm, 256 × 128 matrix (64 phase-encoding steps), pixel 1.25 mm, update 280 ms; flip angle 7° in (A), (B), and (D), 90° in (C) and (E); slice thickness 20 mm in (A) and (B); no slice selection in (C), (D), and (E).

may be removed from the body and the vascular device involved in the procedure is loaded onto the guidewire using the guidewire hole. To achieve this exchange procedure, the proximal end of the guidewire must be free. In the loopless antenna, however, the proximal end of the wire must be connected to the preamplifier of the CMR scanner. In one design, this difficulty was addressed using a special connector that enabled the connection of a magnetic resonance imaging-guidewire (MRIG) to the scanner. When the guidewire was disconnected, the guidewire's connector did not have a bulky piece remaining at the proximal end, and therefore device exchange was easy.[52] The same device can be used to image the coronary vessel wall at high resolution.[53]

An example of the use of these guidewires in guiding transcatheter closure of an atrial septal defect can be found in Figure 20.16.[54] Note that both the guidewire and the anatomy of the heart are visible during the procedure. This capability may be critical for precise placement of catheters in complex locations.

Guiding catheters

Like guidewires, guiding catheters have also been fashioned into the form of MRI antennas. In one study, for example, a loopless antenna was attached to a guiding catheter for complete visualization.[55] Using the combination of an MRIG and an MRI guiding catheter, a complex vascular intervention, namely a coronary balloon angioplasty procedure, was conducted on a dog model.[56] (Figure 20.17).

Stents

Stents can also be converted into the form of RF coils.[57] While maintaining direct contact with the stent during a stent placement procedure is possible, inductive coupling of a stent to an external coil enables excellent visualization of the stent after its deployment.[58] Note that this approach requires changes in the shape of the stent, which is of critical importance for the effectiveness of the stent as a vascular treatment component. Research on stent antennas is in its infancy, and there is a great interest in both the research and clinical communities.

Balloon angioplasty catheters

Balloon angioplasty catheters can also be fashioned into internal RF antennas.[59] As a version of the expandable loop

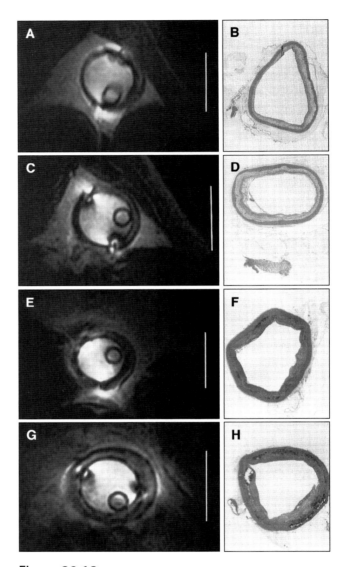

Figure 20.18
High-resolution (117 × 156 μm^2 intravascular T2-weighted images with histopathological correlations (hematoxylin–eosin (H & E) stain; original magnification × 25) transecting the abdominal aorta of four different animals aged 6 months (A, B), 12 months (C, D), 24 months (E, F), and 36 months (G, H) in identical locations (white bar = 5 mm). Wall thickness and plaque area increase with increasing age. Calcified plaque characterized by reduced signal intensity on MR images (arrow in G) was proven in the histological H & E stain (arrow in H). Fibrous tissue containing < 50% fat was easily differentiated from calcification on the basis of higher signal intensity (arrowheads in G and H). The 0.035 in. guidewire lumen is visible inside the inflated balloon (arrow). (Reproduced from Zimmermann-Paul et al. Circulation 1999; 99:1054–61[38] with permission from Lippincott Williams & Wilkins.)

antenna, this design enables imaging of the vessel wall at high resolution (Figure 20.18). One drawback of using the balloon to expand the coil to its best performing stage is that blood flow is blocked. This is especially a problem if

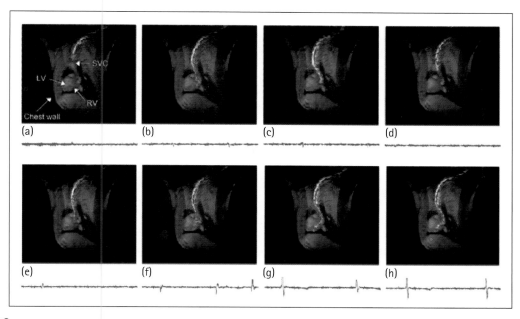

Figure 20.19
Simultaneous catheter function: IEGM recordings concurrent with catheter tracking. Selected images from a 15 s catheter push acquired with a 7 frame/s, real-time gradient-echo sequence: left ventricle (LV), right ventricle (RV), chest wall, and superior vena cava (SVC). The catheter is initially advanced from the jugular vein, down the SVC, toward the right heart **(A,B)**. In **(C)**, the catheter tip hits the right-atrial wall; it is then withdrawn several centimeters **(D)** and torqued. The catheter is advanced again **(E)**, passes through the right atrium **(F)**, and into the RV **(G)**. In **(H)**, the catheter is seated in the RV. Note that a strong bipolar signal is recorded once the catheter tip arrives in the right ventricle (lower-amplitude signal is also seen from the right atrium).

long data acquisitions are planned. As a solution to this problem, blood perfusion catheters were proposed.[59]

Electrophysiology catheters

Another multifunctional device is the electrophysiology (EP) MRI catheter.[60] EP catheters are used in cardiology to measure the pattern of electrical activation in the heart and also for the treatment of atrial fibrillation. In a feasibility study, an EP catheter was modified so that the same device could measure the electrical signal and the MRI signal simultaneously.[60] In the same study, the device was tested on a dog model (Figure 20.19).

Injection catheters

Perhaps the most important impact of CMR will be on new treatment techniques. The current trend in cardiology is toward development of novel agents, such as gene therapy agents, that can be injected directly into the infarcted heart. It is currently believed that this type of

therapy will be most effective when the periphery of the infarcted region is injected. Since the size, shape, and position of the infarction can be accurately determined by CMR, it has been argued that injection of these agents under CMR guidance are of critical importance.[61] An internal MRI coil has been incorporated into an injection catheter to solve the problem of localization of the catheter inside the CMR scanner.[62]

Conclusions

Studies on the development of internal coils are continuing at a high pace. The main design constraints are the flexibility and steerability of the devices. New methods have been developed in order to best utilize these invasive devices. The simplicity of the architecture of some of these internal coils allows their integration into multiple interventional devices. In this chapter, a short review has been given of recent studies on the design and some applications of these internal coils. Currently, internal coils are not used in routine clinical practice in CMR. More studies are necessary to explore their avenues of usefulness in medicine.

References

1. Haake EM, Brown RW, Thompson MR, Venkatesan R. Magnetic Resonance Imaging Physical Principles and Sequence Design. New York: Wiley-Liss. 1999.

2. Kantor HL, Briggs RW, Balaban RS. In vivo P-31 nuclear magnetic-resonance measurements in canine heart using a catheter-coil. Circ Res 1984; 55:261–6.

3. Hurst GC, Hua JM, Duerk JL, et al. Intravascular (catheter) NMR receiver probe – preliminary design analysis and application to canine iliofemoral imaging. Magn Reson Med 1992; 24:343–57.

4. Martin AJ, Plewes DB, Henkelman RM. MR imaging of blood-vessels with an intravascular coil. J Magn Reson Imaging 1992; 2:421–9.

5. Ladd ME, Quick HH, Debatin JF. Interventional MRA and intravas-cular imaging. J Magn Reson Imaging 2000; 12:534–46.

6. Ocali O, Atalar E. Intravascular magnetic resonance imaging using a loopless catheter antenna. Magn Reson Med 1997; 37:112–18.

7. Hofmann LV, Bluemke DA, Lawler B, et al. Intravascular MRI of peripheral arteries – Feasibility study for transvenous imaging of arterial pathology. Circulation 2001; 104(Suppl):1787.

8. Macovski A. Noise in MRI. Magn Reson Med 1996; 36:494–7.

9. Jin J-M. Electromagnetic Analysis and Design in Magnetic Resonance Imaging. Boca Raton, FL: CRC Press, 1998.

10. Vesselle H, Collin RR. The signal-to-noise ratio of nuclear-magnetic-resonance surface coils and application to a lossy dielectric cylinder model. 1. Theory IEEE Trans Biomed Eng 1995; 42:497–506.

11. Hoult DI, Richards RE. Signal-to-noise ratio of nuclear magnetic-resonance experiment. J Magn Reson 1976; 24:71–85.

12. Edelstein WA, Glover GH, Hardy CJ, Redington RW. The intrinsic signal-to-noise ratio in NMR imaging. Magn Reson Med 1986; 3:604–18.

13. Ocali O, Atalar E. Ultimate intrinsic signal-to-noise ratio in MRI. Magn Reson Med 1998; 39:462–73.

14. Edelstein WA. In: Proceedings of 4th Annual Meeting of the Society for Magnetic Resonance in Medicine, 1985:964.

15. Skinner MP, Yuan C, Mitsumori L, et al. Serial magnetic-resonance-imaging of experimental atherosclerosis detects lesion fine-struc-ture, progression and complications in-vivo. Nat Med 1995; 1:69–73.

16. Yuan C, Zhang SX, Polissar NL, et al. Identification of fibrous cap rupture with magnetic resonance imaging is highly associated with recent transient ischemic attack or stroke. Circulation 2002; 105:181–5.

17. Fayad ZA, Fuster V. Clinical imaging of the high-risk or vulnerable atherosclerotic plaque. Circ Res 2001; 89:305–16.

18. Fayad ZA, Hardy CJ, Giaquinto R, et al. Improved high resolution MRI of human coronary lumen and plaque with a new cardiac coil. Circulation 2001; 102(Suppl):1944.

19. Yuan C, Mitsumori LM, Ferguson MS, et al. In vivo accuracy of multispectral magnetic resonance imaging for identifying lipid-rich necrotic cores and intraplaque hemorrhage in advanced human carotid plaques. Circulation 2001; 104:2051–6.

20. Eryaman Y, Yigit H, Hafez I, Atalar E. Evaluation of internal MRI coils using UISNR. Proceedings of ISMRM, Toronto, Canada 2003:2400.

21. Susil RC, Yeung CJ, Atalar E. Intravascular extended sensitivity (IVES) MRI antennas. Magn Reson Med 2003: 50;383–390.

22. Atalar E, Bottomley PA, Ocali O, et al. High resolution intravascular MRI and MRS by using a catheter receiver coil. Magn Reson Med 1996; 36:596–605.

23. Correia LCL, Atalar E, Kelemen MD, et al. Intravascular magnetic resonance imaging of aortic atherosclerotic plaque composition. Arterioscler Thromb Vasc Biol 1997; 17:3626–32.

24. Quick HH, Ladd ME, Zimmermann-Paul GG, et al. Single-loop coil concepts for intravascular magnetic resonance imaging. Magn Reson Med 1999; 41:751–8.

25. Martin AJ, McLoughlin RF, Chu KC, et al. An expandable intra-venous RF coil for arterial wall imaging. J Magn Reson Imaging 1998; 8:226–34.

26. Rogers WJ, Prichard JW, Hu YL, et al. Characterization of signal properties in atherosclerotic plaque components by intravascular MRI. Arterioscler Thromb Vasc Biol 2000; 20:1824–30.

27. Brown RJS, Chandler R, Jackson JA, et al. History of NMR well logging. Concepts Mag Reson 2001; 13:335–413.

28. Kandarpa K, Jakab P, Patz S, et al. Prototype miniature endoluminal MR imaging catheter. J Vasc Interv Radiol 1993; 4:419–27.

29. Scott GC, Hu B. Stub antenna. In: Proceedings of the Annual Meeting of the International Society for Magnetic Resonance in Medicine, 2000.

30. Yung A, Atalar E. SPGR Ghost artifacts in endolumial MRI. Proceedings of ISMRM, Toronto, Canada 2003:1051.

31. Athey TW. A model of the temperature rise in the head due to mag-netic resonance imaging procedures. Magn Reson Med 1989; 9:177–84.

32. Athey TW. Current FDA guidance for MR patient exposure and considerations for the future. Ann NY Acad Sci 1992; 649:242–57.

33. Yeung CJ, Atalar E. A Green's function approach to local rf heating in interventional MRI. Med Phys 2001; 28:826–32.

34. Yeung CJ, Susil RC, Atalar E. RF safety of wires in interventional MRI: using a safety index. Magn Reson Med 2002; 47:187–93.

35. Ladd ME, Quick HH. Reduction of resonant RF heating in intravas-cular catheters using coaxial chokes. Magn Reson Med 2000; 43:615–19.

36. Atalar E. Safe coaxial cables for MRI. Radiology 1998; 209(Suppl):1298.

37. Yeung CJ, Atalar E. RF transmit power limit for the barewire loop-less catheter antenna. J Magn Reson Imaging 2000; 12:86–91.

38. Zimmermann-Paul GG, Quick HH, Vogt P, et al. High-resolution intravascular magnetic resonance imaging – monitoring of plaque formation in heritable hyperlipidemic rabbits. Circulation 1999; 99:1054–61.

39. Martin AJ, Henkelman RM. Intravascular MR-imaging in a porcine animal-model. Magn Reson Med 1994; 32:224–9.

40. Shunk KA, Lima JAC, Heldman AW, Atalar E. Transesophageal magnetic resonance imaging. Magn Reson Med 1999; 41:722–6.

41. Shunk KA, Garot J, Atalar E, Lima JAC. Transesophageal magnetic resonance imaging of the aortic arch and descending thoracic aorta in patients with aortic atherosclerosis. J Am Coll Cardiol 2001; 37:2031–5.

42. Omary RA, Unal O, Koscielski DS, et al. Real-time MR imaging-guided passive catheter tracking with use of gadolinium-filled catheters. J Vasc Interv Radiol 2001; 11:1079–85.

43. Yang XM, Atalar E. Intravascular MR imaging-guided balloon angioplasty with an MR imaging guide wire: feasibility study in rabbits. Radiology 2000; 217:501–6.

44. Burl M, Coutts GA, Herlihy DJ, et al. Twisted-pair RF coil suitable for locating the track of a catheter. Magn Reson Med 1999; 41:636–8.

45. Dumoulin CL, Souza SP, Darrow RD. Real-time position monitoring of invasive devices using magnetic-resonance. Magn Reson Med 1993; 29:411–15.

46. Ladd ME, Zimmermann GG, Quick HH, et al. Active MR visualization of a vascular guidewire in vivo. J Magn Reson Imaging 1998; 8:220–5.

47. Ladd ME, Erhart P, Debatin JF, et al. Guidewire antennas for MR fluoroscopy. Magn Reson Med 1997; 37:891–7.

48. McKinnon GC, Debatin JF, Leung DA, et al. Towards active guidewire visualization in interventional magnetic resonance imaging. Magma 1996; 4:13–18.

49. Atalar E, Kraitchman DL, Carkhuff B, et al. Catheter-tracking FOV MR fluoroscopy. Magn Reson Med 1998; 40:865–72.

50. Aksit P, Derbyshire JA, Serfaty JM, Atalar E. Multiple field of view MR fluoroscopy. Magn Reson Med 2002; 47:53–60.

51. Yang XM, Bolster BD, Kraitchman DL, Atalar E. Intravascular MR-monitored balloon angioplasty: an in vivo feasibility study. J Vasc Interv Radiol 1998; 9:953–9.

52. Serfaty JM, Yang XM, Aksit P, et al. Toward MRI-guided coronary catheterization: visualization of guiding catheters, guidewires, and anatomy in real time. J Magn Reson Imaging 2000; 12:590–4.

53. Yang X, Serfaty J, Quick HH, et al. Intracoronary high-resolution imaging using a 0.032″ MRI-guidewire: an in vivo feasibility study. Radiology 2000; 217(Suppl):355.

54. Rickers C, Jerosch-Herold M, Hu X, et al. Magnetic resonance image-guided transcatheter closure of atrial septal defects. Circulation 2003; 107:132–8.

55. Serfaty JM, Yang X, Quick HH, et al. MR-guided coronary artery intervention. Circulation 2000; 102:II-510.

56. Serfaty JM, Yang X, Foo T, et al. MRI-guided coronary catherization and PTCA: a feasibility study on a dog model. Magn Reson Med 2003; 49:258–63.

57. Quick HH, Ladd ME, Nanz D, et al. Vascular stents as RF antennas for intravascular MR guidance and imaging. Magn Reson Med 1999; 42:738–45.

58. Quick HH, Kuehl H, Kaiser G, et al. Inductively coupled stent antennas in MRI. Magn Reson Med 2002; 48:781–90.

59. Quick HH, Ladd ME, Hilfiker PR, et al. Autoperfused balloon catheter for intravascular MR imaging. J Magn Reson Imaging 1999; 9:428–34

60. Susil RC, Yeung CJ, Halperin HR, et al. Multifunctional interventional devices for MRI: a combined electrophysiology/MRI catheter. Magn Reson Med 2002; 47:594–600.

61. Lederman RJ, Guttman MA, Peters DC, et al. Catheter-based endomyocardial injection with real-time magnetic resonance imaging. Circulation 2002; 105:1282–4.

62. Karmarkar PV, Atalar E, Hofmann L, Kraitchman DL. An active MRI intramyocardial injection catheter. Proceedings of ISMRM, Toronto, Canada 2003:311.

21

The cardiovascular interventional MRI suite: design considerations

Michael A Guttman, Robert J Lederman, Elliot R McVeigh

Introduction

There has been longstanding interest in the use of magnetic resonance imaging (MRI) for feedback during interventional procedures.[1] Soft tissue discrimination, interactively adjustable image contrast and display features, and the more recent ability to produce images in real time have inspired research to evaluate catheter-based cardiovascular procedures that may be enabled or enhanced by MRI. This chapter contains a discussion of the special requirements for a cardiovascular interventional MRI (CV iMRI) suite over and above a standard MRI configuration in terms of room setup, patient monitoring, pulse sequences, computer hardware and software for image reconstruction and display, and interactive features.

Cardiovascular interventional imaging modalities

The modern cardiovascular catheterization lab features multiple imaging modalities for guiding invasive procedures. X-ray fluoroscopy (XRF) and surface ultrasound have long proven useful for introducing devices into the vascular system, both in typical and in difficult cases. However, these modalities both have shortcomings. XRF images exhibit exquisite spatial and temporal resolution, yet soft tissues are nearly impossible to discriminate and radiation dosage is potentially harmful. Ultrasound is a low-cost modality with no siting issues, acquires images with good temporal resolution and visible soft tissues, but image quality can suffer from poor spatial resolution and artifacts. In addition, certain views may not be available, depending on how the transducer can be placed. MRI brings some benefits not offered by the other imaging modalities, such as soft tissue discrimination, different contrast mechanisms, flexible slice orientation, and no harmful radiation, all of which suggest a role for MRI in cardiovascular interventional procedures.

Investigators are planning for interventional procedures to be conducted wholly under MRI guidance. But during early development and deployment, clinical interventional suites should have supplemental imaging modalities beyond MRI to assist the primary procedure or to provide alternative image guidance during an emergency. Investigational and clinical MRI equipment may be prone to computer or other instrumentation failure, and early clinical procedures may be prone to unanticipated catastrophic failure. An analogy can be drawn with the first two decades of coronary artery angioplasty (in the era before coronary stents were widely employed). At the time, standard North American practice was for surgical teams to be kept on standby to respond to the 2–5% likelihood that patients would require emergency coronary artery bypass surgery. At many medical centers, this resulted in an entire operating room, surgeons, perfusionist, and nursing teams remaining on standby.

Even after iMRI applications have become well developed, supplemental imaging modalities may still be required to assist the primary procedure, to provide emergency imaging alternative, or to handle certain difficult cases. For example, image-guided vascular access may prove challenging in even 'short-bore' cylindrical MR systems. Higher-risk therapeutic procedures, such as myocardial or valvular interventions, may be complicated by coronary, rhythm, or other mechanical emergencies that are currently best treated using XRF. Both circumstances would trigger patient egress from the magnet bore and further treatment using alternative imaging modalities.

XMR: the combined X-ray and MRI suite

Although high magnetic fields may significantly distort the X-ray beam of conventional fluoroscopes, high-quality digital C-arm fluoroscopes may be collocated in the MR suite outside the 5 G field line and can provide useful imaging for most traditional or emergency vascular interventions. For myocardial procedures, traditional floor-mounted cardiac fluoroscopy units may be preferable. Solid-state flat-panel X-ray imaging systems are entering the market that, unlike traditional X-ray tube–intensifier systems, can operate satisfactorily even within high magnetic fields. Some proposals to integrate flat-panel X-ray systems into MRI bores may sacrifice craniocaudal angulation, which is important for many cardiovascular interventional procedures.

One cost-effective solution pursued at several medical centers is to install adjacent X-ray interventional and MRI suites separated by a door for patient transport and sharing a single control room. The suites can operate independently and simultaneously for traditional X-ray or MRI procedures or together for combined interventional procedures. An example of one such combined XMR suite in use at the National Institutes of Health is shown in Figure 21.1. A wheel-based trolley is used as a bridge to transport the patient between X-ray and MRI, with rollers on the top surface to facilitate movement of the patient. A sliding door between the rooms saves space while achieving a radiofrequency (RF) seal for MRI when closed.

Patient handling and monitoring

Patient handling and monitoring equipment under XMR needs to have the same intensive care capabilities as an interventional cardiovascular X-ray environment rather than the more limited monitoring available in a non-invasive MRI environment. Transfer between X-ray and MRI lab must be rapid, smooth, and simple in either direction. Even if certain procedures are designed to use MRI alone, rapid transfer into the X-ray lab must be available for emergency imaging alternative in case of device or procedural failure. This capability proves surprisingly difficult to implement.

To avoid disrupting delicate intravascular interventional devices, patients probably should remain attached to a single cradle or shell for both X-ray and MRI environments. This shell needs to have mechanical characteristics suitable to accommodate heavy patients, to be widely radiolucent to permit unattenuated X-ray transmission even at extreme angles, to be nonferrous and nonconducting for safety during MRI, to have a comfort surface (such as thermal memory foam) that awake patients can tolerate throughout interventional procedures lasting many hours, and to be thin enough to accommodate close placement of posterior MRI surface coils. The patient cradle should also have facilities to secure cables, pressure transducers, sterile drapes, intravascular devices, and probably even intravenous medication pumps and power injectors against dislodgement during transfer.

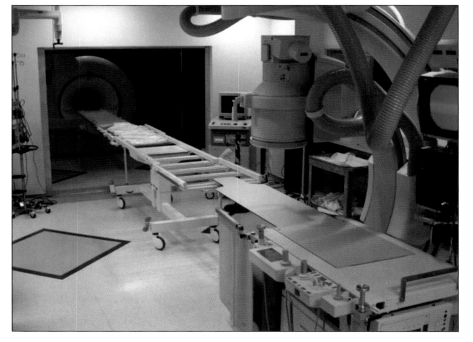

Figure 21.1
The XMR suite at the National Institutes of Health. The equipment shown is a Siemens Multistar X-ray system in the near field within a fully equipped cardiac catheterization laboratory, and a Siemens Sonata 1.5 T MRI scanner in the adjoining room. The shared control room is to the right, behind the C-arm. A wheeled patient trolley is positioned between the X-ray and MRI units. An ultrasound system is located to the right of the patient trolley.

Table 21.1. Devices and cabling/tubing requirements for XMR suites

Type of device	Cable/tube count	Device	Comment
MRI receiver coils	4	Anterior and lateral surface coils	Generally radiopaque; should be removed before X-ray imaging. Secured to torso for imaging or secured to isocenter for 'fluoroscopic' application with moveable table.
	4	Posterior surface coils	Generally radiopaque; should be removed before X-ray imaging.
Monitoring	10	ECG electrodes	For monitoring cardiac rhythm and repolarization: 10 radiolucent nonferrous electrodes desirable for X-ray imaging with ST-segment monitoring; leads must have high impedance. Repolarization cannot currently be monitored in MRI, so only a subset of these electrodes are used for gating and rhythm. Graphite electrodes and lead systems are ideal.
	1	Pulse oximeter	MR-compatible oximeters can be used in both environments to monitor hemoglobin saturation – an index of effective ventilation and oxygenation.
	1	Respiratory bellows	Useful adjunct to monitor diaphragm motion inside MRI bore, and for respiratory gating.
	2	Invasive blood pressure	MR-compatible transducers can be used in both environments. Instantaneous superimposed signal from at least 2 channels used to monitor patients and catheter position (i.e. inflow occlusion, subintimal injection position, myocardial contact).
	1	Noninvasive blood pressure	Remote-controlled MR-compatible cuffs can be used in both X-ray and MRI environments.
Intravenous access	2	Intravenous catheters and extension tubing	For continuous or periodic volume supplementation in response to blood pressure fluctuation. For intravenous sedation and comfort medications. For treatment of life-threatening emergencies.
Supplemental oxygen and other gases	1	Nasal cannula, face mask, or mechanical ventilator	Redundant tubing must be kept tangle-free, especially against accidental dislodgement of endotracheal tubes.
Vascular access	3	Interventional devices	Sheath, guiding catheters, guidewires, balloons, stents, and other devices would resemble X-ray devices, but must be customized for the MRI environment. 'Over-the-wire' devices might extend 1.5 m outside of body, and require sterile containment.
	2	Intravascular MRI receiver coils	Would be applied like interventional devices. Sterile, torque-constrained connectors to MRI receiver chain.
Pacemakers	1	Transvenous	Customized MR-compatible pacemaker leads would resemble steerable or balloon-flotation leads used in X-ray. May be used for pacing as well as for MRI gating.
	1	Transthoracic	Currently a contraindication in the MRI environment.
Video	0	Video camera	Useful for observing patient facial expressions, respiration, and movement inside MRI bore. Widely available. Can be ceiling-mounted.
	1	Patient video headset display or mirrored headset	Available for patient to see outside MRI bore or to watch video programs for calming effect.
Audio	1	Patient audio headset and microphone	For bidirectional communications with nurses and other staff, and to listen to music for calming effect.

Ideally, patient transfer between the two imaging modalities would be as simple as sliding an X-ray table: a low-friction design would permit a single operator to move the shell easily with one hand. However, a bridging mechanism is required in an adjoining-room setup. Existing manufacturer prototypes use either 'tram tracks' in the floor or an interposed trolley to convey the patient-bearing shell between the two modalities. Any such system must protect against rapid deceleration, which can dislodge intravascular equipment and injure the patient.

iMRI procedures such as transcatheter myocardial stem cell delivery would require that a surprisingly large number of devices be secured during transfer between imaging modalities. An example enumeration is shown in Table 21.1. Such a potentially large number of cables and tubes can hinder the movements of personnel, and increases the chance of something being stepped on and damaged. One way to reduce the number of cables is to transmit electrical signals using high-frequency wireless devices. A system could be implemented to maintain wireless connection during the delicate transfer of the patient between X-ray and MRI. Tubes and the equipment to which they are connected still have to be moved in step with the patient; some items require additional hands to move, but other items such as IV poles can be mounted to the patient cradle. Moreover, a sterile field must be maintained over a workspace large enough to accommodate the exchange of long (e.g. 2 m) catheter devices. As a safeguard, the patient and the workspace can be re-draped after every transfer between X-ray and MRI.

An important shortcoming of MRI is the distortion of ECG signals by the Hall effect from blood moving through the magnetic field. The filtered ECG signal is usually satisfactory for QRS detection but not for monitoring repolarization (ST-segment) changes. This limitation has important implications for myocardial or coronary-related interventional procedures. Some surrogate for ST-segment monitoring will need to be developed. Candidate approaches include continuous or intermittent monitoring of myocardial wall motion compared with baseline to detect sudden myocardial ischemia during the procedure.

Room configuration

Several modifications must be made to the design of the typical MRI suite to make it suitable for interventional procedures. Table 21.2 lists essential siting considerations when building an iMRI suite.

Magnet configuration

The basic magnet configurations available today are the cylindrical bore and the parallel plate 'open' magnet design. While the open design is excellent for patient access and comfort, its drawback is relatively low field strength and gradient performance. Side access to the patient afforded by the open design is an advantage for procedures such as image-guided surgery and biopsy. However, groin access may be sufficient for catheter-based procedures, suggesting an advantage with the higher-performance cylindrical bore magnets. Modern 1.5 T magnets are usually less than 90 cm from the front opening to the center of the cylinder, where the imaging takes place. This distance is sufficient for relatively comfortable catheter manipulation using extended-length catheters. Interestingly, the higher-field parallel plate open systems offer no additional groin access, because the distance to the center of the imaging volume is similar to that of the 1.5 T cylinder. When scanning the heart and lower extremities in shorter cylindrical bore models, the patient's face is at least partially out of the bore, reducing the chance of claustrophobia-related complications. While 3 T magnets are becoming widely available, offering imaging with greater signal-to-noise ratio (SNR), a drawback of these systems is the increase in the specific absorption rate of RF energy endured by the patient; restricting the use of short-TR, high-flip-angle sequences for real-time guidance and monitoring. The 1.5 T cylindrical bore magnets offer a good balance between patient accessibility, image quality and speed.

The size of the homogeneous region of static field (i.e. the optimal imaging volume) should be sufficiently large to produce high-quality images over a 30 cm field of view (FOV). While smaller FOV will be used to 'zoom-in' to specific locations, it is important to have images with larger FOV for catheter guidance and to get one's bearings during double oblique scanning. Severe geometric distortion on the fringes of the imaging FOV may cause confusion about the location and orientation of the imaging slice when a 'nonstandard' view is being scanned. At this time, the audible noise level from the switching gradients requires ear protection and/or communication headphones to be worn by the medical personnel performing the procedure; significant reduction in this noise level using quiet gradient technology would be a major development for iMRI.

Communications and image display

During an interventional procedure, the physician requires real-time communication with the MRI scanner,

Table 21.2. Siting considerations for interventional MRI suites

Consideration	Comments
Doors	The suite should have at least two RF-shielded doors: 1. Patient transfer door. This separates the MRI from the X-ray system and may need to contain lead shielding to permit independent X-ray and MRI operation. The door may need to be at least 2 m wide, so 'pocket' or sliding doors may reduce the footprint. Manual operation must be available even if the doors are automated, since motorized systems may fail. 2. Staff door. This door can be foot-operated for passage of scrubbed personnel. Door perimeters must permit adequate cleaning of body fluids and must be kept clean to permit electrical contacts for RF shields.
Sink	A sink in the magnet room is extremely valuable for interventional procedures and experiments, and is extremely difficult to install as an afterthought. Must be located away from magnet bore to reduce effect of RF noise carried in on the pipes.
Sound attenuation	MR gradient noise can be amplified in the confined space of small MRI labs. Moreover, noise transmitted through walls can disrupt neighboring workspaces. Sound-dampening wall and ceiling tile can be well worth the additional expense, but porous materials must be avoided. Sound-dampening magnet pedestals reduce through-floor noise transmission. Nevertheless, patients and staff must wear ear protection.
5 G line	Contemporary high-performance systems generate persistent high magnetic fields and represent a hazard to patients and staff who are not trained in MRI safety. When designing the suite layout, the 5 G magnetic field line should be considered the accepted threshold for safety. A free passage must be designed outside the 5 G line for patients and staff, for example, with implanted defibrillators.
Anesthesia gas lines	These lines are essential to facilitate animal experiments and a range of anticipated clinical procedures. They must be accessible even with the RF doors closed, so interventional suites probably should have at least two sets of gas lines. Typical setups include anesthesia gas exhaust, vacuum, medical air, and oxygen. Consider in advance where ventilators will be positioned for combined X-ray and MRI experiments.
Waveguides and penetration panels	Large-caliber cylinders can be installed through RF shields to permit late additions (such as fiberoptic cables and plethysmography tubing). These should be convenient to open spaces in the MRI control room. Some labs use additional waveguides to transmit images from LCD projectors directly onto screens installed inside the lab, thereby permitting the use of inexpensive unshielded electronics. The location of these waveguides must be planned carefully in advance. Similarly, penetration panels permit late installation of conducting cables, such as for keyboards, mice, and hemodynamics systems. Appropriate RF filters are installed in the penetration panels to prevent RF leaks through these cables.
Power	Numerous RF-filtered power outlets should be available and conveniently located both for routine and for emergency applications, such as hemodynamics systems, intravenous fluid pumps, warmers, ventilators, etc.
Tethers	All ferromagnetic equipment that is installed inside the MRI lab should be tethered, even if loosely, to a wall as a reminder to staff to keep it away from the high magnetic field.
Heating, ventilation, and air-conditioning (HVAC)	The two labs should have independent temperature control and ideally use nonrecirculated air directly vented outside to facilitate sterile patient procedures as well as animal procedures.
Patient orientation	Ideally, the X-ray and MR tables should be colinear, and oriented head-to-foot. Such a facility permits patient transfer along a single line, minimizing potentially disruptive deceleration forces.
Control room	Ideally the X-ray and MRI labs share a common control area with interconnected monitoring equipment.

the other members of the interventional team, and hemodynamic monitoring equipment. These requirements are challenging near the magnet of the MRI scanner, since all equipment must function while immersed in a high magnetic field. In some cases, off-the-shelf equipment will function properly if secured a certain distance from the magnet bore. However, in many cases, equipment must be modified to function properly and not be pulled into the bore by the magnetic field. In this section, we will review potential solutions to these communication and monitoring requirements.

In-room display of computer screens

Much of the information required for monitoring an interventional procedure is displayed on computer screens. For example, the MRI scanner console display and images as well as hemodynamic patient data such as ECG or arterial pressure are typically displayed on flat-panel LCD screens. These displays often operate properly if placed at least 10–15 feet from the magnet bore, but will fail if brought too close. This viewing distance may be acceptable for hemodynamic data, where waveforms are displayed as high-contrast line drawings. However, grayscale images require closer scrutiny, especially given the display sizes commonly available today. MR-compatible LCD monitors are available commercially, which can be located very close to the bore of the magnet (Figure 21.1). Figure 21.2 shows a setup employing two 18-inch units (Aydin Displays, Horsham, PA) mounted on movable aluminum base stands. The units are placed near the bore of a 1.5 T magnet (Signa CV/i, GE Medical Systems, Waukesha, WI), for viewing of real-time image data during a catheterization experiment. In this experimental setup, one monitor replicates the scanner console display and the other replicates the external workstation. Two

keyboards are placed on the patient table, connected to the scanner console and external workstation, respectively. Standard, inexpensive PC-compatible keyboards work from this location, although some models emit RF noise. Aydin Displays sells a shielded keyboard for placement closer to the magnet bore.

Some scanner manufacturers are now providing optional LCD monitors positioned near the magnet. One model from Hitachi Medical Systems America (Twinsburg, OH) has an extensible arm mounted to the top of the magnet, allowing the monitor to be moved to almost any position around the magnet. Other scanner manufacturers are beginning to provide options for an adjustable position monitor in the magnet room.

In Figure 21.3, a rear-projection screen is suspended from the ceiling while the projector, which is not MR-compatible, is positioned away from the 1.5 T magnet (Sonata, Siemens Medical Systems, Erlangen, Germany). The projector can be suspended from the ceiling to assure a clear light pathway to the screen, or can project through glass or a wall opening (e.g. a waveguide) if it is preferred to position the projector outside the magnet room. One advantage of this arrangement is a larger display area that can accommodate more than one projection.

In-room controls

Current MRI scanners have in-room controls for functions such as table positioning, stopping and starting

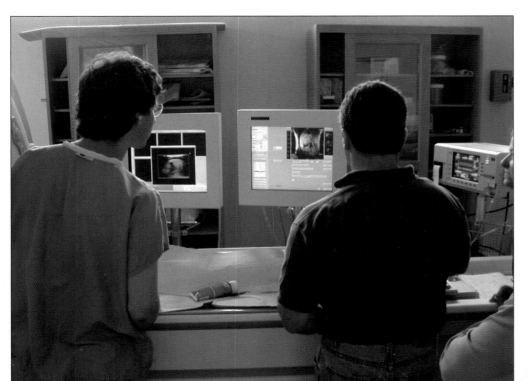

Figure 21.2
Dual-monitor setup for a cardiovascular interventional MRI experiment. The patient table is used as a workspace and monitors for image display and patient monitoring are placed opposite. The patient monitoring unit is not MR-compatible and is tethered to remain outside the 5 G line. The magnet bore is on the left edge of the frame.

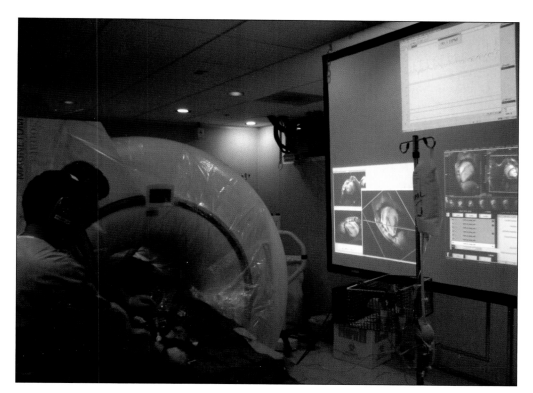

Figure 21.3
Rear-projection screen setup for an interventional MRI suite. A large screen surface is available for viewing the scanner console (shown), with room for additional projections. The LCD rear-projection unit is ceiling-mounted behind the screen, utilizes 'keystone correction', and does not become blocked by in-room personnel.

scanning, and emergency stop. For interventional procedures, more controls are needed for the interactive features of pulse sequences, image reconstruction/display, interventional devices and monitoring equipment. Devices and monitoring equipment have a limited set of interactive features, which can often be controlled by a small number of integrated buttons. On the other hand, the interactive features of pulse sequences and image reconstruction/display are under development with relatively short modification cycles since they are based in software. At the current stage of development, more adaptable and universal user controls are advantageous, such as a general-purpose computer keyboard along with a pointing device such as a mouse, trackball, rocker switch, or joystick. These controls may not need to be placed in the sterile field, but must be cleaned after each procedure. Hence, computer keyboards with membrane panels should be used. For the pointing device, a trackball offers excellent usability for a device that can be adequately cleaned. For those procedures where the keyboard and pointing device are near or in the sterile field, they may be covered with a sterile drape. In this situation, a trackball may be difficult to use and a joystick similar to that used on X-ray tables may be more practical.

In-room audio communication

During a typical MRI scan, enough audiofrequency noise is generated to require hearing protection in the magnet room. The loudness depends on the scanner hardware, pulse sequence, and room configuration. Real-time imaging sequences, which are likely to be used for image-guided interventional procedures, are also the ones that produce the most noise, due to the high slew rates and duty cycles required. As a result, verbal communication between members of an interventional team is nearly impossible in the magnet room without some form of headset-based system.

Several companies manufacture systems that allow the scanner operator in the control room to communicate with the subject lying in the scanner. These systems typically include a patient headset that provides hearing protection and two-way communication as well as music. Some systems provide a headset for a companion to sit near and communicate with the subject in the magnet room. Systems such as these must be expanded to include headsets for all members of the interventional team in the magnet room. The patient should not be able to hear the communication between the team members unless intentionally addressed. Thus, the system must have multiple communications channels and notify the team, perhaps with a chime, when the patient is included. Prototypes for such in-room communication systems are in development by companies such as Magnacoustics (Atlantic Beach, NY), Phone-Or (Glen Head, NY) and Avotec (Stuart, FL), but are not currently available commercially.

Real-time imaging sequences and reconstruction methods

The phrase 'real-time imaging' refers to the ability to depict an event as it happens. Several conditions must be satisfied for an imaging modality to be classified as real-time. Depicting the event requires sufficient contrast-to-noise ratio (CNR) and spatial resolution to distinguish the objects of interest as well as enough temporal resolution to see the motions of interest. Depicting the event 'as it happens' requires low latency, which is the time between an event and its rendering on the computer screen. Exactly what resolution, CNR, and latency are required depends on many factors, including the task to be performed, and the anatomy and devices to be visualized. For tasks requiring image-guided navigation of a device such as a catheter, images should be produced at a rate of at least 5 frames/s with latency no more than one-third of a second. In a procedure requiring more intricate manipulation, or if there is rapid anatomical motion to contend with, as in the heart, at least 10 frames/s with lower latency would be preferable.

Of the large variety of pulse sequences available for MRI, those producing gradient-recalled echoes with short TR offer fairly high efficiency in generating raw k-space data (i.e. more echoes per unit time). This efficiency reduces the imaging time window, which is the time required to generate data for a single image. This in turn reduces the amount of motion that can occur during the acquisition of data for each image, thereby minimizing motion artifacts and blurring. Efficiency can be further increased by acquiring more k-space data for each RF excitation. This can be done by acquiring multiple k-space lines, as in echo-planar imaging (EPI)[2] or increasing the length of each line by covering k-space in a spiral trajectory.[3] However, the longer TR required increases vulnerability to off-resonance effects which can reduce image quality in some situations.

Of the different options for short-TR pulse sequences, the high SNR of steady-state free precession (SSFP),[4] is an attractive choice for real-time imaging. For increased imaging efficiency, multiple-echo implementations of SSFP have been demonstrated.[5] SSFP achieves a high SNR by refocusing the magnetization at the end of each TR, and requires more finely tuned scanner hardware than spoiled sequences (i.e. those in which the magnetization is dephased at the end of each TR). Fortunately,

recent improvements in commercial scanner hardware have increased the availability of SSFP imaging, which is gaining widespread use.

The frame rate may be increased by performing additional image reconstructions using partially updated k-space data, as done in view sharing, or by reconstructing images using undersampled sets of k-space data, as is done in UNFOLD[6] or in so-called parallel imaging methods such as SMASH[7] and SENSE.[8] All of these methods perform imaging with a greatly reduced FOV in the phase-encoding direction and use some form of filtering or other steps to remove the resulting wraparound aliasing artifact. View sharing and UNFOLD employ different forms of temporal filtering, while parallel imaging methods use the independent information from multiple coils (see Chapter 5). Each method has its advantages, and it is important to consider any additional requirements for coils and computer resources. View sharing and UNFOLD work equally well regardless of the number and arrangement of receiver coils. However, it is difficult to achieve an acceleration factor greater than 2. Parallel imaging methods have been shown to achieve greater acceleration factors,[9] and can exhibit decreased motion blurring in real-time imaging,[10] but require multiple coils (from 4 to 8 or more, depending on the desired acceleration). Some disadvantages of parallel imaging are that more receiver channels are required (leaving fewer channels for active devices), image SNR is decreased, and coil arrangement and choice of phase-encoding direction often have a substantial impact on artifact suppression. In addition, updating coil sensitivity maps in parallel imaging methods can be computationally expensive, which is an important consideration when it is desired to perform this update in real time.

Computational resources

The simplest MR image reconstruction typically involves multiplying two-dimensional (2D) k-space data by a windowing function (spatial filter) followed by a fast Fourier transform (FFT), although methods to save time during data acquisition often add steps to the reconstruction task. For example, incomplete k-space coverage can be filled in using homodyne detection, which adds windowing functions, phase corrections, and FFTs. Some methods, such as ramp sampling and spiral and radial k-space trajectories, involve acquisition of data points that do not lie on the rectilinear k-space grid. These data are typically 'regridded' using some form of spatial interpolation before FFT. Parallel imaging methods often update the coil sensitivity maps during scanning, requiring several steps, including window functions, additional FFTs, many small matrix inverses, and temporal filtering in some cases. Further down the processing chain, graphical dis-

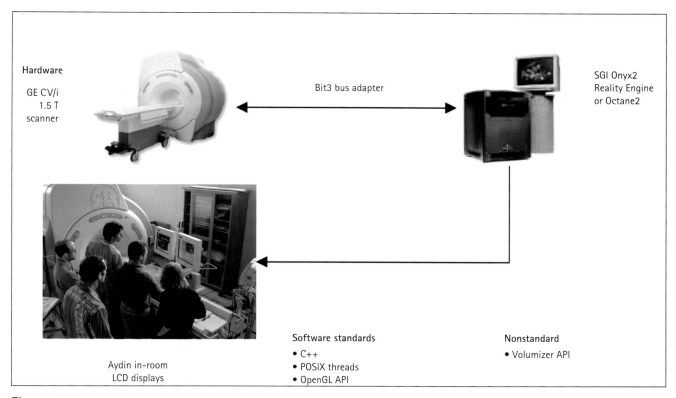

Figure with labels:

Hardware

GE CV/i
1.5 T
scanner

Bit3 bus adapter

SGI Onyx2
Reality Engine
or Octane2

Aydin in-room
LCD displays

Software standards
• C++
• POSIX threads
• OpenGL API

Nonstandard
• Volumizer API

Figure 21.4
Modifications made to a clinical scanner for an experimental CV iMRI lab at the National Institutes of Health. The system is capable of real-time multiplanar imaging with UNFOLD and/or TSENSE acceleration, 3D multiplanar views, and live volume renderings.

plays are becoming more complicated, rendering real-time image planes or volumes[11] in 3D with color guides indicating invasive device positions and user annotations. Factor in the trend towards larger numbers of receiver channels (e.g. 8, 16, or more), and the computational demands of image reconstruction and display become substantial.

Since these techniques are still under development and therefore not commonplace, commercial MRI scanners are not equipped with the high-performance data transfer, image reconstruction, and display hardware capable of the real-time processing described above. As an example of data throughput requirements in a foreseeable configuration, a continuous scan using 256 samples per excitation, 2.5 ms TR, and 16 receiver channels would require a data rate of over 52 Mbits/s, assuming the data are represented as 16-bit complex integers. The need for low latency and high frame rate on this data stream suggests that high-speed data transfer (well in excess of the expected data rate) and a multiple processor configuration should be used in the image reconstruction subsystem.

Several research groups have performed modifications to bypass or supplement the stock reconstruction and display systems. These efforts require the cooperation of the scanner manufacturer, who provides information on how to access the data stream. The typical method used is to add a bus adapter or networking card to the reconstruction subsystem and connect this to a high-speed workstation, where the researchers have complete flexibility in processing the data and displaying the images. One such modification of a GE 1.5 T Signa CV/i scanner is illustrated in Figure 21.4, which was used to perform real-time image reconstructions using view sharing, UNFOLD, and TSENSE,[12] a time-adaptive variant of SENSE. Several other examples of external workstation reconstruction and display have been reported in the literature.[13–15] Some groups have gone further and provided alternate digital receivers, which transform the analog signals from the receiver coils into digital representations.[16,17] This task is more complicated, and has been done to provide more receiver channels, greater receiver bandwidth and to have more control over the receiver electronics. Using such a modification, eight receiver coils were connected to a clinical scanner to demonstrate TSENSE with an acceleration factor of 4;[9] this was not possible on the clinical scanners available at the time.

Research institutions have thus served as valuable proving grounds for new techniques. Depending on the success and promise of a new technique, it can be 'productized', where it is made less expensive, integrated into the scanner environment, and thoroughly tested for FDA approval.

Interactive user features

One of the uniquely useful features of MRI is that the contrast (i.e. which sets of tissues, devices, or agents are bright), content, or spatial and temporal resolution can be changed interactively during imaging. High-end commercial scanners allow real-time control of the pulse sequence through the programming interface. Saturation pulses can be played between excitations, timings within the sequence can be altered, gradient amplitudes can be modified, or k-space trajectories can be changed. Image reconstruction and display can have many interactive features, ranging from changing reconstruction methods and parameters, to adjusting individual channel gains, coloring, thresholds, and display and rendering modes.

Given the many potential features of real-time interactive imaging, a graphical user interface (GUI) must be provided to facilitate adjustments to the pulse sequence, reconstruction, and display during the imaging process. Some scanner manufacturers have introduced GUI products with many features for interactive MRI. These features include 'bookmarking' images for later return to their locations, playing saturation pulses, switching between different but similar types of sequences, providing tools to prescribe new image locations off of the incoming image stream or off previously acquired images, saving sets of images to the scanner database, and adjustment of some MRI parameters such as flip angle, slice thickness, FOV, and triggering. Still more features are required that are not yet available in current products. As iMRI applications become better defined, the GUIs can begin to include protocols that focus on stages of the procedure rather than the technical detail being changed.

Table 21.3. Interactive MRI features

Interactive feature	Potential use
Change slice plane	Navigation, device tracking
Save segments of the image stream	Review and archive
Save individual image frames for quick recall	Bookmarking
Alter slice-select gradient	Change slice thickness
Alter readout and phase-encoding gradients	Change FOV
Alter excitation flip angle, TR, TE	Adjust image contrast
Apply saturation or inversion pulse prior to single or multiple images	Visualization of T1-shortening contrast agent with background suppression
Fat saturation	Suppress bright fat signal from chest wall, pericardium, or other regions
Spatial saturation	Selectively darken inflowing blood
Apply tagging pulses	Observe tissue motion
Partial k-space coverage	Increase temporal or spatial resolution
Enable view sharing, UNFOLD, or parallel imaging	Increase temporal or spatial resolution
Adjust channel gain	Equalize or enhance device signal with respect to surface coil signal
Display selected channels in different colors	Visualize invasive MR-active devices
Display a single channel with no slice-select gradient[18]	See the path of an MR-active device that leaves the imaging slice
Subtract current image from a baseline image	Visualize change in image contrast
Register real-time image with previously acquired volume rendering	Treatment planning or guidance
Display image in 3D, registered with imported markers or contours	Treatment targeting
Multiple parallel slices	Visualize 3D objects
Multiple nonparallel slices	Follow path of tortuous vessel
Acquire high-resolution image at current image location	Perform detailed assessment following navigation or treatment

Table 21.3 lists a variety of interactive MRI features, and a potential use for the interaction. A full-featured interactive MRI interface should provide the user with at least this set of adjustments.

Interventional active devices

In the ideal CV iMRI suite, all of the devices available to the physician in the standard X-ray catheterization lab would be available; however, because of the large static magnetic field, and the exposure to bursts of RF energy, a number of modifications must be made to most devices. First, all ferromagnetic metals used in the construction of the devices must be replaced with nonferromagnetic materials. Materials such as stainless steel will cause large signal voids in the image, and will be subject to substantial forces when brought close to the magnet. (A guidewire or catheter containing steel will be attracted along the direction of the magnetic field lines, causing it to 'straighten out' down the bore of the magnet.) This initially eliminates the majority of the steerable catheters, guidewires, and catheters that are reinforced with metallic braiding. All of these devices can be made from nonferromagnetic materials such as nitinol, or nonferrous stainless steel,[19] but the fact that the existing devices cannot be simply pulled down from the shelf is a constraint on the development of new procedures, and the translation of X-ray guided interventions into the MRI-guided system.

An equally important constraint on interventional devices is electrical isolation and the suppression of currents induced by the transmitted RF and gradient pulses. Significant levels of switching magnetic fields are capable of inducing currents in conducting materials, which can cause heating or high voltages; both of these conditions must be avoided. Modifications to active devices can be made to bring these effects under control.[20–22] Thermal and electronic testing of devices in experimental animals and phantoms need to be carried out to insure that safe operating conditions are always obtained during the procedures.[23,24] For a further description of intraluminal imaging coils, see Chapter 20.

One constraint on the electrical connection of active devices such as guiding catheters and guidewires is that the connections must be easily cycled for device exchange. During the suspension of the electrical connection, the active devices within the patient must remain in a safe configuration with respect to induced currents and voltages. This can be achieved in the device design, or with an interlock on the scanner that does not permit the transmission of RF energy during device exchange. The mechanism for rapid connect and disconnect of active devices should be easily accessible to the physician, and should not present additional distractions from the normal progress of the procedure.

Conclusions

The CV iMRI suite is in a developmental stage. Transforming a standard MRI suite into one for performing interventions requires modifications to the MRI scanner hardware and software, the room (or rooms, for XMR suites), interventional devices, surgical tools, and monitoring equipment. Some progress has been made but mainly in research facilities with customized setups and investigational devices. The work coming out of these efforts is very promising, inspiring further investigation into candidate interventional procedures with new or modified devices. Research in acute animal experiments has been underway for years at several institutions. Trials in human subjects have begun only recently at a small number of facilities. Continued successes should lead to the development of the products required to set up interventional suites in clinical settings.

References

1. Lufkin RB (ed). Interventional MRI. St Louis, MO: Mosby-Year Book, 1999.

2. Mansfield P. Multiplanar image formation using NMR spin echoes. J Phys Colloq 1977; 10:L55.

3. Ahn CB, Kim JH, Cho ZH. High-speed spiral-scan echo planar NMR imaging. IEEE Trans Med Imaging 1986; 5:2–7.

4. Oppelt A. FISP—a new fast MRI sequence. Electromedica 1986; 54:15–18.

5. Herzka DA, Kellman P, Aletras AH, et al. Multishot EPI-SSFP in the heart. Magn Reson Med 2002; 47:655–64.

6. Madore B, Glover GH, Pelc NJ. Unaliasing by Fourier-encoding the overlaps using the temporal dimension (UNFOLD), applied to cardiac imaging and fMRI. Magn Reson Med 1999; 42:813–28.

7. Sodickson DK, Manning W. Simultaneous acquisition of spatial harmonics (SMASH): fast imaging with radiofrequency coil arrays. Magn Reson Med 1997; 38:591–603.

8. Pruessmann KP, Weiger M, Scheidegger MB, Boesiger P. SENSE: sensitivity encoding for fast MRI. Magn Reson Med 1999; 42:952–62.

9. Kellman P, Derbyshire JA, Morris HD, et al. Comparison of several 8-element surface coil configurations for cardiac imaging using SENSE. In: Proceedings of the 10th Scientific Meeting of the International Society for Magnetic Resonance in Medicine 2002; 857.

10. Guttman MA, Kellman P, Dick AJ, Lederman RJ, McVeigh ER. Real-time accelerated interactive MRI with adaptive TSENSE and UNFOLD. Magn Reson Med 2003; 50:315–321.

11. Guttman MA, Lederman RJ, Sorger JM, McVeigh ER. Real-time volume rendered MRI for interventional guidance. J Cardiovasc Magn Reson 2002; 4:431–42.

12. Kellman P, Epstein FH, McVeigh ER. Adaptive sensitivity encoding incorporating temporal filtering (TSENSE). Magn Reson Med 2001; 45:846–52.

13. Wright RC, Riederer SJ, Farzaneh F, et al. Real-time MR fluoroscopic data acquisition and image reconstruction. Magn Reson Med 1989; 12:407–15

14. Hardy CJ, Darrow RD, Nieters EJ, et al. Real-time acquisition, display, and interactive graphic control of NMR cardiac profiles and images. Magn Reson Med 1993; 29:667–73.

15. Kerr AB, Pauly JM, Hu BS, et al. Real-time interactive MRI on a conventional scanner. Magn Reson Med 1997; 38:355–67.

16. Morris HD, Derbyshire JA, Kellman P, et al. A wide-bandwidth multi-channel digital receiver and real-time reconstruction engine for use with a clinical MR scanner. In: Proceedings of the 10th Scientific Meeting of the International Society for Magnetic Resonance in Medicine 2002; 61.

17. de Zwart JA, Ledden PJ, Kellman P, et al. Design of a SENSE-optimized high-sensitivity MRI receive coil for brain imaging. Magn Reson Med 2002; 47:1218–27.

18. Peters DC, Lederman RJ, Dick AJ, et al. Interactive undersampled projection reconstruction for active catheter imaging, with adaptable temporal resolution and catheter-only views. Magn Reson Med 2003; 49:216–222.

19. Melzer A, Stoeckel D, Busch M, et al. MR-compatible instruments for interventional MRI. In: Interventional MRI (Lufkin RB, ed). St Louis, MO: Mosby-Year Book, 1999:55–69.

20. Susil RC, Yeung CJ, Halperin HR, et al. Multifunctional interventional devices for MRI: a combined electrophysiology/MRI catheter. Magn Reson Med 2002; 47:594–600.

21. Atalar E, Ocali O. Enhanced safety coaxial cables. US Patent 6,284,971, September 4, 2001.

22. Tsitlik J, Levin H, Halperin H, Weisfeldt M. ECG amplifier and cardiac pacemaker for use during magnetic resonance imaging. US Patent 5,217,010, June 8, 1993.

23. Yeung CJ, Susil RC, Atalar E. RF heating due to conductive wires during MRI depends on the phase distribution of the transmit field. Magn Reson Med 2002; 48(6):1096–98.

24. Yang X, Yeung CJ, Ji H, et al. Thermal effect of intravascular MR imaging using an MR imaging-guidewire: an in vivo laboratory and histopathological evaluation. Med Sci Monit 2002; 8:MT113–17.

22

Early experience with combined CMR and X-ray suites

Oliver M Weber, Maythem Saeed, Alastair J Martin, Phillip Moore, Randall
Higashida, Simon Schalla, Titus Kuehne, Randall Lee, Charles B Higgins

Introduction

In current clinical practice, X-ray fluoroscopy (XRF) and digital subtraction angiography (DSA) are the modalities of choice for many diagnostic vascular imaging procedures, as well as for monitoring endovascular interventions, such as stent deployment and coil deposition. These methods are based on conventional X-ray projection imaging in combination with X-ray-absorbing materials to mark the interventional devices, and injection of iodinated contrast agent and subsequent image subtraction to outline the vessels. High spatial resolution, high achievable frame rates, and excellent vascular contrast render them excellent modalities for angiographic and interventional purposes, resulting in, for instance, more than a million annual DSA-monitored cardiac catheterization procedures in the USA.[1] However, XRF and DSA suffer from some limitations, including inadequate information on background anatomy, exposure of both patients and physicians to ionizing radiation, and geometrical restrictions due to two-dimensional (2D) projection imaging. The latter may partially be compensated by use of biplanar modalities, at the cost of increased X-ray load.

Magnetic resonance imaging (MRI), on the other hand, provides excellent soft-tissue characterization without exposure to ionizing radiation. In addition to morphology, physiological information can be obtained, such as neuronal activation, blood flow, tissue perfusion, and diffusion coefficients. It also provides cross-sectional or 3D image acquisition in arbitrary orientations. However, it generally suffers from poorer resolution and slower acquisition speed than X-ray imaging. Recent progress in both hardware (mainly faster magnetic gradients and improved reconstruction boards) and methodology (e.g. parallel imaging techniques such as SENSE[2] and fully refocused steady-state free precession (SSFP; also known as balanced

FFE, TrueFISP, and FIESTA) sequences) has considerably accelerated acquisition speed, allowing one either to reduce acquisition time per image, reaching fluoroscopic frame rates with online display, or to increase spatial resolution, depicting also submillimeter structures.

These technical advances have led MR angiography (MRA) to rival X-ray angiography for diagnostic imaging of vasculature in several body areas, including the aorta, extremities,[3] and head,[4] and also in even smaller vessels such as the coronary arteries.[5]

Cardiovascular MRI (CMR)-guided interventional procedures have recently been shown to be feasible. However, the tradeoff in spatial resolution against temporal resolution has made interventional CMR difficult in comparison with XRF for guiding endovascular interventional procedures. Furthermore, direct CMR guidance requires endovascular devices that have been customized to be safe and easily visualized in the CMR environment. Such devices are still in the developmental stages, lack widespread availability, and are limited to a small subset of device designs. In the setting of CMR-guided endovascular interventions, catheter-directed contrast-enhanced (CE)-MRA offers many of the same capabilities as conventional X-ray DSA. Local injections permit rapid delineation of blood vessels, generate rapid vascular road maps, and help guide interventions. It has been shown that the primary benefit of intraarterial injections is a significant reduction in the administered dose compared with clinically approved dose for intravenous injection.[6]

Based on the recognition that X-ray and CMR provide information that is over a wide range complementary, prototype combined 'XMR' suites have been installed, placing an X-ray modality in the vicinity of an MRI system with the goal of exploring the benefit of combined procedures. The main goals are (1) to perform correlative and comparative studies between the two modalities; (2) to enhance the vascular information obtained using X-ray by combining it with the soft-tissue information of CMR; and (3) to explore the possibilities of using CMR fluoroscopy for guiding cardiovascular interventions, while using X-ray for steps that are not safe or not accurate enough under CMR control. This chapter will provide an overview of XMR concepts and early applications.

XMR Systems

Open MRI scanners, without an XRF system, have been used for interventional procedures since about 1995.[7,8] These scanners have operated at a field strength of ≤0.5 T. It has been shown, however, that vascular interventional procedures, such as transarterial embolization, percutaneous transluminal angioplasty, or stenting, require high spatial resolution and optimized real-time imaging to monitor the procedure, rendering inadequate such open systems with lower field strength.[9,10]

Currently, two different philosophies have been applied in the construction of XMR systems: (1) to combine fully featured, state-of-the-art X-ray and CMR systems close to each other, with easy patient transport between the two systems on a traveling table; and (2) to implant the X-ray modality into a low-field open CMR system, combining the two modalities in a single system of lower performance, but without the requirement of physical movement of the patient. Both approaches will be briefly discussed here. Separating the two modalities allows a choice of the individual systems without restrictions. The systems used are thus basically state-of-the-art systems with minor modifications. Our installation at the Department of Radiology, University of California San Francisco (Figure 22.1) includes a 1.5 T short-bore (1.57 m) magnet (Intera I/T; Philips Medical Systems, Best, the Netherlands) with full cardiovascular features (gradient strength 30 mT/m; gradient slew rate 150 mT/m/ms). To facilitate interaction with the scanner during CMR-guided interventions, in-room active matrix liquid crystal displays and an operator system are attached to the magnet. Thus, the system can be operated by the interventionalist in a manner akin to XRF. The X-ray side consists of a catheterization (interventional) laboratory equipped with a fluoroscopy C-arm (Integris V5000; Philips Medical Systems) and a number of in-room displays. In addition to the ability to acquire 30 frames/s, the catheterization laboratory provides a 3D rotational angiography (3DRA) feature. During 3DRA, the C-arm swings around the body during injection of contrast agent, allowing for a 3D reconstruction of vascular structures. The only modification necessary to the catheterization laboratory was mu-metal shielding of the image intensifier, which was shown to eliminate residual image distortions caused

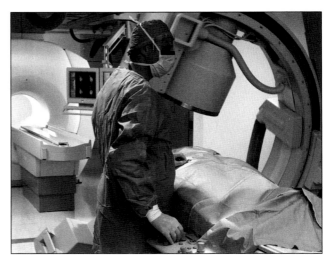

Figure 22.1
Collinear arrangement of a 1.5 T short-bore MR imager (background) and a catheterization laboratory (foreground). The two systems can be connected to facilitate easy patient transport between the two systems using a floating tabletop. Note the two in-room flat panels next to the MR scanner, enabling interactive MR operation from a position next to the patient and display of additional images, such as X-ray images or processed data.

by the effect of the fringe field of the neighboring MR imager (the distance from the magnet's isocenter to the C-arm center is 6 m) on the accelerated electrons in the intensifier.[11] Alternatively, a flat-panel detector may be used, which is inherently insensitive to the magnetic field.

The two modalities are connected by a moving tabletop, allowing transport of the patient smoothly from one system to the other. Transferring the patient from the angiographic suite to the MRI scanner is typically achieved in <2 min. In order to extend system usage, a sliding door between the two systems, shielding against both X-radiation and radiofrequency (RF) leakage, allows the two systems to be used independently.

A similar hybrid system has recently been developed by Siemens Medical Solutions (Erlangen, Germany).[12]

In an alternative concept,[13] a flat-panel X-ray system was placed at the center of a low-field open system (Signa SP; GE Medical Systems, Milwaukee, WI) in a fixed position above the imaging volume (Figure 22.2). To prevent electrons in the X-ray source from missing their target, the anode–cathode axis of the X-ray tube was aligned with the static magnetic field. Only minor further adaptations to the X-ray component were required. The presence of the X-ray detector decreases magnetic field homogeneity and thus MR image quality. Increasing its distance from the magnet by lowering it during MR imaging can reduce this problem. Furthermore, RF leakage of the X-ray systems, when left on, increases noise in the MR images. Both problems seem not to be insurmountable, and improve-

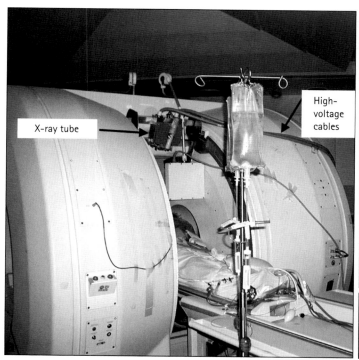
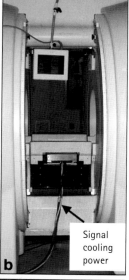
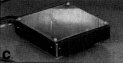

Figure 22.2
(a) Photograph of the hybrid XMR system with static-anode X-ray tube and flat panel detector during a transjugular intrahepatic porosystemic shunt (TIPS) procedure, with the X-ray tube in position above the patient table. (b) View of the system taken from the opposite side, showing the standard location of the flat-panel detector below the patient table. This geometry allows acquisition of projections at ~ 18° to the vertical. (c) The 20 cm × 20 cm flat panel detector. (Courtesy of Rebecca Fahrig, Norbert J Pelc, Kim Butts, Bruce L Daniel, Stephen T Kee, Daniel Y Sze, and Zhifei Wen, Stanford University.)

ments may be expected in future installations. This setup allows X-ray and CMR without the need to move the patient between the two modalities. However, this is achieved at the cost of reduced MR field strength and gradient performance, reducing achievable image quality and imaging speed, and of an immobile X-ray system, allowing projection X-ray imaging in one direction only.

The combination of CMR with an X-ray modality offers an optimal platform for interventional procedures requiring high spatial and temporal resolutions as well as morphological or physiological information on surrounding tissue. Thus, complementary diagnosis and therapeutic procedures can be performed in one session, saving time and permitting various selective arterial and venous catheterizations.

In the following sections, our initial experience with a hybrid XMR installation is described, illustrating both early clinical and experimental applications.

Stent repair of aortic coarctation in pediatric patients

Coarctation of the aorta, a congenital anomaly not uncommon in pediatric patients, usually causes reverse flow in the intercostal arteries and other thoracic arterial branches constituting collateral flow, substituting

for reduced aortic flow through the coarctation. Consequently, blood flow is lower immediately distal to the coarctation than in more distal segments of the descending aorta. After coarctation repair by transcatheter balloon angioplasty and deployment of a stent over the affected aortic segment, immediate reduction in collateral flow is expected. Since phase contrast CMR can estimate collateral flow,[14] the XMR facility can be employed to guide transcatheter therapy and to demonstrate the functional effect of the treatment.

An example of this use of XMR involves CMR before and after stent placement. Before the intervention, black blood imaging in axial and sagittal orientations, as well as a 3D CE-MRA, were performed to visualize anatomy. Quantitative flow measurements (phase contrast cine CMR) were performed distal to the coarctation and at the level of the diaphragm (Figure 22.3) in order to quantify collateral flow. The patient was then transferred to the X-ray side, where X-ray thoracic angiography and pressure measurements were performed. Treatment consisted of percutaneous balloon angioplasty and subsequent deployment of a stainless steel stent (Genesis, Cordis, Warren, NJ). After successful intervention, the patient was transferred back to the CMR side, where black-blood imaging and flow measurements were repeated at identical positions. A fully refocused steady-state sequence was applied for bright-blood imaging.

CMR and X-ray depiction of the coarctation before intervention were in agreement (Figure 22.4, top row), illustrating a narrowing of aortic diameter of 51% on

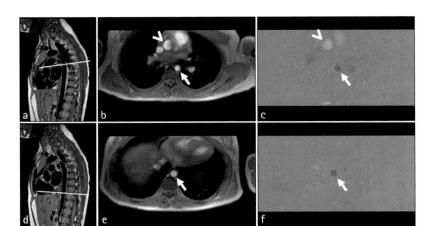

Figure 22.3

Flow measurements were performed at two cross-sections of the aorta: proximal to the stenosis (top) and at the level of the diaphragm (bottom). Shown are modulus images (b, e) and phase images (c, f) at both levels. In the (flow-encoded) phase images, middle gray means no flow. Brighter colors reflect flow towards the head (as, for instance, in the ascending aorta; arrowhead), whereas darker colors reflect flow in the opposite direction (descending aorta; arrows).

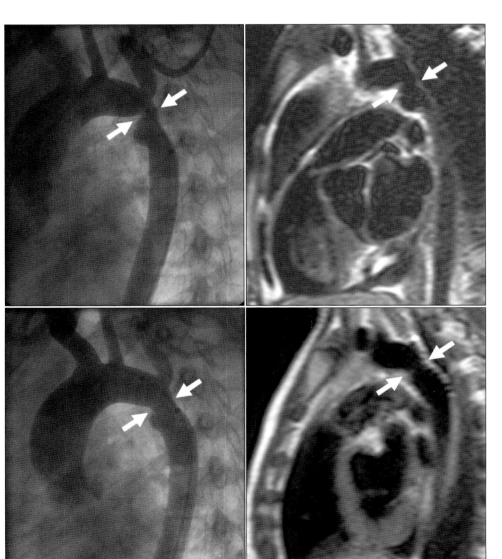

Figure 22.4

X-ray (left) and black-blood (right) MR images, acquired before (top) and after (bottom) stent repair of arotic coarctation in a 14-year-old patient. Note the increased diameter at the location of the coarctation (arrows) after intervention. An aneurysm distal to the coarctation was seen with both modalities.

X-ray angiography and 58% on MRA. Distal to the coarctation segment, an aneurysm was found with both modalities. After placement of the stent, the pressure gradient was reduced from 20 to 0 mmHg. Flow measurements before intervention showed that 20% of total aortic flow at the level of the diaphragm were contributed through collateral vessels. After intervention, this fraction was reduced to 2%, reflecting a physiologic improvement after stent placement (Figure 22.5). Despite the presence of a

stent, altered vessel geometry could also be visualized on the black-blood images, which again corresponded well to X-ray angiography (Figure 22.4, bottom; diameter narrowing, 30% with X-ray, 32% with CMR). On the other hand, bright-blood imaging was not able to visualize the stented segment of the aorta because of the artifact caused by the stent (Figure 22.6).

Immediate functional assessment of the interventional procedure provides an additional confirmation of success-

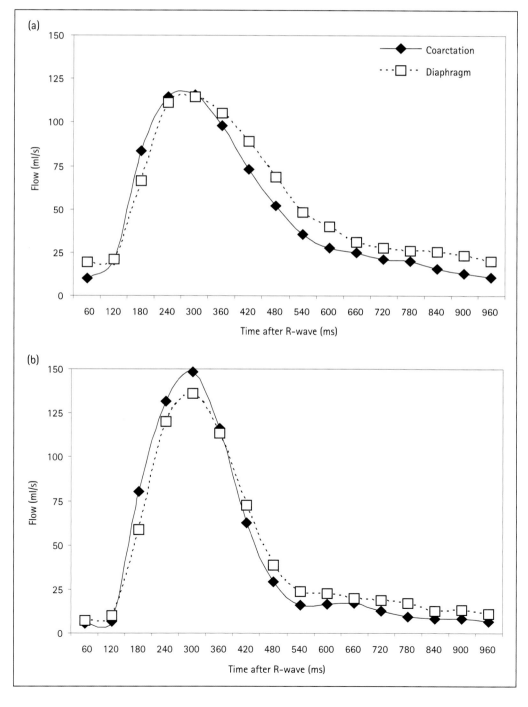

Figure 22.5
Flow values immediately distal to the coarctation and at the level of the diaphragm obtained prior to (a) and following (b) aortic stent deployment in the coarctation of a patient. Prior to the intervention, 20% of aortic flow at the diaphragm level were contributed by means of collaterals; this value was reduced to 2% after intervention. Note the increased peak flow and the narrower flow curve in the stented vessel, caused by less resistance in the aorta.

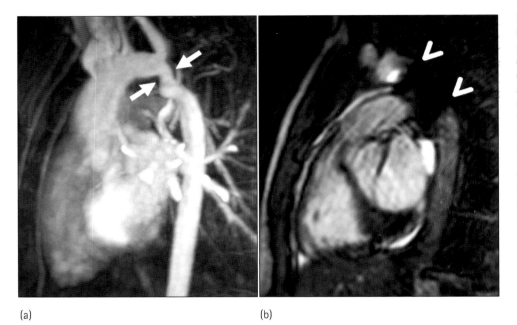

(a)   (b)

Figure 22.6
(a) Maximum-intensity projection in sagittal orientation through a three-dimensional MRA data set, acquired during first pass of contrast agent. Arrows indicate the position of the coarctation. (b) Refocused SSFP image, acquired after stainless steel stent placement. Note the signal void at position of the stent (arrowheads) due to susceptibility artifacts caused by the metal.

ful treatment and, if indicated, offers the opportunity for further treatment without the need for additional setup and anesthesia. It also offers the additional benefit of serving as baseline anatomical information for late follow-up comparison evaluation of aneurysm or stenosis formation.

Stent repair of carotid stenosis

Stenting of the carotid artery is becoming an increasingly popular alternative to carotid endarterectomy as a therapy

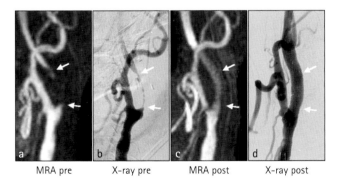

MRA pre   X-ray pre   MRA post   X-ray post

Figure 22.7
Maximum-intensity projections of three-dimensional contrast-enhanced MRA in comparison with projection X-ray imaging in a 87-year-old patient. Both modalities show a severe stenosis (99%) in the left internal carotid artery (a, b; arrows) with good correlation in stenosis length. After stent placement, both modalities demonstrate restoration of vessel lumen (c, d). Note the signal reduction in the MRA in the stent region due to RF shielding.

for moderate to severe atherosclerotic disease.[15,16] In many cases, stenting is the only viable alternative because the lesion cannot be accessed from an operative approach. Concerns remain regarding the effect of such therapy – most notably the release of microemboli to distal brain tissue. MRI can potentially augment such procedures with information on the status of the plaque, flow conditions within neck vessels, and the presence or absence of regions of distal ischemia. Correlation of this data with the eventual outcome of the procedure may provide key insights regarding what circumstances are most amenable to stenting over endarterectomy.

Patients with severe stenosis of the internal carotid artery (ICA) undergoing carotid stent placement have had CMR (Figure 22.7) before and immediately after transcatheter therapy (Figure 22.8). Phase contrast CMR flow measurements were performed in the carotid and vertebral arteries. Additionally, brain perfusion imaging and diffusion imaging were performed. 3D CE-MRA was compared with 3DRA, which was performed at the time of intervention. Stent (Smart Stent, Cordis, Warren, NJ) delivery was performed in a conventional fashion under X-ray guidance.

In the presence of severe stenosis of the ICA, stenting of the lesion resulted in a substantial increase in flow (from 1.4 ± 0.9 ml/heartbeat to 4.6 ± 0.8 ml/heartbeat), as demonstrated by quantitative MRI flow data. Perfusion and diffusion assessments did not reveal any foci of acute ischemia immediately following therapy in these patients. CE-MRA reliably defined the location and extent of stenotic disease, although it tended to overestimate the severity of stenosis and underestimate vessel diameters.

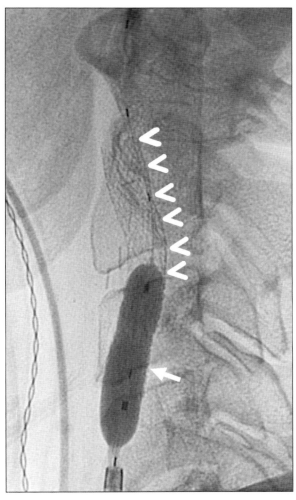

Figure 22.8
X-ray, acquired during stent deployment in the internal carotid artery. A balloon (arrow) is used to dilate the stent (arrowheads) and the vessel wall. The procedure improved flow from 0.4 ml/heartbeat prior to the intervention to 4.4 ml/heartbeat after the intervention.

monary valve.[20] The guiding catheter and stent were inserted into the femoral vein using X-ray fluoroscopic guidance. The animals were then directly moved to the MR imager, and advancement of the stent delivery system to the heart and into the main pulmonary artery was monitored under real-time CMR. Passive tracking was dependent upon the artifact caused by the stent. Once an optimal delivery position had been achieved, the stent was deployed. Stent position was verified on multiphase bFFE images (Figure 22.9). Subsequently, phase contrast CMR was used to assess flow volumes both within and just distal to the stent. After completion of the CMR, the animals were brought back to the X-ray system to confirm stent position, to assess valve functionality qualitatively, and to assess potential complications or arterial injuries occurring during the CMR procedure. Findings confirmed the successful stent deployment, functionality of the valve, and the absence of complications. The animals were then sacrificed and stent position was verified in the excised heart.

In this application, CMR provided immediate postinterventional evaluation of stent position, patency, morphology, and function. Additionally, the procedure itself was performed under CMR guidance. Alternatively, the procedure could be performed under X-ray control, using the CMR for quantitative evaluation of valve functionality.

Previous studies have indicated that CMR provides no visualization of the stent lumen and therefore is unable to detect stent stenosis or occlusion.[21,22] The limitation of visualization of the stent lumen placed in the pulmonary system using CMR has been partially resolved by adding MR contrast media.[23,24] A blood pool agent injection (NC100150; Amersham Health, Buckinghamshire, UK) provided persistent enhancement of the signal within the lumens of nitinol and platinum stents, but not of stainless steel stents.[24] Accordingly, administration of MR contrast media might be useful for the MR detection of stent stenosis.

Deployment of valve stents in the pulmonary artery

Transcatheter placement of valved stents for treatment of pulmonary insufficiency has been shown to be feasible.[17] Real-time CMR-guided stent placement with radial scanning and passive visualization was first demonstrated in 1998.[18] Later, passive visualization was used for CMR-guided stent placement in humans.[19]

We have recently evaluated the delivery of valve stents to the region of the pulmonary annulus and its effects on flow values in a swine model. Self-expanding nitinol stents (Memotherm; Angiomed, Karlsruhe, Germany) were placed in the main pulmonary artery over or near the pul-

Closure of atrial septal defects

Atrial septal defects (ASD) are common congenital heart lesions that often require surgery or transcatheter intervention in pediatric and adult patients. They are associated with stroke, heart failure, and pulmonary hypertension. Transcatheter delivery of ASD closure devices using XRF has become an attractive and effective alternative to surgery. A hybrid XMR system has also been employed to guide placement of ASD closure devices.[25]

In our laboratory, an ASD was created in a swine model under XRF. CMR was used to monitor the advancement of the catheter and closure device using real-time SSFP imaging (300 ms/image, reconstructed at 10 frames/s).

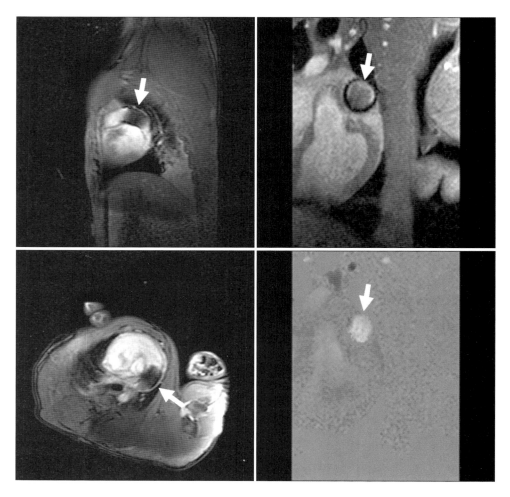

Figure 22.9
Stent placement in the pulmonary artery in a pig model. SSFP imaging is used to verify the position of the stent (left; arrows). Valve function is confirmed by means of flow measurements immediately adjacent to the stent (right: top, modulus image; bottom, phase image during maximal systolic flow).

Figure 22.10 illustrates some steps of the placement of the closure device under CMR guidance. Before and after delivery of the ASD closure device, flow in the pulmonary artery and in the ascending aorta was assessed to estimate the shunt volume. In this example, closure of the ASD reduced pulmonary flow (pre, 5.81 l/min; post, 4.75 l/min) and left-to-right shunt volume (pre, 1.81 l/min; post, 0.41 l/min) considerably, whereas aortic flow changed only to a minor degree (pre, 4.00 l/min; post, 4.34 l/min).

The hybrid XMR system provides a new monitoring method for delivery of ASD closure devices and assessment of the alterations in flow after closure of the defect.

Myocardial injection of therapeutic solutions

New therapeutic frontiers employing gene therapies hold great promise, but will need an appropriate means of tissue delivery and monitoring. The treatment of ischemic portions of the myocardium with angiogenic growth factors (AGF) is an early example of this emerging field. MRI is an ideal means of delivering such therapy, since it can delineate the ischemic territory, as well as guide and monitor the injection of AGF into the ischemic portions of the myocardium.

CMR guidance of myocardial injections requires that the distribution volume of AGF corresponds well with the MR-detected volume. Tagging of therapeutic agents with MR-visible agents such as Gd-DTPA permits optimal depiction of the distribution pattern of the injectate. To confirm that the MR-indicated distribution volume corresponds to the true area of delivery, we have been studying injections of dilute gadolinium contrast, iodinated contrast, and blue dye. It has proved possible to guide catheters into the left ventricle and monitor transcatheter injection of these agents into the myocardium both using X-ray and CMR guidance. There has been close correspondence between locations and volumes of the injectate as indicated by X-ray and CMR and the histologically determined distribution volumes (Figure 22.11). This intriguing early application of XMR should encourage further development of CMR guidance of transcatheter delivery of therapeutic solutions to the myocardium.

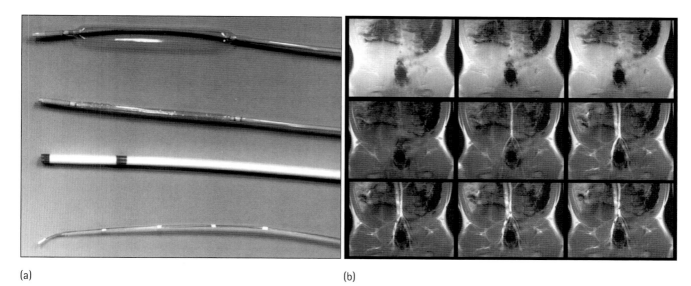

(a)   (b)

Figure 23.2

(a) Photograph of a 0.035 in. fiberglass-based guidewire with five Dy_2O_3 markers indicating the tip segment (bottom), a 7F introducer sheath with two Dy_2O_3 markers at the tip (lower middle), a 5F nylon balloon catheter with two Dy_2O_3 markers indicating the outer margins of the deflated balloon (upper middle), and a 6 mm-diameter inflated balloon (top). (b) Non-enhanced (top row) and contrast-enhanced (middle and bottom row) images obtained during MRI-guided placement of a guidewire with four paramagnetic markers into the abdominal aorta of a pig. The middle row shows a baseline image (left), an image obtained during the first pass of Gadomer-17 through the aorta (middle), and an image obtained during the first pass through the vena cava (right). The bottom row represents three consecutive contrast-enhanced images that were acquired while pushing the guidewire across the aortoiliac bifurcation into the aorta. The top row shows the corresponding non-enhanced images. ((a) Reproduced from Bakker et al. Magn Reson Med 1998; 8:245–50[19] and (b) from Bakker et al. Magn Reson Med 2001; 45:17–23.[121])

thus a signal loss around the catheter. Through this, the entire catheter can be visualized. The strength of the current varies between 50 and 150 mA, and increasing the current increases the effect, making the catheter blacker and larger. The movement of the catheter in the main magnetic field due to the forces on the wires is a drawback, which can be minimized by an antiparallel configuration of the wires.[17] The inhomogeneity catheter also presents visualization problems in small and tortuous vessels.[18]

A susceptibility-based device is designed by constructing paramagnetic materials, such as dysprosium oxide rings, into the wall or onto the surface of a conventional catheter or guidewire. These dysprosium oxide rings produce susceptibility artifacts, which then can be passively tracked under MRI (Figure 23.2).[15,19] In an appropriate design, the susceptibility artifact must be small enough not to obscure the surrounding anatomy, and therefore compromise the ability to perform the intervention.

Coating the surface or filling the guidewire lumen of an interventional device with gadolinium is an alternative method to monitor catheter positioning, which can display signal enhancement of such a device with T1-weighted, 2D, spoiled gradient-recalled echo MRI sequences (Figure 23.3).[20,21] This technique combines high temporal resolution, independence of orientation within the magnetic field, and visibility of the entire length of a conventional angiographic catheter. The ability to passively track various commercially available interventional devices with four different pulse sequences has been tested.[22] It was found that cobalt/nickel/steel alloy wires give the best and most consistent results.

Passive tracking offers some advantages, such as allowing visualization of the entire device as well as no safety or maneuverability problems with the catheters.[15] However, because of the dependence of the passive tracking technique on field strength, device orientation, and the particular pulse sequence parameters, susceptibility artifacts are often inconsistent and the temporal resolution is usually inadequate.[16,19]

Active MR tracking

The active tracking technique is achieved by visualizing a signal from a miniature radiofrequency (RF) coil that is incorporated into the commercially available interventional devices such as embolization catheters and balloon catheters.[14,16,23,24] The miniature coils are connected, through a fully insulated coaxial cable embedded in the catheter wall, onto the surface coil reception port for signal reception. The improved SNR characteristics of

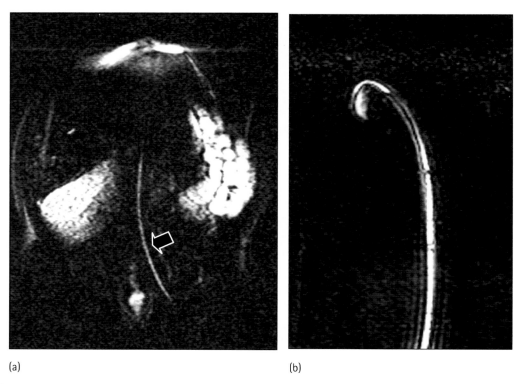

(a)   (b)

Figure 23.3
(a) MRI-guided passive catheter tracking. An 8F sheath filled with 4% gadolinium is placed via a percutaneous left common femoral artery approach. Inversion recovery FLASH gradient-echo imaging. (b) MRI-guided passive/active catheter tracking. A 7F catheter placed into the thoracic aorta via a percutaneous common femoral artery approach. The same pulse sequence was used, but this time the 4% Gd-filled catheter also had the MR imaging-guidewire (MRIG) (Surgi-Vision, Inc.) located within it. The MRIG was used as a receiver coil to visualize the adjacent Gd-filled catheter lumen. (Images courtesy of Dr RA Omary.)

these miniature coils not only permit visualization of microscopic anatomic details of vessels but also allow fast high-resolution imaging.[14]

A coil-tipped catheter is made by winding the miniature coil, which is a copper wire spiral, for 16–20 turns, around the tips of an interventional device to actively identify its position.[16,23] The miniature coil detects MR signals from only those spins near the coil, so that a single sharp peak is observed in the power spectrum and is indicative of the location of the coil in real space.[25] The coil-tipped catheter allows both real-time imaging and active tip localization within a single fluoroscopic mode sequence, and provides adequate temporal resolution.[26] The primary drawback with this catheter is the fact that only the tip of the device can be seen on the MR image.[15,27] Visualization of only a single point may not be sufficient for steering a device in complex vascular territory.[28]

In conventional cardiovascular interventional procedures, a guidewire is usually placed first either to guide interventional devices or to directly recanalize severely stenotic or occluded vessels. There have been attempts to make the guidewire visible under MR fluoroscopy.[28,29] Investigators initially tested electrically coupled antennas

with either loop or stub shapes, which offered the potential to incorporate these antennas into conventional sterile guidewires.[29] Efforts have also been made to build miniature coils with different geometries onto the tips of commercially available guidewires (Figure 23.4).[27,30] The miniature coil is attached to a coaxial cable running through the center of the guidewire, and the entire assembly is enclosed in a sheath of polyfluoroethylenepropylene (FEP) to protect the coil and make the guidewire smooth.[28] The miniature RF coil delivers a high-contrast signal over its full length, enabling visualization of the position and curvature of the tip of the guidewire.[30] Since a guidewire has limited space to place a tuning and coupling component at the distal (neck) portion (between the coil and the long coaxial cable), the coil-tipped guidewire is tuned and matched at its proximal end (at the interface between the coaxial cable and the surface coil input of the scanner).[28] As with coil-tipped catheters, the problems with coil-tipped guidewires are that the signal is limited to the coil at the guidewire tip and that there is a possible local heating risk from the coils attached to the tip.[30]

In the active tracking technique, the position of the device is derived from the signal received by a miniature RF coil that is attached to the instrument itself.[16,26,28] The

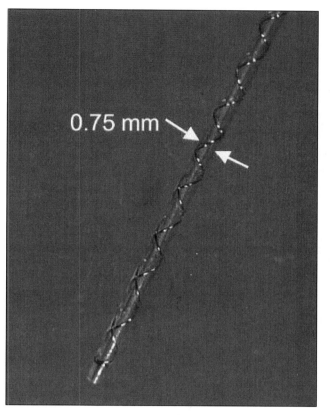

(a)

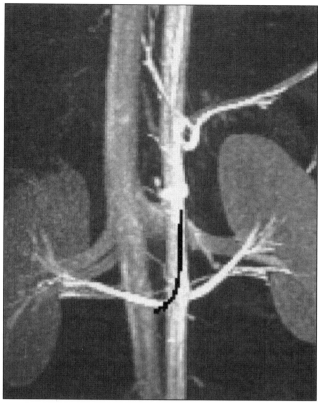

(b)

Figure 23.4

(a) An MR profiling coil in the tip of a 0.035 in. guidewire. (b) MR profiling in a swine, showing the curvature of the guidewire as it is steered into the right renal artery. (Reproduced with permission from Ladd et al. J Magn Reson Imaging 2000; 12:534–46.[120])

position of the coil is used to control the motion of a cursor over a scout (roadmap) image. Active MR tracking provides a high-contrast signal, robust determination of device position, and higher tracking speeds, but requires hardware modification of the MRI scanner and seems to be limited to roadmap techniques.[26,31,32] The miniature coils and electric wires may reduce the maneuverability of an interventional device,[19] and active tracking of coil-tipped guidewires and microcatheters remains challenging because the SNR decreases as the size of the miniature RF coil is decreased.[27]

Loopless antenna MR tracking

For effective manipulation, a guidewire needs to be visualized along its entire length. Subsequent development on MR tracking devices produced an alternative to active MR tracking guidewire – a loopless antenna (Figure 23.5a).[33] The loopless antenna is made from a coaxial cable, consisting of a conducting wire that is an extended inner conductor from the coaxial cable. The tip of the loopless

antenna is essentially a dipole, which makes a very small-diameter antenna possible. The characteristics of the loopless antenna include: (1) high sensitivity to the MR signal along the entire length of the antenna; (2) sensitivity inversely proportional to distance from the antenna; (3) production of very high signal around the antenna when it is used as a transmitter/receiver probe; and (4) creation of a projection image, since the antenna localizes the MR signal around itself and does not require slice selection.[34]

Unlike the coil-tipped guidewire, in which only a spot signal from the miniature RF coil can be visualized, the entire body of the loopless antenna can be observed under MRI (Figure 23.5b). In addition, since the electronic circuits are placed at the proximal end of the coaxial cable (and therefore outside the vessels), the physical dimensions of the loopless antenna can be constructed without limitations. Currently, the thinnest loopless antenna that can be manufactured easily is 0.014 in. in diameter. Analogous to a conventional guidewire, the thin antenna can be either directly inserted into small or tortuous vessels or placed into the central channel of interventional devices. Since the loopless antenna is expected to function not only as an intravascular MR receiver probe for IVMRI

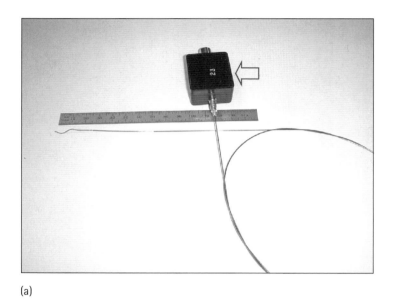

(a)

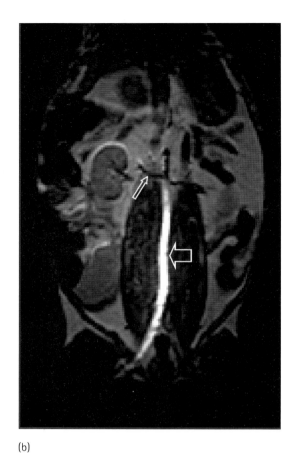

(b)

Figure 23.5
(a) A 0.032 in. MR imaging-guidewire (MRIG) connected to a turning/decupling box (arrow). (b) The MRIG (large arrow) is placed in the aorta of a rabbit. The entire length of the MRIG can be visualized under MRI. The small arrow indicates the right renal artery. (Reproduced from (a) Serfaty et al. J Magn Reson Imaging 2000; 12:590–4[81] and (b) Yang et al. Med Sci Monitor 2002.[109])

and for intravascular MR fluoroscopy but also as a conventional guidewire for interventional MRI, it is called an MR imaging-guidewire (MRIG).[35] Indeed, for reasons of safety and for technical purposes, such as torque control and subselective placement as well as negotiation of hard atherosclerotic lesions, this antenna/guidewire must also function as an imaging receiver probe when performing IVMRI-guided interventional procedures. The MRIG has been tested in vivo and found to be useful for both IVMRI and interventional CMR.[36,37] A study has also demonstrated the possibility of 3D visualization of the MRIG by depth reconstruction from projection MR images.[38]

A new MR tracking technique, loopless antenna-tracking FOV MR fluoroscopy, has been subsequently presented.[34] In this study, by using a very narrow rectangular field of view (FOV) combined with roadmap 3D image data, the authors acquired a movie of the percutaneous placement procedure of the loopless antenna at a rate of 7.3 frames/s. The advantage of this tracking technique is that the surrounding tissue as well as the antenna is visible during the tracking procedure. Using this tracking technique, investigators have successfully

performed an entire procedure of MRI-guided balloon angioplasty in vivo.[35,37]

Intravascular MRI-guided interventional procedures

To date, different MRI-guided cardiovascular interventional procedures, including balloon angioplasty, endovasuclar stenting, arterial embolization, transjugular intrahepatic portocaval shunt procedures (TIPS), vena cava filter placement, and vascular gene delivery/tranfection, have been tested and evaluated in various arteries of both animals and humans.

MRI-guided balloon angioplasty

To test and validate the new techniques of MRI-guided balloon angioplasty, the creation of a stenotic, balloon-inflatable vessel is essential. Currently, different methods are available to create experimental vascular stenosis. Artificial stenoses have been created using a plastic cable tie to tighten the surgically exposed aorta of a rabbit (Figures 23.6–23.8).[35,36] The cable tie was reversed such that it would slide easily as the balloon inflated. MR-compatible ameroid constrictors have also been used to create renal artery stenosis (Figures 23.9 and 23.10). These devices are constructed with an inner hydrogel ring, which can automatically expand to narrow the target vessel lumen. Other methods to create experimental stenoses of vessels include using a titanium clip or a suture to tighten

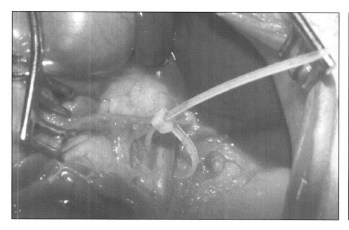

(A)

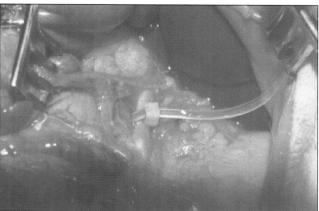

(B)

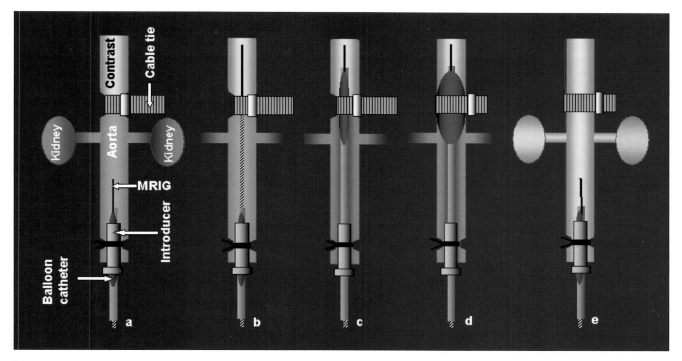

(C)

Figure 23.6

Surgery on a rabbit for creation of an aortic stenosis. The cable tie is placed (A) and bound (B) around the exposed portion of the upper abdominal aorta. (C) Illustration of in vivo experimental design for intravascular MR-guided balloon angioplasty in the rabbit aorta. (a) An artificial aortic stenosis is created by binding a plastic cable tie at the upper abdominal aorta, while a 7 Fr introducer is inserted into the lower abdominal aorta. (b) The stenosis is located by tracking an MR imaging-guidewire (MRIG) under intravascular MR fluoroscopy. (c) Along with the MRIG, a balloon catheter is tracked into the stenosis. (d) The stenosis is dilated by inflating the balloon with MR contrast agent. (e) The stenosis is completely opened. (Part (B) reproduced from Yang et al. J Vasc Interv Radiol 1998; 9:953–9[36] with permission from Lippincott Williams & Wilkins.)

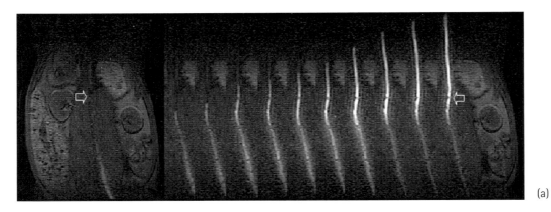

(a)

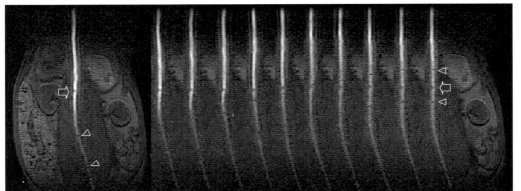

(b)

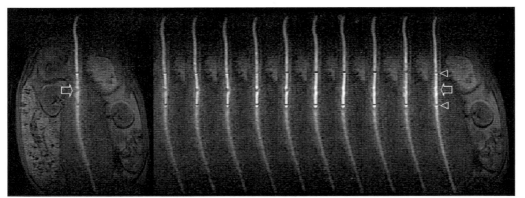

(c)

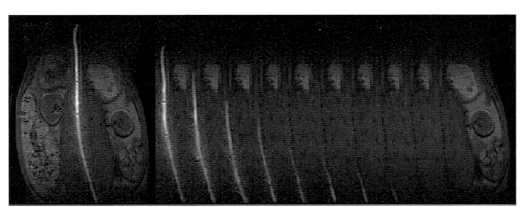

(d)

Figure 23.7

Intravascular MRI-guided balloon angioplasty in the rabbit aorta. Coronal projection MR image of the MR imaging-guidewire (MRIG) overlaid on a roadmap image. The intensity of the roadmap image is intentionally decreased for better visualization of the MRIG. (a) The aortic stenosis (arrows) is located by tracking the MRIG. (b) The balloon is delivered into the aortic stenosis (arrows). Arrowheads indicate two alloy rings of the balloon. (c) Dilation of the aortic stenosis (arrows) by inflation of the balloon with an MR contrast agent. (d) Withdrawing the MRIG and the balloon catheter from the treated stenotic aorta. (Reproduced from Yang and Atalar. Radiology 2000; 217:501–6[35] with permission from the Radiological Society of North America.)

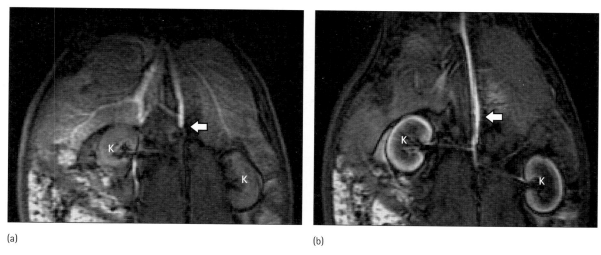

(a)

(b)

Figure 23.8

Contrast-enhanced MR aortography and renal MR perfusion imaging in a rabbit. **(a)** Before balloon angioplasty, even in the venous phase, no significant enhancement of either kidney is observed, due to the aortic stenosis (arrow). There is a small amount of distal flow into the downstream aorta and the right renal artery (K). **(b)** After balloon angioplasty, blood flows through the stenosis (arrow) and both kidneys are enhanced immediately. (Reproduced from Yang and Atalar. Radiology 2000; 217:501–6[35] with permission from the Radiological Society of North America.)

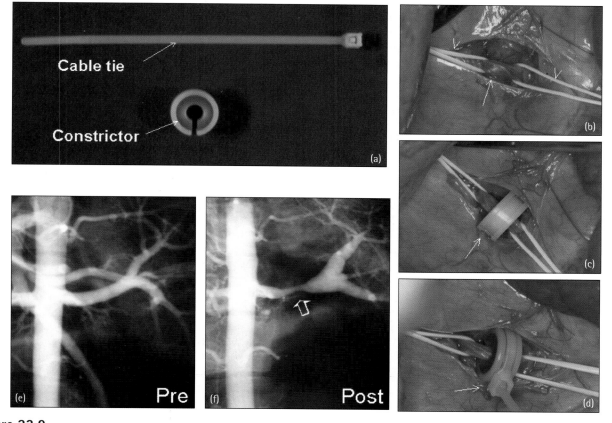

Figure 23.9

Creation of an experimental stenosis in the left renal artery of a pig. **(a)** An MR-compatible ameroid constrictor. **(b–d)** Placement of the ameroid constrictor around the renal artery to create stenosis. After expositing the left renal artery (arrow in b) via a lamarotomy, the constrictor (arrow in c) is placed around the target renal artery, and subsequently, the cable tie (arrow in d) is placed around the constrictor. **(e,f)** X-ray angiography obtained before (e) and after (f) the placement of the ameroid constrictor. A stenosis is detected in the left renal artery (arrow in f).

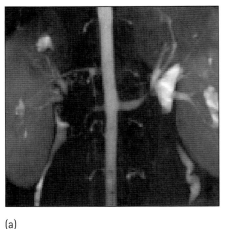 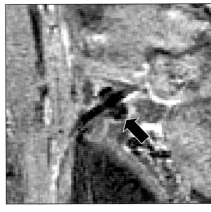 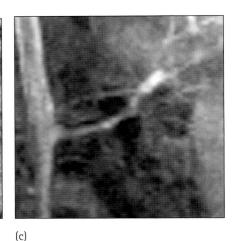

(a)   (b)   (c)

Figure 23.10
MRI-guided angioplasty of renal artery stenosis in a pig. (a) 3D intravenous gadolinium-enhanced preliminary MR image demonstrating occlusion of right renal artery and 90% stenosis of left renal artery from bilateral ameroid constrictor placement. The pigtail catheter is seen within infrarenal abdominal aorta. (b) 3D gradient recalled echo MR image showing balloon catheter across left renal artery stenosis. The arrow highlights the ameroid constrictor. (c) 3D intraarterial gadolinium-enhanced MR image after balloon angioplasty to 4 mm. The residual stenosis measures 50%. (Reproduced from Omary et al. J Vasc Intern Radiol 2000; 11:373–81.[41])

the target vessels.[39] Using these mechanical approaches with different tightening devices, one can quickly obtain stenotic models for laboratory studies. The balloon overdilation and de-endothelialization methods have been used for many years and still represent the best means to provide excellent animal models with near-real stenotic arteries for preclinical validation of new endovascular interventional techniques.[40]

Using the cable-created stenotic model, initial investigations tested the possibility of monitoring inflation/deflation of an angioplasty balloon catheter when opening an experimentally created stenosis of a rabbit aorta. A subsequent study with the same stenotic model demonstrated the feasibility of performing intravascular MRI-guided balloon angioplasty in vivo. This technical development provides an online methodology to (i) adequately monitor the entire process of selective catheterization and the dilation of stenotic vessels and (ii) provide immediate confirmation of the success of the primary balloon angioplasty treatment by assessing distal organ function using MR perfusion imaging (Figures 23.6–23.8).[35] In these studies, balloons were inflated using a gadolinium-based MR contrast agent (14 mg Gd/ml) to monitor balloon inflation/deflation in a 1.5 T MRI scanner using a fast spoiled gradient-echo (SPGR) pulse sequence and short repetition time (TR)/echo time (TE).

The feasibility of using MRI to guide balloon angioplasty of renal artery stenosis generated by a constrictor has been demonstrated using a passive tracking approach with MR angiography (MRA) (Figure 23.10).[41]

Recently, the success of MRI-guided percutaneous transluminal coronary angioplasty (PTCA) in living animals has been reported. Using active tracking methods,

investigators performed the entire process, including: (i) catheterization of the targeted coronary artery; (ii) generation of selective coronary MRA; (iii) creation of high-resolution MR images of the target coronary arterial wall; and (iv) positioning and inflation/deflation of an angioplasty balloon, under MRI guidance (Figure 20.17).[42]

Endovascular stent imaging and placement

The common occurrence of restenosis following balloon-assisted angioplasty has led to the development of new catheter-based therapies designed to limit vascular injury and achieve long-term vessel patency. Of these, endovascular stents have been shown to reduce restenosis by limiting the postintervention inflammatory response to intimal and medial damage, and have become front-line therapy for the treatment of obstructive peripheral and coronary disease.[43–45] X-ray angiography is currently used to both detect the presence of vascular obstruction and guide the stent to this focal location for deployment. The well-known limitations of 2D X-ray angiography, however, often result in underestimation/nondetection of potentially dangerous, non-flow-limiting soft plaques. Over the past several years, it has been shown that high-resolution atherosclerosis imaging of the vessel wall can be performed using noninvasive MRI, including the ability to detect various components of complex plaques.[46,47] This feature, combined with the recent success of coronary MRA to detect critical stenosis[48] and the advent of fast imaging techniques that permit real-time imaging[49,50] and catheter tracking, have opened new prospects for MRI to guide stent placement. This section will provide a brief review of MRI of vascular stents and recent studies that use MRA in combination with real-time MRI to perform stent placement.

MRI of vascular stents

In 2002, over 900 000 endovascular stents were placed in the USA alone. This number, combined with the rapid growth and acceptance of CMR in the clinic, have set the table for an enormous increase in the number of CMR examinations performed in patients with endovascular stents. Numerous studies have been performed in phantoms and in patients with coronary/peripheral stents to characterize artifacts, address heating and safety issues, and confirm stent patency.[51] In general, while the safety profile appears favorable, traditional stainless steel stents generate significant susceptibility artifacts that preclude reliable imaging of the vessel wall. This has lead many stent manufacturers to develop stents with new MRI-compatible materials that eliminate torque and aim to permit assessment of the vessel wall. Artifact-free luminal stent imaging would indeed be useful for assessment of in-stent restenosis, which is reported to occur in 10–30% of patients at 6 months post implantation.[52] In-stent restenosis is the result of the formation and unregulated and growth of a composition of smooth muscle-like cells in a collagen matrix (neointima) within the stent lumen that eventually results in a flow restriction through the vessel. While intravascular radiation therapy[53] and drug-eluting stents[54] have shown promise to greatly reduce neointimal proliferation and improve patency rates, in-stent restenosis remains a major problem that requires patients to undergo repeat percutaneous coronary interventions. The ability to assess in-stent restenosis using noninvasive MRI may greatly reduce the need for coronary catheterization in these patients.

Stent artifacts

Traditional stainless steel stents become significantly magnetized during MRI and generate large circular or eccentric black signal voids (susceptibility artifacts) that preclude reliable vascular MRI. In general, these artifacts appear much larger than the actual physical size of the device and often obliterate the vessel wall and nearby structures. In addition to the stent material, several other parameters modulate the size, shape, and extent of susceptibility-based artifacts, including pulse sequence type, specific parameters of the pulse sequence (e.g. TR and flip angle), orientation of the stent with the main magnetic

field, presence and nature of flow, and stent strut design.[51] RF-based artifacts, including the generation of eddy currents and RF shielding (Faraday effect), serve to further decrease the signal inside the stent lumen, independent of susceptibility effects. More MRI-compatible metals (those metals with lower magnetic susceptibility values) such as nitinol and tantalum have shown great promise, since they greatly reduce susceptibility artifacts and possess favorable mechanical properties.[55] From the experience in our laboratory and others, materials with lower conductivity have a better imaging profile during MRI, since strut susceptibility artifacts are small and largely reflect the true physical cross-section of the stent. Further, the signal inside the stent improves greatly in materials with lower conductivity compared with stents with more conductive materials.

MRI-guided stent placement and imaging

Improvements in MRA techniques, real-time imaging/tracking, and MRI-compatible materials have made it particularly attractive to place peripheral and coronary stents using MRI guidance. To date, however, there has been only limited experience in animals and humans. The first reported MRI-guided stent graft deployment in vivo was in 1996 using spin-echo imaging.[56] Buecker et al[32] demonstrated the feasibility of MRI-guided iliac nitinol stent placement in pigs using radial scanning together with a sliding window reconstruction technique. After placement of an introducer sheath using X-ray guidance, the animal was brought to the MRI scanner. Dysprosium markers placed on guidewires and balloon catheters were used for passive tracking and monitoring of devices in space and time. All stents were well visualized and successfully placed using the real-time radial imaging technique.

Stainless steel balloon expandable coronary stents have recently been placed in animals under real-time MRI guidance using a newly developed real-time steady-state free procession sequence with radial k-space sampling.[57] During free breathing and without cardiac gating, this sequence allowed for real-time fluoroscopy imaging at 15 frames/s with reasonable spatial resolution and coronary lumen contrast without the need for exogenous contrast injection. In a porcine model, 10 of 11 stents were successfully placed in the left main coronary artery without complication.

Manke et al[58] described the first human MRI-guided stent placement study in 13 patients with iliac artery stenosis.[58] Passive gradient-echo imaging was used to track the guidewires, balloon catheters, and nitinol stents used in the study. For enhanced visualization during imaging, the angioplasty balloon was inflated with a water/gadolinium solution. Images were evaluated with both digital subtraction angiography and contrast-enhanced MRA. Ten of 13 patients were treated successfully by MRI-guided intervention alone and 11 of 12 stents were placed correctly. Three patients required additional procedures with fluoroscopic guidance due to complications (panic attack, subintimal dissection, and stent misplacement). The mean MRI-guided procedure time was 74 min (range 47–122 min). The investigators reported a steep learning curve, and attributed the relatively high complication rate and long procedure time to the lack of real-time monitoring during the procedure. Furthermore, stent artifacts and signal loss inside the stent lumen were reported to resemble lumen narrowing.

Lardo et al[59] have performed MRI-guided stent placement in the iliac arteries of pigs with the assistance of an intravascular MRIG.[59] Following real-time monitoring of a self-expandable biliary stent (Guidant) using a steady-state fast precession sequence, an intravascular MRI coil was placed inside the stent lumen and high-resolution in-stent imaging performed (Figures 23.11 and 23.12). The increased signal generated by the local intravascular coil greatly improved visualization of the stent wall and vessel compared with external coil imaging of the same vascular segment.

Other MRI-guided endovascular interventions

MRI technology has also been tested and evaluated to guide other conventional endovascular interventional procedures. One study has demonstrated the in vivo placement of a temporary vena cava filter using a passive tracking technique, which is preferred in pregnant patients with deep vein thrombosis before Cesarean section.[31] The alloy (e.g. tantalum) rings on the surfaces of balloon catheters, dilators, and Wallstents produce significant image artifacts, which function as excellent markers for monitoring the delivery of these devices. Other studies have shown the feasibility of

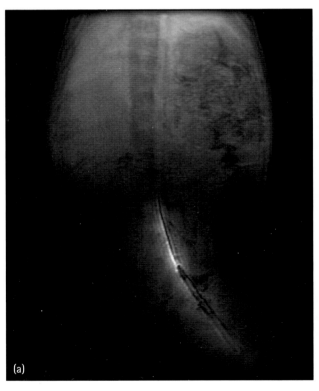
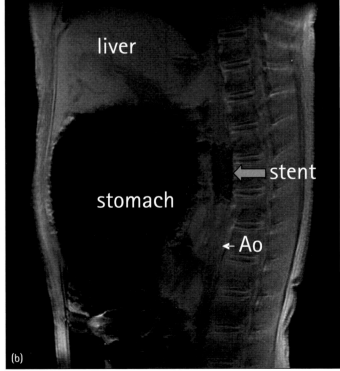

Figure 23.11
MRI-guided stent placement. An intravascular imaging catheter was placed in the lumen of a nitinol self-expanding bilary stent applicator and (a) inserted into a femoral sheath under real-time MRI and positioned in the aorta for (b) stent deployment. (Reproduced from Lardo et al. Circulation 2001; 104 (abstract supplement); 11–764.)

MRI of phenotypic consequences of vascular gene therapy

Conventional vascular radiological techniques, such as digital subtraction angiography (DSA) and ultrasound imaging, associated with advanced MRA and CT angiography, still play a primary role in the assessment of the phenotypic success of vascular gene therapy. These imaging methods enable convenient assessment of reperfusion of the vasculature in the tissues/organs distal to the gene-targeted vessels. For example, gene transfer of plasmid DNA encoding vascular endothelial growth factor (VEGF) brings about clinical benefits, such as the abolition of rest pain, limb salvage, and the healing of ischemic ulcers. These benefits are associated with angiographic evidence of new collateral vessels as well as improved leg blood flow as monitored by MRA.[91]

Functional MRI, such as perfusion MRI, provides a unique and sensitive imaging method to evaluate the circulatory improvement in tissues/organs.[92,93] Future applications of MRI technology in the genetic management of cardiovascular diseases should focus on not only identifying artery disease at an early stage with high-spatial-resolution MRA, but also on assessing the beneficial effects of vascular gene therapy using functional MRI.[94]

Real-time MRA

Central to the success of vascular interventional procedures, such as transluminal angioplasty and embolization, is the accurate depiction of the vascular tree and interventional instruments. Such depiction has been accomplished by means of X-ray fluoroscopy. The potential to perform accurate two-dimensional (2D) and three-dimensional (3D) angiography,[95] obtain high-spatial-resolution MR images with excellent soft tissue contrast,[96,97] and track interventional devices[79] make MRA potential alternative to conventional X-ray angiography. However, conventional 2D and 3D MRA sequences (time-of-flight (TOF) angiography, phase-contrast angiography, and contrast medium-enhanced angiography), when used for the guidance of vascular intervention devices through the arterial tree,[98,99] have general limitations. First, acquisition times are >1 s, which precludes the gathering of information about local hemodynamic conditions. Second, long postprocessing analysis is required to generate roadmaps. Third, contrast-enhanced angiography necessitates the use of large amounts of contrast medium, which precludes the possibility of multiple injections, because of increased background signal intensity. Some authors have reported that 2D projection techniques, coupled with intravenous injections of gadopentetate dimeglumine, can depict

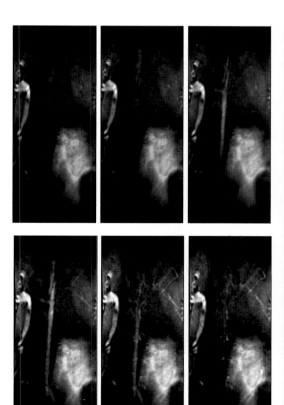

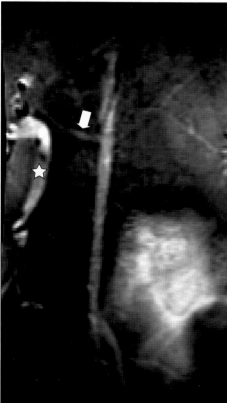

Figure 23.15
Real-time projection MRA of a pig aorta after intraarterial injection of gadolinium. Selection of coronal projection images acquired at 300 ms each, separated by 300 ms to better appreciate bolus tracking. Enhancement is first seen in the aorta, then the right renal artery (white arrow) and the iliac arteries. The left renal artery is experimentally occluded. Note the high signal intensity in the right renal pelvis and ureter (white star).

arterial flow in large arteries.[100,101] Subsequently, a new method, real-time projection MRA, has been developed.[102] This technique combines selective intraarterial injections of small doses of gadopentetate dimeglumine with a fast 2D gradient-echo sequence, and is used to avoid problems relative to arterial localization and to enable imaging of a tortuous vessel in a single image (Figure 23.15). The term 'projection' refers to 2D imaging over a thick-imaging slab, generally 5–20 cm, similar to 2D X-ray fluoroscopy.[103]

To perform real-time projection coronary MRA, a cardiac phased array coil needs to be placed on the surface under which the target vessel is located. After positioning angiography catheters into the target arteries, intracatheter administration of 1 ml gadopentetate dimeglumine at 62.50 mmol/l concentration into canine coronary arteries and 3 ml gadopentetate dimeglumine at 31.25 mmol/l concentration into the rabbit aorta can satisfactorily generate a roadmap of the target arteries in a 1.5 T MR imager (Signa, GE Medical Systems, Milwaukee, WI) (Figure 23.16). The parameters of MR imaging include a fast spoiled gradient-echo (SPGR) sequence, 4.4/1.4 ms TR/TE, 12 or 24 cm FOV for rabbit aorta and 16 or 20 cm FOV for canine coronary arteries, 90° flip angle (FA), bandwidth 64 kHz, 1 signal acquired, and 300 ms imaging time per image. These parameters allowed imaging at a rate of 3.5 frames/s.[102]

To perform real-time MRA with intraaortic injection of an MR contrast agent, time-resolved 2D and single-phase 3D techniques are used.[104] The parameters for time-resolved 2D angiography include 5.7/1.4 ms TR/TE, 30° FA, 24 cm × 18 cm FOV, 40 mm slice thickness, 256 × 192 acquisition matrix, 32.7 s duration with 30 frames at 1.09 s/frame. The parameters for single-phase 3D angiography include 6.2/1.6 ms TR/TE, 45° FA, 24 cm × 12 cm FOV, 1.0 mm slice thickness, 256 × 144 acquisition matrix, and 21.4 s duration.

Gadolinium-enhanced MRA is based on the T1-shortening effect of gadolinium in blood, and T1 shortening increases MR signal.[103] The optimal arterial gadolinium range is shown between 1% and 6%, depending on the selected imaging parameters. To obtain a desired arterial gadolinium, one needs to either (a) increase the injection rate and reduce the injected gadolinium or (b) increase the injected gadolinium and reduce the injection rate.

In the setting of MRI-guided endovascular interventions, catheter-directed gadolinium-enhanced MRA offers many of the same capabilities as conventional X-ray DSA.[103] Intraarterial local injections of gadolinium permit rapid depiction of blood vessels and help to guide interventions. The primary benefit of intraarterial injections of gadolinium is a significant reduction in administered contrast agent dose compared with conventional intravenous injections. Another major benefit is facilitated background suppression, including that of adjacent vascular beds. The reader is referred to an excellent review for a more detailed discussion about how to perform catheter-directed gadolinium-enhanced MRA during MRI-guided interventions.[103]

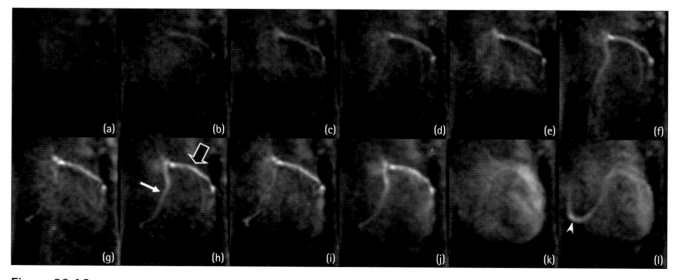

Figure 23.16
Real-time projection MRA of the left coronary artery of a dog with successive images acquired at 300 ms each. (a)–(j): right anterior oblique caudal view (RAO caudal) showing the left anterior descending coronary artery (LAD, open arrow) and the circumflex coronary artery (CCA, white arrow) at different arterial phases. (k) Left-ventricular myocardial perfusion phase. (l) Venography of the great cardiac vein (arrowhead). (Reproduced from Serfaty et al. Radiology 1999; 217:290–5.[102])

Advantages of MRI guidance for cardiovascular interventions

MRI guidance of cardiovascular interventions offers several advantages over conventional X-ray fluoroscopic guidance: (i) elimination of radiation exposure to both the patient and the operator; (ii) minimization of the risks for those patients who suffer from nephropathy and allergic reaction to iodinated contrast agents; (iii) provision of 3D information regarding the relationship of blood vessels to the organ of interest; and (iv) immediate feedback regarding the success of the primary interventional procedure and the status of the end-organ function, such as glomerular filtration rate, cerebral blood flow, and diffusion/perfusion.[21,35]

Currently, various cardiovascular interventional techniques (e.g. balloon angioplasty and endovascular stenting) are widely used in clinical practice. The classification of atherosclerotic plaques using IVMRI before an interventional procedure may provide predictive indicators for the most appropriate clinical methodology.[16,97,105] For example, balloon angioplasty is most often indicated in cases where the plaque is 'soft' (as in fibromuscular dysplasia and in fatty atheromas), and endovascular stenting is most often indicated in cases where the plaque is 'hard' (as in calcified atheromas).[106] In conjunction with conventional MRA and noninvasive flow quantification, these possibilities constitute a fascinating, integrative MR-based approach to percutaneous transluminal angioplasty.[24]

Safety

An important concern for performing IVMRI or IVMRI-guided interventions is the potential for local heating resulting from exposed conductive device components such as wires, electrodes and shielding. The thermal effect is produced by the electric field of the RF excitation of the body coil.[107] If the transmit coil couples with the receiver probe or with the cables of the probe, the electric field around the probe increases and may cause excessive heating. The temperature rises due to currents flowing in the coil and could lead to patient burns, especially when using RF-intense imaging sequences, such as fast spin-echo.[28] Even when a conventionally used Terumo guidewire (with a titanium core) is inappropriately placed into the vessel during MR scanning, heating may occur, with evidence of increased signal around the titanium core. The degree of heating at the RF coils equipped at the tip of the active tracking catheters is directly proportional to the power of the RF pulses. RF coil-induced heating is negligible with MR tracking, conventional spin-echo, and low-flip-angle gradient-echo sequences.[24] It has also been found that sequences with higher duty cycles, such as fast spin-echo sequences, produce harmful heating effects when RF coil-equipped active tracking devices are used.

To avoid the RF heating problem, decoupling circuitry is frequently used. With appropriate imaging sequence restrictions (e.g. no fast spin-echo, limited flip angle, and longer TR), the temperature can be limited and therefore tissue damage can be avoided.[30,108] Some investigators find that when operating built-in guidewires in a transmit/receive mode, no temperature rise can be detected.[30]

There are limited reports on the safety of intravascular MR technology, although there have not been any reports of RF-related damage.[18,109] In one study, by testing a field inhomogeneity catheter with a current induction, investigators found no evidence of electrically induced damage to the vessel wall.[18] The local thermal safety of the loopless antenna has also been evaluated in a normal rabbit aorta.[109] The authors investigated three issues concerning thermal safety, including the possibility of blood coagulation (particularly disseminated intravascular coagulation (DIC)), histopathologic changes in the target vessels and their adjacent tissues, and discoloration of the antenna surface. The study showed no evidence of local thermal injury when using the loopless antenna for IVMRI of normal vessels.[109] The authors believe that there are clinically relevant situations where an MRIG can be used safely in humans. However, further studies are required to precisely define the boundaries of these safe operating situations.

Clinical applications

To date, clinical MRI-guided therapies and applications have been limited to nonvascular interventions, such as discectomy, laser ablation of breast cancer, laser or RF ablation of head and neck tumors, monitoring of prostate cancer therapy, interstitial cryotherapy, interstitial focused ultrasound surgery, and needle biopsies.[110–113] Although MRI of the cardiovascular system has some prominent advantages, cardiovascular interventional MRI is still in the developmental phase. During the last decade, most of the investigations on IVMRI-guided interventions were carried out either in vitro using phantoms or in vivo in animals. In recent years, however, the application of intravascular MR technology in humans has been initiated.

One study demonstrated the safe intravascular MR tracking of a susceptibility-based catheter within the basilic vein in a 47-year-old healthy male volunteer with no complications.[15] A subsequent report demonstrated the successful monitoring of balloon dilation of an iliac and femoral artery stenosis in six patients, using coil-tipped catheters under MRI guidance.[114] Some authors validated the feasibility of both active and passive tracking in six patients.[115] They positioned successfully both active and passive tracking catheters into the superior mesenteric artery (SMA) in a 0.2 T open MRI scanner and a 1.5 T MRI scanner. Others demonstrated the success of MRI-guided stent placement to treat iliac arterial stenosis in 13 patients.[58] A recent study also reported using MRI to monitor accurate catheter position during endovascular embolization of liver tumors in 23 patients.[116] In addition, an alternative method for imaging the aortic wall using an intraesophageally placed loopless antenna has been also performed in a number of human cases, with no abnormal events to date.[117]

Use of IVMRI in conjunction with other MR techniques

Currently, the initial puncture and placement of introducer sheaths are performed using conventional X-ray fluoroscopy rather than MR fluoroscopy due to access problems and the inability to position the region of puncture close enough to the magnet center for scanning.[32] This encouraged the development of a hybrid interventional x-ray/MRI system.[118] This hybrid system is capable of MRI and X-ray imaging of the same field of view without patient movement. With this system, investigators successfully performed TIPS and chemoembolization.[119] Another combination of X-ray fluoroscopy with MRI is to set up a movable patient table between the X-ray machine and the magnet.[116] This allows interventional radiologists to first insert the introducer sheath or place the guidewire into the target under X-ray, and then move the patient to the magnet and position the endovascular interventional devices through the introducer sheath in the groin while monitoring these devices in the pelvic and abdominal vessels under MR fluoroscopy.[32] Several studies have demonstrated the performance of MRI-guided interventional procedures, such as TIPS placement,[61] vascular gene delivery,[69] and endovascular stent placement,[32] by combining conventional X-ray fluoroscopy and MRI techniques.

Significance of MRI-guided cardiovascular interventions

MRI is capable of providing useful functional information, such as quantification of flow data and capillary perfusion, pressure-gradient calculations using appropriate phase-contrast pulse sequences, and tissue metabolism. The use of functional MRI and 2D or 3D MRA, pre and post therapeutic interventions, is a current reality. The

online monitoring of the effectiveness of such interventions to guide the next therapeutic step is an important feature that may significantly improve patient care. Advanced MR techniques, such as MR perfusion imaging and MRA, as well as interventional MRI, may become essential imaging modalities for the online management (the early diagnosis followed by the prompt treatment and immediate postoperative evaluation at the same facility) of vascular ischemic diseases. For example, one may use the MR perfusion technique to functionally evaluate early vascular insufficiency of organs and MRA to locate the diseased arteries. MRI-guided interventional therapy could then be carried out in the same MR facility without moving the patient. After treatment, postoperative MR perfusion imaging and MRA could be performed to immediately confirm the reperfusion status of the organs, to assess the effectiveness of the interventions, and to determine the next steps necessary for further treatment.[37]

Conclusions

Cardiovascular MRI has some prominent advantages, including the ability to image the vessel wall and atherosclerotic plaque, obtain multiple diagnostic evaluations of organ function and morphology, avoid the potential hazards of iodinated contrast agents, provide multiple image planes with no risk of ionizing radiation. Intravascular MR technology, including IVMRI and IVMRI-guided interventions, represents a new and promising imaging modality with unique properties for characterizing atherosclerotic plaque structures and guiding vascular interventional therapy. The use of intravascular MR techniques, combined with other advanced MRI techniques, such as MRA and functional MRI, will open up new avenues for the future comprehensive management of cardiovascular atherosclerotic disease. The further improvements in MR fluoroscopy with true real-time display (analogous to X-ray fluoroscopy), open high-field-strength MRI units, and faster pulse sequences, will establish the role of intravascular MR technology in modern medicine.

References

1. American Heart Association. 2001 Heart and Stroke Statistical Update. Dallas: American Heart Association.

2. Spears JR, Marais HJ, Serur J, et al. In vivo coronary angioscopy. J Am Coll Cardiol 1983; 1:1311–14.

3. Isner JM, Rosenfield K, Losordo DW, et al. Percutaneous intravascular US as adjunct to catheter-based interventions: preliminary experience in patients with peripheral vascular disease. Radiology 1990; 175:61–70.

24

MRI-guided drug and cell injection therapies for heart disease

Alexander J Dick, Venkatesh K Raman, Michael A Guttman, Dana C Peters, Elliot R McVeigh, Robert J Lederman

Introduction: surgical exposure without surgery

Surgical therapy implies effective mechanical treatment by direct access to diseased tissue. *Exposure* is the term surgeons use to describe the visibility and accessibility of tissue to image guidance and manipulation. Wide surgical dissection is attractive because of the excellent *exposure* but is unattractive because of the exposure-related morbidity to the patient. Minimally invasive procedures, such as laparoscopic surgery or transcatheter angioplasty, may be more technically challenging or even less effective than conventional open surgery, but are widely employed because of the reduced exposure-related morbidity.

Magnetic resonance imaging (MRI) is attractive to guide catheter-based procedures precisely because of the wide *exposure* offered by the ability to visualize soft tissue and blood space in vivo in any arbitrary orientation. This chapter focuses on nonsurgical delivery of therapeutic agents into the beating heart using MRI.

Why inject the heart?

Myocardial disease is widely prevalent and is primarily related to atherosclerotic coronary artery disease and to hypertension.[1] A large number of patients suffer angina pectoris, congestive heart failure, and reduced survival despite the best available therapy, including surgery, angioplasty, electrophysiologic interventions, and a wide array of pharmacologic and rehabilitative treatments.

In ischemic heart disease, several novel biologic agents are being developed for direct myocardial delivery, such as protein or gene angiogenic agents to improve local blood flow, receptor kinases to improve pump function, and stem cells to regenerate damaged heart muscle. *Local* delivery is attractive because of the high concentrations that may be necessary for a biological effect while avoiding toxicities associated with comparable systemic levels. Intracoronary artery or retrograde venous infusion may not work well in patients with extensive vascular obstruction, or without maneuvers to enhance first-pass extraction or extravasation. Intrapericardial drug depots allow only epicardial access, and may not be feasible in patients after cardiac surgery. The most intuitively effective means of local drug or cell delivery to the heart may be direct injection into the heart muscle. The myocardium can be accessed directly with surgical visualization, although adjunctive imaging may be necessary to observe the distribution and retention of drugs within the myocardium. Direct heart muscle injections can be achieved using catheter-based techniques, although available image guidance modalities have important limitations discussed below.

One attractive investigational application that we have investigated is precise targeting and local delivery of cells having cardiomyogenic potential[2] into myocardial infarct borders, in an attempt to regenerate heart tissue. This border zone between normal and infarcted tissue may be the best microenvironment for engraftment and milieu-specific differentiation. Here pluripotent cells may be exposed to local cytokine inflammatory signals in the absence of triggers for differentiation into fibroblast scar. Similarly, we seek to treat chronic myocardial ischemia by targeting and local delivery of angiogenic or chemotactic agents into specific upstream (donor) and downstream (recipient) zones of the heart.

Myocardial injection without MRI

Contemporary cardiovascular interventional procedures are widely and successfully guided by projection X-ray fluoroscopy. Spatial and temporal resolution are excellent, but soft tissue contrast is poor and blood space imaging requires exposure to toxic radiocontrast agents. X-ray-guided injection into heart muscle from within the ventricular cavity ('endomyocardial injection') is straightforward; however, the exact anatomic placement of injections cannot be assured, and inadvertently overlapping injections are common. Moreover, the needle position relative to the endomyocardial surface cannot be determined accurately. Nevertheless, these systems are attractive in their simplicity and rapidity of use.[3–5]

An electromechanical navigation and injection system has been developed (NOGA with Myostar injection catheter, Cordis-Webster), which overlays a real-time magnetically guided three-dimensional (3D) position sensor onto a previously acquired electromechanical anatomic roadmap. This and related systems have been used successfully, alone or in combination with X-ray, in preclinical and clinical investigation of 'direct' ablative laser 'revascularization' and of gene and cell transfer for putative angiogenic or regenerative therapeutic investigation.[6–13] While this catheter guidance system is clearly effective for myocardial drug delivery, there are important potential limitations. The spatial precision of injection sites is controversial, especially in light of the 'roadmapping' over previously acquired geometric data in the face of periodic and nonperiodic cardiac and respiratory motion. The baseline roadmaps themselves are relatively time-consuming to acquire. In addition, there is no capability to monitor success of drug delivery or intramyocardial distribution of injectate. Finally, the system has performed poorly in distinguishing subtle wall motion abnormalities as manifestations of local myocardial ischemia.[14] Nevertheless, electromechanical navigation remains attractive because it exploits a preexisting physician skill-set and requires less capital outlay in combination with an existing X-ray fluoroscopic laboratory than would an interventional MRI system.

Ultrasound has the ability to distinguish soft tissue from blood space, and several investigators have attempted to apply transthoracic, transesophageal, intravascular, or intracardiac transducer systems to guide transcatheter procedures in the heart.[15–18] In addition, gas bubbles and other contrast mechanisms can aid in demonstrating successful drug delivery.[19] Overall, the constraints in obtainable planar imaging views, and 'blackout' shadows created by intracardiac devices, make 2D sonography suboptimal to guide many transcatheter proce-

dures. 3D ultrasound systems with extremely rapid image reconstruction and even surface rendering have been developed, but frequently poor transthoracic imaging windows limit their application to therapeutic myocardial procedures.[20] After further miniaturization, these approaches may prove useful.

Ultrafast multidetector X-ray computed tomography (CT) can provide very rapid 3D images of cardiac soft tissues. Unfortunately, the whole-body radiation doses required for these imaging methods may be prohibitive for wholly CT-guided interventional procedures on the heart. Conceivably a system combining projection and tomographic image guidance may have cardiac applications in the future.

The appeal of real-time MRI for myocardial drug and cell injection

'Real-time' MRI means rapid image acquisition with immediate reconstruction and display to the operator, sufficiently fast to facilitate application of therapeutic devices despite normal cardiac and respiratory motion. For our purposes, real-time MRI means acquisition of approximately five or more frames per second and subsequent display of reconstructed images within 250 ms of acquisition. Heart rates faster than approximately ~80 beats/min require even faster imaging.

Even at this early stage, real-time MRI appears an important advance over existing technologies for local myocardial drug delivery. Any myocardial segment is available for anatomic characterization, in any user-selectable imaging plane or 3D volume, independent of interposed air or bone that might interfere with sonography. Whether the heart, valves, lungs, or catheters move, synchronously or independently, real-time MRI can offer nearly instantaneous image updates, in contrast to 'roadmapped' techniques such as NOGA electromechanical guidance. Myocardial thickness can readily be determined in both systole and diastole, so that injections may be delivered at a suitable depth. Qualitative or even quantitative perfusion abnormalities can be demonstrated using local or systemic contrast administration. Tissue viability can be assessed by gadolinium accumulation, so-called 'delayed hyperenhancement', which can even be demonstrated in real time, as described below. Ischemic wall-motion responses to pacing, catecholamine, or vasodilator stress can be demonstrated online. All of these modalities can be used to identify myocardium that might be suitable, or unsuitable, for novel biological treatments (Figure 24.1).

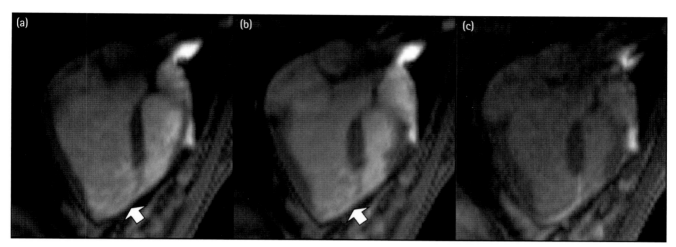

Figure 24.1
Anatomic, functional and tissue characterization of myocardium using real-time MRI. **(a)** Diastolic frame of real-time steady-state free precession (SSFP) delayed hyperenhancement, showing thinned apical infarction (arrow). **(b)** Systolic frame of same sequence shows noncontractile apical infarction. **(c)** Inversion recovery SSFP shows delayed hyperenhancement by gadolinium contrast, characteristic of myocardial infarction.

Table 24.1 compares real-time MRI with alternative image guidance modalities. Only MRI offers multidimensional anatomic imaging from any arbitrary perspective, online functional, and viability testing, combined with the possibility of instantaneous monitoring of successful injection.

The challenge of interventional cardiac MRI

As in any developing field, there are many challenges yet to be fully overcome. The first and most important is patient safety. The high-magnetic-field environment poses unique challenges. Members of the clinical team are unfamiliar with working in a magnetic field and must be carefully trained in MR safety to protect both themselves and their patients.

We have come to take for granted the excellent electrocardiographic (ECG) and hemodynamic monitoring provided in interventional cardiac catheterization laboratories. In an MR environment, there are significant impediments to obtaining comparable patient monitoring. Hemodynamic monitoring with pressure manometers can currently be performed in an MR environment, but ECG monitoring has proven to be more challenging. The magnetic field itself affects the ability to discern changes in depolarization as represented by fluctuations in the ST segments.[21] The high and rapidly changing levels of radiofrequency (RF) energy required for imaging are a tremendous source of electronic noise. Robust filtering

techniques and potential surrogates for ST segment changes are still being developed.

Communication and hearing protection within the noisy MR environment is also a challenge for interventional procedures. It is necessary for the interventionist to be in constant communication with the patient, MR technologist, and other members of the team. MR-compatible headsets are necessary.

All interventional devices used in the magnetic field must be MR-compatible: that is, they should not be affected by the magnetic field and should not heat up due to absorption of RF energy. Fortunately, there are materials and methods to assure the safety of these devices within the MRI environment.[22] A significant challenge to this field, however, is the small number of these devices currently available. There is a tremendous opportunity for development of interventional devices to help move this field forward.

In vivo experience with real-time MRI-guided myocardial injection in swine

We have been conducting endomyocardial injection experiments since early 2001 in healthy and postinfarction swine. Elements of these procedures include development of catheter devices that can be visualized under MRI, visualization and navigation of catheter devices, selection of myocardial targets, interactive scan prescriptions, and therapy delivery.

Table 24.1. Comparison of image-guidance modalities for endomyocardial injection

Modality/Feature	X-ray fluoroscopy	Intracardiac or extracardiac 2D or 3D ultrasound	Electromechanical mapping	Real-time MRI
Imaging commercially available in USA?	Yes	Yes	Yes	Yes
Catheters commercially available in USA?	No[a]	No[a]	No[a]	No[a]
Rapid to use?[b]	Yes	Yes	No	Yes
Imaging dimensions	2D projections[c]	2D sectors	3D acquisitions	2D projections, 2D thin slice, or 3D acquisitions
Images in any arbitrary plane?	No	No	Yes	Yes
Soft-tissue imaging?	No	Yes	No	Yes
Targeting to online viability maps?	No	Yes (combined with dobutamine administration)	Yes	Yes (delayed hyperenhancement of gadolinium contrast)
Targeting feasible to wall-motion abnormalities, resting or induced?	Maybe: images from ventriculography can be superimposed on injection images	Yes	Maybe: baseline abnormalities only	Yes
Confirmation of needle purchase in myocardial wall?	Yes, after contrast injection or endocardial electrogram	Yes, visual or after contrast injection	Yes, based on endocardial electrogram	Yes, visual or after contrast injection or endocardial electrogram
Instantaneous monitoring of drug or contrast delivery?	Yes	Yes	No	Yes
Approximate cost	$1M	$0.25M + X-ray lab	$0.25M + X-ray lab	>$1–2M + X-ray lab

[a] X-ray-guided and NOGA-guided injection needles are commercially available for investigational use; however, they are not approved for general marketing in the absence of an approved biological or pharmacologic agent for intramyocardial administration.
[b] NOGA mapping requires baseline mechanical mapping before injections can begin.
[c] Biplane X-ray systems can be modified in investigational laboratories to provide 3D catheter mapping, or can be used by experienced operators to provide 3D data.

Catheter adaptation to the MR environment

Catheter systems for endomyocardial injection all have elements that enable percutaneous arterial access, transvascular access to the left ventricle, facilities to permit device steering, and facilities to enable delivery of therapy through the length of the catheter into the myocardium.

Most contemporary X-ray diagnostic and therapeutic catheters and guidewires have metallic components to impart desirable characteristics such as radiopacity, axial rigidity, torque transmission, flexibility, ability to navigate tortuous vasculature, kink resistance, etc. When ferrous, these components compromise MR images by disrupting local magnetic fields, and they risk inductive heating.[23] Unfortunately, catheters without ferrous markers and braids usually not only are invisible under MRI but also can be difficult to manipulate. Fortunately, alternative materials are available.[24]

There are two general approaches to rendering catheter devices visible under MRI. *Active* MRI catheters and guidewires contain elements that serve as MRI 'antennas' or receiver or navigation coils. These coils either receive signal from locally excited spins,[25] resulting in images with bright signals near the catheter, or are used to compute catheter position through some other independent mechanism.[26] *Passive* MRI catheters are visualized either through susceptibility-induced signal voids (dark spots generated by disruption of the local magnetic field) or through T1-shortening signal enhancement (bright spots generated by gadolinium-based markers).[27–29] In our experience, passively visualized catheters are readily obscured because of volume-averaging effects within the imaging slabs. We have had more favorable experience

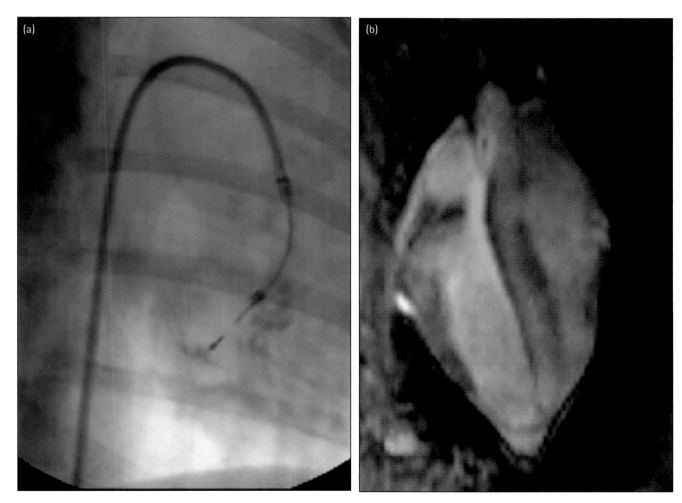

Figure 24.2
Comparison of X-ray and MRI-guided myocardial injection catheters. **(a)** X-ray Stiletto injection into posterobasal myocardium. Note the 'sharp' contrast of the catheter. **(b)** MRI Stiletto engaging apical myocardium. Note the 'hazy' appearance of the catheter signal in this implementation.

with active catheter and guidewire designs. However, as discussed in Chapter 21, active catheter designs are both more cumbersome and consume more computational and system resources. In addition, using our image-based catheter navigation approach, catheter images are 'hazy' because catheter-based receiver coils detect a local cloud of excited spins. These images are very different from the high-contrast shadows of catheters on X-ray projection imaging, and require operator re-education (Figure 24.2).

Percutaneous arterial access in patients with normal peripheral arteries is generally obtained by guiding needle entry through palpation. Once endoluminal, guidewires are used to introduce a valved 'sheath' device that permits device exchanges without blood loss or blood vessel trauma. In patients with peripheral artery disease, vascular entry often requires adjunctive imaging such as X-ray or ultrasound. MRI guidance is feasible; however, the distance to the isocenter of the magnet bore can make the procedure logistically difficult. MR-compatible vascular sheaths are commercially available, but none are readily visualized in present form.

Endomyocardial injection systems can readily be introduced into the left ventricle either retrograde from the femoral or brachial artery across the aortic valve, or antegrade from the venous system after puncturing the interatrial septum and crossing the mitral valve. Catheter systems are usually steered through the vasculature and within the left-ventricular cavity based on remote tip deflection or based on manipulation of two or more coaxial curved guiding catheters. Finally, once these catheters are manipulated near the target tissue, they are used to deliver or deploy an injection needle, usually with a long externalized central lumen for drug delivery. Other therapeutic devices can be substituted for or introduced alongside the needle, such as RF or cryoablation devices. It is useful for the catheter devices to include a lumen for monitoring of intravascular or intraventricular pressure, or a conductive lead for monitoring intracardiac electrograms.[30]

Boston Scientific Scimed (Plymouth, MN) has developed a Stiletto X-ray-guided endomyocardial injection system modified for operation in an MR environment. The Stiletto system uses a guide-in-guide steering design with a 9 Fr outer diameter to deliver a 27 G spring-loaded needle. The MR-modified system has some materials substitutions for MR compatibility. The MRI guiding catheter has a receiver coil integrated into its shaft. The first generation MR Stiletto injection catheter relied on passive susceptibility characteristics; a second-generation MR Stiletto has a small receiver coil just proximal to the needle tip. With different device components attached to different MR receiver channels, signal from the pig, from the guiding catheter, and from the Stiletto needle can be assigned different colors.[31,32] As described below, this color highlighting has proven extremely useful to guide

targeted injections. Finally, the MR Stiletto has facilities to attenuate potential inductive heating.

Rapid imaging

Real-time MRI guidance of catheter navigation within the left ventricle requires rapid image acquisition and reconstruction. We have used a 1.5 T MRI scanner (CV/i, General Electric, Waukesha, WI), customized[33] with an external workstation for real-time reconstruction of raw data transferred from the scanner, a pair of in-room keyboards and shielded liquid crystal displays with 1280×1024 pixels (Aydin Displays, Horsham, PA) and four independent high-impedance surface coils (Nova Medical, Wakefield, MA).[33,34] The active receiver catheter coils are connected in place of one or more elements of the surface phased array. A real-time MRI steady-state free precession sequence[35] (RT-SSFP, referred to by scanner manufacturers as TrueFISP, ASSET, or Balanced FFE) with either rectilinear or radial k-space trajectories is used to guide the catheter stiletto delivery system. Image-acceleration techniques are applied, such as echo sharing, where acquisitions are alternated between even and odd phase-encoding lines, or UNFOLD.[36] In radial trajectories, acceleration is also achieved using undersampling of projection views.[37] This implementation permits the user to adjust the compromise between temporal resolution and image quality by varying the amount of undersampling.[38] New 1.5 T MRI hardware systems are capable of even faster imaging.

Selection of myocardial targets for injection

Selection of injection sites includes consideration of anatomy, regional myocardial thickness, regional wall thickening, and myocardial viability. MRI permits ready identification of all of these characteristics.

In order to identify contractile abnormalities warranting transcatheter treatment, conventional cardiac MRI has required electrocardiographic gating combined with breathholds to generate segmented cinematic representations of heart function over as many as 20 heartbeats.[39] Recent advances in rapid cardiac image acquisition and reconstruction (see Chapter 21) now generate this information for the interventionist instantaneously, without the need for gating or breathholding.

In our laboratory, current accelerated image acquisition protocols using echo-sharing or UNFOLD provides 8 frames/s of SSFP images. At heart rates up to 90 beats/min, this amounts to 4–5 frames per cardiac cycle, which, when observed over several cardiac cycles, allowed satisfactory differentiation of akinetic and normal segments in swine after anterior myocardial infarction. Assessment of average thickening of the septum, lateral wall, and apical infarcted region compared favorably with that of standard gated and breathheld SSFP protocols.[40] Hypokinetic or akinetic regions are then examined for regional extent of infarction (tissue viability). Delayed hyperenhancement of the infarcted region can be created by injecting Gd-DTPA (Magnevist, Berlex, Montville, NJ) 0.2 mmol/kg via a peripheral IV 20 to 30 minutes before imaging. This is typically visualized using ECG-gated, breathheld inversion-recovery gradient-recalled echo imaging. However, the infarcted tissue can often be seen in the real-time SSFP images and can be enhanced using intermittent inversion pulses (Figure 24.1B, C).[41] Real-time inversion recovery SSFP images compare favorably with conventional segmented, ECG-gated, breathheld inversion recovery gradient delayed hyperenhancement imaging.[40] Using these techniques, three distinct regions have easily been targeted in real time in swine: normal myocardium, infarct border region, and infarcted nonviable myocardium.

Interactive scan/image prescription

We have been successful in navigating injection catheters and in targeting and guiding injections using real-time interactive graphical slice prescription in the GE *i-Drive* application. Slices only 6–8 mm thick can be used to guide catheters only 2–3 mm thick without difficulty. The color-highlighted sensitivity profiles of the catheter channels have proven very helpful when devices are out of plane yet nearby, in which care faint color is seen.

In our laboratory, one operator moves the catheter and the other, side-by-side, simultaneously controls the interactive scan plane prescription. We have found it useful to base our real-time prescriptions on a long-axis left-ventricular view derived from axial localizers. The image is rotated around the long axis to reveal the ascending aorta, and then 'centered' on the aortic valve. The image is then further rotated and/or tilted to reveal the aortic arch and brachiocephalic vessels. In this view, the catheter is navigated across the aortic valve. From this position, the catheter can be best visualized as it traverses the arch and enters the left ventricle. Once the catheter is in the ventricle, its distal extent is kept in view primarily by rotation and to a lesser extent by through-plane translation ('pushing/pulling') of the imaging slice. Scan plane 'bookmarks' are useful to store useful slice prescriptions for rapid recall. When the injection needle is deployed, short-axis slices in plane with the distal curvature of the catheter and needle can be useful to confirm needle position. We have also found interactive 'thick-slab' or projection images to be useful when the catheter inadvertently appears outside of the selected scan plane[38] (Figure 24.3). Another

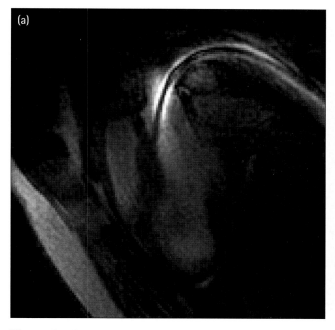
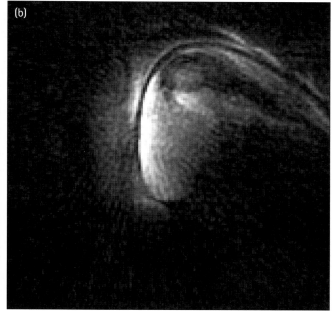

Figure 24.3
Thick-slab MRI helps to 'find' an out-of-plane catheter. Still frames from catheter tracking using a real-time radial *k*-space trajectory sequence showing **(a)** Thin slab of catheter within the left ventricle. The distal tip is outside of the scan plane and therefore not visible. **(b)** By switching to a catheter-only thick-slab mode, the entire catheter becomes visible, analogous to X-ray projection.

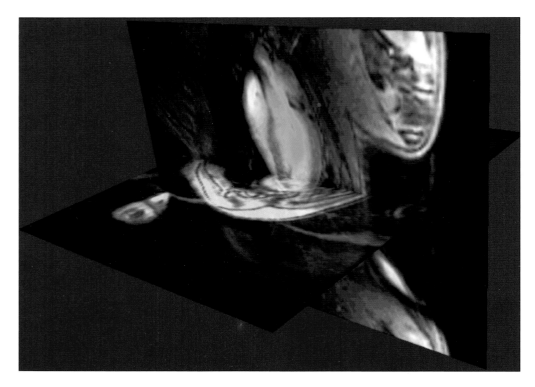

Figure 24.4
Multislice real-time MRI monitoring of cardiac injection. Two orthogonal real-time slices are rendered in three dimensions online, permitting simultaneous long- and short-axis views of the injection site. The injection needle channel is colored red.

feature that we have found useful is the ability to have interleaved real-time orthogonal multiple slice views. In the case of endomyocardial injection, this allows for combined display of the long-axis and short-axis views during injection[32,40] (Figure 24.4). This proves invaluable in confirming needle purchase on the endocardial surface.

Therapy delivery

Injectate must be appropriately prepared. Injection systems must be designed with biocompatibility in mind, since prototypes from several manufacturers have proved destructive to a variety of genes, viral vectors, and cellular preparations. Optimal endomyocardial injection volumes

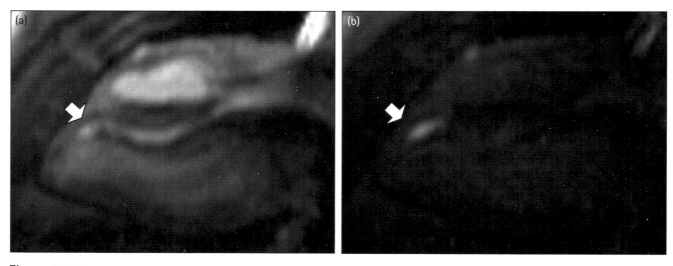

Figure 24.5
Saturation preparation to enhance visualization of test injections. **(a)** Real-time test injection of Gd–DTPA (30 mM) into the anterior apical septum. **(b)** Saturation preparation enhances the appearance of the test injectate compared with black myocardium and blood.

are uncertain, and range among investigators from 10 to 1000 μl. There is some evidence that higher injection volumes are associated with increased early injectate loss,[3] as myocardial contraction 'squeezes' injectate out of the myocardial interstitium through the injection hole or into the cardiac veins.

Successful injection requires successful needle engagement with the endocardial surface. The modification of the MR Stiletto to add an MRI receiver coil near the needle tip enabled better tip visualization and had a significant impact on device performance. The incidence of successful injections rose from 84% to almost 100%.[40]

Confirmation of successful delivery of potential therapeutic agents can be accomplished in several ways. The injectate can be doped with dilute iso-osmolar Gd-DTPA (~10–30 mmol/l) to give a transient bright signal at the injection location. The contrast between the surrounding tissue and this Gd-DTPA-doped injection can be further enhanced by the application of an interactive saturation prepulse (Figure 24.5). Many cell preparations, including mesenchymal stem cells, can be labeled with MR contrast agents such as particulate iron oxide.[42] This permits imaging delivery of the cells in real time and then serial in vivo surveillance in subsequent imaging sessions (Figure 24.6). It remains to be demonstrated, however, whether

gadolinium chelates or intracellular iron labels will interact with putative biologic therapies or will prove safe in clinical use.

Finally, injectate labeling techniques also permit for the first time in vivo visualization of the exact intramyocardial distribution of the delivered therapy. Using the 3.5 mm spring loaded needle of the Stiletto system, ~1.0 ml endomyocardial injections had an average depth of 4.0 ± 1.4 mm and appeared to spread circumferentially along midmyocardial fiber directions to a maximum of 4.2 mm × 10.8 mm.[34] In vivo visualization is further enhanced by an interactive increase in the number of projections or decrease of the field of view in radial trajectory imaging techniques.[38] In this way, higher temporal and lower spatial resolution are used during catheter and needle positioning, but as injection begins, a smaller field of view and better spatial resolution imaging are seamlessly employed so as to visualize carefully the injectate as it enters the myocardium. The gross location of the injectate can be marked and used to create a 'therapeutic map' that can be overlaid on all subsequent images. This facilitates complete therapeutic coverage while preventing overlap of injection delivery sites (Figure 24.7).

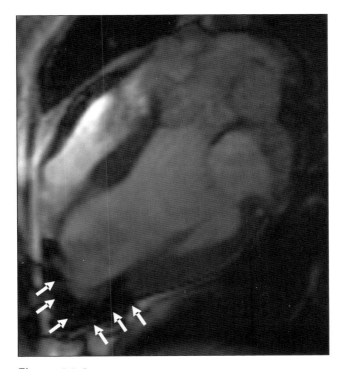

Figure 24.6
Long-term surveillance of injected mesenchymal stem cells (MSCs). Multiple large signal voids are apparent at sites 4 weeks after iron-labeled MSCs (arrows) were injected into an apical myocardial infarction.

Future directions

MRI-guided injection of drugs and cellular agents is feasible in both healthy and postinfarction swine. Imaging and catheter technology are maturing to the point that clinical deployment is now foreseeable.

Other catheter-based cardiac treatments could benefit from the MRI guidance. In electrophysiologic disorders of the heart such as atrial fibrillation, precise and complete electrical isolation of arrhythmic triggers is necessary for successful treatment. The ability to visualize all four pulmonary veins and to confirm the extent and continuity of tissue ablation is very important in the success of catheter-based cardiac electrophysiologic ablation procedures and is feasible using MRI.[43] In hypertrophic cardiomyopathy, catheter-based noncoronary myocardial chemoablative therapies to reduce the dynamic outflow obstruction might benefit from similar exposure, confirmation of delivery, and verification of its effect. Also, future putative transcatheter therapies for valvar disease, such as mitral valve regurgitation, may become feasible because of improved visualization both of the target tissues and of the mechanical therapeutic devices used in annuloplasty, leaflet reapposition, and papillary muscle modification. In summary, the future of MRI guidance and determination of efficacy will allow the development of therapies that currently are not possible or not even conceived.

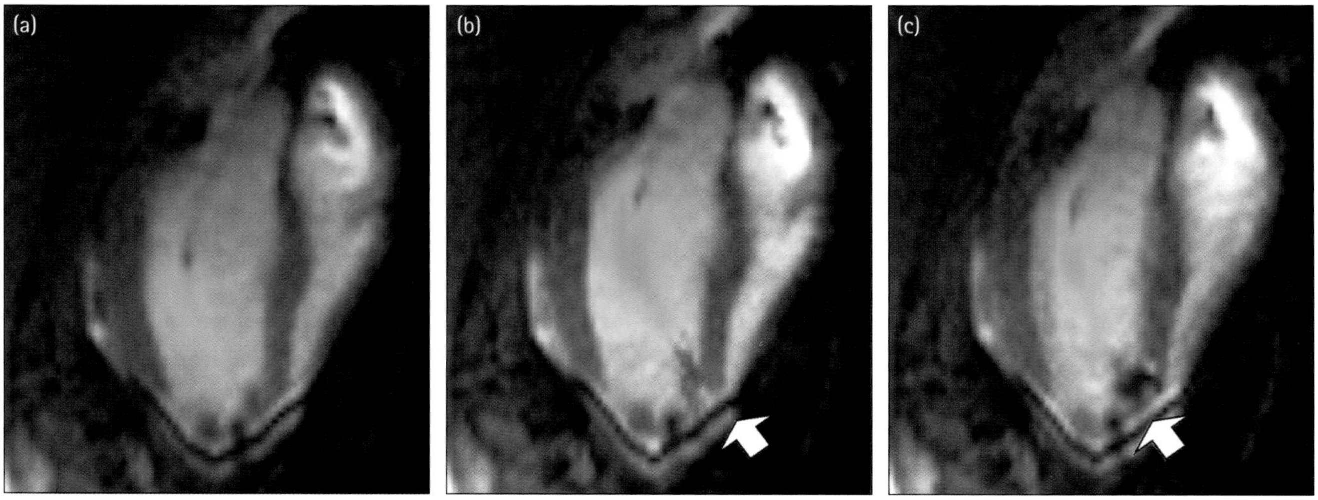

Figure 24.7

A sequence illustrating stem cell injection using real-time MRI. **(a)** Guiding catheter (colored green) is navigated within the left ventricle to the apical region of myocardial infarction. **(b)** Stiletto (colored red) is engaged at the border between normal myocardium and infarcted tissue. A 150 μl test injection of Gd-DTPA (white) confirms needle engagement (arrow). **(c)** Iron-labeled mesenchymal stem cells (MSCs) are injected into the same spot, which now appears black (arrow). Two other black spots reflect previous labeled-MSC injections.

References

1. American Heart Association. Heart Disease and Stroke Statistics – 2003 Update. Dallas: American Heart Association 2002.

2. Orlic D, Kajstura J, Chimenti S, et al. Bone marrow cells regenerate infarcted myocardium. Nature 2001; 410:701–5.

3. Grossman PM, Han Z, Palasis M, et al. Incomplete retention after direct myocardial injection. Catheter Cardiovasc Interv 2002; 55:392–7.

4. Sanborn TA, Hackett NR, Lee LY, et al. Percutaneous endocardial transfer and expression of genes to the myocardium utilizing fluoroscopic guidance. Catheter Cardiovasc Interv 2001; 52:260–6.

5. Rezaee M, Yeung AC, Altman P, et al. Evaluation of the percutaneous intramyocardial injection for local myocardial treatment. Catheter Cardiovasc Interv 2001; 53:271–6.

6. Oron U, Halevy O, Yaakobi T, et al. Technical delivery of myogenic cells through an endocardial injection catheter for myocardial cell implantation. Int J Cardiovasc Intervent 2000; 3:227–30.

7. Kamihata H, Matsubara H, Nishiue T, et al. Improvement of collateral perfusion and regional function by implantation of peripheral blood mononuclear cells into ischemic hibernating myocardium. Arterioscler Thromb Vasc Biol 2002; 22:1804–10.

8. Losordo DW, Vale PR, Hendel RC, et al. Phase 1/2 placebo-controlled, double-blind, dose-escalating trial of myocardial vascular endothelial growth factor 2 gene transfer by catheter delivery in patients with chronic myocardial ischemia. Circulation 2002; 105:2012–18.

9. Vale PR, Losordo DW, Milliken CE, et al. Randomized, single-blind, placebo-controlled pilot study of catheter-based myocardial gene transfer for therapeutic angiogenesis using left ventricular electromechanical mapping in patients with chronic myocardial ischemia. Circulation 2001; 103:2138–43.

10. Kornowski R, Fuchs S, Epstein SE, et al. Catheter-based plasmid-mediated transfer of genes into ischemic myocardium using the pCOR plasmid. Coron Artery Dis 2000; 11:615–19.

11. Vale PR, Losordo DW, Milliken CE, et al. Left ventricular electromechanical mapping to assess efficacy of phVEGF^{165} gene transfer for therapeutic angiogenesis in chronic myocardial ischemia. Circulation 2000; 102:965–74.

12. Kornowski R, Fuchs S, Tio FO, et al. Evaluation of the acute and chronic safety of the biosense injection catheter system in porcine hearts. Catheter Cardiovasc Interv 1999; 48:447–53; discussion 454–5.

13. Leon M. DMR in regeneration of endomyocardial channels trial. In: American College of Cardiology Annual Scientific Sessions, Orlando, FL, 2001.

14. Mayes CE Jr, Bashore TM. Biosensibility of viability: NOGA or no good? Catheter Cardiovasc Interv 2001; 52:348–50.

15. Hung JS, Fu M, Yeh KH, et al. Usefulness of intracardiac echocardiography in transseptal puncture during percutaneous transvenous mitral commissurotomy. Am J Cardiol 1993; 72:853–4.

16. Ren JF, Marchlinski FE, Callans DJ, Herrmann HC. Clinical use of AcuNav diagnostic ultrasound catheter imaging during left heart radiofrequency ablation and transcatheter closure procedures. J Am Soc Echocardiogr 2002; 15:1301–8.

17. Epstein LM, Mitchell MA, Smith TW, Haines DE. Comparative study of fluoroscopy and intracardiac echocardiographic guidance for the creation of linear atrial lesions. Circulation 1998; 98:1796–801.

18. Tamborini G, Pepi M, Susini F, et al. Comparison of two- and three-dimensional transesophageal echocardiography in patients undergoing atrial septal closure with the amplatzer septal occluder. Am J Cardiol 2002; 90:1025–8.

19. Lederman RJ, Richards M, Avelar E, et al. Intracardiac echocardiography permits high spatial resolution for percutaneous local

myocardial delivery using a needle injection catheter. J Am Coll Cardiol 2000; 5:5A (abst).

20. Szili-Torok T, Kimman GJ, Scholten MF, et al. Interatrial septum pacing guided by three-dimensional intracardiac echocardiography. J Am Coll Cardiol 2002; 40:2139–43.

21. Weikl A, Moshage W, Hentschel D, Schittenhelm R, Bachmann K. [ECG changes caused by the effect of static magnetic fields of nuclear magnetic resonance tomography using magnets with a field power of 0.5 to 4.0 tesla]. Z Kardiol 1989; 78:578–86.

22. Ladd ME, Quick HH. Reduction of resonant RF heating in intravascular catheters using coaxial chokes. Magn Reson Med 2000; 43:615–19.

23. Yang X, Yeung CJ, Ji H, et al. Thermal effect of intravascular MR imaging using an MR imaging-guidewire: an in vivo laboratory and histopathological evaluation. Med Sci Monit 2002; 8:MT113–17.

24. Melzer A, Stoeckel D, Busch M, et al. MR-compatible instruments for interventional MRI. In: Interventional MRI. St Louis, MO: Mosby-Year Book 1999:55–69.

25. Atalar E, Bottomley PA, Ocali O, et al. High resolution intravascular MRI and MRS by using a catheter receiver coil. Magn Reson Med 1996; 36:596–605.

26. Dumoulin CL, Souza SP, Darrow RD. Real-time position monitoring of invasive devices using magnetic resonance. Magn Reson Med 1993; 29:411–15.

27. Unal O, Korosec FR, Frayne R, et al. A rapid 2D time-resolved variable-rate k-space sampling MR technique for passive catheter tracking during endovascular procedures. Magn Reson Med 1998; 40:356–62.

28. Bakker CJ, Bos C, Weinmann HJ. Passive tracking of catheters and guidewires by contrast-enhanced MR fluoroscopy. Magn Reson Med 2001; 45:17–23.

29. Omary RA, Unal O, Koscielski DS, et al. Real-time MR imaging-guided passive catheter tracking with use of gadolinium-filled catheters. J Vasc Interv Radiol 2000; 11:1079–85.

30. Susil RC, Yeung CJ, Halperin HR, et al. Multifunctional interventional devices for MRI: a combined electrophysiology/MRI catheter. Magn Reson Med 2002; 47:594–600.

31. Aksit P, Derbyshire JA, Serfaty JM, Atalar E. Multiple field of view MR fluoroscopy. Magn Reson Med 2002; 47:53–60.

32. Quick HH, Kuehl H, Kaiser G, et al. Interventional MRA using actively visualized catheters, TrueFISP, and real-time image fusion. Magn Reson Med 2003; 49:129–37.

33. Guttman MA, McVeigh ER. Techniques for fast stereoscopic MRI. Magn Reson Med 2001; 46:317–23.

34. Lederman RJ, Guttman MA, Peters DC, et al. Catheter-based endomyocardial injection with real-time magnetic resonance imaging. Circulation 2002; 105:1282–4.

35. Oppelt A. FISP – a new fast MRI sequence. Electromedica 1986; 54:15–18.

36. Madore B, Glover GH, Pelc NJ. Unaliasing by fourier-encoding the overlaps using the temporal dimension (UNFOLD), applied to cardiac imaging and fMRI. Magn Reson Med 1999; 42:813–28.

37. Peters DC, Korosec FR, Grist TM, et al. Undersampled projection reconstruction applied to MR angiography. Magn Reson Med 2000; 43:91–101.

38. Peters D, Lederman R, Dick A, et al. Interactive undersampled projection reconstruction for active catheter imaging, with adaptable temporal resolution and catheter-only views. Magn Reson Med 2003; 49:216–22.

39. Carr JC, Simonetti O, Bundy J, et al. Cine MR angiography of the heart with segmented true fast imaging with steady-state precession. Radiology 2001; 219:828–34.

40. Dick AJ, Guttman MA, Raman VK, et al. Magnetic resonance fluoroscopy enables targeted delivery of mesenchymal stem cells to infarct borders in swine. Circulation 2003 (in press).

41. Guttman MA, Dick AJ, Raman VK, et al. Imaging of myocardial infarction for diagnosis and intervention using real-time interactive MRI without ECG-gating or breath holding. Magn Reson Med 2003 (in press).

42. Hill JM, Dick AJ, Raman VK, et al. Serial in vivo magnetic resonance imaging of mesenchymal stem cells using intracellular iron-fluorophore labeling. Circulation 2003; 108:1009–14.

43. Lardo AC, McVeigh ER, Jumrussirikul P, et al. Visualization and temporal/spatial characterization of cardiac radiofrequency ablation lesions using magnetic resonance imaging. Circulation 2000; 102:698–705.

25

MRI-guided interventional electrophysiology

Albert C Lardo, Timm Dickfeld, Henry Halperin

Introduction

Since its initial description in 1982, catheter-based radiofrequency (RF) ablation (Figure 25.1) has evolved from a highly experimental technique to its present role as a first-line and highly successful therapy for most supraventricular arrhythmias, including atrioventricular nodal reentrant tachycardia and Wolff–Parkinson–White syndrome.[1] In current practice, these arrhythmias are identified and targeted for therapy by manipulating intracardiac mapping catheters while viewing a real-time, two-dimensional (2D) silhouette of the heart as provided by X-ray fluoroscopy. More recently, the clinical indications for RF ablation have expanded to include more

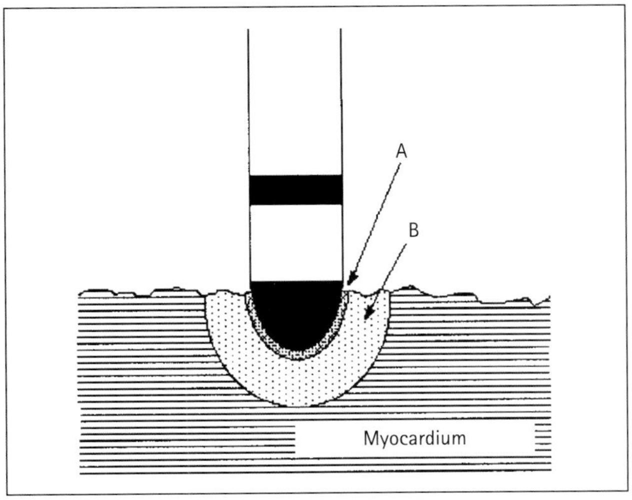

Figure 25.1
Mechanism of heating during RF catheter ablation. Because current density drops off rapidly as a function of distance from the electrode surface, only a small shell of myocardium adjacent to the distal electrode (A) is heated directly. The majority of the lesion (B) is produced by conduction of heat away from the electrode-tissue interface into the surrounding tissue. (Reproduced from Zipes D. Cardiac Electrophysiology. Philadelphia: Saunders, 1995: 1435.)

complex tachycardias such as atrial fibrillation, atrial flutter, and scar-mediated ventricular tachycardia. For these arrhythmias, appropriate sites for energy delivery are identified almost entirely on an anatomic basis and thus have placed a great emphasis on three-dimensional (3D) anatomic imaging/information to help guide therapy. While the feasibility of X-ray-guided anatomy-based RF ablation has been demonstrated for these more complex arrhythmias, the fundamental limitations of X-ray fluoroscopy limit precise targeted catheter movements, do not allow for visualization of critical anatomic landmarks, and do not permit visualization of ablated or infarcted regions of the myocardium. Such limitations, in part, lead to long procedure times, prolonged fluoroscopy exposure and a high frequency of complications and recurrences. For these reasons, there is general agreement that new approaches to facilitate anatomic-based catheter ablation are needed.

Magnetic resonance imaging (MRI)-based intervention is a rapidly evolving field that offers a number of unique advantages for delivering RF endomyocardial therapy. This chapter will provide an overview of the most recent experience with MRI-guided electrophysiologic intervention and will identify arrhythmia applications most likely to benefit from MRI-based therapy.

Anatomically based treatment of cardiac arrhythmias

Atrial fibrillation – chronic reentrant

Moe and Abildskov[2] proposed that atrial fibrillation results from multiple, independent wavelets that wander through the myocardium around islets or strands of refractory tissue. Each of these wavelets may accelerate or

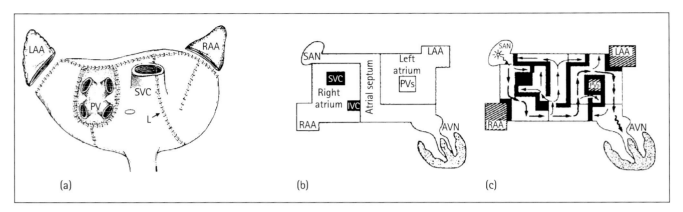

Figure 25.2
(a) Posterior heart showing incision lines (L) of the maze procedure. LAA, left-atrial appendage; RAA, right-atrial appendage; PVs, pulmonary veins; SVC, superior vena cava. (Reproduced from Cox. Semin Thorac Card Surg 1989; 1:67.) (b, c) Schematic of activation sequence of atrium following the maze procedure: (b) atrial structures; (c) lines of block (thick lines) with activation (arrows). Insufficient atrial tissue remains contiguous to sustain reentrant rotors. IVC, inferior vena cava; SAN, sinoatrial node; AVN, atrioventricular node. (Modified from Cox. J Thorac Card Surg 1991; 101:406–26.)

decelerate as it encounters tissue in a more or less advanced state of recovery of excitability, and may extinguish, divide, or combine with neighbor wavelets as they continuously fluctuate in size and change direction of propagation. A major factor needed for the wavelets to propagate is a critical mass of atrial tissue in electrical contact.[3] In patients with drug-refractory chronic atrial fibrillation, attempts have been made to eliminate the reentrant substrate for atrial fibrillation by surgically compartmentalizing the atria with incision lines of conduction block[4] (Figure 25.2). While the surgical maze procedure has proven to be highly effective treatment,[5] recovery times are long and the procedure includes all the inherent risks of open heart surgery. A less invasive catheter-based alternative to compartmentalize the atria was introduced by Haissaguerre et al.[6] In this fluoroscopy-guided tech-

nique, strategic lines of RF ablation lesion, delivered via a catheter, mimic the scalpel incisions of the surgical maze procedure and generate lines of conduction block (Figure 25.3). Although several small series have been reported with 90% success,[7–9] the procedure is arduous and requires general anesthesia and procedure durations often greater than 12 hours, with 2-hour cumulative X-ray exposure. One of the main limitations of the procedure is the difficulty associated with precise anatomic placement, delivery, and confirmation of continuous linear atrial lesions due to the inability of X-ray fluoroscopy to visualize anatomic landmarks or ablated regions of the myocardium. If the linear lesions have critical gaps, then activation can pass through the gap and complete a reentrant circuit, thereby sustaining atrial fibrillation or flutter.

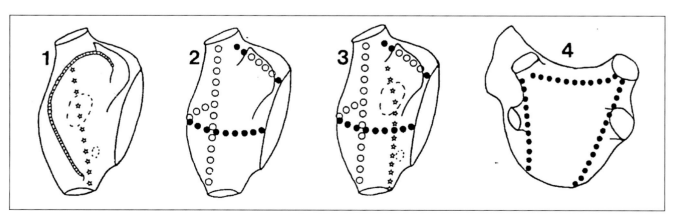

Figure 25.3
Lines of RF ablation attempted in the right atrium (RA) (1–3) and in the left atrium (LA) (4) for control of atrial fibrillation. Shown are RA septal lines (1), longitudinal and transverse RA lines (2), combinations (3), and LA lines (4). (Reproduced from Haissaguerre J Cardiovas Electrophysiol 1996; 7:1132–44.)

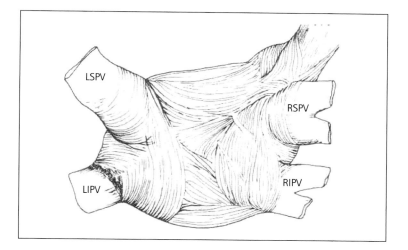

Figure 25.4
Diagram showing the location of atrial myocardium in the pulmonary veins (PVs). LS, left superior; LI, left inferior; RS, right superior; RI, right inferior. (Reproduced from Nathan and Eliakim. Circulation 1966; 34:412–22 with permission from Lippincott Williams & Wilkins.)

Atrial fibrillation – paroxysmal focal

In the last few years, investigators have realized that many patients with paroxysmal atrial fibrillation may have episodes of arrhythmia triggered by a focal source of rapid ectopic activity.[10] Intracardiac mapping has demonstrated that these ectopic foci are most often located in the pulmonary veins.[11] The source of these ectopic foci has been determined to be sleeves of atrial myocardial tissue that extend several centimeters from the left-atrial insertions and encircle the outer aspects of the pulmonary veins (Figure 25.4).[11] Histologic analysis of the venoatrial junction suggests an asymmetric circumferential spiraling distribution of myocardial tissue that decreases in thickness as a function of distance from the ostium (Figure 25.5). While the presence of atrial myocardium in the pulmonary veins was suggested in illustrations nearly 150 years ago,[12] the role of this tissue in initiating and sustaining atrial fibrillation has been studied and appreciated only recently.[13] Since the first report of a possible electrophysiologic role of pulmonary vein myocardial sleeves in 1998, over 350 publications have addressed their role in the mechanism and treatment of atrial fibrillation. This work has lead to two fluoroscopy-guided catheter-based ablation approaches for treating atrial fibrillation originating in the pulmonary veins: (1) electrical map-guided focal ablation, whereby specific sites that trigger or sustain atrial fibrillation are identified and ablated; (2) anatomically based circumferential ostial ablation, whereby the pulmonary veins are electrically disconnected from the pulmonary veins (pulmonary vein isolation) using an energy source transmitted through a balloon catheter that is inserted into the pulmonary vein.[14] While catheter ablation at the focal source of ectopic activity has produced promising cure rates,[15,16] focal ablations are complicated by the inability to determine the amount and distribution of atrial myocardium present in any pulmonary vein. The

pulmonary vein isolation approach is attractive in this regard, since it does not require knowledge of the distribution of atrial tissue in the venoatrial junction because the entire circumference of the ostium is ablated. While promising acute results have been noted, post-ablation stenosis of the pulmonary veins has been reported in several series,[17] and is thought to he attributable to a cascade of vascular inflammatory responses to high-temperature injury and necrosis. It is possible that visualizing the pulmonary vein ostium during the ablation procedure will allow for more precise therapy titration and thus help avoid 'overtreating' the ablation site at the venoatrial junction, which may reduce the occurrence of pulmonary vein stenosis.

Scar-mediated ventricular tachycardia

Myocardial scar resulting from a previous myocardial infarction consists of dense, unexcitable fibrotic segments distributed throughout normal myocardium that generate a potential path of reentry.[18] Numerous studies have confirmed this mechanism for ventricular tachycardia between the infarct scar and normal tissue. Currently, complex and detailed mapping is required to determine the precise location of myocardial scar such that targeted RF therapy can be delivered to interrupt the reentry circuit. One of the key problems limiting the success of standard RF ablation of ventricular tachycardia is the presence of scar located deep in subendocardial segments. This is due to the limited penetration depth of standard RF without generating prohibitive increases in impedance. This particular issue has been addressed by saline-irrigated, large-electrode catheters that discharge a constant stream or spray of saline at the distal end of the catheter during RF delivery to eliminate coagulum

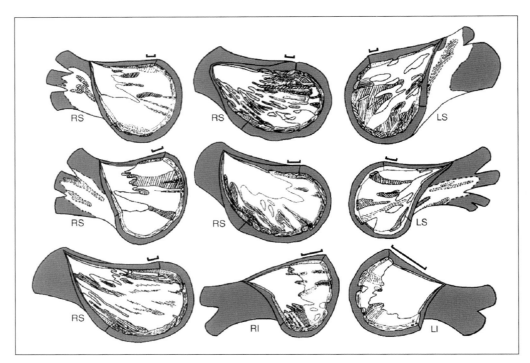

Figure 25.5
Graphic reconstructions of nine pulmonary veins with the venous wall (white) removed from the endothelial aspect to show the extensions of the muscular sleeves (pale gray). The bars represent 2 mm along the length of each vein. The unhatched areas of pale gray represent circularly or spirally arranged myocytes; hatched areas represent longitudinal or oblique myocytes. Dark gray areas represent the fibrofatty tissues of the adventitia, the layer that is external to the sleeves. White areas among pale gray areas represent gaps in the venous wall that were without the outer myocardial sleeve. LI, left inferior pulmonary vein; LS, left superior pulmonary vein; RI, right inferior pulmonary vein; RS, right superior pulmonary vein. (Reproduced from Ho et al. Heart 2001; 86:265–70.)

formation on the electrode surface, which allows greater energy deposition and electrode cooling.[19] Along with these techniques for generating larger lesions and deeper penetration of energy comes an increase in the risk of complications such as damage to functional myocardium and ventricular rupture. The ability to visualize the location of myocardial scar would be of great value in the successful ablation of ventricular tachycardia, since the optimal site for therapy can be targeted anatomically rather than depending upon detailed and complex mapping studies.

Potential role of interventional MRI in arrhythmia therapy

Interventional MRI may be a logical alternative to X-ray fluoroscopic techniques, since it offers several specific practical advantages over X-ray fluoroscopy for guiding and monitoring catheter-based arrhythmia therapy, including: (1) real-time catheter placement with detailed endocardial anatomic information; (2) rapid high-

resolution 3D visualization of cardiac chambers and pulmonary vein anatomy; (3) generation of true 3D electroanatomic data; (4) the potential for real-time spatial and temporal lesion monitoring during therapy; (5) high-resolution functional atrial imaging to evaluate atrial function and flow dynamics during therapy; (6) elimination of patient and physician radiation exposure.

Our laboratory at the Johns Hopkins School of Medicine has described the use of a novel MRI-compatible interventional electrophysiology hardware system in conjunction with a real-time interactive cardiac MRI (CMR) system to perform the first ever comprehensive cardiac RF ablation study.[20] Using a standard external surface coil, it was shown that: (1) MR images and intracardiac electrograms could be acquired *during* RF ablation therapy using special filtering techniques; (2) nonmagnetic MR-compatible catheters could be successfully visualized and placed at right-atrial and right-ventricular targets using real-time MRI sequences with interactive scan plane modification; (3) regional changes in ablated cardiac tissue are detectable and can be visualized using T1-weighted fast gradient-echo and T2-weighted fast spin-echo images; (4) the spatial extent of tissue damage by MR correlates well with the histologic necrosis area.

These results may have significant implications for the guidance, delivery, and monitoring of cardiac ablation therapy for a number of arrhythmias.

MRI catheterization suites and scanners

One of the key requirements of MRI-guided interventional cardiovascular procedures is direct unhindered access to the groin and neck for manipulation of catheters and devices. In recent years, several exciting short-bore interventional MRI magnet designs have been described that emphasize patient access for therapy delivery and anesthesia. These designs are available from most MR manufacturers and can be used both for high-quality diagnostic imaging and as interventional procedures. The primary limitation of open systems is the use of relatively low magnetic field strengths (0.21–0.6 T), which leads to lower signal-to-noise ratios (SNRs) and longer scan times compared with higher-strength systems (1.5 T). Interventional MRI catheterization laboratories will require a new generation of monitoring hardware. Special RF-shielded displays are currently available, and can be used in close proximity to the magnet for guiding and monitoring the intervention (Figure 25.6). MR-compatible equipment – such as pulse oximeters, ECG monitors, respirators, anesthesia apparatus contrast injectors, and infusion pumps – can all be safely operated outside the 5 G line in the scanner room, provided that the correct filtering and grounding systems have been employed. Furthermore, special filters must be employed to suppress radiation from monitoring equipment to avoid image distortion, as well as to protect the electronics of monitoring equipment from malfunctioning due to the high static and dynamic electromagnetic fields generated by the scanner. Due to the growing promise and interest in interventional MRI, the number of manufacturers offering MR-compatible equipment has expanded dramatically over the past 5 years, and this trend is expected to continue as further experience is gained. A comprehensive and detailed description of requirements for interventional MRI laboratories is presented in Chapter 21 of this book.

MRI-guided catheter tracking and localization

Accurate atrial catheter placement is of growing clinical importance for the study of a variety of supraventricular arrhythmias as the relationship between endocardial

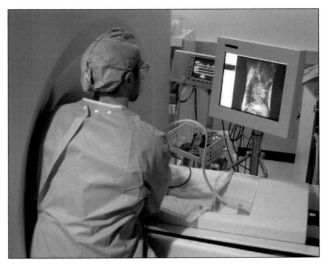

(a)

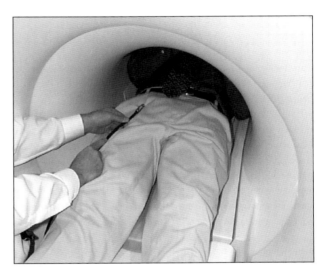

(b)

Figure 25.6
(a) In-room display used for performing real-time cardiovascular interventions in a short-bore 1.5 T scanner. The operator has access to interactive slice prescription features and scanner functions from inside the scan room, as well as (b) reasonable groin access for catheter manipulation and positioning.

anatomy and arrhythmia substrate becomes increasingly appreciated. Current catheter-based techniques to map and identify arrhythmogenic foci are based upon low-resolution voltage maps generated by point-by-point catheter movements under X-ray fluoroscopy. In addition to the limited anatomic information provided by X-ray, catheter manipulation under X-ray fluoroscopy can be arduous and poorly reproducible. Non-contact mapping catheters that provide electroanatomic information have shown promise in guiding ablation therapy for anatomically based procedures,[21–24] although these systems require

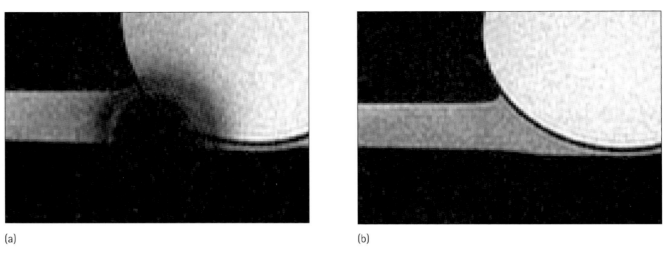

(a)   (b)

Figure 25.7
Phantom showing (a) susceptibility artifact generated by a standard ablation catheter with nonmagnetic materials and (b) the catheter removed.

a high degree of user training and do not appreciation of structural/functional changes to the myocardial tissue post therapy.

Performing accurate positioning of interventional devices to intracardiac locations of interest under MRI guidance requires visual and positional updates of the catheter/device at a reasonable spatial and temporal resolution. Methods have been developed over the past several years to improve the localization of catheters, and can be categorized into two primary tracking methods: *passive tracking* and *active tracking* (see Chapter 23 of this book for a detailed discussion of this topic). Passive tracking techniques are based upon device visualization due to magnetic susceptibility artifacts or signal voids generated by the physical displacement of protons. The ideal passive tracking material produces an artifact that is visible enough to track, yet small enough so as not to obscure underlying anatomy. Materials such as titanium and nickel alloys have magnetic susceptibility close to that of tissue and therefore are ideal materials for the construction of catheters and needles. However, the artifact generated by a particular material is dependent upon several factors, including the magnetic field strength, the spatial orientation of the device with respect to the main magnetic field, the physical cross-section of the device, the pulse sequence, and the imaging parameters. Therefore, careful attention must be given to both material selection and sequence parameters to achieve the optimal tracking artifact. Many standard cardiac ablation catheters have stainless steel mesh bodies and generate large susceptibility artifacts and torques that preclude their use in an MRI scanner (Figure 25.7). Ablation catheters can be constructed without metal braiding and with copper trans-

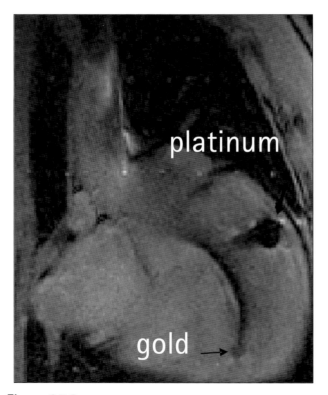

Figure 25.8
MR image showing passive visualization of two cardiac ablation/mapping catheters in the right-ventricular apex and right atrium in a canine model. The catheter in the right-ventricular apex has a 4 mm gold electrode tip, while the atrial catheter has a 4 mm platinum electrode tip. Note the distinct difference in susceptibility artifact between the materials, since the right-atrial catheter artifact obscures some of the anatomic features of the image.

mission wires and MR-compatible electrode materials such as platinum and gold (Figure 25.8). A limitation of passive tracking methods is that many polymeric materials used for catheters and intravascular sheaths have very low magnetic susceptibilities and therefore are difficult to visualize. To improve the visualization of these devices, paramagnetic materials such as dysprosium oxide can be incorporated into the walls of the catheter or sheath to increase magnetic susceptibility without altering the mechanical properties of the device.[25]

Active tracking methods require the creation of a signal that is actively detected or emitted by the device to identify its location. While several techniques have been described, the most popular active tracking technique uses a small RF coil consisting of an untuned loop attached to the tip of the interventional device that provides 3D numeric space coordinates of the coil in real time with a spatial positional resolution of ~1 mm.[26] The position of the coil can then be superimposed upon a previously acquired 2D or 3D 'roadmap' image in real time and thus allow direct visualization of the catheter position. A limitation of this approach is the inability to simultaneously image the region of interest and track the trajectory of the device, as can be done using X-ray fluoroscopy. Another limitation is that the position is known only for the tip of the catheter/guidewire. This may complicate placement at the target location, since device navigation through tortuous vessels often involves the formation of loops. Multiple RF sensing coils may help in this respect to give positional information along the axis of the device/catheter. Active tracking can be also be reliably performed using coupled antenna guidewire coils[27,28] that allow active visualization of the entire trajectory of a catheter/device. This approach helps simplify complex catheter navigations, particularly in cardiac chambers.

Experience with MRI-guided interventional electrophysiology studies

Passive ablation catheter placement and localization

In our laboratory, passively tracked custom MR-compatible catheters are used routinely to successfully target atrial and ventricular structures for ablation therapy under MRI guidance with fast gradient-echo sequences (Figure 25.9).[20] In more recent studies, we have performed catheter placement using a real-time steady-state free precision (SSFP) sequences that provide both higher spatial and higher temporal resolution. In addition to accurate placement within the atria, an important advantage of MRI-guided navigation is the ability to visualize the electrode–endocardial tissue interface (Figure 25.10). The

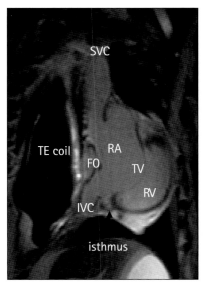

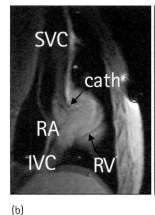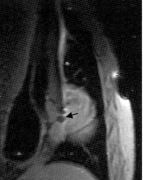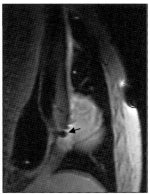

(a)

(b)

Figure 25.9

(a) MRI of the canine right heart showing several anatomic landmarks critical for catheter navigation. (b) Passive visualization of an MR-compatible ablation catheter (cath) in the right atrium of a canine model using a real-time gradient-echo fluoroscopy sequence. SVC, superior vena cava; TE, transesophageal; FO, fossa ovalis; RA, right atrium; TV, tricuspid valve; IVC, inferior vena cava; RV, right ventricle.

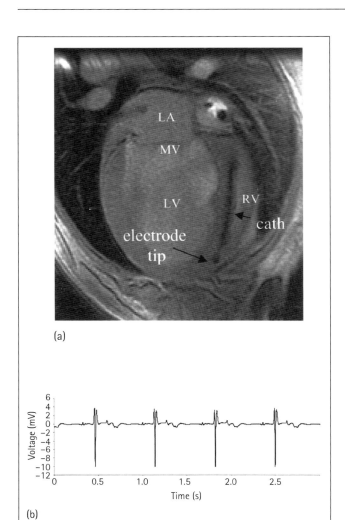

(a)

(b)

Figure 25.10

(a) Preablation fast spin-echo image showing electrode–tissue interface in the right-ventricular (RV) apex, with (b) the corresponding high-amplitude intracardiac electrogram acquired during imaging. Low-amplitude, high-frequency deflections surrounding the R-wave represent low-level electromagnetic interference from the scanner excitation pulse. LA, left atrium; cath, catheter; MV, mitral valve; LV, left ventricle. (Reproduced from Lardo et al. Circulation 2000; 102:698–705 with permission from Lippincott Williams & Wilkins.)

ability to visualize the electrode–tissue interface and acquire simultaneous intracardiac electrograms helps ensure good electrical contact and efficient RF energy transfer from the electrode to the tissue. One limitation of this navigation approach is the requirement to manipulate the catheter within the imaging slice (typically 5–10 mm wide), which may be especially difficult during catheter placement in geometrically complex vessels and cardiac chambers, where catheter curvature and loops are common. To help with this problem, we have used projection MRI, which essentially provides a large/thick-slice slab for navigation (we turn off the slice-select gradient). While this is useful to maintain visualization of the catheter, a great deal of anatomic information can be lost, which in turn complicates the navigation. We have found that a combination of both 'thick-slice' projection imaging and real-time interactive slice prescription provides the optimal solution for passive tracking approaches.

Active catheter placement and localization

We have also used active tracking methods to perform real-time catheter navigation studies with a specially designed multifunctional catheter[29] (Figure 25.11). The catheter body acts as a long loop receiver to allow active tracking and complete visualization of the entire catheter length while simultaneously behaving as a traditional two-wire electrophysiology catheter for intracardiac electrogram recording and ablation (Figures 25.12 and 25.13). We are currently adapting this basic design to include multiple sensing and RF-transmitting electrode arrays for both linear lesion generation and pulmonary vein isolation procedures.

In our experience with both passive and active tracking, the most time-consuming and tedious component of the catheter navigation is localization of the tip in a slice that allows visualization of the electrode and an appropriate segment of myocardial tissue simultaneously to allow monitoring of therapy. To help overcome this difficulty, we have used an additional active tracking approach that involves the placement of 3D microsensing coils (Figure 25.14a) at the tips of the passive MR-compatible ablation catheters described above. Using this approach, the catheter body is tracked passively, while the catheter tip or electrode is tracked actively and can be superimposed both visually and quantitatively on cardiac structures (Figure 25.14b). An added feature of this approach is the ability to direct the 3D positional information of the sensor back to the rotation matrix of the scanner for the automatic prescription of a series of orthogonal slices around the tip. This feature is especially valuable for guiding and monitoring ablation therapy, since it allows instant automatic visualization of myocardium in direct contact with the catheter/device without manual sweeping and empirical determination of the correct imaging slice.

Active transseptal needle localization

Transseptal catheterization has experienced a revival recently due to the development of curative left-sided

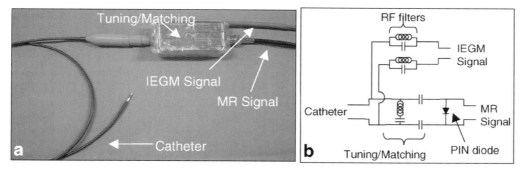

Figure 25.11

Electrical connections of the catheter. (a) The 100 cm modified electrophysiology catheter is interfaced with the tuning, matching, and signal-splitting circuit. The intracardiac electrogram (IEGM) and MR signal are connected to their respective receivers. (b) Electrical diagram of the catheter and related circuits. The catheter signal is passed through a tuning/matching network to the MR receiver. The IEGM signal is passed to its receiver through RF filters (parallel *LC* circuits tuned to 64 MHz). Reproduced from Susil RC et al. Magn Reson Med, 2002; 47:594–600.

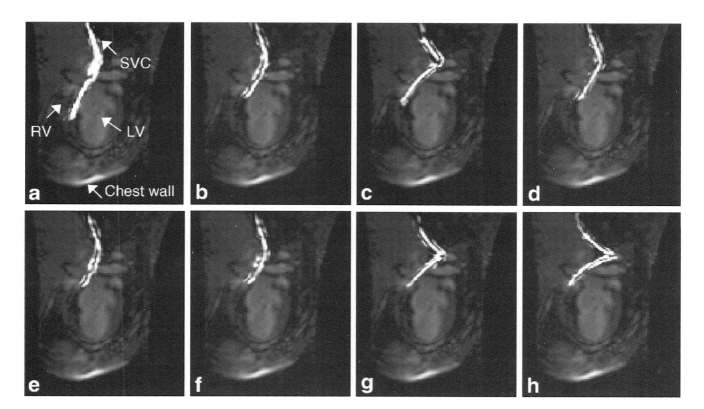

Figure 25.12

High-frequency catheter function: catheter visualization and tracking. Selected images from a 10 s catheter push acquired with a 10 frame/s, real-time SSFP sequence. Projection images of the catheter are overlaid on a static, slice-selective roadmap image. LV, left ventricle; RV, right ventricle; SVC, superior vena cava. The catheter starts in the right ventricle and is then pulled up into the right atrium (a,b). As the catheter is subsequently pushed, the tip stays in the atrium and the catheter body flexes (c). The catheter is pulled back further (d,e). In (f) and (g), the catheter is pushed once again, the tip stays in the right atrium, and the catheter shaft flexes. Note that the full length of the catheter can be easily visualized. (Reproduced from Susil et al. Magn Reson Med 2002; 47:594–600.)

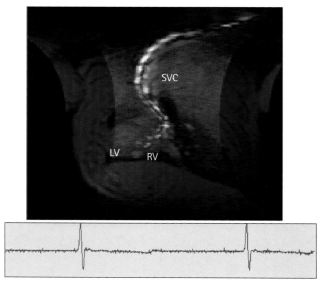

Figure 25.13

Simultaneous catheter function: intracardiac electrogram recordings concurrent with catheter tracking. Selected image from a 15 s catheter push acquired with a 7 frame/s, real-time gradient-echo sequence. LV, left ventricle; RV, right ventricle; SVC, superior vena cava. The catheter is initially advanced from the jugular vein, down the superior vena cava, toward the right heart. Note that a strong bipolar signal is recorded once the catheter tip arrives in the right ventricle. (Modified from Susil et al. Magn Reson Med 2002; 47:594–600.)

atrial RF catheter ablation procedures. Fluoroscopy-guided transseptal catheterization remains a technically difficult procedure, particularly in the setting of conditions that distort the normal atrial anatomy and the fluoroscopic position of the interatrial septum. Improvements in the technique and apparatus have yielded lower complication rates; however, even when performed by experienced operators, improper positioning of the needle can result in cardiac or aortic perforation. These complications can, in part, be attributed to the inability to directly visualize the fossa ovalis and other critical endocardial landmarks using 2D projection X-ray fluoroscopy. We have recently designed a multifunctional transseptal needle antenna that receives MR signals and permits active tracking of the entire needle shaft and tip (Figure 25.15). This device can also be equipped with the 3D microposition sensors mentioned above and the needle tip position superimposed upon 2D or 3D images of the right atrium, intraatrial septum, and fossa ovale. Such an approach may substantially improve the safety of this common and technically changing procedure that is commonly performed to achieve left-heart access for ablation therapy.

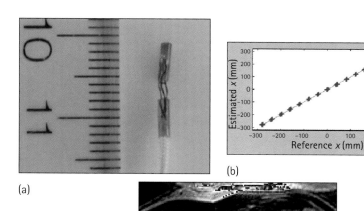

(a)

(b)

(c)

Figure 25.14

(a) Photograph of a 3D active tracking sensor. (b) Positions estimated from the gradient field measurements were compared with the real (reference) positions for each position in the scanner. (c) Once the quantitative position of the coil has been determined, it can then be superimposed on 2D images of cardiac anatomy (represented by the cursor).

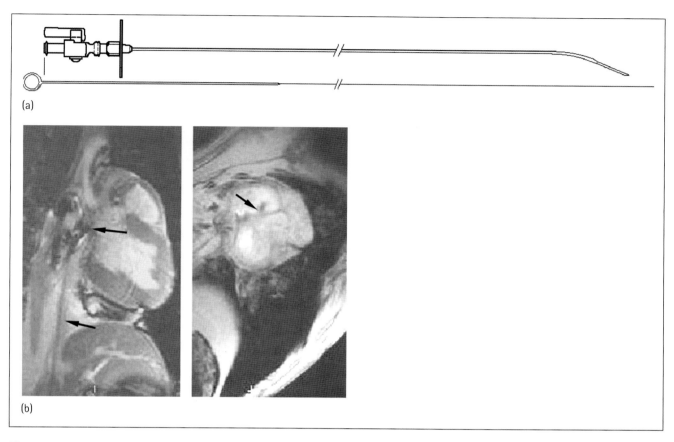

Figure 25.15
(a) MRI compatible Brockenbrough needle and (b) FIESTA imaging showing the needle in the inferior vena cava and approaching the interatrial septum in a dog.

MR imaging of RF lesions

T2-weighted fast spin-echo imaging

Perhaps the unique and most valuable advantage of MRI-guided ablation therapy is the ability to visualize and monitor lesion formation with high temporal and spatial resolution. Lardo and colleagues showed that RFA lesions in the right-ventricular apex could be reliably visualized as hyperintense areas with T2-weighted fast spin-echo sequences (Figures 25.16 and 25.17). In this study, catheters were placed in the right-ventricular apex under MRI guidance and RF energy was delivered for 70 s at 60 W. Imaging was performed at 30 s intervals post ablation. The lesion signal intensity increased in a linear faction, and then reached a plateau at 12.2 ± 2 min. The lesion size reached a maximum ~3 min post ablation (Figure 25.18). More recently, MRI of epicardial lesions has been evaluated in a dog model. In an open chest preparation, RF lesions were created on the epicardial surface and imaged over several hours of follow-up. In T2-weighted images, the ablation lesion is visible as an area of increased signal intensity with a small rim of decreased signal. This allows the identification of the lesion in comparison with the healthy surrounding myocardium in all three imaging planes (Figure 25.19). These lesions can be reliably followed for several hours, and show similar imaging characteristics up to 15 hours post ablation. The lesion size correlated well with the pathologic findings.

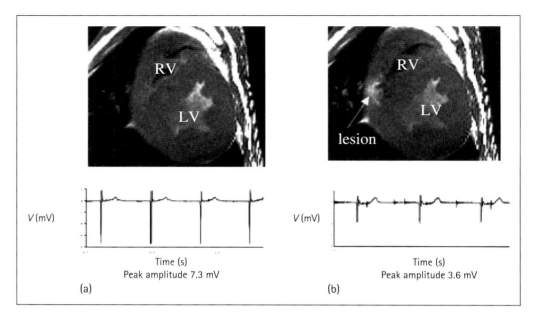

Figure 25.16
Fast spin-echo images of right-ventricular (RV) free wall (a) before and (b) 10 min after ablation, with the corresponding intracardiac electrode tracings. A transmural lesion directly adjacent to the catheter tip could be visualized 4 min after RF delivery. The intracardiac ECG amplitude decreased 50% after ablation. LV, left ventricle. (Reproduced from Lardo et al. Circulation 2000; 102:698–705 with permission from Lippincott Williams & Wilkins.)

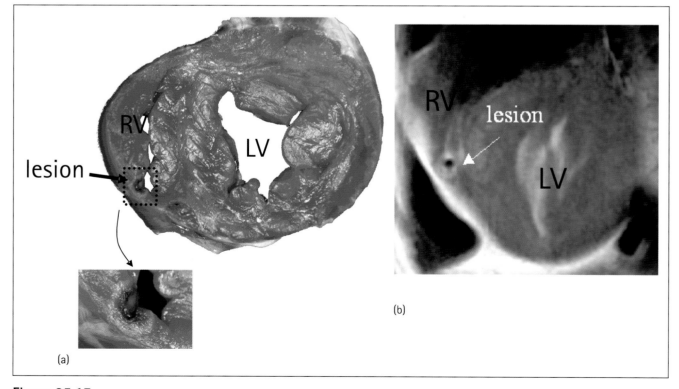

Figure 25.17
(a) Gross exam and (b) FSE MRI appearance of a right ventricular (VR) radiofrequency lesion (arrow). (Reproduced with permission from Lardo et al., Circulation, 2000; 102:698–705).

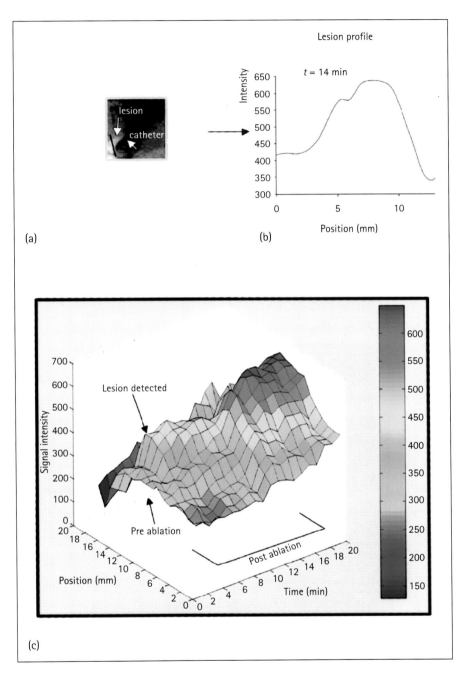

(a)

(b)

Lesion profile

Intensity

$t = 14$ min

Position (mm)

(c)

Figure 25.18
(a) Right-ventricular apex lesion showing spatial location of the intensity profile line and (b) the resulting intensity-versus-location data for a single point in time during temporal assessment of the lesion. (c) 3D surface plot showing temporal and spatial development of right-ventricular lesions, created by plotting several intensity profiles in time. The maximum lesion size and peak signal intensity occurred 5 and 12 min after ablation, respectively. (Reproduced from Lardo et al. Circulation 2000; 102:698–705 with permission from Lippincott Williams & Wilkins.)

T1-weighted gradient-echo imaging

Imaging of RF lesions is also possible with T1-weighted images. In these images, the lesions appear as areas of increased signal intensity. They are visible during follow-up over several hours, and were visible in some experiments over a follow-up period of 12 hours (Figure 25.20). The lesion size correlated well with histologic findings.

Delayed enhancement lesion imaging

Gadolinium has been used for many years to evaluate myocardial scarring after myocardial infarction, where the infarct zone exhibits early hypoenhancement, which is frequently explained by the microvascular obstruction with delayed hyperenhancement, thought to be due to an increased volume of distribution. The inflow and outflow

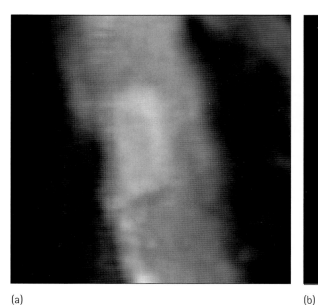

(a)

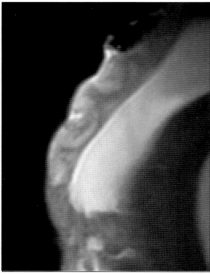

(b)

Figure 25.19
(a) Fast spin-echo images of right-ventricular epicardial RF ablation lesions (a) premortem and (b) postmortem. The lesions consist of an outer rim of low signal and a central region of high signal intensity. TE = 68 ms, ELT = 16, 256 × 128 matrix.

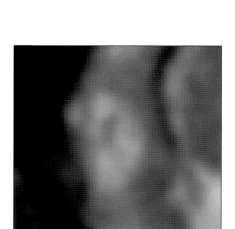

(a)

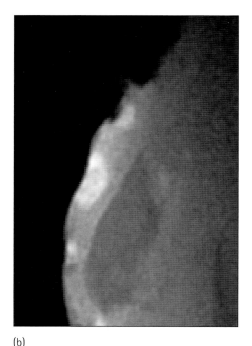

(b)

Figure 25.20
Spoiled gradient-echo images of right-ventricular epicardial RF ablation lesions (a) premortem and (b) postmortem. Gradient-echo-derived lesions consisted of a homogenous region of hyperintensity compared with normal untreated myocardium. TE = 12 ms, TR = 1000 ms, FA = 20°, 5 mm thickness, 256 × 256 matrix.

kinetics for RF ablation lesions were examined in a model of epicardial and endocardial ablations, which were followed over a time course of several hours using an open chest preparation to allow imaging with high-resolution coils. Preliminary results suggest that RF ablations may exhibit an even longer time for hyperenhancement (Figure 25.21). This process lasted 1–2 hours in some experiments. Once enhanced, the lesion could be seen in some experiments up to a follow-up of 12 hours.

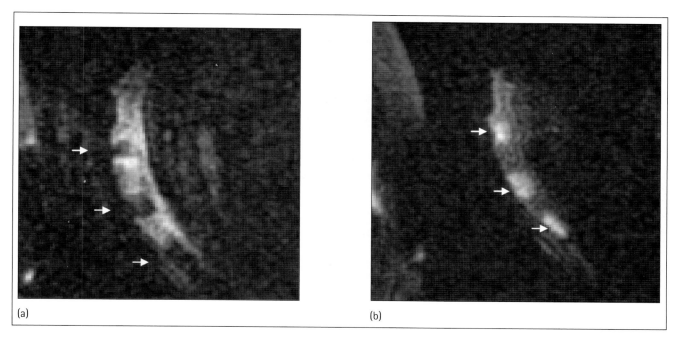

(a)   (b)

Figure 25.21
Epicardial radiofrequency ablation lesions (a) 1 min, (b) 1h post gadolinium injection and (c) 5 h post ablation at gross exam. Note that treated regions of the myocardium early following injection display as areas of lower signal intensity compared with untreated regions due to a contrast void in the lesion, likely due to microvascular obstruction. One hour post injection, lesions exhibit delayed enhancement and display as homogenous hyperintense regions.

Mechanism of detection by MRI

Lesions can be visualized since MRI is able to detect one or more specific changes in T1 and T2 relaxation parameters resulting from heat-induced biophysical changes in cardiac tissue, such as interstitial edema, hyperemia, conformational changes, cellular shrinkage, and tissue coagulation. Reviewing this general inventory of effects in the context of parameters detectable by MRI, acute interstitial edema is most likely responsible for the hyperintense regions representing the area of damage observed by T2-weighted fast spin-echo imaging. The edema response is mediated by thermal injury that cause water and proteins to escape through gaps in the endothelial cells lining the vessel and enter the interstitial space. This near-instantaneous local increase in the number of unbound protons increases the T2 relaxation constant of the tissue and gives rise to the hyperintense regions that appear to represent the spatial extent of the anatomic lesion. Additionally, lesion detection 1–2 min following ablation, with subsequent formation over 10–15 min, is consistent with the temporal physiologic response of local acute interstitial edema.

Lesion visualization and 3D imaging in humans

We have obtained encouraging results detecting atrial lesions in patients following standard X-ray fluoroscopy-guided ablation procedures. Figure 25.22 represents a series of images from a patient following a right-sided atrial fibrillation ablation procedure using a new experimental linear array catheter and RF generator system. The procedure consisted of an isthmus ablation and a line of ablation along the lateral wall of the right atrium, starting at the superior vena cava and extending to the inferior vena cava. Figure 25.22a shows a short-axis fast spin-echo image post ablation, while Figure 25.22b represents the post-ablation 3D reconstruction of the right atrium, consisting of a total of eight slices, each 6 mm thick. The depth

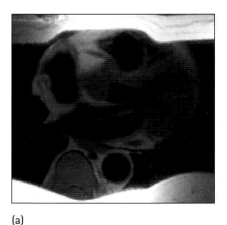

(a)

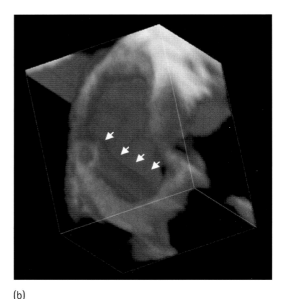

(b)

Figure 25.22
(a) 2D and (b) 3D images following atrial fibrillation catheter ablation in a human subject. The ablated area of the myocardium appears as a hyperintense swollen region along the lateral wall of the right atrium (arrow). The 3D reconstruction of the atrium and lesion (total of eight slices, 6 mm thick) provides information regarding the extent and depth of thermal damage along the right-atrial lateral wall (arrows).

and extent of RF-induced damage on the lateral wall can be clearly visualized (arrows). A large lesion on the lateral wall of the right atrium is clearly identified, as indicated by the swollen appearance of the atrial myocardium.

Use of local receiver coils and antennas

While ventricular lesions can be visualized using a standard cardiac phased array thoracic coil, lesions on thin-walled atrial structures are significantly more difficult to image due to a decrease in SNR with decreasing voxel volume (field of view). Recently developed intravascular antennas produce a very high signal close to the coil and thus make it possible to image thin-walled atrial structures with near-microscopic resolution. We have demonstrated the feasibility of transesophageal imaging for the visualization of left-atrial RF lesions in a canine model. Following the creation of a line of ablation on the posterior wall of the left atrium using standard techniques, imaging was performed using an internal imaging coil placed in the esophagus (Figure 25.23). The lesions appeared as hyperintense regions in the left atrium; discontinuous lesions could be identified and the interlesion gap width could be identified and quantified. The lesion length and width measured by MRI correlated strongly with those parameters measured at histologic analysis, and correlated well with direct measurements at gross examination.

Arrhythmia-specific advantages of MRI

Chronic atrial fibrillation

RF catheter manipulation and localization in geometrically complex cardiac chambers is hindered by the large degree of anatomic ambiguity inherent to X-ray fluoroscopy. With the advent of ultrafast imaging sequences, MRI can be used to perform real-time catheter placement and can quantitatively target key anatomic landmarks for ablation. The ability to image RF damage to the myocardium facilitates the creation and confirmation of complete linear lesions, which may allow for a reduction in the number of lesions and may reduce recurrence. Lesion visualization may allow (1) precise titration of therapy, (2) the ability to test the length and depth of lesions from new ablation-energy sources, (3) accurate assessment of the success of making lines of ablation, and (4) the study of hybrid therapy, since the contribution of ablation can be quantified.

Another important and practical advantage of MRI-guided ablation therapy is the potential to perform functional imaging post therapy. In patients with dilated left atria secondary to mitral regurgitation undergoing right- and/or left-sided atrial fibrillation ablation, high-resolution cine atrial imaging can be easily performed to assess atrial mechanical function and flow dynamics pre- and post ablation, which may provide useful information regarding the future risk of embolization.

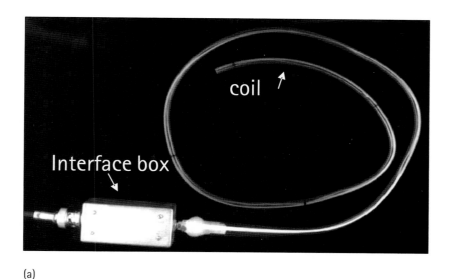

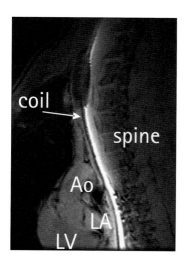

(a)

(b)

Figure 25.23

(a) Transesophageal MRI coil and (b) its placement in a canine model. Signal is generated both by a cardiac phased array coil and the esophageal coil. Due to the close proximity of the esophagus to the posterior wall of the left atrium, high-resolution imaging (~150 μm) is possible.

Ablation of focal atrial fibrillation

MRI can help facilitate ablation of the pulmonary veins by providing detailed pulmonary vein anatomy prior to fluoroscopy-guided ablation procedures. At our institution, 3D pulmonary vein angiography has been used successfully as a preplanning tool to determine pulmonary vein ostial diameters and branching patterns prior to X-ray-guided pulmonary vein isolation procedures (Figure 25.24).[30] This detailed information allows for appropriate device sizing and accurate catheter navigation. When performing pulmonary vein ablation under MRI guidance, the ability to image the pulmonary vein ostium (Figure 25.25) and myocardial pulmonary vein sleeves while simultaneously acquiring electrical information may help facilitate therapy titration and thereby eliminate excess energy delivery and pulmonary vein injury. It is likely that visualization of the anatomic structures combined with electrical activity can aid in the understanding of the roles of these structures in governing cardiac electrical function, as well as leading to optimal techniques to ablate in the pulmonary vein to reduce or eliminate complications (Figure 25.26).

Ablation of scar-mediated ventricular tachycardia

Recent studies have shown that ischemic regions of myocardium can be noninvasively identified using delayed contrast enhancement MRI techniques.[31,32] Thus, it is possible to visualize myocardial scars from prior cardiac ischemic events and thereby help better localize a relevant and effective target for catheter-based RF therapy. Our laboratory has begun extensive work in this area.

Limitations of MRI-guided interventional electrophysiology

Safety

The most important consideration with any new diagnostic or therapeutic approach is safety. While a number of studies have been performed to determine the safety of

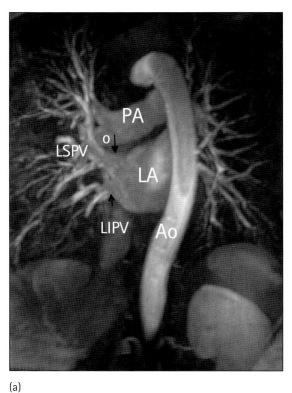
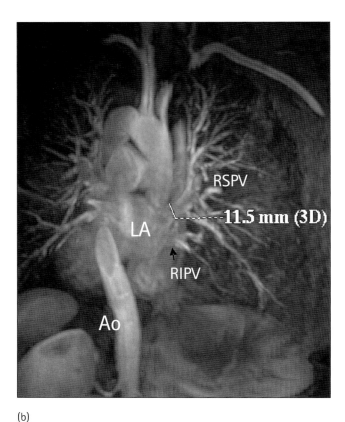

(a)   (b)

Figure 25.24

3D pulmonary vein MR angiography in a patient before undergoing a pulmonary vein isolation procedure. Ostial diameters, pulmonary vein anatomy, and branching details are used in preplanning of the procedure. PA, pulmonary artery; o, ostium; LSPV, left superior pulmonary vein; LA, left atrium; LIPV, left inferior pulmonary vein; Ao, aorta; RSPV, right superior pulmonary vein; RI, right inferior pulmonary vein.

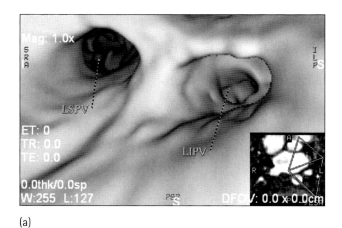

(a)   (b)

Figure 25.25

3D endoscopic views of the left atrium and pulmonary veins (a) pre ablation and (b) following pulmonary vein isolation in a human. Note that the left inferior and left superior pulmonary ostia diameters are greatly reduced post ablation. This view allow a fly-through mode that is helpful to provide an understanding of the branching network of the pulmonary veins pre ablation for planning purposes.

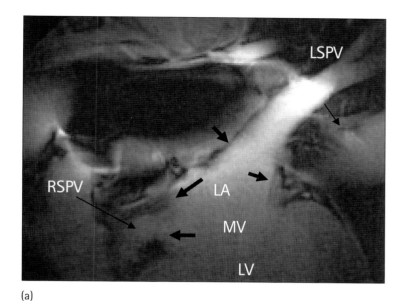

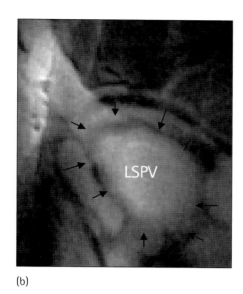

(a)

(b)

Figure 25.26
(a) Gradient-echo transesophageal image of the left atrium (LA), the left superior pulmonary vein (LSPV), and the right superior pulmonary vein (RSPV). MV, mitral valve. (b) High-resolution cross-sectional image through the LSPV showing the various vascular and atrial tissue segments (arrows); resolution 250 μm.

conventional MRI with regard to electromagnetic energy exposure and internal heating,[33–35] interventional procedures present additional unique parameters that raise new safety concerns. Besides the obvious hazards of placing incompatible monitoring equipment and surgical instruments in close proximity to a high static magnetic field, the in vivo placement of long conductive wires and electrical components within rapidly changing magnetic and electric fields may result in local heating. This effect is primarily due to coupling of the body coil RF excitation (which is on the order of kilowatts) with any conductive wire or component in the RF field. This transfer of energy from the body coil to the device increases the electric field around the device and can cause localized concentrated heating. Indeed, previous work has confirmed substantial local heating with straight copper wires, tracking catheters, and guidewires in place.

Such heating effects can be minimized and/or eliminated by incorporating decoupling circuitry into the device and thereby limiting the amount of energy transfer through the probe/wire by the transmit coil. Additionally, the judicious use of imaging sequences that limit RF power deposition and duration (i.e. gradient-echo sequences with high repetition times and low flip angles) greatly reduces the possibility of excessive heating. The propensity for heating is also affected by the magnetic field strength, since the power of an RF pulse is proportional to the square of the magnetic field. Few studies have been performed to determine the complex local heating effects of catheters and probes placed in vivo during inter-

ventional MRI. While more comprehensive studies are certainly required, existing studies appear promising, and adverse effects from heating have not been reported in any clinical interventional MRI studies.

Specialty training

In addition to the very specific and demanding training requirements for performing electrophysiologic interventions, the use of MRI as a guidance modality introduces new complexities and challenges. Thus, the future of MRI-guided interventional cardiology lies not only within the rapid technological advances in the field, but also with the willingness of fellowship programs to establish specific training initiatives for performing MRI guided procedures.

Future of MRI-guided electrophysiologic intervention

Real-time MRI, combined with recent advances in internal coil technology, represents an exciting new approach for performing electrophysiologic interventions. While the basic science and potential clinical applications are exciting, the field is in its very earliest stages of development. The continued refinement of MRI in this regard is dependent upon a collaborative effort from a multidisciplinary team of basic scientist, engineers, and clinicians. A wealth of information is quickly emerging and approaching a critical mass that has placed us at the threshold of a revolutionary approach for diagnosing and treating the most debilitating cardiac arrhythmias. Intracardiac MRI techniques – combined with other advanced MRI techniques, such as MR angiography and functional MRI – will undoubtedly open up new avenues for the future comprehensive management of complex arrhythmias.

References

1. Calkins H, et al. Catheter ablation of accessory pathways, atrioventricular nodal reentrant tachycardia, and the atrioventricular junction: final results of a prospective, multicenter clinical trial. The Atakr Multicenter Investigators Group. Circulation 1999; 99:262–70.

2. Moe GJ, Abildskov J. Atrial fibrillation as a self-sustaining arrhythmia independent of focal discharge. Am Heart J, 1959; 58:59–70.

3. Moe GJ. On the multiple wavelet hypothesis of atrial fibrillation. Arch Int Pharmacodyn Ther 1962; 140:183–99.

4. Cox JL. The surgical treatment of atrial fibrillation. IV. Surgical technique. J Thorac Cardiovasc Surg 1991; 101:584–92.

5. Cox JL. Evolving applications of the maze procedure for atrial fibrillation. Ann Thorac Surg, 1993; 55:578–80.

6. Haissaguerre M, Gencel L, Fischer B, et al. Successful catheter ablation of atrial fibrillation. J Cardiovasc Electrophysiol 1994; 5:1045–52.

7. Maloney JD, Milner L, Barold S, et al. Two-staged biatrial linear and focal ablation to restore sinus rhythm in patients with refractory chronic atrial fibrillation: procedure experience and follow-up beyond 1 year. Pacing Clin Electrophysiol 1998; 21:2527–32.

8. Haissaguerre M, Shah DC, Jais P, et al. Role of catheter ablation for atrial fibrillation. Curr Opin Cardiol 1997; 12:18–23.

9. Haissaguerre M, Jais P, Shah DC, et al. Right and left atrial radiofrequency catheter therapy of paroxysmal atrial fibrillation. J Cardiovasc Electrophysiol 1996; 7:1132–44.

10. Haissaguerre M, Jais P, Shah DC, et al. Spontaneous initiation of atrial fibrillation by ectopic beats originating in the pulmonary veins. N Engl J Med 1998; 339:659–66.

11. Jais P, Haissaguerre M, Shah DC, et al. A focal source of atrial fibrillation treated by discrete radiofrequency ablation. Circulation 1997; 95:572–6.

12. Walmsley R. The Heart. Quian's Elements of Anatomy (Sharpey-Schafer E, Brice TH, eds). London: Longmans, Green, 1929.

13. Lesh MD, Diederich C, Guerra PG, et al. An anatomic approach to prevention of atrial fibrillation: pulmonary vein isolation with through-the-balloon ultrasound ablation (TTB-USA). Thorac Cardiovasc Surg 1999; 47(Suppl 3):347–51.

14. Shah DC, Haissaguerre M, Jais P. Catheter ablation of pulmonary vein foci for atrial fibrillation: PV foci ablation for atrial fibrillation. Thorac Cardiovasc Surg 1999; 47(Suppl 3):352–6.

15. Chen SA, et al. Radiofrequency catheter ablation of atrial fibrillation initiated by pulmonary vein ectopic beats. J Cardiovasc Electrophysiol 2000; 11:218–27.

16. Scanavacca MI, Kajita LJ, Vieira M, et al. Pulmonary vein stenosis complicating catheter ablation of focal atrial fibrillation. J Cardiovasc Electrophysiol 2000; 11:677–81.

17. Stevenson WG, Delacretaz E. Strategies for catheter ablation of scar-related ventricular tachycardia. Curr Cardiol Rep 2000; 2:537–44.

18. Soejima K, Stevenson WG. Ventricular tachycardia associated with myocardial infarct scar: a spectrum of therapies for a single patient. Circulation 2002; 106:176–9.

19. Lardo AC, McVeigh ER, Jumrussirikul P, et al. Visualization and temporal/spatial characterization of cardiac radiofrequency ablation lesions using magnetic resonance imaging. Circulation 2000; 102:698–705.

20. Duru F. CARTO three-dimensional non-fluoroscopic electroanatomic mapping for catheter ablation of arrhythmias: a useful tool or an expensive toy for the electrophysiologist? Anadolu Kardiyol Derg 2002; 2:330–7.

21. Bhuripanyo K, Raungratanaamporn O, Sriratanasathavorn C, et al. Biosense mapping for ablation of ventricular tachycardia in cardiomyopathy. J Med Assoc Thai 2000; 83(Suppl 2):S206–13.

22. Worley SJ. Use of a real-time three-dimensional magnetic navigation system for radiofrequency ablation of accessory pathways. Pacing Clin Electrophysiol 1998; 21:1636–45.

23. Callans DJ, Ren JF, Michele J, et al. Electroanatomic left ventricular mapping in the porcine model of healed anterior myocardial infarction. Correlation with intracardiac echocardiography and pathological analysis. Circulation 1999; 100:1744–50.

24. Bakker CJ, Hoogeveen RM, Weber J, et al. Visualization of dedicated catheters using fast scanning techniques with potential for MR-guided vascular interventions. Magn Reson Med 1996; 36:816–20.

25. Dumoulin CL, Souza SP, Darrow RD. Real-time position monitoring of invasive devices using magnetic resonance. Magn Reson Med 1993; 29:411–15.

26. Ladd ME, Zimmermann GG, Quick HH, et al. Active MR visualization of a vascular guidewire in vivo. J Magn Reson Imaging 1998; 8:220–5.

27. Ladd ME, Erhart P, Debatin JF, et al. Guidewire antennas for MR fluoroscopy. Magn Reson Med 1997; 37:891–7.

28. Susil RC, Yeung CJ, Halperin HR, et al. Multifunctional interventional devices for MRI: a combined electrophysiology/MRI catheter. Magn Reson Med 2002; 47:594–600.

29. Yamane T, Shah DC, Jais P, et al. Pseudo sinus rhythm originating from the left superior pulmonary vein in a patient with paroxysmal atrial fibrillation. J Cardiovasc Electrophysiol 2001; 12:1190–1.

30. Lardo AC, Halperin H, McVeigh ER. Magnetic resonance imaging transseptal needle antenna. US Patent # 6606513 2003.

31. Kato R, Lickfett L, Meininger G, et al. Pulmonary vein anatomy in patients undergoing catheter ablation of atrial fibrillation: lessons learned by use of magnetic resonance imaging. Circulation 2003; 107:2004–10.

32. Kim RJ, Wu E, Rafael A, et al. The use of contrast-enhanced magnetic resonance imaging to identify reversible myocardial dysfunction. N Engl J Med 2000; 343:1445–53.

MRI imaging: overview of physical principles

A brief review of MRI physical principles clarifies the multiple choices that enable targeting of MRI to different key questions relating to angiogenesis. Tissue in a strong applied magnetic field develops net magnetization vectors in each volume element (voxel) of interest. The longitudinal magnetization develops with time constant T1, and may be converted all or in part to transverse magnetization, which decays with time constant T2* (Figure 26.1). The oscillating transverse magnetization generates signal detectable with an antenna coil receiver. T2* can be increased by arrival of a magnetic susceptibility contrast agent to zones of new vessel development, due to increased heterogeneity of precession frequencies. During the tens of milliseconds that the transverse (xy-plane) magnetization is present, magnetic field gradients may be applied to modify the resonance frequencies in a pattern called a k–t trajectory so that the signal will report information corresponding to different patterns that transform to images (Figures 26.2 and 26.3).

The most common k–t trajectory is rectilinear, sweeping left to right, row by row, by stepwise application of magnetic field gradients. The second most common pattern is spiral,[1,2] achieved by changing x- and y-gradients simultaneously, in decelerating or accelerating sinusoidal patterns. Spiral is commonly used for echo-

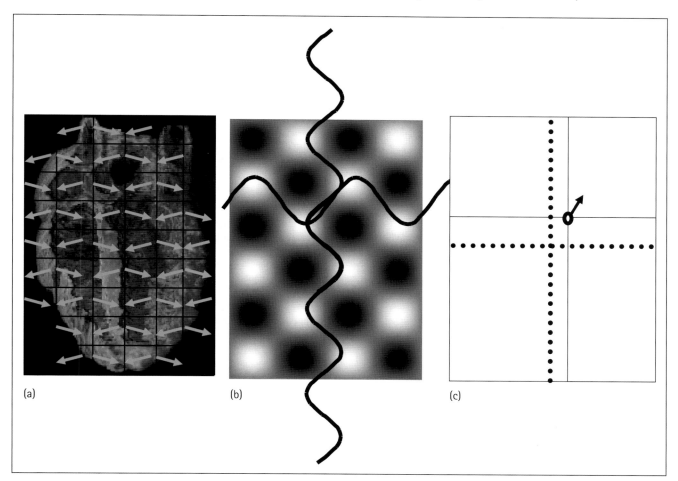

(a)   (b)   (c)

Figure 26.2

k-space. (a) The target region is divided into volume elements called voxels based on choices of field of view, matrix, and slice thickness. Each voxel has a magnetization vector whose length will determine the brightness at a corresponding location in the image. (b) Magnetic field gradients in various combinations impose patterns of cycles of advancement of vector direction in the transverse (xy) plane. This example shows 2 cycles horizontally and 3 cycles vertically. (c) Each pattern of cycles (spatial frequencies) can be represented as a single point in 'k-space'. The point (2,3) represents the pattern shown of 2 cycles horizontally and 3 vertically. k-space is a grid in which the 'goodness of fit' of each pattern will be recorded as a complex number. k–t-space explicitly tracks the time of putting data in k-space. Most MRI aims to fill out k-space with a particular contrast method. Collateral neovascular-sensitive imaging (CS-MRI) acquires different parts of k-space with different contrast mechanisms, as a hybrid. The edges of k-space are acquired with T2* contrast, while the center is acquired with T1 contrast.

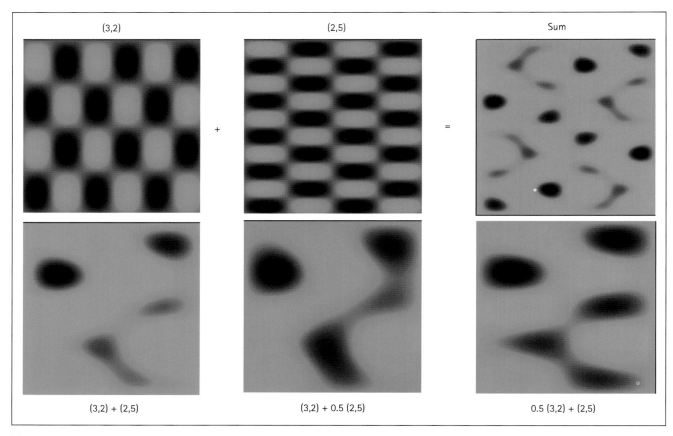

Figure 26.3
k-space sums. This figure illustrates what happens when two patterns of cycles (two points in k-space) are combined. Adding the pattern represented by the point (3,2) (upper left) to that of (2,5) (upper center) yields the sum shown in the upper right. Images are constructed from the magnitude of the right upper quadrant. Adding different strengths of each of the two patterns produces several different image patterns (bottom row). Using appropriate strengths for all the different points in k-space produces the desired image. The appropriate strengths are in essence the goodness of fit of each pattern to the pattern of magnetization in the tissue at the time of imaging.

planar imaging (EPI), in which all of k-space is covered following a single excitation. Other trajectories are possible.[3,4] Creative use of gradients during excitation,[5] as well as during data collection, enables other imaging opportunities, such as real-time (60 frames/s) blood velocity assessment,[6] or real time M-mode MRI.[7] The various combinations of magnetization preparation, k–t trajectory, data collection, and image reconstruction result in a myriad imaging methods that are typically summarized by various acronyms.[8,9]

We have applied MRI to achieve the following goals: (1) scout imaging, to determine cardiac orientation for precise image alignment with the heart in its own coordinates for accurate measurements and valid comparisons over time; (2) dynamic bright-blood imaging in biplane long-axis views, to determine the timing of systole and diastole and the concomitant changes in base and apical endpoint positions of the heart; (3) angiogenesis-sensitive T2*,T1 hybrid imaging, to identify and measure neovascular development; (4) perfusion-sensitive bright-blood

imaging, to identify and quantify impaired blood delivery, at rest, and at peak vasodilation or stress; (5) SMART motion-tracked wall thickness change and radial motion, to assess accurately the local impact of angiogenesis on wall mechanics;[10] (6) assessment of global cardiac function via end-diastolic and peak systolic volumes (ejection fraction, stroke volume, cardiac output, and end-diastolic dimensions); (7) strain maps, to identify partial thickness functional improvements; (8) metabolic imaging (simultaneous ^{1}H and ^{31}P), to identify changes in the utilization and recovery of high-energy phosphates (by monitoring relative concentrations of regional phosphocreatine, adenosine triphosphate, inorganic phosphate concentrations, and intracellular pH); (9) incipient efforts applying T2*,T1 hybrid imaging, to identify molecular targets.[11]

MRI provides a means for identifying good candidates for therapeutic angiogenesis by demonstrating the presence of myocardial zones of impaired blood delivery. Importantly, in our experience, MRI provides quantitative dose–response evidence of neovascularization in double-blinded placebo-controlled therapeutic angiogenesis trials using a technique that we call collateral neovascular sensitive MRI (CS-MRI). The observed improvement ranges from small reductions in the size of territory demonstrating delayed contrast arrival (ischemic zone) and minimal appearance of CS-MRI signal, to full restoration of flow and function in the target area with an appearance of large CS-MRI signal.[12–17]

Scout imaging

Scout imaging determines the unique orientation of the heart and timing of contraction for each individual, so that subsequent imaging is performed in views that relate to the orientation of the organ of interest. Scout imaging does not require maximal image quality, or any particular mechanism for contrast. The data for scout imaging should simply be acquired quickly. There are a number of ways to image quickly.[18] One of the simplest takes advantage of conjugate symmetry (half of k-space can be approximated as a reflection of the other half) to gain a factor of nearly 2 by collecting data for little more than half of k-space, filling in the rest of the data array by estimation. The data for half of k-space can be acquired rapidly without waiting for T1 recovery ($< \frac{1}{2}$ second total imaging time) following a single 90° excitation pulse, by using gradient reversals or 180° radiowave refocusing pulses to recover signal, repeatedly, until half of k-space is covered.[19–21] Refocusing pulses invert the magnetization vectors, a technique called spin-echo, which recovers the signal losses of coherence due to local field strength differences. A popular example method, HASTE, is an acronym for the descriptive phrase 'half-Fourier acquisition single-shot turbo spin-echo'. Additional opportunities for accelerated imaging include the use of multiple detectors on the chest that enable estimation of multiple points in k-space at the same time: SENSE,[22–25] SMASH,[26–33] and variants,[34–36] offering an acceleration factor of 2–4 with current detectors, discriminant orchestrated time series or DOTS (an acceleration factor of 8–12), and variants of UNFOLD[37,38] (a factor of 2 or 3).

Scout imaging of the left ventricle identifies the orientation of the long axis. Typically, this is achieved sequentially by bisecting the visible portion of the long-axis view of the left ventricle, first to determine in-plane tilt, then out-of-plane tilt. A third image prescription perpendicular to the double-oblique long axis produces a view in the true short axis.

From the short-axis view, cardinal long-axis views may be prescribed (Figure 26.4). A line from the center of the left ventricle that passes perpendicular to the septum, dividing both the right and left ventricles in half, generates a view that echocardiographers call the 'four-chamber

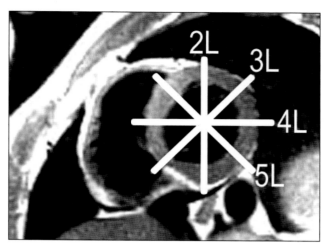

Figure 26.4
Scout imaging. Dark-blood MR image of a middle level in the heart in short-axis view. The lines indicate prescription planes, perpendicular to the view shown, intersecting the image along the drawn lines. In particular, 2L is parallel to the septum, and results in a two-chamber view (left atrium and left ventricle); 4L provides a four-chamber view atria (both atria and both ventricles). 3L and 5L are intermediate views that provide a three-chamber view (left atrium, left ventricle, and part of the right ventricle) and five-chamber view (atria, ventricles, and aortic root), respectively. The terms 'two-chamber', 'three-chamber', 'four-chamber', and 'five-chamber' are commonly used in echocardiography and are familiar to most cardiologists.

view' because it shows left and right ventricles and atria (Figure 26.5). We call that view '4L'. The line through the center of the left ventricle that runs parallel to the septum, perpendicular to the 4L prescription, shows only the left ventricle and left atrium. Echocardiographers call that the 'two-chamber view' and we call it '2L'. Between 2L and 4L, there are two more views that we call '3L' and '5L'. The 5L view corresponds to what the echocardiographers call the 'five-chamber view' (it includes both atria and both ventricles, and is angled to include the aortic root as a 'fifth chamber'). The 5L view shows anteroseptal and posterolateral wall motion, and the aortic valve leaflets. The 2L view shows anterior and inferior walls. The 3L shows anterolateral and inferoseptal motion and thickness. The 4L view shows the lateral wall, mid septum, and mitral and tricuspid valve leaflets. The hinge points of the mitral valve define the base of the left ventricle. Target short-axis slices followed over time are located by their percentage distance from base to apex of the left ventricle.

Cine imaging

The simplest approach to image the beating heart is to collect the data for k-space coverage of an image plane in

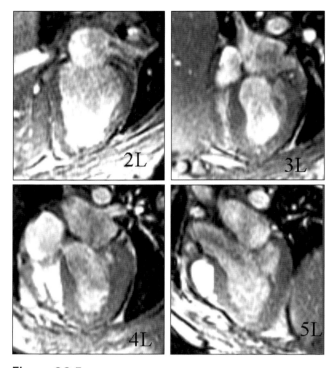

Figure 26.5

Long-axis chamber views. (2L) Left ventricle and left atrium; of the left ventricle, it shows anterior and inferior walls. (3L) Left and right ventricles and left atrium; of the left ventricle it shows anterolateral and inferoseptal walls. (4L) Both atria and both ventricles; of the left ventricle, it shows the lateral wall and mid septum, and also mitral and tricuspid valves. (5L) Both atria and both ventricles; this view is angled to include the aortic root as a 'fifth chamber'; of the left ventricle, it shows anteroseptal and posterolateral walls, and also the aortic valve.

short windows of opportunity, at a fixed delay after the R-wave of the ECG, across multiple heartbeats. That reproduces the stroboscopic effect of freezing the motion of the heart to build a coherent image at a particular phase in the cardiac cycle. Display of a series of such images representing different portions of the cardiac cycle nets a cine motion series (Figure 26.6). Long-axis views provide information for separate accurate motion-tracked prescription of the true short axis at end-diastole and at peak systole (Figure 26.7), depending on the time delay after the R-wave at which the definitive data are generated. As discussed below, in a separate heading.

First, a series of long-axis views are obtained in two perpendicular views (2L and 4L), each with 20 mm slice thickness, each spanning the cardiac cycle in 50 ms increments. Rather than trigger the data collections from the ECG, the data are collected continuously and the collection time relative to the ECG R-wave is recorded. Subsequently, the data are sorted into bins that correspond to progressive fractions of the cardiac cycle, each

made precise by interpolation of observed nearest pairs of k–t data at appropriate spatial frequencies, with respect to the requisite time delays after the R-wave. That approach enables coverage of the entire cardiac cycle uniformly. If the imaging is collected by setting a progressive delay after the R-wave as a trigger to acquisition (e.g. in increments of 50 ms), the results are fairly good, but late phases in the cardiac cycle are difficult to image because of variable cardiac cycle lengths. Expressing the portions of the cardiac cycle as fractions of each observed cardiac cycle lengths solves that problem. We obtain cine image series in two perpendicular long-axis views (e.g. 2L and 4L), each during an end-expiration breathhold. We ask the patient to hyperventilate for four breaths ('Deep breathe in, hard out, deep in, hard out, deep in, hard out') and then come to resting position ('Relax out. Don't move, don't breathe.'). End-expiratory breathhold provides a reproducible position of the diaphragm, and thus of the heart, which is essential. Examination of the resultant image series shows us the correct time delays for end-diastole (largest left-ventricular volume) and peak systole (smallest left-ventricular volume). For accuracy, we interpolate the timing for these two crucial moments: end-diastole, peak systole. Also, the two perpendicular thick-slice long-axis views determine the 3D tilt of the heart at end-diastole and at peak systole, important information for accurate measurements of wall thickness changes and radial wall motion.[10]

MR angiography

Many different MRI methods have been developed to examine arterial blood supply. In general, such methods take advantage of the fact that arterial blood moves and carries the magnetization of the blood with it. Imaging of arteries by magnetic resonance is called magnetic resonance angiography (MRA), a topic covered in Chapters 9 and 15. The usual approaches aim to produce signal from arteries and suppress signal from stationary tissues. That can be achieved by generating signal proportional to velocity along a series of magnetic field gradients, a technique known as phase contrast.[39] Another method relies on the use of an intravascular contrast agent to generate distinct magnetization characteristics for the blood, combined with imaging in a manner that generates signal only from the changed magnetization character, for example shortened T1 relaxivity.[40–44] The typical resolution of MRA is >0.5 mm, several times the diameter of the microvessels produced by angiogenesis. Thus, MRA is useful for identifying arterial obstructions responsible for tissue jeopardy, and may be useful to identify arteriogenesis and collaterals, but it cannot identify angiogenesis per se.

Base   Middle   Apex

Diastolic

Systolic

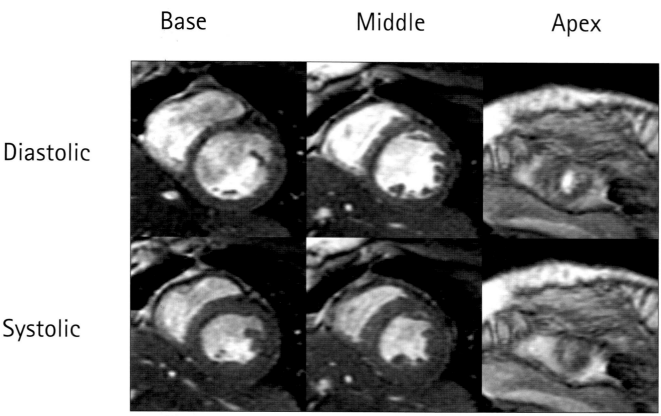

Figure 26.6
Short-axis cine (stack) view. A cine stack consists of a series of image frames in a particular view, repeated at different time delays, spanning the cardiac cycle. The images shown are a subset, showing the end-diastolic frame (maximal dilation of the heart) and the peak systolic frame (maximal contraction of the heart) at each of three short-axis levels from base to apex.
Left: Short-axis views near the base of the heart. Middle: Short-axis views at the middle level of the heart. Right: Short-axis views near the apex of the heart.

We apply two basic methods to assess changes in vascular development by MRA, especially for peripheral angiogenesis and arteriogenesis in ischemic limbs. First, by examining images perpendicular to the general direction of the major blood supply, the vascular volume fraction can be computed by tallying vascular signal area versus tissue area over a series of consecutive slices. Signal separability statistics[45] provide an objective means of performing this computation. Second, 3D MRA reconstructions are examined pairwise for qualitative assessment of changes, blinded to order and treatment, to identify marked increase, mild increase, no significant change, mild decrease, marked decrease. The latter assessment is performed independently by three different observers, with interactive control over 3D displays to enable detailed comparisons of comparable views with adjustable matched cut-away for regional inspection.

Delayed blood arrival

Although many MRI methods are described as methods of perfusion imaging, that is a convenient but inaccurate shorthand. Properly speaking, perfusion represents the bulk volume rate of movement of nutrient fluid through a tissue, whereas MRI generally examines the arrival of agents. Typically a blood-borne contrast agent increases the MRI signal from a contrast-labeled bolus of blood, and its arrival to tissue is marked by increased signal intensity in the region of interest.

Blood arrival is examined by injection of a contrast agent. Imaging the heart as a bolus of contrast agent arrives to the myocardium was first applied to computed tomography (CT) by Leon Axel[46] and then to MRI.[40,41,47–54] In MRI, the effect of contrast arrival on images depends on the contrast agent and the pulse sequence. Susceptibility contrast agents[55] and T2 contrast

Diastolic   # Systolic

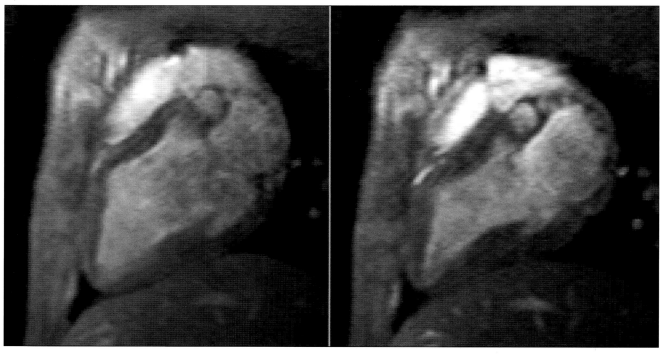

Figure 26.7
Long-axis views. Left: Diastolic long-axis view (3L). Right: Systolic long-axis view (3L). Long-axis views measure changes in tilt and motion of the base towards the apex, and are used for motion-tracked prescription of the true short-axis views for SMART measurements.

agents darken the surrounding tissue in T2*-sensitive imaging techniques (Figure 26.8), while T1 contrast agents brighten the adjacent tissue in T1-sensitive images (Figure 26.9). An important consideration for contrast MRI is the time required to image, which does not ordinarily allow imaging at every level of the heart for every heartbeat during a single injection. For that reason, we developed methods that improve the imaging time 20-fold. Simultaneously, we substantively improved the contrast effect for the time–intensity curves over the myocardium, by discriminate-orchestrated time series. These improvements may be applied to virtually any pulse sequence and any method of calculating perfusion. We have since evaluated multiple outcome measures and derived novel parameters for the assessment of local perfusion by MRI.

Investigation of the contrast arrival is facilitated by creating space–time maps (Figure 26.10) and time–intensity curves (Figure 26.11).[56,57] As illustrated in Figure 26.10, the image of the myocardium undergoes a virtual operation. Cutting the myocardium at the junction of the anterior two-thirds and posterior one-third of the septum reduces the left-ventricular myocardium in a short-axis view to a strip of muscle. That strip of muscle is effectively straightened by remapping its signal intensities to form a vertical slab, with endocardium to the left. Similar slabs from the diastolic images from consecutive heartbeats are placed next to each other in sequence to form a space–time map. Our software automates this, and maintains linkage to the original source images, such that pointing to any location brings up the corresponding image frame and marks the corresponding location in the wall of the heart in the original blood arrival image series. The space–time map is dark to the left and bright to the right, demonstrating contrast arrival. A zone of impaired blood delivery with delayed blood arrival is visually evident as persisting darkness indenting into the bright signal (Figures 26.9 and 26.10).

The half-height width of the indentation reports the spatial extent of the zone with impaired blood arrival. Infarctions have persisting impaired arrival, resulting in a dark band across the space–time map. The inverse of the delay is proportional to flow per gram of tissue.[56]

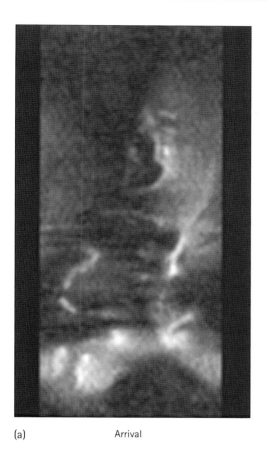

(a)   Arrival

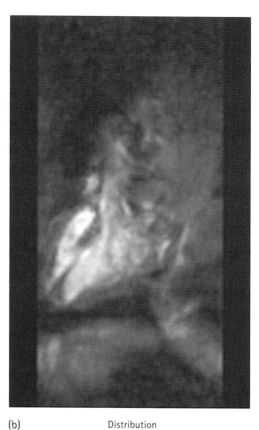

(b)   Distribution

Figure 26.8
T2*-MRI (EPI). Echo-planar imaging eliminates T1 contrast because all signal is fully recovered for the images. T2* contrast dominates. Image quality is low because the total data collection is fast (50 ms) and limiting. (a) The image at time of contrast arrival to the left ventricle shows black-out of the heart. (b) There is resolution of the heart black-out after contrast has distributed into tissue. (Reprinted from Pearlman et al. Radiology 2000; 214:801–7.[12])

First-pass fast MRI after bolus injection of intravenous contrast agent detects regional impairment of blood delivery to the myocardium[40,43,52,58–65] as the agent first passes through the circulation. Different approaches have been proposed for perfusion measures from contrast-enhanced MRI; however, none is established as a standard for perfusion-impairment detection. On a simple descriptive basis, first-pass perfusion has two phases: wash-in and wash-out (Figure 26.12). Uncleared blood-borne contrast agent recirculates and arrives in the left-ventricle on a second pass through the circulation. Thus a time–intensity curve (TIC, a graph of the time course of signal intensity changes due to passage of blood-borne contrast agent through the heart) can show a second peak after the wash-in phase.[43] Stenosis of a coronary artery grossly impairs both wash-in and wash-out from the affected myocardial region. Based on these observations, regional impairment of blood supply can be determined descriptively by examining signal intensity changes from different regions of interest (ROI) or by computing a map for each point in the myocardium showing blood arrival time, relative blood flow, or other measures derived from the TICs.[42,66] Conversion of data to concentration of agent coupled with mathematical

modeling offers physiologic parameters reporting what happens in more detail. Model-independent descriptive measures avoid assumptions but have numerous confounding factors and complex interpretation, whereas physiologic modeling offers potentially greater insight into the biological changes associated with the disease and response to treatment.

The delivery of contrast-labeled blood may be analyzed as the transfer of contrast agent between multiple compartments (e.g, right ventricle, left ventricle, large arterial vessels, myocardial microvessels, extracellular space, intracellular space, and veins). Each compartment has volume, transit times, and fractional turnover or exchange rates. Signal intensity bears a nonlinear relation to the concentration of contrast agent. Using T1-weighted imaging, one may estimate tissue relaxivities (R1 = 1/T1), which, after accounting for hematocrit and compartment effects, approximates a linear relation to the concentration of contrast agent.[44,67] That offers a substantive theoretical advantage toward converting observed signal to physiologically meaningful parameters, but there remain significant issues. Conversion of signal intensities to concentrations of the contrast agent requires knowing the hematocrit not just in large vessels but also in the

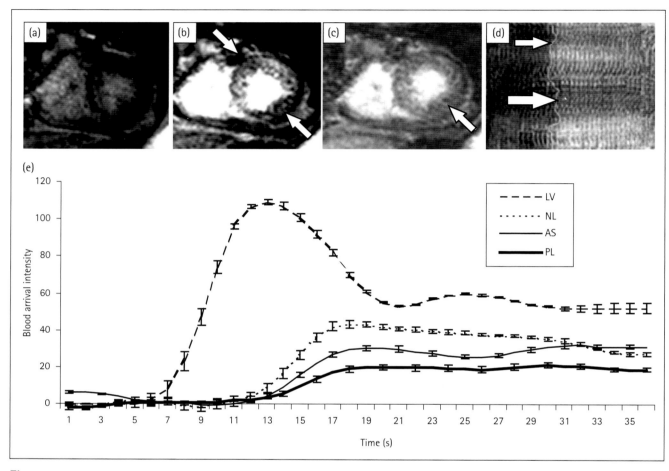

Figure 26.9

Perfusion-sensitive MRI. A series of images are obtained, one per heartbeat, in diastole, to observe the effects of a bolus of T1 contrast agent arriving in the myocardium. (a) Imaging at the time of zero-crossing of magnetization in the resting myocardium shows heart muscle as dark. (b) Imaging when contrast agent arrives in the myocardium under the same imaging conditions illuminates normal areas ahead of impaired areas. (c) Later, all perfused regions enhance. (d) Time–space map of myocardial strips from sequential heartbeats including the myocardium in (a–c) (see Figure 26.10 for an explanation). The top arrow corresponds to a small anteroseptal defect (delayed arrival), and the lower arrow corresponds to the posterolateral wall defect. (e) Time–intensity curves. The horizontal rows in the space–time map (d) correspond to time–intensity curves at different locations, reporting signal brightness versus time, which may be converted to contrast agent concentration versus time. LV, left ventricle, NL, normal wall; AS, anteroseptal defect; PL, posterolateral defect.

microcirculation. It also requires determination of the T1 relaxivity in different compartments. Simple use of FLASH to assess relaxivities can introduce 10–25% error.[44,68] With complex pulse sequences, there arises also a need to address different T1 dependences of different spatial frequencies. Also, one must consider the influence of timing in the method of observation on the net time–intensity curve. For example, a basic inversion recovery TurboFLASH sequence applies multiple low-tip excitations after the inversion pulse, each extracting a portion of the remaining longitudinal magnetization to generate gradient echoes for different phase modulations relating to spatial frequencies. As the acquisition pro-gresses, T1 recovery proceeds, so different phase-encoded spatial frequencies have differences in T1 contrast. Furthermore, accelerated imaging of a time series involves changes in timing of k-space components that also affect the T1 contrast. The hybrid technique[12,69] is based on differences in the relaxivity effects at different spatial frequencies. That method introduces the ability to adjust relaxivity sensitivity in relation to spatial frequency – a complexity that carries the substantive advantage of enabling reduction in signal from the left ventricle to avoid saturation, while enabling higher contrast in the myocardium. Such effects must also be examined with respect to converting signal changes to concentrations.

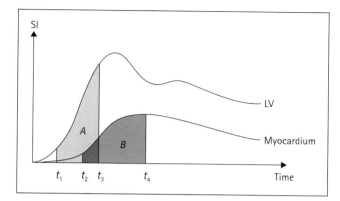

Figure 26.14

Equitime measure of perfusion. *A* is the area under the left-ventricular time–intensity curve from 10% to 90% of maximum (t_1 to t_3). *B* is the area under the time–intensity curve for a location of interest, integrated from 10% rise (t_2) until the area equals *A* (t_4). Then t_4-t_2, computed automatically, reports the arrival time of contrast-labeled blood.

produce inaccuracies, so it is beneficial to suppress blood pool signal by using dark-blood imaging, such as double inversion recovery. However, such measurements are flawed due to the fact that the apex approaches the base during the cardiac cycle, so the observed image plane does not represent the same muscle in both diastole and systole. The heart undergoes multiple complex motions summarized by the acronym STTART: shortening, thickening, twisting, accordian, rotation, and translation. Those issues are addressed by making SMART measurements.[10] Using SMART instead of fixed-plane measurements doubles the sensitivity to ischemic impairment.[92]

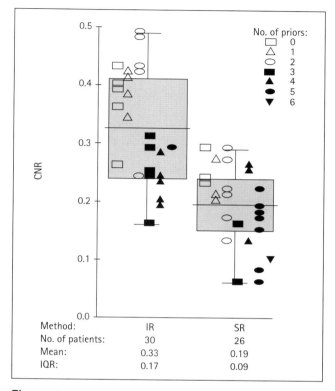

Method:	IR	SR
No. of patients:	30	26
Mean:	0.33	0.19
IQR:	0.17	0.09

Figure 26.15

Inversion recovery versus saturation recovery. This box-and-whisker plot shows that the contrast-to-noise ratio (CNR) is significantly higher for inversion recovery (IR) than for saturation recovery (SR): IR 33%, SR 19%, SE 3%, $p<0.001$. The order of performing IR versus SR was randomized, with sufficient time between for signals to return to baseline.

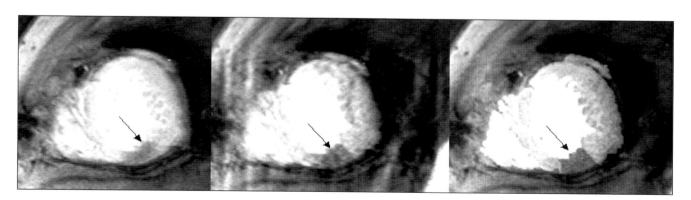

Keyhole   Dither   DOTS-M

Figure 26.16

Discriminant orchestrated time series (DOTS-M) versus keyhole and dither. Using only 12 lines of k-space per heartbeat, an inversion recovery T1-sensitive image obtained every heartbeat delineates a perfusion defect (arrow) better with DOTS-M. These methods differ in the pattern of k–t-space coverage, with keyhole obtaining high-frequency data only at the start of the series, and dither and DOTS-M distributing the coverage. Dither is similar to TRICKS. DOTS-M is optimized for contrast-to-noise ratio (CNR) of the defect.

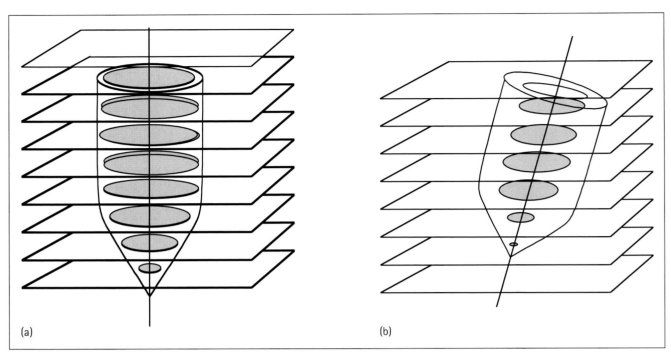

Figure 26.17
Serial motion assessment by reference tracking (SMART): tilt and length correction. (a) Alignment of short-axis image stack with the long axis of the left ventricle at end-diastole. (b) Motion from diastole to systole includes tilt, accordian, and other motions such that the diastolic prescriptions no longer match the corresponding parts of the heart. Accurate measurement of radial wall motion and wall thickening needs to account for these changes. Such correction is achieved by the SMART prescription so that systolic images correspond to the same portions of the heart as the diastolic images.

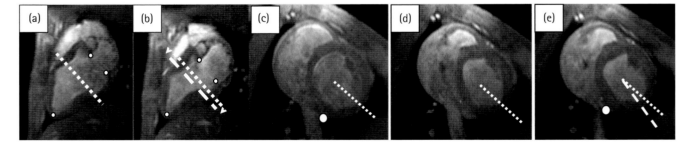

Figure 26.18
SMART measurements of wall thickness change and radial motion change. SMART accounts for various motions of myocardium that affect proper comparison of condition in diastole versus systole. (a) Long-axis L3 view at end-diastole, with a target level shown by the dotted line, the base by two points at the mitral hinge points, and the apex by a single dot. (b) View at peak systole. The base (two dots) has moved towards the apex (one dot), and the target level has moved down towards the apex, as indicated by the dashed line. (c) End-diastole with a dotted radial line to the center of the target region. (d) The same slice prescription, but at a different level of the heart at peak systole. (e) Tracked level (lower slice, centered on the target) at peak systole. In addition to shifting towards the apex, the heart has rotated and tilted, among other changes. The white dots mark the junction of right and left ventricles. The dotted lines mark the position of the radial through the center of the maximum perfusion deficit in diastole. The dashed line in (c) shows where the corresponding radial moved. SMART tracking accounts for these changes in position so that thickness and radial measurements correspond to the target tissue even though the target moved. Technique: TR/TE= 228/6.1 ms, 100 × 256 matrix, FOV=188 × 250 mm^2. (Reprinted from Pearlman et al. J Comput Assist Tomogr 2001; 25:558–62.[10])

Of the cine series, key frames are peak systole (maximal contraction) and end-diastole (maximal dilation). Accurate capture of peak systole may require interpolation from observed images followed by adjustment of timing. While motion tracking may be applied to an entire set of short-axis image slices spanning base to apex, we illustrate the concept by focusing on a particular target level, for example a level with dramatic flow impairment or greatest inducible ischemia. Using the SMART prescription, the out-of-plane motion and tilt of the target slice (translation, tilt, accordion) are determined from a pair of perpendicular long-axis views at end-diastole and at peak systole. The twist is determined by examining fiduciary markers within the target slice, for example anterior and posterior attachment points of right ventricle to left ventricle.[10] Alternatively, or in addition, slice selection may be performed immediately after the R-wave for both peak systolic and end-diastolic frames, with delayed image acquisition of the selected slice accommodating the subsequent out-of-plane motion and tilt of the selected slice.

Figures 26.19 and 26.20 compare SMART measurements with FIXED (nontracked) measurements of wall thickness and radial motion. The data were obtained using a porcine model of left circumflex chronic ischemia induced by Ameroid, resulting in impaired wall motion and wall thickening in the posterolateral wall.[10] SMART measurements identify twice the deficit in radial motion and twice the impairment in wall thickening as FIXED measurement. Thus, SMART measurements can double

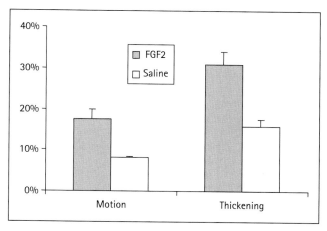

Figure 26.20
Wall motion and thickening three weeks after treatment, measured by SMART. The bar graph shows wall motion (left pair) and wall thickening (right pair). Within each pair, the left reports the response to FGF2, and the right reports the response to saline (control). The FGF2 elicited significantly better results in both measures of cardiac function.

the power to discern health from disease.[10] We then examined the ability to distinguish angiogenesis effect from placebo in a double-blinded analysis.[92] SMART clearly distinguished fibroblast growth factor 2 (FGF2) improvement of wall thickening and radial motion, where as FIXED did not. Thus, SMART measurements enable accurate detection of the functional benefits of angiogenesis.

The common measurements of local wall function are radial shortening and wall thickening. Radial shortening is the distance from centroid to endocardium at end-diastole minus the distance at peak systole, divided by the diastolic length. Radial thickening applies the same formula to wall thickness. The values are normalized to the resting condition to mitigate the influence of volume loading. Recall that the metabolically active component of the cardiac cycle is not contraction (systole) but rather relaxation (diastole). In principle, the relevant consequence of angiogenesis is wall thickness release, not wall thickening. More importantly, in all measurements, it is important to control noise. Noise propagation of a ratio is minimized by using the larger denominator ($f(x) = x/y$ propagates error by $df = \pm dx\, y^{-1} \pm xy^{-2}\, dy$). Therefore, the assessment of wall thickness change should include reporting the wall thickness release (change in tracked radial thickness divided by the systolic value).

The SMART methods of measurement also promote accurate volume measurements (end-diastolic volume (EDV), peak-systolic volume (PSV), and left-ventricular mass), and derived clinical values (stroke volume = EDV − PSV, cardiac output = stroke volume times heart rate, and ejection fraction = (EDV − PSV)/EDV). Examination of

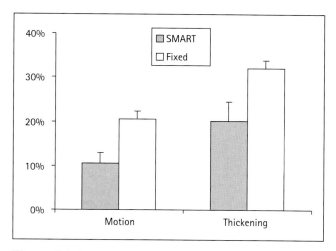

Figure 26.19
Wall motion and thickening for fixed versus SMART measurements. The bar graph shows motion (left pair) and thickening (right pair) from SMART measurements of ischemic myocardium (left bar of each pair) versus fixed-plane, fixed-radial measurements (right bar of each pair). SMART reports significantly lower values, providing a greater distinction from normal myocardium. (Reprinted from Pearlman et al. J Comput Assist Tomogr 2001; 25:558–62.[10])

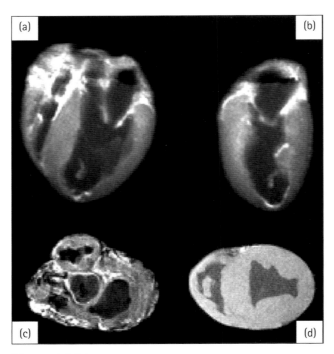

Figure 26.21

Agar casts for validation of accurate volume assessment. Fresh ex vivo hearts are filled with 5 g/dl molten agar under appropriate distending pressures. After imaging, the volume of agar is determined by weight and by displacement volumes after dissecting away the tissue. Custom software that corrects for partial-volume effects achieves <2% error for chamber volumes and muscle mass. (a) Long-axis image of a heart filled with 5 g/dl agar (L4). (b) Perpendicular long-axis image (L2). (c) Short-axis image at the level of the aortic valve. (d) Short-axis image halfway down the ventricle, at the base of the papillary muscles. Interior slice accounting (not recommended) would include (d) but none of (c). Partial-volume correction includes the partial contributions to the volume appropriately.

fresh ex vivo hearts casted full of agar (Figure 26.21) provided means to measure these volumes with an error under 2% by combining data from the biplane long-axis cine with short-axis cine stacks of contiguous 5 mm-thick short-axis slices spanning apex to base. The analysis takes into account changes in tilt, translation, accordian, and partial-volume corrections.[10]

Molecular MR imaging

Molecular imaging by MRI is a nascent technology that is not yet clinically applicable to angiogenesis studies. The basic idea is to combine molecular targeting by antibodies, peptidomimetics, or ligands with a source or modulator of MRI signal that can be amplified so that events on the molecular level can be identified at available imaging reso-

lution. Signal changes may identify location and/or amount of target per unit volume. For angiogenesis, suitable targets include the growth factor receptors that are upregulated in ischemic tissue, such as vascular endothelial growth factor (VEGF) receptors or a fibroblast growth factor receptor. Other relevant targets may include other cell surface proteins involved in angiogenesis signaling, such as α_v integrin,[93] syndecan-4,[94] and CD13.[95]

Contrast label

In view of concern that indiscriminant administration of growth factors can stimulate cancer growth, a number of researchers have investigated localized delivery.[16,96-98] Inclusion of an MRI contrast agent in the injectate can mark the region of injection. For example, if Magnevist or Omniscan are included in the injectate, then T1-sensitive imaging will delineate the area infused with injectate due to the T1-shortening effects of those agents that result in markedly increased MRI signal in T1-sensitive images. The localization will only be approximate if the contrast agent is not bound to the treatment agent, because it may have higher or lower dispersion into the tissue.

Collateral sensitive MRI (CS-MRI)

In the course of performing MRI for a preclinical angiogenesis study,[13] we encountered the case of the 'missing heart' (Figure 26.22). Evidently, the animal (a pig) had previously swallowed something that erased MRI signals from the abdomen and chest. We determined subsequently that the pig had ingested a magnetic beebee, a small sphere of metal 2 mm in diameter. Magnetic field lines emanating from that small source erased image-encoding information from the abdomen and heart. Removal of the beebee resolved the problem and we were able to complete the acute study. We reasoned that if a small source can erase signal from the entire chest, then similar field lines might be able to flag the presence of molecular targets or neovascular development too small to see directly. The idea is similar to an isolated soldier sending up a large flare, or setting a campfire – only our dark flare would consist of magnetic field disturbance due to the arrival of a contrast agent into a territory of sparse new microvessels.

Minimal detected spot size can be augmented by generating a dark flare of magnetic field disturbance that amplifies a microscopic target, making it visible at available image resolutions. In particular, the arrival of a magnetic susceptibility contrast agent to the microvessel products of angiogenesis nets a high magnetic field within

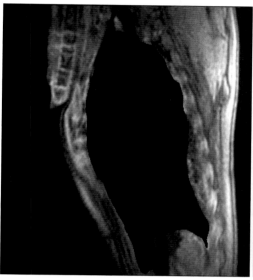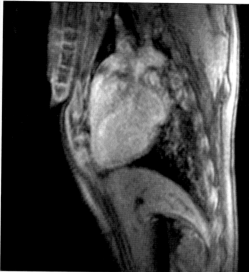

Figure 26.22
The case of the missing heart. In the course of a perfusion study on a pig, MRI failed to show the heart in the chest. A 2 mm magnetic beebee in the stomach blacked out the heart and upper abdomen. Removal of the beebee restored the heart. This observation stimulated thinking of how small targets such as neovascular microvessels can be identified even if the targets are smaller than the image resolution.

the sparse newly connected vascular elements and not between them. This inhomogeneity of magnetic field can be exploited to dephase magnetization vectors so that they oppose and cancel. This principle can also be applied to molecular imaging, identifying molecules expressed under specific conditions by generating a dark flare whose scope of influence is controlled by hybrid imaging.

We tested first the concept on a phantom that contained microtubules in a surrounding bath (Figure 26.23). We adjusted the T1 and T2 values with manganese and copper sulfate[99] in order to match those encountered in the heart and vessels, and observed a regional blackout marking arrival of contrast agent to the microvessels by T2* imaging (a method that causes blackout from magnetic field inhomogeneity). The distinction between regions of neovascular development and normal capillaries is based on the fact that the former engender sparse tubular elements that are not completely connected to rapid blood delivery, such that arrival of contrast creates a disparity of high magnetic field where the susceptibility effect of contrast increases magnetic field strength, and relatively low magnetic field where contrast agent is not rapidly delivered. The effect is ephemeral, vanishing when the contrast agent disperses on a unifrom basis in the tissue. At the moment of contrast arrival, and persisting for a second, there is a heterogeneous magnetic field strength when contrast agent arrives in a neovascular development zone. In a normal capillary bed, the contrast agent is delivered to the tissue and the blackout from marked heterogeneity of field strength is not seen.

Next we applied the T2* imaging by echo-planar imaging[18] to a porcine model of chronic ischemia known to activate angiogenesis (Figure 26.8). There was a notable blackout of the heart region when contrast agent (Gd-DPTA, Magnevist) filled the left ventricle, and after that

resolved we could briefly identify the region where angiogenesis was induced. Thus we had a partial success – angiogenesis could be detected as long as the blood arrival to that region proved sufficiently late that the left-ventricular blackout resolved first. That partial success was not satisfactory, because effective angiogenesis would, in principle, resolve delayed blood arrival, and mask itself in the blackout period.

The problem of blackout from the left-ventricular filling was solved by the invention of T2*, T1 spatial frequency hybrid imaging.[69] Noting that the left-ventricular filling occupies a large portion of the field of view, whereas neovascular blackout is confined to within the left-ventricular wall, which is less than a twentieth of the field of view, we determined that restriction of the T2* effect to positive and negative frequencies corresponding to the higher 1/16th of k-space would limit the blackout to neovascular zones within the left-ventricular wall and mitigate the blackout from left-ventricular filling. That approach proved successful.[69] Magnetization preparation using a 90°, –90° excitation pair reduces magnetization by T2*. Following the T2* preparation with Turbo-FLASH imaging[18] provides progressive T1 weighting. Ordering of the spatial frequencies (phase-encoding sequence positive and negative highest 1/16th first, then lowest in increasing order) leads to the desired T2*–T1 spatial frequency hybrid.

Contrast arrival to the left ventricle yields minimal effect (no blackout), but blackout within the heart wall (signal differences confined to high spatial frequencies) is preserved. Figures 26.24 and 26.25 show an early example of partial neovascular blackout, demonstrating that the ventricular blackout problem is solved. This enables one to identify neovascular blackout even while angiogenesis matures and the blackout transpires relatively soon after ventricular filling. Figure 26.26 shows that mild

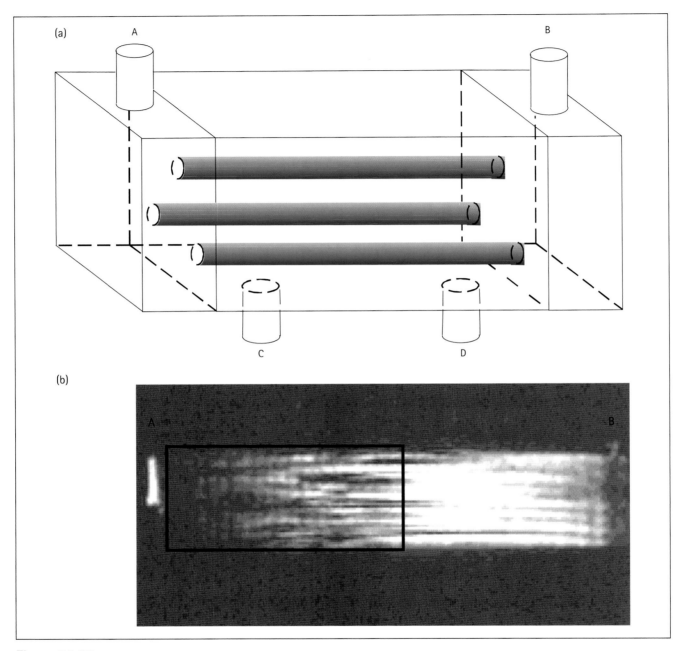

Figure 26.23

Phantom collateral neovascular-sensitive MRI (CS-MRI). (a) Microtubules in a dialysis filter provide a model for contrast arrival in microvessels. Contrast passes from port A to port B. Doped saline passed from port C to port D fills the tissue compartment with relaxivity appropriate for tissue. (b) As contrast enters the microtubules, there is an MRI blackout due to inhomogeneous magnetic fields producing dephasing that is most evident on T2*-weighted imaging. (Reprinted from Pearlman et al. Radiology 2000; 214:801–7.[12])

neovascular blackout also occurs following reduction in angina by transmyocardial laser, but the result is much more focal and limited. Following therapeutic angiogenesis over a longer period of time suggests that neovascular development following intracoronary administration of growth factors begins at the juncture of normal and ischemic tissue, and progresses inwards to cover the zone

with impaired blood delivery; and as neovascular development progresses, impaired blood delivery improves inwards in the same pattern (Figure 26.27).

To validate neovascular blackout as a marker of the location and extent of neovascular development, we examined microsphere distributions, X-ray angiography results, and histology. A most effective microsphere

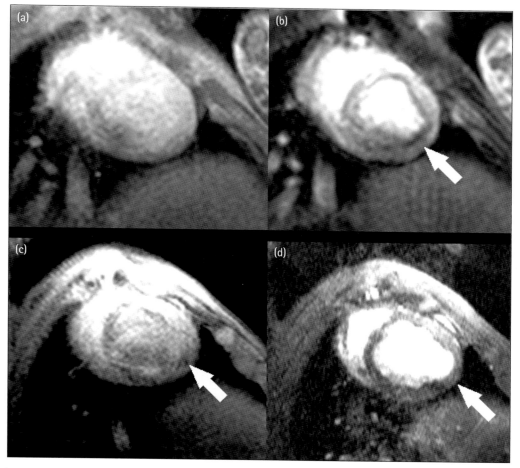

Figure 26.24

Collateral neovascular-sensitive MRI (CS-MRI) versus Delayed-arrival MRI (DA-MRI). (a) CS-MRI showing no evidence of neovascular development of a pig with an occluder on the left circumflex supply to the posterolateral wall. (b) Corresponding DA-MRI showing impaired blood delivery to the posterolateral wall, 12% of the myocardium; this defines the target region. (c) CS-MRI after pericardial FGF2, showing posterolateral neovascular development, 5% of the myocardium (arrow), in the center of the target region. (d) Corresponding DA-MRI showing improved blood delivery in the center of the defect, reducing the extent to 6%. This central effect of FGF2 is observed with pericardial delivery; with intracoronary delivery of growth factor, the CS-MRI response occurs at the outer borders of the target zone.

method for identifying angiogenesis is the shadow microsphere method,[100] which documents the location and extent of collateral-dependent myocardium. In this method, small particles are injected under different conditions: one in which blood distributes into the collateral-dependent myocardium and one in which flow into the collateral-dependent region happens to be inhibited. Microsphere distributions have a limited spatial accuracy, so, in addition, we developed a more precise method based on CT.[101] Submillimeter-resolution three-dimensional (3D) imaging is performed during a contrast agent injection in a contralateral artery in a heart that has the proximal left circumflex artery occluded. One condition has a high-pressure saline infusion in the cannulated left circumflex beyond the occlusion, to reduce the pressure gradient for collateral filling. The other condition has

no backpressure. This allows the contrast agent to become free, to follow collateral and microvascular channels and he delivered to the collateral-dependent myocardium. In order to generate an accurate image of the collateral-dependent myocardium, we developed an elastic match technique.[69,101,102]

Elastic Match compares two volumes to identify what is distinct, allowing for biological elastic shifts.[101,102] Contrasting contralateral contrast injection with backpressure to contralateral contrast injection without backpressure identifies the zone that fills from contralateral injection only without backpressure. By definition, that process identifies the collateral-dependent tissue (Figures 26.28 and 26.29). We later studied a series of animals in which chronic ischemia leads to collateral-dependent myocardium protected by angiogenesis.[12] We compared

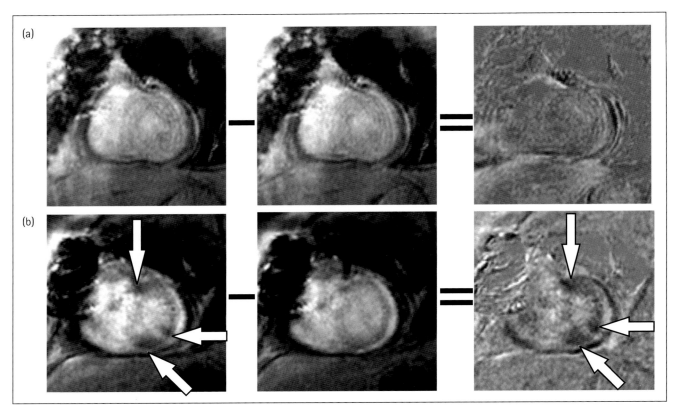

Figure 26.25
Collateral response to intracoronary FGF2 in a patient with a large posterolateral and small anteroseptal zones of inducible ischemia. (a) Collateral neovascular-sensitive MRI (CS-MRI) in a patient with chronic angina after bypass surgery, at peak contrast arrival (left), minus baseline (middle), shows no neovascular development zones (right). (b) CS-MRI 64 days after FGF2 treatment shows zones of neovascular development in the target zones. The larger posterolateral zone clearly shows that the neovascular development is occurring at the outer borders of the zone of inducible ischemia.

angiogenesis-sensitive MRI, in vivo, to Elastic Match, in the same set of animals, fresh ex vivo. There was excellent correspondence of the extent and location of angiogenesis localized blackout and collateral-dependent myocardium ($r = 0.90$; Figures 26.29 and 26.30). As an extra benefit, application of the Elastic Match method to electron-beam tomography data at rest and during arterial phase of a venous injection of iodinated contrast delineates coronary anatomy (Figure 26.31) as that which is different between the baseline volume data and the arterial phase data (aorta and vena cava are clipped out and the results are then 3D-rendered, superimposed on a simulated hologram of the resting data).

Metabolic markers: PCr, γ-ATP, pH

Protons (^{1}H) in a 1.5 T magnet respond selectively to radiowaves at 63.87 MHz. In the same magnet, examina-

tion at 25.88 MHz will identify MR responses from phosphorus-31 (^{31}P). While the signal strength from ^{31}P is not as strong as that from ^{1}H, it is quite informative because the relative concentrations of phosphocreatine (PCr), adenosine triphosphate (ATP), and inorganic phosphate (P$_i$) are readily discerned (Figure 26.32). The weaker signal is compensated by using larger volume elements and/or collecting data over multiple cardiac cycles, ECG-triggered for stroboscopic effect. Within every heartbeat, PCr becomes depleted and P$_i$ rises. We have studied the kinetics of PCr and P$_i$ recovery noninvasively by MR, and the recovery rates are highly sensitive to even mild ischemia. These different metabolites are distinguished by differences in the electron cloud density around the ^{31}P nuclei in these different chemical forms. Those differences result in shifts in the resonance frequency of just a few parts per million, but are readily identifiable with proper experimental design. We used a dual-tuned coil that picked up resonance signal both from ^{1}H and from ^{31}P. We used the ^{1}H signals to adjust magnetic field uniformity, image the heart, and identify regions of interest. We then colorized the myocardium based on regional

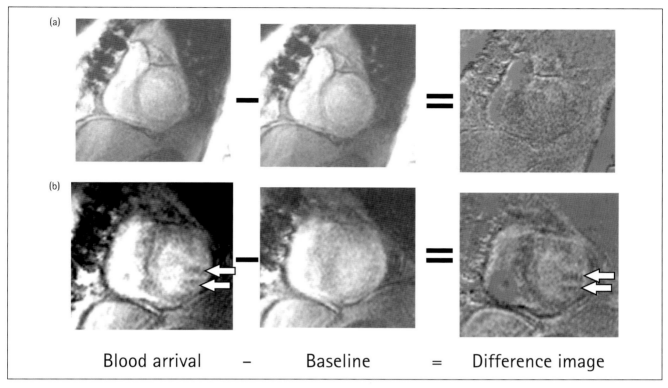

Blood arrival   –   Baseline   =   Difference image

Figure 26.26

Collateral neovascular-sensitive MRI (CS-MRI) before and after laser myocardial revascularization. (a) Prior to treatment, the baseline images show no dark flare of neovascular development. Subtraction of baseline from contrast arrival produces a difference image that makes the dark flare of neovascularization more conspicuous if present. (b) Thirty-six days after laser treatment, CS-MRI was repeated. The arrival image (left) and the subtracted image (right) show stripes of dark flare indicating focal neovascular development of limited scope.

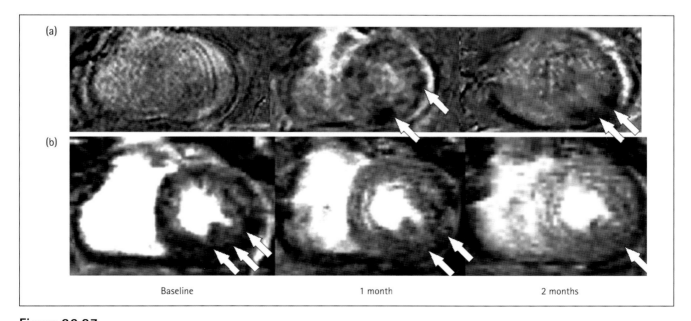

Baseline   1 month   2 months

Figure 26.27

Collateral neovascular-sensitive MRI (CS-MRI) dark flare predicts improved blood arrival. (a) CS-MRI shows no zones of neovascular development at baseline (left), large zones at the outer borders of a large posterolateral zone of inducible ischemia 1 month after treatment with FGF2 (middle), and migration of neovascular development to the center of the target zone at 2 months (right). (b) Delayed-arrival imaging (DA-MRI) shows a large posterolateral target zone at baseline (left), that is decreased at 1 month after treatment (middle), and further decreased at 2 months (right).

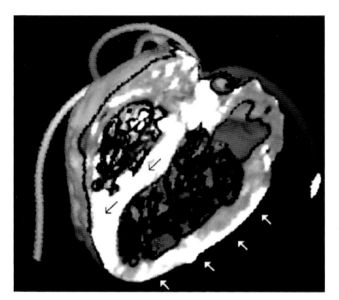

Figure 26.28
3D CT of collateralization. In a porcine model of chronic ischemia, an Ameroid occluder is placed on the proximal left circumflex coronary artery. The slow progressive occlusion allows time for collaterals to develop to protect myocardium distal to the occluder. After CS-MRI and DA-MRI, the heart was freshly excised, and the vessels were cannulated proximally and also distal to the occluder. Injection of contrast in the left anterior descending and right coronary arteries supplies contrast also to the posterolateral wall distal to the occluder, via collaterals, as shown above. By first imaging while infusing high-pressure (200 mmHg) saline distal to the occluder, a baseline volume image does not supply contrast agent to the collateral bed because the perfusion gradient is abolished. Elastic match of these two volumes identifies the collateral-dependent myocardium.

responses of ^{31}P subselected to identify PCr, the γ peak of ATP, and P_i. Saturation of blood pool was applied to suppress signal from 2,3-diphosphoglycerate in the blood. A resonance shift between PCr and P_i occurs that directly reports the intracellular pH. Due to a change in the dominant metabolic pathways, even mild ischemia results in a detectable pH shift, as well as a slowing of PCr and P_i recovery rates. Impaired ability to regenerate high-energy phosphates is a key component of the pathophysiology of myocardial stunning and hybernation. Evaluation of this ability directly tracks the linkage between angiogenesis and functional benefits. However, the ability to perform

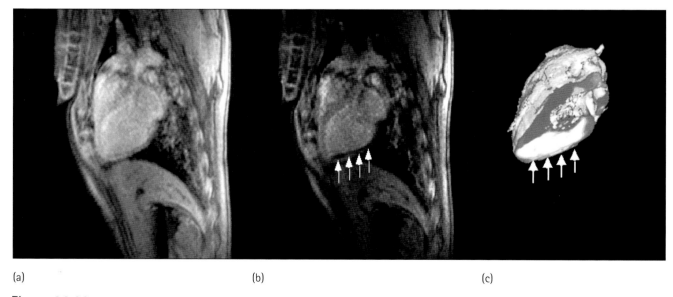

(a)   (b)   (c)

Figure 26.29
Comparison of collateral neovascular sensitive MRI (CS-MRI) with elastic match. (a) Baseline CS-MRI prior to contrast arrival. (b) CS-MRI at the time of contrast arrival shows a zone of neovascular development in the posterolateral wall of the heart (arrows). (c) Elastic match CT shows collateral-dependent myocardium in the same region. The location and extent of collateral-dependent myocardium agree well between CS-MRI in vivo and the elastic match CT fresh ex vivo (r=0.90, p<0.001). (Reprinted from Pearlman et al. Radiology 2000; 214:801–7.[12])

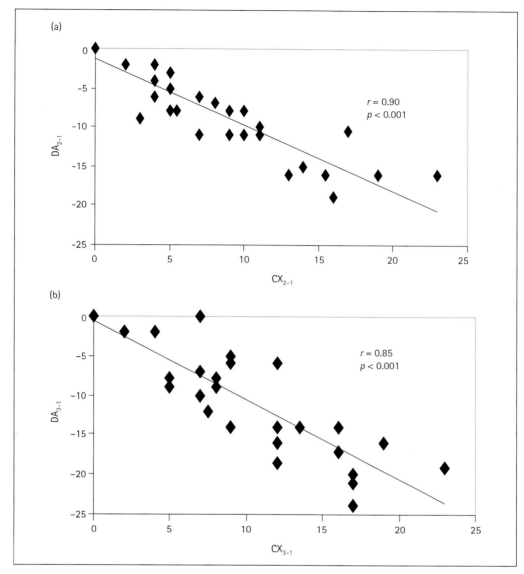

Figure 26.30

Changes in delayed arrival versus collateral extent. (a) The decrease in delayed arrival from the first visit (baseline) to the second (DA_{2-1}) is inversely related to the increase in collateral extent (CX_{2-1}). The Pearson correlation $r = -0.90$; $p<0.001$. (b) The change in delayed arrival from the first to third (60-day) visits (DA_{3-1} versus CX_{3-1}) is also inversely related to the concurrent change in collateral extent ($r = -0.85$; $p<0.001$).

^{1}H- and ^{31}P-MR with a dual-tuned coil is not widely available.

Conclusions

MRI is very adaptable, and offers methods for evaluation of every step of therapeutic angiogenesis, from vascular occlusion, to tissue jeopardy, to molecular upregulation and treatment delivery, through microvascular development and its consequences. A key advantage of such detailed investigation of angiogenesis is the ability to recognize a benefit that may not include abolition of inducible ischemia. Other advantages include mechanistic data and the ability to adjust therapy to individual needs.

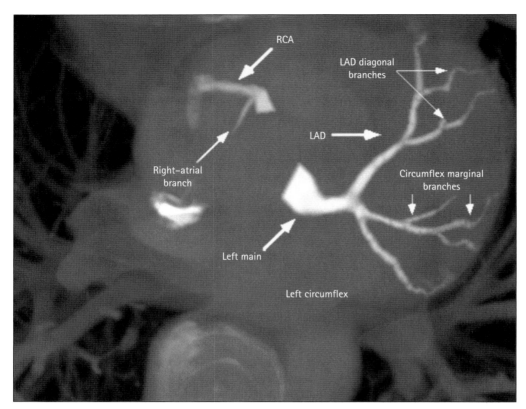

Figure 26.31
Elastic match automated coronary artery imaging. Elastic match automatically compares two volumes in order to identify what is distinct. Comparing a baseline volume with the arterial phase of contrast automatically identifies the arterial tree. The image shown here additionally used software to eliminate the aorta, solid-render the coronary arteries, and superimpose the results on a simulated hologram of the region for context.

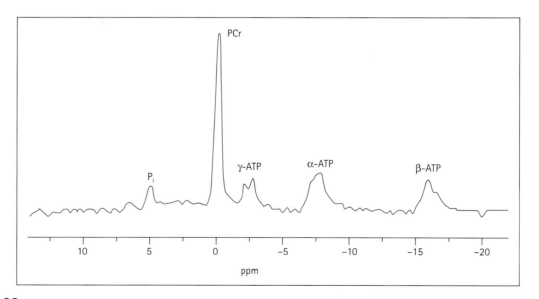

Figure 26.32
Phosphorus-31 magnetic resonance spectrum (^{31}P-MRS) from resting muscle. With exercise demand in excess of supply, the phosphocreatine peak (PCr) decreases and the inorganic phosphate (P$_i$) increases. The intracellular pH can be estimated from the relative distance between the P$_i$ and the PCr peaks. The selected volume from which signal is obtained must avoid blood pool, otherwise 2,3-diphosphoglycerate (DPG) would mask the γ-ATP resonance peak. A dual-tuned ^{1}H and ^{31}P coil was used, so that image data guided shimming and the selection of the volume of interest for MRS.

References

1. Ding X, Tkach J, Ruggieri P, et al. Improvement of spiral MRI with the measured *k*-space trajectory. J Magn Reson Imaging 1997; 7:938–40.

2. Bornert P, Aldefeld B, Eggers H. Reversed spiral MR imaging. Magn Reson Med 2000; 44:479–84.

3. Reese TG, Pearlman JD. MR gradient response modeling to ensure excitation coherence. J Magn Reson Imaging 1994; 4:569–76.

4. Mason GF, Harshbarger T, Hetherington HP, et al. A method to measure arbitrary *k*-space trajectories for rapid MR imaging. Magn Reson Med 1997; 38:492–6.

5. Pearlman JD, Wieczorek TJ. Relaxivity corrected response modulated excitation (RME): a T2-corrected technique achieving specified magnetization patterns from an RF pulse and a time-varying magnetic field. Magn Reson Med 1994; 32:388–95.

6. Pearlman JD, Moore JR, Lizak MJ. Real-time NMR beam-directed velocity mapping. V-mode NMR. Circulation 1992; 86:1433–8.

7. Pearlman JD, Hardy CJ, Cline HE. Continual NMR cardiography without gating: M-mode MR imaging. Radiology 1990; 175:369–73.

8. Brown MA, Semelka RC. MR imaging abbreviations, definitions, and descriptions: a review. Radiology 1999; 213:647–62.

9. Nitz WR. MR imaging: acronyms and clinical applications. Eur Radiol 1999; 9:979–97.

10. Pearlman JD, Gertz ZM, Wu Y, et al. Serial motion assessment by reference tracking (SMART): application to detection of local functional impact of chronic myocardial ischemia, J Comput Assist Tomogr 2001; 25:558–62.

11. Weissleder R, Mahmood U. Molecular imaging. Radiology 2001; 219:316–33.

12. Pearlman JD, Laham RJ, Simons M. Coronary angiogenesis: detection in vivo with MR imaging sensitive to collateral neocirculation – preliminary study in pigs. Radiology 2000; 214:801–7.

13. Sato K, Laham RJ, Pearlman JD, et al. Efficacy of intracoronary versus intravenous FGF-2 in a pig model of chronic myocardial ischemia. Ann Thorac Surg 2000; 70:2113–18.

14. Laham RJ, Chronos NA, Pike M, et al. Intracoronary basic fibroblast growth factor (FGF-2) in patients with severe ischemic heart disease: results of a phase I open-label dose escalation study. J Am Coll Cardiol 2000; 36:2132–9.

15. Laham RJ, Rezaee M, Post M, et al. Intrapericardial delivery of fibroblast growth factor-2 induces neovascularization in a porcine model of chronic myocardial ischemia. J Pharmacol Exp Ther 2000; 292:795–802.

16. Sellke FW, Laham RJ, Edelman ER, et al. Therapeutic angiogenesis with basic fibroblast growth factor: technique and early results. Ann Thorac Surg 1998; 65:1540–4.

17. Pearlman JD, Gao L, Wu Y, et al. Collateral-sensitive cardiac MRI shows a dose-dependent angiogenic response to fibroblast growth factor in the pig ameroid model. In: Proceedings of the Annual Scientific Section of the American Heart Association, Chicago. November 15–20, 2002.

18. Pearlman JD, Edelman RR. Ultrafast magnetic resonance imaging. Segmented turboflash, echo-planar, and real-time nuclear magnetic resonance. Radiol Clin North Am 1994; 32:593–612.

19. Semelka RC, Kelekis NL, Thomasson D, et al. HASTE MR imaging: description of technique and preliminary results in the abdomen. J Magn Reson Imaging 1996; 6:698–699.

20. Imura C. [HASTE: features and clinical applications]. Nippon Rinsho 1998; 56:2778–82.

21. Tang Y, Yamashita Y, Abe Y, et al. Experimental study on HASTE sequences: impacts of parameters on liver imaging. Comput Med Imaging Graph 1999; 23:227–34.

22. Pruessmann KP, Weiger M, Boesiger P. Sensitivity encoded cardiac MRI. J Cardiovasc Magn Reson 2001; 3:1–9.

23. Pruessmann KP, Weiger M, Bornert P, Boesiger P. Advances in sensitivity encoding with arbitrary *k*-space trajectories. Magn Reson Med 2001; 46:638–51.

24. Pruessmann KP, Weiger M, Scheidegger MB, Boesiger P. SENSE: sensitivity encoding for fast MRI. Magn Reson Med 1999; 42:952–62.

25. Weiger M, Pruessmann KP, Osterbauer R, et al. Sensitivity-encoded single-shot spiral imaging for reduced susceptibility artifacts in BOLD fMRI. Magn Reson Med 2002; 48:860–6.

26. Sodickson DK, McKenzie CA, Ohliger MA, et al. Recent advances in image reconstruction, coil sensitivity calibration, and coil array design for SMASH and generalized parallel MRI. Magma 2002; 13:158–63.

27. Sodickson DK, McKenzie CA. A generalized approach to parallel magnetic resonance imaging. Med Phys 2001; 28:1629–43.

28. Sodickson DK. Tailored SMASH image reconstructions for robust in vivo parallel MR imaging. Magn Reson Med 2000; 44:243–51.

29. Sodickson DK, Manning WJ. Simultaneous acquisition of spatial harmonics (SMASH): fast imaging with radiofrequency coil arrays. Magn Reson Med 1997; 38:591–603.

30. Sodickson DK, Griswold MA, Jakob PM, et al. Signal-to-noise ratio and signal-to-noise efficiency in SMASH imaging. Magn Reson Med 1999; 41:1009–22.

31. Sodickson DK, Griswold MA, Jakob PM. SMASH imaging. Magn Reson Imaging Clin North Am 1999; 7:237–54, vii–viii.

32. McKenzie CA, Yeh EN, Sodickson DK. Improved spatial harmonic selection for SMASH image reconstructions. Magn Reson Med 2001; 46:831–6.

33. Madore B, Pelc NJ. SMASH and SENSE: experimental and numerical comparisons. Magn Reson Med 2001; 45:1103–11.

34. Kellman P, Epstein FH, McVeigh ER. Adaptive sensitivity encoding incorporating temporal filtering (TSENSE). Magn Reson Med 2001; 45:846–52.

35. Larkman DJ, deSouza NM, Bydder M, Hajnal JV. An investigation into the use of sensitivity-encoded techniques to increase temporal resolution in dynamic contrast-enhanced breast imaging. J Magn Reson Imaging 2001; 14:329–35.

36. Larkman DJ, Hajnal JV, Herlihy AH, Coutts GA, et al. Use of multi-coil arrays for separation of signal from multiple slices simultaneously excited. J Magn Reson Imaging 2001; 13:313–17.

37. Madore B. Using UNFOLD to remove artifacts in parallel imaging and in partial-Fourier imaging. Magn Reson Med 2002; 48:493–501.

38. Madore B, Glover GH, Pelc NJ. Unaliasing by Fourier-encoding the overlaps using the temporal dimension (UNFOLD), applied to cardiac imaging and fMRI. Magn Reson Med 1999; 42:813–28.

39. Silverman JM, Raissi S, Tyszka JM, et al. Phase-contrast cine MR angiography detection of thoracic aortic dissection. Int J Card Imaging 2000; 16:461–70.

40. Atkinson DJ, Burstein D, Edelman RR. First-pass cardiac perfusion: evaluation with ultrafast MR imaging. Radiology 1990; 174:757–62.

41. van Rugge FP, Boreel JJ, van der Wall EE, et al. Cardiac first-pass and myocardial perfusion in normal subjects assessed by subsecond Gd-DTPA enhanced MR imaging. J Comput Assist Tomogr 1991; 15:959–65.

42. Canet E, Revel D, Forrat R, et al. Superparamagnetic iron oxide particles and positive enhancement for myocardial perfusion studies assessed by subsecond T1-weighted MRI. Magn Reson Imaging 1993; 11:1139–45.

43. Wilke N, Simm C, Zhang J, et al. Contrast-enhanced first pass myocardial perfusion imaging: correlation between myocardial blood flow in dogs at rest and during hyperemia. Magn Reson Med 1993; 29:485–97.

44. Cullen JH, Horsfield MA, Reek CR, et al. A myocardial perfusion reserve index in humans using first-pass contrast-enhanced magnetic resonance imaging. J Am Coll Cardiol 1999; 33:1386–94.

45. Pearlman J. Proposal of methods to tag harmlessly and transiently label myocardial segments during NMR imaging based on selective saturation and inversion recovery. Presentation at Johns Hopkins University, 1986.

46. Axel L. Tissue mean transit time from dynamic computed tomography by a simple deconvolution technique. Invest Radiol 1983; 18IS:94–9.

47. Chenevert TL, Pipe JG, Williams DM, Brunberg JA. Quantitative measurement of tissue perfusion and diffusion in vivo. Magn Reson Med 1991; 17:197–212.

48. van Rossum AC, Visser FC, Hofman MB, et al. Global left ventricular perfusion: noninvasive measurement with cine MR imaging and phase velocity mapping of coronary venous outflow. Radiology 1992; 182:685–91.

49. Walsh EG, Doyle M, Lawson MA, et al. Multislice first-pass myocardial perfusion imaging on a conventional clinical scanner. Magn Reson Med 1995; 34:39–47.

50. Williams DS, Grandis DJ, Zhang W, Koretsky AP. Magnetic resonance imaging of perfusion in the isolated rat heart using spin inversion of arterial water. Magn Reson Med 1993; 30:361–5.

51. Larsson HB, Fritz-Hansen T, Rostrup E, et al. Myocardial perfusion modeling using MRI. Magn Reson Med 1996; 35:716–26.

52. Lauerma K, Virtanen KS, Sipila LM, et al. Multislice MRI in assessment of myocardial perfusion in patients with single-vessel proximal left anterior descending coronary artery disease before and after revascularization. Circulation 1997; 96:2859–67.

53. Miller DD, Holmvang G, Gill JB, et al. MRI detection of myocardial perfusion changes by gadolinium-DTPA infusion during dipyridamole hyperemia. Magn Reson Med 1989; 10:246–55.

54. Schaefer S, van Tyen R, Saloner D. Evaluation of myocardial perfusion abnormalities with gadolinium-enhanced snapshot MR imaging in humans. Work in progress. Radiology 1992; 185:795–801.

55. Weisskoff R, Kiihne S. MRI susceptometry: image-based measurement of absolute susceptibility of MR contrast agents and human blood. Magn Reson Med 1992; 24:375–83.

56. Pearlman JD, Hibberd MG, Chuang ML, et al. Magnetic resonance mapping demonstrates benefits of VEGF-induced myocardial angiogenesis. Nat Med 1995; 1:1085–9.

57. Pearlman J, Yaseen Z. Multiplexed space–time maps for time-series data visualization: application to 4-D cardiac imaging, The International Society for Optical Engineering: Visual Data Exploration and Analysis V, San Jose, CA, January 26, 1998:3298–321.

58. Vallee JP, Sostman HD, MacFall JR, Coleman RE. Quantification of myocardial perfusion with MRI and exogenous contrast agents. Cardiology 1997; 88:90–105.

59. Vallee JP, Sostman HD, MacFall JR, et al. Quantification of myocardial perfusion by MRI after coronary occlusion. Magn Reson Med 1998; 40:287–97.

60. Vallee JP, Lazeyras F, Kasuboski L, et al. Quantification of myocardial perfusion with FAST sequence and Gd bolus in patients with normal cardiac function. J Magn Reson Imaging 1999; 9:197–203.

61. Miller DD, Johnston DL, Dragotakes D, et al. Effect of hyperosmotic mannitol on magnetic resonance relaxation parameters in reperfused canine myocardial infarction. Magn Reson Imaging 1989; 7:79–88.

62. Fritz-Hansen T, Rostrup E, Sondergaard L, et al. Capillary transfer constant of Gd-DTPA in the myocardium at rest and during vasodilation assessed by MRI. Magn Reson Med 1998; 40:922–9.

63. Fritz-Hansen T, Rostrup E, Ring PB, Larsson HB. Quantification of gadolinium-DTPA concentrations for different inversion times using an IR-turbo flash pulse sequence: a study on optimizing multislice perfusion imaging. Magn Reson Imaging 1998; 16:893–9.

64. Beache GM, Kulke SF, Kantor HL, et al. Imaging perfusion deficits in ischemic heart disease with susceptibility-enhanced T2-weighted MRI: preliminary human studies. Magn Reson Imaging 1998; 16:19–27.

65. Lima JA, Judd RM, Bazille A, et al. Regional heterogeneity of human myocardial infarcts demonstrated by contrast-enhanced MRI. Potential mechanisms. Circulation 1995; 92:1117–25.

66. Penzkofer H, Wintersperger BJ, Knez A, et al. Assessment of myocardial perfusion using multisection first-pass MRI and color-coded parameter maps: a comparison to ^{99m}Tc sestaMIBI SPECT and systolic myocardial wall thickening analysis. Magn Reson Imaging 1999; 17:161–70.

67. Kraitchman DL, Young AA, Bloomgarden DC, et al. Integrated MRI assessment of regional function and perfusion in canine myocardial infarction. Magn Reson Med 1998; 40:311–26.

68. Jivan A, Horsfield MA, Moody AR, Cherryman GR. Dynamic T1 measurement using snapshot-FLASH MRI. J Magn Reson 1997; 127:65–72.

69. Pearlman J. MRI imaging method and apparatus. US Patent No. 6,121,775 (September 19, 2000).

70. Rausch M, Scheffler K, Rudin M, Radu EW. Analysis of input functions from different arterial branches with gamma variate functions and cluster analysis for quantitative blood volume measurements. Magn Reson Imaging 2000; 18:1235–43.

71. Benner T, Heiland S, Erb G, et al. Accuracy of gamma-variate fits to concentration–time curves from dynamic susceptibility-contrast enhanced MRI: influence of time resolution, maximal signal drop and signal-to-noise. Magn Reson Imaging 1997; 15:307–17.

72. Machnig T, Koroneos A, Engels G, et al. [Quantitative evaluation of myocardial perfusion with ultrafast magnetic resonance tomography]. Z Kardiol 1994; 83:840–50.

73. Larson KB, Perman WH, Perlmutter JS, et al. Tracer-kinetic analysis for measuring regional cerebral blood flow by dynamic nuclear magnetic resonance imaging. J Theor Biol 1994; 170:1–14.

74. Larsson HB, Stubgaard M, Sondergaard L, Henriksen O. In vivo quantification of the unidirectional influx constant for Gd-DTPA diffusion across the myocardial capillaries with MR imaging. J Magn Reson Imaging 1994; 4:433–40.

75. Tofts PS. Modeling tracer kinetics in dynamic Gd-DTPA MR imaging. J Magn Reson Imaging 1997; 7:91–101.

76. Diesbourg LD, Prato FS, Wisenberg G, et al. Quantification of myocardial blood flow and extracellular volumes using a bolus injection of Gd-DTPA: kinetic modeling in canine ischemic disease. Magn Reson Med 1992; 23:239–53.

77. Bassingthwaighte JB, Sparks HV. Indicator dilution estimation of capillary endothelial transport. Annu Rev Physiol 1986; 48:321–34.

78. Bassingthwaighte JB, Knopp TJ, Anderson DU. Flow estimation by indicator dilution (bolus injection). Circ Res 1970; 27:277–91.

79. Bassingthwaighte JB, King RB, Sambrook JE, van Steenwyk B. Fractal analysis of blood–tissue exchange kinetics. Adv Exp Med Biol 1988; 222:15–23.

80. Bassingthwaighte JB, Ackerman FH. Mathematical linearity of circulatory transport. J Appl Physiol 1967; 22:879–88.

81. Bassingthwaighte JB. Physiology and theory of tracer washout techniques for the estimation of myocardial blood flow: flow estimation from tracer washout. Prog Cardiovasc Dis 1977; 20:165–89.

82. Sapirstein LA. The indicator fractionation technique for the study of regional blood flow. Gastroenterology 1967; 52:365–71.

83. Zierler KL. Equations for measuring blood flow by external monitoring of radioisotopes. Circ Res 1965; 16:309–21.

84. Kroll K, Wilke N, Jerosch-Herold M, et al. Modeling regional myocardial flows from residue functions of an intravascular indicator. Am J Physiol 1996; 271:H1643–55.

85. Qian H, Bassingthwaighte JB. A class of flow bifurcation models with lognormal distribution and fractal dispersion. J Theor Biol 2000; 205:261–8.

86. Beard DA, Bassingthwaighte JB. Advection and diffusion of substances in biological tissues with complex vascular networks. Ann Biomed Eng 2000; 28:253–68.

87. Beard DA, Bassingthwaighte JB. The fractal nature of myocardial blood flow emerges from a whole-organ model of arterial network. J Vasc Res 2000; 37:282–96.

88. Pearlman JD. Nuclear magnetic resonance spectral signatures of liquid crystals in human atheroma as basis for multi-dimensional digital imaging of atherosclerosis. PhD Dissertation, School of Engineering and Applied Science Thesis, University of Virginia. 1986

89. Akaike H. [Data analysis by statistical models]. No To Hattatsu 1992; 24:127–33.

90. Hanley JA, McNeil BJ. A method of comparing the areas under receiver operating characteristic curves derived from the same cases. Radiology 1983; 148:839–43.

91. Song HH. Analysis of correlated ROC areas in diagnostic testing. Biometrics 1997; 53:370–82.

92. Pearlman JD, Gao L, Leiner T, et al. Therapeutic angiogenesis induces regional functional changes in the myocardium detectable with serial motion assessment by reference tracking (SMART) MRI. Academy of Molecular Imaging, San Diego, CA, October 23–27, 2002.

93. Eliceiri BP, Cheresh DA. Role of α_v integrins during angiogenesis. Cancer J 2000; 6(Suppl 3):S245–9.

94. Simons M, Horowitz A. Syndecan-4-mediated signalling. Cell Signal 2001; 13:855–62.

95. Bhagwat SV, Lahdenranta J, Giordano R, et al. CD13/APN is activated by angiogenic signals and is essential for capillary tube formation. Blood 2001; 97:652–9.

96. Laham RJ, Sellke FW, Edelman ER, et al. Local perivascular delivery of basic fibroblast growth factor in patients undergoing coronary bypass surgery: results of a phase I randomized, double-blind, placebo-controlled trial. Circulation 1999; 100:1865–71.

97. Lee LY, Patel SR, Hackett NR, et al. Focal angiogen therapy using intramyocardial delivery of an adenovirus vector coding for vascular endothelial growth factor 121. Ann Thorac Surg 2000; 69:14–23; discussion 23–4.

98. Huwer H, Welter C, Ozbek C, et al. Simultaneous surgical revascularization and angiogenic gene therapy in diffuse coronary artery disease. Eur J Cardiothorac Surg 2001; 20:1128–34.

99. Mathur-De Vre R, Grimee R, Parmentier F, Binet J. The use of agar gel as a basic reference material for calibrating relaxation times and imaging parameters. Magn Reson Med 1985; 2:176–9.

100. Hirzel HO, Nelson GR, Sonnenblick EH, Kirk ES. Redistribution of collateral blood flow from necrotic to surviving myocardium following coronary occlusion in the dog. Circ Res 1976; 39:214–22.

101. Pearlman JD. Imaging apparatus and method with compensation for object motion. 1997.

102. Pearlman JD, Laham RJ, Simons M, et al. Extent of myocardial collateralization: determination with three-dimensional elastic-subtraction spiral CT. Acad Radiol 1997; 4:680–6.

27

Molecular imaging

Gregory M Lanza, Shelton D Caruthers, and Samuel A Wickline

Introduction

Advances in molecular and cell biology are unraveling the mysteries of the genome and creating new insights with extraordinary ramifications for diagnosis and therapy. These developments in molecular science are pushing the temporal detection horizon of medical diagnosis and therapy back from the anatomical sequellae of disease to its earliest physiological and biochemical manifestations. The emerging field of 'molecular imaging' has been variously defined and broadly envisioned by many investigators, and in general may be expressed as the in vivo diagnosis of complex pathological processes by detection of unique biochemical signatures.

Molecular imaging is being pursued in all arenas of noninvasive medical imaging, initially with nuclear and magnetic resonance imaging (MRI) approaches, and more recently with ultrasound and optical techniques. Each noninvasive modality has unique advantages and disadvantages and ultimately, the best approach is dependent upon the specific question being addressed. However, molecular imaging with MRI is emerging as a particularly advantageous modality, given its high spatial resolution and the unique opportunity to extract both anatomical and physiological information simultaneously. MRI molecular imaging agents have many forms, but most often are site-directed agents that specifically enhance the contrast from pathological tissue, which would otherwise be difficult to distinguish from surrounding normal tissue. Unlike blood pool agents (e.g. Gd-DTPA and MS-325), which highlight the entire vasculature and to varying extents the tissue interstitium, most ligand-targeted contrast agents seek to illuminate tissues expressing pathognomonic biomarkers. The concept is analogous to microscopic detection of specific epitopes with immunohistochemistry techniques translated into a complex and hostile in vivo environment and detected with noninvasive medical imaging systems. Assessment of molecular information in vivo requires high-affinity target-specific probes, a robust signal amplification strategy, and a sensitive high-resolution imaging modality.[1] These requirements are met through optimization of the image acquisition and process methods and by the development of sensitive and specific molecular contrast agents.

MRI issues

In addition to the issues of target specificity and biological barriers that a molecular imaging agent must overcome, MR detection of a bound contrast agent is a function of many factors, including the number of contrast units localized within a voxel, the paramagnetic influence of each unit of contrast, the local environment of the target, the magnetic field strength, and the voxel volume. In all instances, the net signal intensity for a given voxel equates to the summation of the magnetic signals derived from all tissues, the contrast agent, and other effects occurring within that imaging element. In simplistic terms, a weak contrast agent, such as a typical gadolinium blood pool agent, must occupy a large portion of the voxel to exert a significant influence on net signal intensity. At the opposite extreme, molecular imaging agents are bound to biomarkers in the nanomolar and picomolar concentration range. These agents must exert an enormous effect to overcome the partial volume dilution of the voxel. One approach is to use a susceptibility agent with wide-ranging effects, for example USPIO or MION. These agents elicit strong signal effects, which appear as dark or negative contrast. Against the proper background, such agents provide clear contrast and are very illustrative of disease. Another approach has been to develop 'ultraparamagnetic' nanoparticles, which exert a tremendous influence on T1-weighted images when bound to a target, usually due to high paramagnetic payloads. In the earlier years of MR molecular imaging, inability of targeted MR contrast agents to overcome partial-volume dilution effects led to numerous failures.[2]

Partial-volume effects can be addressed from the hardware perspective by utilizing smaller imaging voxels, which decrease signal dilution and increase molecular contrast influence (this assumes that the target is heterogeneously distributed and can be further localized into a smaller volume). However, this approach of reducing slice thickness or in-plane field of view (FOV) places increasing demands on the MR system. High-performance radio-frequency (RF) transmitters are required to achieve narrow-bandwidth excitation in concert with strong imaging gradients to reduce slice-selection thickness while maintaining short timing parameters. The increasing necessity for strong gradients is particularly evident when sampling FOV <3–5 cm with high spatial resolution. Reducing pixel volume to increase contrast-to-noise ratio (CNR) implies that location of the molecular imaging target is reasonably well defined within the patient a priori and that a coil sensitive to the target area or a strategy for controlling 'foldover' artifacts is available. Another common approach is to utilize three-dimensional (3D) acquisition techniques rather than 2D approaches to achieve thinner slices, again at the expense of longer scan times. Regardless of the approach, small voxels have inherently low signal-to-noise ratios (SNR), which translate into a need for longer scan times, better-optimized coils to avoid noisy images, or higher magnetic field strengths.

The commercial availability of higher-magnetic-field systems (3.0 T) is considered by many to be a boon to molecular imaging by allowing reduced voxel sizes and providing higher resolution images. Theoretically, SNR is directly related to the strength B_0 of the static magnetic field. However, these benefits may be mitigated by various factors[3] including: increased susceptibility artifacts, reduced T2*,[4] increased T1, RF field distortions,[5] and changed tissue dielectric constants or body dielectric resonances.[6] Unfortunately, these effects (e.g. T1 and T2* variations) are not constrained to a simple linear relationship across field strengths, and prediction of image quality is more difficult. An additional key advantage to higher field strength is the potential to utilize MR spectroscopy (MRS) in concert with imaging to confirm and quantify contrast delivery to a specific target site. Although spectroscopy is itself a form of molecular or physiological interrogation, its conjunctive use with proton MRI adds exciting potential for some molecular imaging contrast agents, in particular perfluorocarbon nanoparticle systems.

'Statistical' imaging techniques may be considered to improve image quality. BOLD imaging ('blood oxygenation level-dependent'), as an example, relies on the inherent difference in T2 signal between oxygenated and deoxygenated hemoglobin. In neurological applications, functional MRI has utilized this slight effect to register 5% or smaller changes within focal regions of the brain. BOLD imaging applications achieve these sensitive effects by robust postprocessing and statistical analysis of multiple images to designate where functional changes are occurring. Like BOLD imaging, molecular imaging may benefit from digital subtraction or other statistical techniques, which can accentuate subtle contrast effects. However, motion artifacts can diminish the utility of these approaches. In normal clinical imaging, 1 mm of motion may be inconsequential, but for molecular imaging applications, where in-plane voxel dimensions are 0.1–0.5 mm and the target tissue itself is only a few millimeters, subtle motion might create severe misregistration artifacts. To avoid ambiguity secondary to motion artifacts, robust image alignment techniques both in- and through-plane may be required to implement statistical molecular imaging strategies.

Contrast-targeting approaches

Contrast agents may accumulate at a pathological site by passive or active targeting mechanisms. Passive targeting systems take advantage of the body's inherent defense mechanisms to highlight phagocytic cells naturally responsible for particle clearance. Macrophages are among the most important components of the immune defense system and play a major role in clearance of particulate contrast media. These cells originate as premonocytes in bone marrow, circulate as monocytes, and localize to connective tissue (histiocytes), liver (Kupffer cells), lung (alveolar and intravascular macrophages), spleen and lymph nodes (free and fixed macrophages), bone (osteoclasts) and bone marrow, the peritoneum, and nerve tissue (microglia) creating the monocyte phagocytic system (MPS), also known as the reticuloendothelial system (RES). Phagocytosis by macrophages at all of these sites can occur, but typically particulate contrast agents are cleared from circulation by cells in the liver, spleen, and bone marrow.

On a molecular level, contrast clearance is facilitated by opsonization with blood proteins followed by macrophage uptake of these biologically tagged particles. Opsonins may be immune – immunoglobulins and complement proteins – or nonimmune serum factors, such as fibronectin or thrombus, which bind to foreign particles and promote phagocytosis.[7] In general, liver sequestration appears to be complement-mediated while the spleen removes foreign particulate matter via antibody Fc receptors.[8]

Active targeting refers to ligand-directed, site-specific accumulation of contrast and/or therapeutic agents. A wide variety of ligands, including antibodies, peptides, polysaccharides, aptamers, and drugs, may be utilized to target agents specifically to cellular biomarkers. These ligands may be attached covalently (direct conjugation) or noncovalently (indirect conjugation) to the contrast agent. In this chapter, focus has been placed upon ligand-directed targeting agents, and the reader is referred elsewhere for recent examples of passive targeting contrast research with USPIO.[9–12]

Ligand-coupling strategies

Avidin–biotin interactions

Avidin–biotin interactions are extremely useful, noncovalent targeting systems that have been incorporated into many biological and analytical systems and selected in vivo applications. Avidin has a high affinity for biotin (K_d ~10^{-15} M), facilitating rapid and stable binding under physiological conditions. Targeted contrast systems utilizing this approach are administered in two or three steps, depending on the targeting strategy. Typically, a biotinylated ligand, such as a monoclonal antibody, is administered first and 'pretargeted' to the unique molecular epitopes. Next, avidin is administered, which binds to the biotin moiety of the 'pretargeted' ligand. Finally, the biotinylated contrast agent (e.g. a nanoparticle), is added and binds to the unoccupied biotin-binding sites remaining on avidin, thereby completing the ligand–avidin–contrast 'sandwich'. The sequential avidin–biotin approach avoids accelerated, premature clearance of contrast agents by the MPS secondary to the presence of targeting antibody on its surface. Additionally, avidin, with four independent biotin-binding sites, provides signal amplification and improves detection sensitivity.

Sequential avidin–biotin strategies have been employed extensively for targeted imaging, particularly in the field of nuclear medicine,[13–15] with limited success for several reasons. First, the prerequisite multistep method is time-consuming and inconvenient to implement in a clinical environment. Next, endogenous biotin competes with the biotinylated ligand for avidin-binding sites, which must be compensated with a marked excess of avidin. Avidin and its natural analogues are immunogenic foreign proteins derived from egg white or bacterial sources that may have clinical implications, particularly when used repeatedly over time. Furthermore, avidin, a cationic macromolecule, rapidly binds and concentrates at anionic sites within the renal glomerulus basement membrane, forming in situ immunocomplexes.[16] Investigators often utilize streptavidin in vivo to avoid kidney sequestration. Avidin–biotin conjugation techniques are ideally suited for in vitro and limited in vivo contrast research. For robust clinical applications, a simpler, 'one-step' conjugated ligand system is preferred.

Avidin–biotin interactions may be used to create a 'one-step' system by performing the avidin–biotin conjugations in vitro prior to injection. Investigators have used this approach to successfully target vascular epitopes in vivo.[17,18] The key to this coupling mechanism is control of the polymerization rate of the ligand with contrast agent by the addition of exogenous free biotin. Free biotin is added in sufficient quantity to occupy approximately half of the avidin-binding sites, which slows the crosslinking reaction and reduces the formation of high-molecular-weight aggregates.

Covalent ligand coupling techniques

For in vivo use, targeting ligands are preferably attached chemically to the contrast agent by a variety of methods, depending upon the nature of the particle surface.[19] Conjugations may be performed before or after the particle is created, depending upon the ligand employed and its tolerance to the chemical processing conditions required. Direct chemical conjugation of ligands to proteinaceous agents often take advantage of numerous amino groups (e.g. lysine) inherently present within the surface. Alternatively, functionally active chemical groups, such as pyridyldithiopropionate, maleimide, amino or aldehyde, may be incorporated into the surface as chemical 'hooks' for ligand conjugation after the particles are formed. Another common postprocessing approach is to activate surface carboxylates with carbodiimide prior to ligand addition. The selected covalent linking strategy is primarily determined by the chemical nature of the ligand. Monoclonal antibodies and other large proteins may denature under harsh processing conditions, whereas the bioactivity of carbohydrates, short peptides, aptamers, drugs, or peptidomimetics can often be preserved. To ensure high ligand-binding integrity and maximize targeted particle avidity, flexible polymer spacer arms (e.g. polyethylene glycol or simple caproate bridges) can be inserted between an activated surface functional group and the targeting ligand. These extensions can be ≥10 nm and minimize interference of ligand binding by particle surface interactions.

Candidate ligands

Monoclonal antibodies and fragments

Rapid expansion of the monoclonal antibody industry has prepared the stage for the clinical success of site-targeted contrast agents by providing a plethora of ligands that can be directed against a wide spectrum of pathological molecular epitopes. Immunoglobin-γ (IgG) class monoclonal antibodies have been conjugated to particles to provide active, site-specific targeting. These proteins are symmetric glycoproteins (molecular weight ~150 kDa) composed of identical pairs of heavy and light chains. Hypervariable regions at the end of each of two arms provide identical antigen-binding domains. A variably sized branched carbohydrate domain is attached to complement-activating regions, and the hinge area contains particularly accessible interchain disulfide bonds that may be reduced to produce smaller fragments.

Bivalent $F(ab')_2$ and monovalent F(ab) fragments are derived from selective cleavage of the whole antibody by pepsin or papain digestion, respectively. Elimination of the Fc region greatly diminishes the immunogenicity of the molecule, diminishes nonspecific liver uptake secondary to bound carbohydrate, and reduces complement activation and resultant antibody-dependent cellular toxicity. Complement fixation and associated cellular cytotoxicity can be detrimental when the targeted site must be preserved or beneficial when recruitment of host killer cells and target cell destruction is desired (e.g. with antitumor agents).

Most monoclonal antibodies are of murine origin and are inherently immunogenic to varying extents in other species. Humanization of murine antibodies through genetic engineering has led to the development of chimeric ligands with improved biocompatibility and longer circulatory half-lives. The binding affinity of recombinant antibodies to targeted molecular epitopes can be occasionally improved with selective site-directed mutagenesis of the binding idiotype.

Phage display

Phage display techniques are now used to produce homing ligands against a large range of different antigens without involving antibody-producing animals. In general, cloning creates large genetic libraries of corresponding DNA (cDNA) chains deducted and synthesized by means of the enzyme reverse transcriptase from total messenger RNA (mRNA) of human B lymphocytes. Immunoglobulin cDNA chains are amplified by PCR (polymerase chain reaction), and light and heavy chains specific for a given antigen are introduced into a phagemid vector. Transfection of this phagemid vector into the appropriate bacteria results in the expression of numerous single-chain immunoglobulin fragments (scFv) or short peptide sequences on the surface of the bacteriophage. Bacteriophages expressing specific targeting fragments are selected by repeated immunoadsorption/phage multiplication cycles against desired antigens (e.g. proteins, peptides, nuclear acids, and sugars). Bacteriophages

strictly specific to the target antigen are introduced into an appropriate vector (e.g. *Escherichia coli* or yeast, cells) and amplified by fermentation to produce large amounts of targeting ligands. This technology has already permitted the production of unique ligands for targeting and therapeutic applications.[20–27]

Peptides

Peptides, like antibodies, may have high specificity and epitope affinity for use as vector molecules for targeted contrast agents. These may be small peptides (5–10 amino acids) specific for unique receptor sequences (e.g. the RGD epitope of the platelet GP IIbIIIa receptor)[28] or larger, biologically active hormones such as cholecystokinin.[29] Smaller peptides potentially have less inherent immunogenicity than antibodies and are more tolerant of chemical processing conditions.

Peptidomimetics

Peptidomimetics are small organic molecules, often ~1 kDa, which bind to targets with the affinity of an antibody. They have been frequently used in nuclear medicine conjugated to radionuclide chelates, but often fail for this application because their small size leads to rapid renal clearance. With falling serum concentrations, the targeted mimetics frequently dissociate from their target and the contrast signal fades. However, coupled to particles with prolonged circulatory half-lives, peptidomimetics may be among the best targeting moieties available. They are typically tolerant of chemical processing procedures and usually resistant to denaturation with terminal heat sterilization. Many new chemical entities developed within pharmaceutical companies, which fail to undergo complete therapeutic development for pharmacokinetic, bioavailability, or physical–chemical reasons, represent a potential treasure-trove of targeting ligands for molecular imaging applications.

Asialoglycoproteins and polysaccharides

Asialoglycoproteins (ASG) have been used for liver-specific applications due to their high affinity for ASG receptors located uniquely on hepatocytes.[30,31] ASG-directed agents (primarily MR agents conjugated to iron oxides) have been used to detect primary and secondary hepatic tumors as well as benign, diffuse liver diseases such as hepatitis.[32,33] The ASG receptor is highly abundant on hepatocytes (~500 000 per cell), rapidly internalizes, and is subsequently recycled to the cell surface. Polysaccharides such as arabinogalactan may also be utilized to localize contrast agents to hepatic targets. Arabinogalactan has multiple terminal arabinose groups that display high affinity for ASG hepatic receptors.[31,34]

Aptamers

Aptamers are high-affinity, high-specificity RNA- or DNA-based ligands produced by in vitro selection experiments (SELEX: systematic evolution of ligands by exponential enrichment).[34] They are generated from random sequences of 20–30 nucleotides, selectively screened by absorption to molecular antigens or cells, and enriched to purify specific high-affinity binding ligands. To enhance in vivo stability and utility, aptamers are generally chemically modified to impair nuclease digestion and to facilitate conjugation with drugs, labels, or particles. Other, simpler chemical bridges often substitute nucleic acids not specifically involved in the ligand interaction. In solution, aptamers are unstructured, but can fold and enwrap target epitopes, providing specific recognition. The unique folding of the nucleic acids around the epitope affords discriminatory intermolecular contacts through hydrogen bonding, electrostatic interaction, stacking, and shape complementarity. In comparison with protein-based ligands, aptamers are stable, are more conducive to heat sterilization, and have lower immunogenicity. Aptamers are currently used to target a number of clinically relevant pathologies, including angiogenesis,[35] activated platelets,[36] and solid tumors,[37] and their use is increasing. The clinical effectiveness of aptamers as targeting ligands for particles may be dependent upon the impact of the negative surface charge imparted by nucleic acid phosphate groups on contrast clearance rates. Previous research with lipid-based particles suggest that negative zeta potentials markedly decrease liposome circulatory half-life, whereas neutral or cationic particles have similar, longer systemic persistence.

Targeting valency

The concept of agent valency is very important to the efficacy and utility of targeted contrast agents. Valency, in this context, refers to the number of binding sites each unit of contrast agent presents for target interaction. In the case of an IgG antibody, the valency is 2 whereas its F(ab) fragment has a valency of 1. The functional combination of ligand valency and binding affinity is often referred to as avidity, or, in conceptual terms, its 'stick and stay' quality. The higher the avidity of a contrast agent for its target, the more rapidly and tenaciously the agent will bind to the intended biomarker(s).

Extending this concept are the terms 'multivalency' and 'polyvalency'. Although both terms are sometimes used interchangeably within the literature, 'multivalency' usually refers to an agent presenting many binding moieties specific for the same biochemical epitope. A natural example of this is an IgM immunoglobulin, a pentamer construct with 10 identical binding sites. This class of immunoglobulin can have high affinity (i.e. the dissociation constant K_d, of each binding region) and high avidity (i.e. the propensity for multiple binding sites of the IgM to interact with the target tissue).

The term 'polyvalency' is frequently used to refer to contrast designs that bear ligands with specificities towards multiple epitopes (e.g. a particle bearing ligands for two different cell surface adhesion molecules). Polyvalency, like multivalency, can increase avidity, but may be most usefully employed to increase contrast sequestration at target tissues when the concentration of a single biomarker is too low. Polyvalent systems inherently have a greater propensity for nonspecific targeting, and their effectiveness can be dependent upon the relative spatial distribution of the epitopes.

Polyvalency may also be achieved by combining single or multivalent contrast agents into a composite system. Targeting of multiple epitopes increases the total payload of magnetic label deliverable to a given site, which increases the total signal and improves detectability. However, polyvalency applied in this manner may also be used to allow noninvasive molecular phenotyping by formulating each agent to have a distinguishable MR signature. For example, a mixture of targeted perfluorocarbon nanoparticles (see the next section) that incorporate different perfluorocarbon cores (e.g. perfluorodecalin or perfluorooctyl bromide) could be distinguished in vivo with high-field MRS by their unique fluorine-19 (^{19}F) signatures (Figure 27.1). Deconvolution of these ^{19}F-MR spectra could provide the relative ratio of two biomarkers within the sampling voxel. In theory, this approach could be extended to several perfluorocarbons, allowing several epitopes to be detected and quantified. Molecular phenotyping may be utilized to diagnose and stage disease, characterize and segment patient populations for risk or therapeutic stratification, or provide a metric for longitudinally assessing disease progression or treatment efficacy.

Contrast agent platforms

Molecular imaging with MRI has until recently been fraught with over a decade of failure. Partial-volume

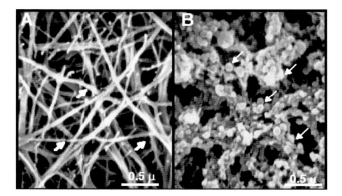

Figure 27.1
Scanning electron micrographs (30 000 ×) of a control fibrin clot (A) and fibrin-targeted paramagnetic nanoparticles bound to the clot surface (B). Thick arrows indicate fibrin fibrils. Thin arrows indicate fibrin-specific nanoparticle-bound fibrin epitopes. (Reprinted from Flacke et al. Circulation 2001; 104:1280–5[55] with permission from Lippincott Williams & Wilkins.)

dilution, inherent in MRI, mandates robust cellular amplification strategies for sensitive detection. These amplification strategies may be chemically mediated through contrast agent design or biologically implemented through contrast–cellular interactions.

Monoclonal antibody-based systems

Initially, target-specific contrast agents evolved from the coupling of a magnetic label (i.e. paramagnetic lanthanides and superparamagnetic iron oxides) to an antibody. This approach to MR molecular imaging was analogous to prior efforts in nuclear medicine. Nuclear medicine efforts benefited from high sensitivity but were often plagued by low spatial resolution and poor target-to-background ratios. The converse was true for MRI, which provided higher spatial resolution and tomographic imaging but lower contrast signal sensitivity due to partial-volume dilution effects. Antibodies conjugated to 2–4 gadolinium chelates provided inadequate signal when interrogated at physiological biomarker concentrations and density. Coupling of antibodies or other proteins to superparamagnetic agents was better, but produced a negative contrast signal (e.g. CCK-MION), and has not been widely adopted for general clinical use.[29]

The success of any targeted MR contrast agent design is highly dependent upon solution of the signal amplification issue. Molecular epitopes expressed at nanomolar or picomolar concentrations must be detected at clinical imaging field strengths within voxels optimistically sized between 2.0×10^7 μm^3 and 5.0×10^9 μm^3. As a result, the most successful examples of targeted MR agents to date involve nanoparticulates with high paramagnetic or superparamagnetic properties. Examples of nanoparticulate constructs include liposomes, dendrimers, emulsions, polymerics, and recently fullerenes. The particulate nature of these platforms provides a natural scaffold to couple targeting ligands, which provide the 'molecular zip-codes' to deliver the agent to the desired site. Macromolecular contrast agent constructs may be sterically inhibited from free access to biochemical epitopes deep within the parenchyma of target organs or even within cells. However, for specific targets expressed on the luminal aspect of vascular endothelium in a variety of important diseases, for example inflammation (i.e. rheumatoid arthritis or atherosclerosis), angiogenesis (i.e. neoplasia, atherosclerosis, ischemic diseases, or wound-healing), or thrombosis (i.e. unstable angina, stroke, or pulmonary embolism), nanoparticulate agents have demonstrated great potential.

Liposomes

Liposomes are vesicles in which an aqueous volume is entirely enclosed by a bilayer membrane(s) composed of lipid molecules, which is in principle identical to the lipid portion of natural cell membranes. Univesicular liposomes entrap the aqueous medium within a single bilayer membrane, whereas multivesicular liposomes feature multilayered membranes organized concentrically (i.e. 'onion-like') or heterogeneously within an encapsulating membrane envelope. Interest in liposomes as MR contrast agents was propelled by a need to amplify target signal and overcome partial-volume dilution effects at the pathological area of interest.

Initially, liposomes were used to entrap gadolinium chelates, (e.g. Gd-DTPA) and increase chelate concentration in the pathological area.[38,39] However, the limited diffusive permeability to water molecules of stabilized lipid vesicles with entrapped paramagnetic solute ions greatly diminished the effectiveness of such formulations, particularly those constructs incorporating cholesterol for increased bilayer rigidity and in vivo survival.[40–42] Subsequently, investigators explored the incorporation of amphipathic paramagnetic chelates into the lipid bilayer membrane of liposomes,[43–45] which provided improved relaxivity relative to entrapment. However, at least 50% of the amphipathic chelate was incorporated into the internal leaflet of the bilayer membranes and remained poorly accessible to water. Increasing liposome vesicle size as a means to increase signal did not further improve the relaxivity of particles.[46,47] Nevertheless, liposomal particles bearing metal chelates on the membrane surfaces have had success as MR contrast agents.

In early work reported by Sipkins et al,[17] an $\alpha_v\beta_3$-targeted paramagnetic polymerized liposome was employed to detect angiogenesis in the Vx-2 tumor model 24 hours after injection. Paramagnetic Gd-DTPA complexed to lipid monomers was spontaneously intercalated into the self-assembly bilayer.[48] A unique feature of this liposomal construct was the use of ultraviolet polymerization to stabilize the lipid bilayer membrane from rapid in vivo destruction. The targeting ligand, a monoclonal antibody, was coupled to the polymerized vesicle through avidin–biotin interactions.

Perfluorocarbon nanoparticulate emulsions

Emulsion technology is very old, and distinct from the more modern liposome systems. Emulsions are heterogeneous systems, consisting of at least one immiscible liquid intimately dispersed in another in the form of droplets, whose diameters, in general, exceed 0.1 μm. The prolonged stability of such systems is mediated through the addition of surface-active components, the most common being phospholipids for targeted agents. The dispersed or internal phase consists of finely divided droplets, whereas the continuous or external phase forms the matrix in which these droplets are suspended.

Liquid perfluorocarbon emulsions are specialized formulations with various medical applications, most notably oxygen transport or 'artificial blood'. Paramagnetic perfluorocarbon emulsions for intravenous administration have an average particle size of ~0.2–0.3 μm. A novel ligand-targeted, lipid-encapsulated, liquid perfluorocarbon emulsion useful across the medical imaging spectrum (i.e. ultrasound, MR, and nuclear imaging applications) has been demonstrated for MR molecular imaging, and provides an excellent illustration of the concepts presented within this chapter.

The perfluorocarbon emulsion, produced through microfluidization techniques, is robustly stable to handling, pressure, atmospheric exposure, heat, and shear. During early phases of this research, biotinylated ligands were coupled to a biotinylated nanoparticle through avidin–biotin interactions either in vivo[49] or prior to injection.[18] Subsequently, a covalent ligand conjugation approach using monoclonal antibodies, F(ab) fragments,[50] or peptidomimetics[51–53] was adopted to facilitate future clinical implementations.

All targeted contrast agents must have appropriate pharmacokinetics, which are affected by many factors, including surface chemistry, in vivo stability, and size. Perfluorocarbon nanoparticle distribution and clearance data fit well into a biexponential function with an esti-mated circulatory half-life in excess of 1 hour. Moreover, preliminary data suggest that these nanoparticles persist bound to tissues for hours, and (depending upon location and perfluorocarbon composition) even days.[54]

The effectiveness of perfluorocarbon nanoparticles as a molecular imaging platform reflects their capacity to transport enormous paramagnetic payloads to target sites.[55] Rather than the 2–4 gadolinium ions that might be transported with an antibody or peptide, perfluorocarbon nanoparticles can deliver 50 000–90 000 gadolinium ions with each bound particle – and all of these paramagnetic ions are positioned along the outer particle interface in contact with the aqueous external phase.

The classic description of relaxivity, calculated with respect to the absolute Gd-DTPA concentration, is typically used for blood pool agents. However, for targeted paramagnetic agents, which depend upon the payload of gadolinium delivered to each molecular epitope bound, a relaxation rate may be estimated relative to units of contrast agent and referred to as the particulate or molecular relaxivity. Nanoparticle particulate relaxivities were calculated, and increased up to 0.54 s^{-1} $pmol^{-1}$ for formulations with >50 000 Gd^{3+}/particle.[55]

We have discovered that the position of gadolinium relative to the particle surface can dramatically influence the nanoparticle molecular relaxivity. Substitution of one form of lipophilic chelate (e.g. Gd-DTPA bisoleate, Gd-DTPA-BOA) with another (e.g. Gd-DTPA phosphatidylethanolamine, Gd-DTPA-PE) that chemically positions the Gd-DTPA moiety slightly beyond the lipid surface more than doubled the molecular relaxivity of the nanoparticles. The relaxivity of paramagnetic contrast agents is well known to depend upon the effective correlation time τ_c, a composite function of the rotational correlation time τ_r, the electron spin relaxation time τ_s, and the water exchange time τ_M, with the overall effect being dominated by the fastest process. The rotational correlation time of lipid particles is reported to be independent of size from 50 to 400 nm, minimizing any relaxivity effects attributable to the small differences in the particle size. Temperature-dependent relaxivities, obtained at 3°C and 37°C with field cycling relaxometry, suggest that closer proton–gadolinium interaction was achieved with the Gd-DTPA-PE nanoparticle, which was in part responsible for marked increases in ionic and molecular relaxivities.[56]

Although the size of nanoparticulates may limit access to intracellular or parenchymal sites, vascular targets offer a rich field of opportunity for these molecular imaging agents. Paramagnetic perfluorocarbon nanoparticles have been employed for molecular imaging of important vascular epitopes, including fibrin (i.e. thrombosis) and integrins (i.e. angiogenesis). For example, fibrin, a prevalent component of thrombus, is a biochemical signature of ruptured atherosclerotic plaques, which are well recognized as the thromboembolic source of unstable angina, myocardial infarction, transient ischemic attacks, and stroke.[57] Early detection of rupturing atherosclerotic plaques in arteries with modest 40–60% stenosis[58] remains diagnostically elusive despite the use of routine angiography or duplex ultrasound techniques. Recent studies reveal a window of opportunity extending from days to months in which to intercede and prevent the progression of vulnerable plaque rupture and microthrombus formation to more serious clinical sequelae.[59]

Fibrin-targeted nanoparticles

Sensitive molecular imaging and detection of microthrombi along the intimal surface of vulnerable plaques require a high-avidity, target-specific probe with robust signal amplification compatible with a sensitive high-resolution imaging modality. Scanning electron micrographs of clots exposed to control and fibrin-targeted nanoparticles reveal nanoparticles densely and specifically adhered to the fibrin fibrils along the clot surface, with each bound complex delivering tens of thousands of gadolinium atoms (Figure 27.1). MRI demon-

strates the significant contrast enhancement produced by the fibrin-specific nanoparticles targeted to human plasma clots in vitro at a clinically relevant field strength (1.5 T Intera CV, Philips Medical Systems, Best, Netherlands). Using a typical low-resolution clinical imaging protocol, the fibrin clots targeted with nanoparticles provide homogeneous T1-weighted contrast enhancement that improves with increasing gadolinium level (0, 2.5 and 20 mol% Gd^{3+}, i.e. as a percentage of the encapsulating lipid monolayer) (Figure 27.2A). However, higher-resolution MRI (Figure 27.2B) and scanning electron microscopy (Figure 27.1) indicated that the nanoparticles are present only as a thin layer bound to the outer surface of the dense fibrin clot. The large number of nanoparticles bound in conjunction with the high payloads of gadolinium each carries overcome the partial-volume, signal-dilution effect of the low-resolution voxel and appear as an area completely filled with signal.

The magnitude of contrast enhancement expected in vivo under open circulation conditions was evaluated in dogs. Control or antifibrin paramagnetic nanoparticles were targeted to thrombus created within the external jugular vein (Figure 27.3A). Phase-contrast angiography showed that the clots produced obstructing flow deficits

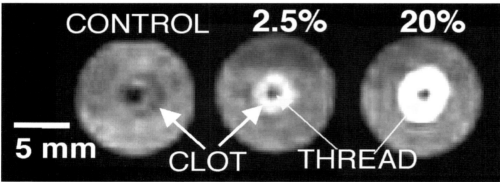

(a)

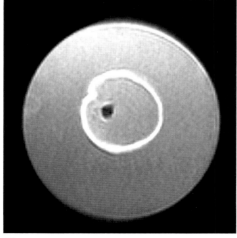

(b) (c)

Figure 27.2
(A) Low-resolution images (3D GRASE) of fibrin clots targeted with nanoparticles presenting a homogeneous, T1-weighted enhancement that improves with increasing gadolinium level (0, 2.5, and 20 mol%). (B) High-resolution scans of fibrin clots (3D T1-weighted gradient recalled echo sequence) revealing thin layer of nanoparticles along the surface. (C) Histogram of signal intensity across the high-resolution fibrin clot scan. (Modified and reprinted from Flacke et al. Circulation. 2001; 104:1280–5[55] with permission from Lippincott Williams & Wilkins).

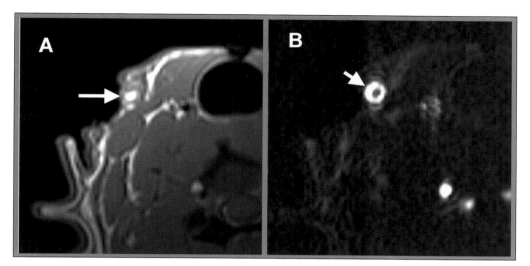

Figure 27.3
(A) Thrombi in the external jugular vein targeted with fibrin-specific paramagnetic nanoparticles demonstrating dramatic T1-weighted contrast enhancement in the gradient-echo image (arrow). (B) Flow deficit (arrow) of thrombus in the corresponding phase-contrast image (3D phase-contrast angiogram). (Modified and reprinted from Flacke et al. Circulation 2001; 104:1280–5[55] with permission from Lippincott Williams & Wilkins).

in both external jugular veins (Figure 27.3B). Fibrin-specific paramagnetic nanoparticles markedly enhanced the detectability of thrombus relative to control when imaged with a 3D T1-weighted, fat-suppressed, fast gradient-echo sequence (GRASE). Corresponding gradient-echo images revealed a selective enhancement of the treated clot yielding a signal intensity (1780 ± 327) that was higher than the bright fat signal (1360 ± 140), whereas the control clot had a signal intensity (815 ± 41) that was similar to that of the adjacent muscle (768 ± 47). On T1-weighted gradient recalled echo images with fat suppression, the targeted clot showed the brightest image signal. The CNR between the targeted clot and blood using paramagnetic nanoparticles measured with this sequence was $\sim 118 \pm 21$. The CNR between the targeted clot and the control clot was 131 ± 37.

As a further conceptual example, carotid artery endarterectomy specimens from a symptomatic patient was exposed to either targeted or control paramagnetic nanoparticles and imaged with a T1-weighted, GRASE sequence similar to that used in the canine experiments (Figure 27.4). The enhancement of the small fibrin deposits along the ruptured 'shoulders' of the carotid plaque treated with targeted paramagnetic nanoparticles was readily apparent, in contradistinction to control specimens. Similar direct molecular imaging of intimal fibrin deposition in a patient with moderate carotid stenosis may one day prompt acute surgical or interventional therapy.

Molecular imaging of angiogenesis

Detection of angiogenesis and its therapy are of key interest to scientists and physicians involved with cardiovascular, oncological and rheumatological disease. One molecular signature, $\alpha_v\beta_3$-integrin[60–64] has attracted significant interest for angiogenic targeting applications. $\alpha_v\beta_3$-Integrin is expressed on activated endothelial cells, but not on mature quiescent cells. We have developed and employed an $\alpha_v\beta_3$-integrin-targeted nanoparticle to detect angiogenic endothelium with a clinical 1.5 T MRI scanner (Intera CV, Philips Medical Systems, Best, Netherlands). The sensitivity and specificity of this agent was demonstrated in New Zealand White rabbits bearing Vx-2 tumors implanted into the hindlimb. Dynamic T1-weighted MRI was used to spatially and temporally determine nanoparticle deposition within the tumor and

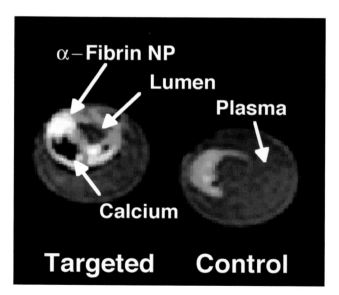

Figure 27.4
Color-enhanced MR images (3D fat-suppressed, T1-weighted fast gradient-echo) of fibrin-targeted and control carotid endarterectomy specimens revealing contrast enhancement (white) of a small fibrin deposit on a symptomatic ruptured plaque. A calcium deposit appears black. (Reprinted from Flacke et al. Circulation. 2001; 104:1280–5[55] with permission from Lippincott Williams & Wilkins).

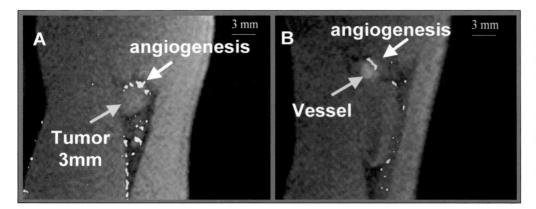

Figure 27.5
(A) T1-weighted, fat-suppressed baseline image of a 3 mm Vx-2 tumor with overlay of regions of contrast enhancement at 2 h (yellow pixels). (B) T1-weighted, fat-suppressed baseline image of a large vein adjacent to the Vx-2 tumor with overlay of regions of contrast enhancement at 2 h (yellow pixels).

adjacent skeletal muscle. The $\alpha_v\beta_3$-integrin was observed by MRI in an asymmetrical distribution along the outer tumor capsule (Figure 27.5A), within connective tissue interface between tumor and muscle, and within the adventitia of neighboring vessels (Figure 27.5B). Two hours post injection, $\alpha_v\beta_3$-targeted nanoparticles enhanced MR signal in the tumor by 126%, which was 56% greater than the enhancement produced by neovascular leakage alone. In vivo competition studies confirmed the specificity of the $\alpha_v\beta_3$-targeted paramagnetic agent, decreasing the signal enhancement by more than 50%. Hindlimb muscle did not enhance with either the $\alpha_v\beta_3$-targeted or the nontargeted agents. Immuno-histochemistry of $\alpha_v\beta_3$-integrin corroborated the extent and asymmetrical distribution of neovascularity observed by MRI (Figure 27.6).

In a similar study, $\alpha_v\beta_3$-integrin-targeted or control nanoparticles were administered by jugular vein injection into athymic mice subcutaneously implanted with human melanoma (C-32, ATCC) over the left flank or right inguinal area. Mice 12 days post tumor implantation received $\alpha_v\beta_3$-targeted or control nanoparticles and were

MR-imaged at 1.5 T (Intera CV) using a T1-weighted, fat-suppressed, 3D spoiled gradient-echo technique (TR/TE/α = 46/6.5/65°), a standard 5 cm diameter circular surface coil, with ~10 min acquisition times. The in-plane image resolution was 200 μm, with a 500 μm slice thickness and 55 mm FOV.

Native angiogenesis was detected with $\alpha_v\beta_3$-targeted nanoparticles along tumor borders with muscle, fat, and skin. The angiogenic vasculature was visually enhanced by the paramagnetic nanoparticles bound to $\alpha_v\beta_3$-integrin in 30 min and became progressively more prominent through 120 min (Figure 27.7). At 120 min post injection, $\alpha_v\beta_3$-targeted nanoparticles increased MR signal from tumor angiogenic vasculature by 177%, which was 82% greater than the nontargeted nanoparticle control ($p<0.05$). Surrounding muscle tissue showed no significant change in signal intensity with either targeted or nontargeted nanoparticles. As noted for the Vx-2 tumor studies, histology correlated well with MRI. Molecular imaging of natural $\alpha_v\beta_3$-integrin expression by proliferating mouse endothelial cells within the ~100 μm connective tissue tumor capsule reflects the dramatic

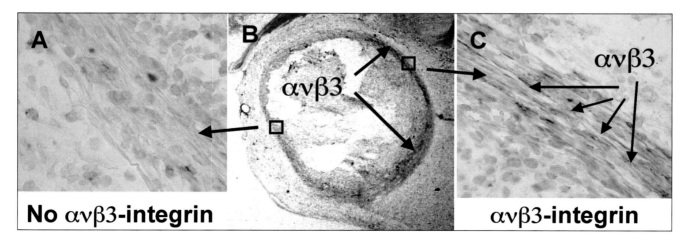

Figure 27.6
A 3 mm Vx-2 tumor with asymmetrically distributed peripheral angiogenesis. This tumor histology corresponds to the MRI images in Figure 27.5.

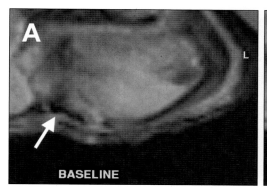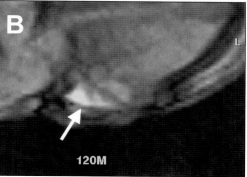

Figure 27.7
High-resolution MR images of a 2 mm human melanoma xenograft implanted into athymic nude mouse flank at baseline (A) and 120 min after intravenous injection of $\alpha_v\beta_3$-targeted paramagnetic nanoparticles (B).

paramagnetic impact of the nanoparticles, i.e. particulate relaxivity $>10^6$ s^{-1} mM^{-1}. Molecular imaging data such as these may one day provide important metrics in the early detection of atherosclerosis or cancer, the characterization and segmentation of patient populations for antiangiogenic therapies, or as a sensitive means to longitudinally follow the effectiveness of treatments.

RGD-USPIO

Ultrasmall superparamagnetic iron oxide (USPIO) particles have been used to detect GP IIbIIIa receptors present on platelets in thrombi in vitro and in vivo.[65] In these experiments, an RGD peptide (i.e. a cyclic arginine–glycine–aspartic acid) was coupled to the surface carbohydrate of the USPIO (partially oxidized to the aldehyde with sodium periodate) via an oxime linkage (RGD–USPIO). T1-weighted imaging of targeted clots was per-

formed at 1.5 T on a Gyroscan ACS-NT system (Philips Medical Systems, Best, Netherlands), using spoiled 3D gradient-echo sequences at varying in-plane spatial resolutions.

Thrombus targeting with RGD–USPIO was studied in vitro and in vivo. In vitro, whole human blood clots created around glass tubes were targeted with RGD-USPIO at 1.0 mM Fe or comparable levels of nontargeted USPIO. Imaging was performed using an 80 mm surface coil with graduated in-plane resolutions (0.31×0.31, 0.62×0.62, and 1.25×1.25 mm^2). Other scan parameters included TR/TE/α = 29/2.7/35° and a slice thickness of 1 mm (Figure 27.8). In vivo, clots were induced in the jugular veins of domestic pigs, and RGD–USPIO (1.0 mM Fe) was administered. Imaging was performed 5 hours post injection (when the background signal in blood returned to baseline values), with saturation slabs to eliminate in-flow effects, a 22 mm surface coil, and graduated in-plane resolutions, TR/TE/α = 35/8/35°, and a slice thickness of 0.8 mm (Figure 27.9).

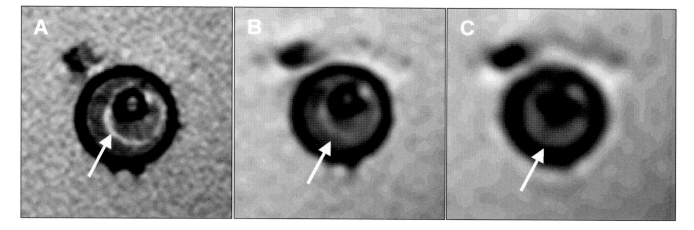

0.31 x 0.31 mm²   0.62 x 0.62 mm²   1.25 x 1.25 mm²

Figure 27.8
T1-weighted image of a phantom containing clots exposed to 1.0 mM RGD–USPIO at varying in-plane resolutions. The dark circular object with a white center is the hollow glass tube plus glass fiber filter.

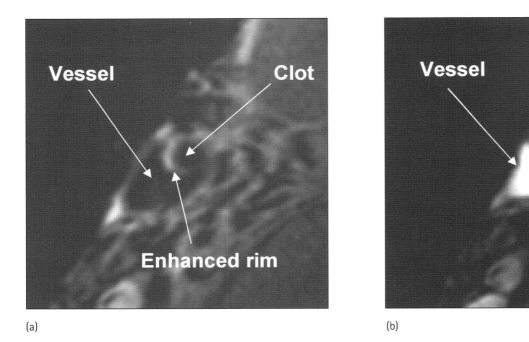

(a)   (b)

Figure 27.9
Black–blood (A) and bright–blood (B) T1-weighted images of jugular vein thrombi targeted in vivo with RGD–USPIO.

The contrast-enhanced clots were well visualized under ideal imaging conditions, but thrombus detection sensitivity diminished rapidly with decreasing spatial resolution (Figure 27.10). Maximum contrast and SNR were achieved with an in-plane resolution of 0.2 × 0.2 mm.[2] Further increases in resolution caused a significant reduction in SNR, illustrating the tradeoffs discussed earlier (see the section above on 'MRI issues'). These investigators also noted confounding the effect of physiological motion, which limits spatial resolution to the magnitude of the motion during the acquisition period.

Tat-CLIO

Peptides with membrane translocating properties include Tat peptides from the HIV Tat protein, polyarginyl peptides, and penetrin (the third helix homeodomain of antennapedia). Wunderbaldinger et al[66] have shown that the attachment of Tat peptides to a superparamagnetic iron oxide known as Tat–CLIO (Tat-crosslinked iron oxide) facilitates the intracellular accumulation of iron oxide and makes cells detectable by MRI.[67] Uses of Tat–CLIO, a prominent T2 contrast agent, include label-

T1w bright-blood   T1w black-blood

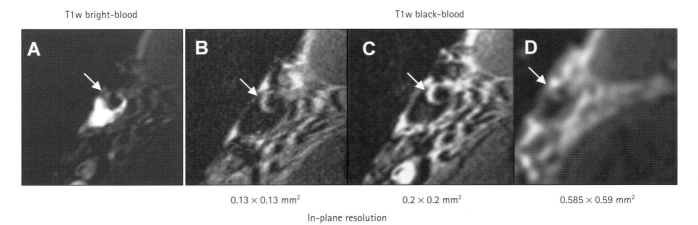

0.13 × 0.13 mm²   0.2 × 0.2 mm²   0.585 × 0.59 mm²
In-plane resolution

Figure 27.10
(A) Bright-blood T1-weighted image of jugular vein thrombi targeted in vivo with RGD–USPIO. (B–D) Effect of increasing resolution on clot visualization in vivo. Sequence parameters (except for in-plane resolution) were constant for all three images.

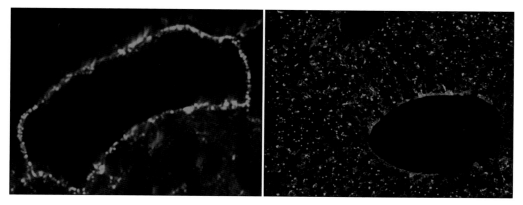

Figure 27.11
Fluorescence microscopy of livers of mice injected with amino-CLIO (A) and Tat–CLIO (B). Note that the fluorescent staining of amino-CLIO is restricted to the perivascular cuff, while Tat–CLIO has a marked intraparenchymal distribution.

ing stem cells homing to bone marrow[68] and labeling T cells homing to the spleen.[69] These topics of cell tracking represent an emerging area of interest by these and other investigators,[70] which are introduced here for the reader but which are beyond the scope of this chapter.

Tat–CLIO has been used in vivo to target the hepatic parenchyma in contradistinction with two other iron oxide nanoparticles, MION-47 and amino-CLIO. Amino-CLIO is synthesized by crosslinking MION-47 in strong base followed by a reaction with ammonia to provide primary amino groups.[67] Tat–CLIO (modified with a fluorescent marker) is formed through a stable thioether linkage between Tat peptide (i.e. GRKKRRQR-RRGYK(FITC)C-NH$_2$) and amino-CLIO.

Fluorescence microscopy of rat liver, following injection of Tat–CLIO or amino-CLIO, reveals that amino-CLIO concentrates, like other nanoparticles, along the hepatic vessels in endothelial cells and/or Kupffer cells, whereas Tat-CLIO is found in numerous discrete foci throughout the parenchyma and is notably absent around blood vessels (Figure 27.11). These data suggest that Tat peptides may be used to channel ligand-directed magnetic contrast agents from the vascular compartment, through cells surrounding blood vessels, and into a parenchymal distribution. Coupling Tat peptides to ligand-directed magnetic nanoparticles may allow nanoparticles to deliver high therapeutic or genetic payloads specifically to nuclei.

Conclusions

Targeted contrast agents take several physical forms, and can accomplish site-directed imaging or therapy by a variety of active and passive mechanisms. Ligand-targeted particles provide the opportunity to detect the expression of pathognomonic cell-surface molecular signatures

present in nano- or picomolar quantities. These agents have been conceptually demonstrated to improve the diagnosis of early atherosclerosis, vulnerable plaques, intracardiac thrombus, and angiogenesis, and could be studied in clinical trials for these applications within the next few years. Although not fully addressed here, the particulate nature of these agents creates an ideal platform for targeted drug delivery of steroids, antineoplastics, and oligonucleotides with the opportunity for rational therapeutic dosing, a feature unique to drug delivery coupled with molecular imaging.[66,71] Molecular imaging, possibly in conjunction with rational targeted therapies, will likely change the future of clinical medicine as these technologies continue to mature.

References

1. Weissleder R. Molecular imaging: exploring the next frontier. Radiology 1999; 212:609–614.

2. Gupta H, Weissleder R. Targeted contrast agents in MR imaging. Magn Reson Imaging Clin North Am 1996; 4:171–84.

3. Wen H, Denison TJ, Singerman RW, Balaban RS. The intrinsic signal-to-noise ratio in human cardiac imaging at 1.5, 3, and 4 T. J Magn Reson 1997; 125:65–71.

4. Noeske R, Seifert F, Rhein KH, Rinneberg H. Human cardiac imaging at 3 T using phased array coils. Magn Reson Med 2000; 44:978–82.

5. Dougherty L, Connick TJ, Mizsei G. Cardiac imaging at 4 tesla. Magn Reson Med 2001; 45:176–8.

6. Wen H, Jaffer FA, Denison TJ, et al. The evaluation of dielectric resonators containing H$_2$O or D$_2$O as RF coils for high-field MR imaging and spectroscopy. J Magn Reson 1996; 110:117–23.

7. Moghimi S, Patel H. Serum opsonins and phagocytosis of saturated and unsaturated phospholipid liposomes. Biochim Biophys Acta 1989; 984:384–7.

8. Moghimi S, Patel H. Differential properties of organ-specific serum opsonins for liver and spleen macrophages. Biochim Biophys Acta 1989; 984:379–83.

9. Schmitz S, Taupitz M, Wagner S, et al. Iron-oxide-enhanced magnetic resonance imaging of atherosclerotic plaques: postmortem analysis of accuracy, inter-observer agreement, and pitfalls. Invest Radiol 2002; 37:405–11.

10. Sigal R, Vogl T, Casselman J, et al. Lymph node metastases from head and neck squamous cell carcinoma: MR imaging with ultrasmall superparamagnetic iron oxide particles (Sinerem MR) – results of a phase-III multicenter clinical trial. Eur Radiol 2002; 12:957–8.

11. Dardzinski B, Schmithorst V, Holland S, et al. MR imaging of murine arthritis using ultrasmall superparamagnetic iron oxide particles. Magn Reson Imaging 2001; 19:1209–16.

12. Kanno S, Wu Y, Lee P, et al. Macrophage accumulation associated with rat cardiac allograft rejection detected by magnetic resonance imaging with ultrasmall superparamagnetic iron oxide particles. Circulation 2001; 104:934–8.

13. Paganelli G, Magnani P, Zito F, et al. Three-step monoclonal antibody tumor targeting in carcinoembryonic antigen-positive patients. Cancer Res 1991; 51:5960–6.

14. Dosio F, Magnani P, Paganelli G, et al. Three-step tumor pretargeting in lung cancer immunoscintigraphy. J Nucl Biol Med 1993; 37:228–32.

15. Modorati G, Brancato R, Paganelli G, et al. Immunoscintigraphy with three step monoclonal pretargeting technique in diagnosis of uveal melanoma: preliminary results. Br J Ophthalmol 1994; 78:19–23.

16. Kaseda N, Uehara Y, Yamamoto Y, Tanaka K. Induction of in situ immune complexes in rat glomeruli using avidin, native cation macromolecule. Br J Exp Pathol 1985; 66:729–35.

17. Sipkins DA, Cheresh DA, Kazemi MR, et al. Detection of tumor angiogenesis in vivo by $\alpha_v\beta_3$-targeted magnetic resonance imaging. Nat Med 1998; 4:623–6.

18. Anderson SA, Rader RK, Westlin WF, et al. Magnetic resonance contrast enhancement of neovasculature with $\alpha_v\beta_3$-targeted nanoparticles. Magn Reson Med 2000; 44:433–9.

19. Hermanson GT. Bioconjugate Techniques. San Diego: Academic Press, 1996.

20. de Bruin R, Spelt K, Mol J, et al. Selection of high-affinity phage antibodies from phage display libraries. Nat Biotechnol 1999; 17:397–9.

21. Stadler B. Antibody production without animals. Dev Biol Stand 1999; 101:45–8.

22. Wittrup K. Phage on display. Trends Biotechnol 1999; 17:423–4.

23. Pasqualini R, Koivunen E, Kain R, et al. Aminopeptidase N is a receptor for tumor-homing peptides and a target for inhibiting angiogenesis. Cancer Res 2000; 60:722–7.

24. Ruoslahti E. Targeting tumor vasculature with homing peptides from phage display. Semin Cancer Biol 2000; 10:435–42.

25. Ruoslahti E, Rajotte D. An address system in the vasculature of normal tissues and tumors. Annu Rev Immunol 2000; 18:813–27.

26. Arap W, Haedicke W, Bernasconi M, et al. Targeting the prostate for destruction through a vascular address. Proc Natl Acad Sci USA 2002; 99:1527–31.

27. Essler M, Ruoslahti E. Molecular specialization of breast vasculature: a breast-homing phage-displayed peptide binds to aminopeptidase P in breast vasculature Proc Natl Acad Sci USA 2002; 99:2252–7.

28. Wright WJ, McCreery T, Krupinski E, et al. Evaluation of new thrombus-specific ultrasound contrast agent. Acad Radiol 1998; 5(Suppl 1):S240–S242.

29. Reimer P, Weissleder R, Shen T, et al. Pancreatic receptors: initial feasibility studies with a targeted contrast agent for MR imaging. Radiology 1994; 193:527–31.

30. Reimer P, Bader A, Weissleder R. Preclinical assessment of hepatocyte-targeted MR contrast agents in stable human liver cell cultures. J Magn Reson Imaging 1998; 8:687–9.

31. Leveille-Webster C, Rogers J, Arias I. Use of an asialoglycoprotein receptor-targeted magnetic resonance contrast agent to study changes in receptor biology during liver regeneration and endotoxemia in rats. Hepatology 1996; 23:1631–41.

32. Reimer P, Kwong K, Weisskoff R, et al. Dynamic signal intensity changes in liver with superparamagnetic MR contrast agents. J Magn Reson Imaging 1992; 2:177–81.

33. Reimer P, Weissleder R, Wittenberg J, Brady T. Receptor-directed contrast agents for MR imaging: preclinical evaluation with affinity assays. Radiology 1992; 182:565–9.

34. Small W, Nelson R, Sherbourne G, Bernardino M. Enhancement effects of a hepatocyte receptor-specific MR contrast agent in an animal model. J Magn Reson Imaging 1994; 4:325–30.

35. Blank M, Weinschenk T, Priemer M, Schluesener H. Systematic evolution of a DNA aptamer binding to rat brain tumor microvessels. Selective targeting of endothelial regulatory protein pigpen. J Biol Chem 2001; 276:1664–8.

36. Boncler M, Koziolkiewicz M, Watala C. Aptamer inhibits degradation of platelet proteolytically activatable receptor, PAR–1, by thrombin. Thromb Res 2001; 104:215–222.

37. Kim E, Serur A, Huang J, et al. Potent VEGF blockade causes regression of coopted vessels in a model of neuroblastoma. Proc Natl Acad Sci USA 2002; 99:11 399–404.

38. Devoisselle J, Vion-Dury J, Galons J, et al. Entrapment of gadolinium-DTPA in liposomes. Characterization of vesicles by P-31 NMR spectroscopy. Invest Radiol 1988; 23:719–24.

39. Navon G, Panigel R, Valensin G. Liposomes containing paramagnetic macromolecules as MRI contrast agents. Magn Reson Med 1986; 3:876–80.

40. Fossheim S, Fahlvik A, Klaveness J, Muller R. Paramagnetic liposomes as MRI contrast agents: influence of liposomal physicochemical properties on the in vitro relaxivity. Magn Reson Imaging 1999; 17:83–9.

41. Koenig SH, Ahkong QF, Brown RD, et al. Permeability of liposomal membranes to water: results from the magnetic field dependence of T1 of solvent protons in suspensions of vesicles with entrapped paramagnetic ions. Magn Reson Med 1992; 23:275–86.

42. Tilcock C, Unger E, Cullis P, MacDougall P. Liposomal Gd-DTPA: preparation and characterization of relaxivity. Radiology 1989; 171:77–80.

43. Grant C, Karlik S, Florio E. A liposomal MRI contrast agent: phosphatidylethanolamine-DTPA. Mag Reson Med 1989; 11:236–43.

44. Kabalka G, Davis M, Moss T, et al. Gadolinium-labeled liposomes containing various amphiphilic Gd-DTPA derivatives: targeted MRI

contrast enhancement agents for the liver. Magn Reson Med 1991; 19:406–15.

45. Kabalka G, Davis M, Holmberg E, et al. Gadolinium-labeled liposomes containing amphiphilic Gd-DTPA derivatives of varying chain length: targeted MRI contrast enhancement agents for the liver. Magn Reson Imaging 1991; 9:373–7.

46. Tilcock C, Ahkong QF, Koenig SH, et al. The design of liposomal paramagnetic MR agents: effect of vesicle size upon the relaxivity of surface-incorporated lipophilic chelates. Magn Reson Med 1992; 27:44–51.

47. Rebizak R, Schaefer M, Dellacherie E. Polymeric conjugates of Gd^{3+}-diethylenetriaminepentaacetic acid and dextran. 2. Influence of spacer arm length and conjugate molecular mass on the paramagnetic properties and some biological parameters. Bioconjugate Chem 1998; 9:94–9.

48. Li K, Bednarski M. Vascular-targeted molecular imaging using functionalized polymerized vesicles. J Magn Reson Imaging 2002; 16:388–93.

49. Lanza G, Wallace K, Scott M, et al. A novel site-targeted ultrasonic contrast agent with broad biomedical application. Circulation 1996; 94:3334–40.

50. Lanza G, Abendschein D, Hall C, et al. Molecular imaging of stretch-induced tissue factor expression in carotid arteries with intravascular ultrasound. Invest Radiol 2000; 35:227–34.

51. Winter P, Caruthers S, Schmieder A, et al. Molecular imaging of angiogenesis in atherosclerotic rabbits by MRI with $\alpha_v\beta_3$-targeted nanoparticles. Mol Imaging 2002; 1:218.

52. Winter P, Caruthers S, Schmieder A, et al. Molecular imaging of angiogenesis by MRI with $\alpha_v\beta_3$-targeted paramagnetic nanoparticles. Mol Imaging 2002; 1:78.

53. Schmieder A, Winter P, Caruthers S, et al. Molecular imaging of angiogenesis in human melanoma xenografts in nude mice by MRI (1.5 T) with $\alpha_v\beta_3$-targeted nanoparticles. Mol Imaging 2002; 1:190.

54. Krafft M. Fluorocarbons and fluorinated amphiphiles in drug delivery and biomedical research. Adv Drug Del Rev 2001; 47:209–28.

55. Flacke S, Fischer S, Scott M, et al. A novel MRI contrast agent for molecular imaging of fibrin: implications for detecting vulnerable plaques. Circulation 2001; 104:1280–5.

56. Winter P, Chen J, Song S-K, et al. Relaxivities of paramagnetic nanoparticle contrast agents for targeted molecular imaging. In: Proceeding of the Annual Meeting of the International Society for Magnetic Resonance in Medicine, 2001:54.

57. Constantinides P. Plaque fissuring in human coronary thrombosis. J Atheroscler Res 1966; 6:1–17.

58. Ambrose J, Tannenbaum M, Alexopoulos D, et al. Angiographic progression of coronary artery disease and the development of myocardial infarction. J Am Coll Cardiol 1988; 12:56–62.

59. Ojio S, Takatsu H, Tanaka T, et al. Considerable time from the onset of plaque rupture and/or thrombi until the onset of acute myocardial infarction in humans: coronary angiographic findings within 1 week before the onset of infarction. Circulation 2000; 102:2063–9.

60. Falcioni R, Cimino L, Gentileschi M, et al. Expression of β_1, β_3, β_4, and β_5 integrins by human lung carcinoma cells of different histotypes. Exp Cell Res 1994; 210:113–22.

61. Brooks P, Stromblad S, Klemke R, et al. Antiintegrin $\alpha_v\beta_3$ blocks human breast cancer growth and angiogenesis in human skin. J Clin Invest 1995; 96:1815–22.

62. Felding-Habermann B, Mueller B, Romerdahl C, Cheresh D. Involvement of α_v gene expression in human melanoma tumorigenicity. J Clin Invest 1992; 89:2018–22.

63. Natali P, Hamby C, Felding-Habermann B, et al. Clinical significance of $\alpha_v\beta_3$ integrin and intercellular adhesion molecule-1 expression in cutaneous malignant melanoma lesions. Cancer Res 1997; 57:1554–60.

64. Gladson C, Cheresh D. Glioblastoma expression of vitronectin and the $\alpha_v\beta_3$ integrin. J Clin Invest 1991; 88:1924–32.

65. Johansson LO, Bjornerud A, Ahlstrom HK, et al. A targeted contrast agent for magnetic resonance imaging of thrombus: implications of spatial resolution. J Magn Reson Imaging 2001; 13:615–18.

66. Wunderbaldinger P, Josephson L, Weissleder R. Tat peptide directs enhanced clearance and hepatic permeability of magnetic nanoparticles. Bioconjugate Chem 2002; 13:264–8.

67. Josephson L, Tung CH, Moore A, Weissleder R. High efficiency intracellular magnetic labeling with novel superparamagnetic–Tat peptide conjugates. Bioconjugate Chem 1999; 10:186–91.

68. Lewin M, Carlesso N, Tung CH, et al. Tat peptide-derivatized magnetic nanoparticles allow in vivo tracking and recovery of progenitor cells. Nat Biotechnol 2000; 18:410–14.

69. Dodd CH, Hsu HC, Chu WJ, et al. Normal T-cell response and in vivo magnetic resonance imaging of T cells loaded with HIV transactivator-peptide-derived superparamagnetic nanoparticles. J Immunol Methods 2001; 256:89–105.

70. Bulte JW, Duncan ID, Frank JA. In vivo magnetic resonance tracking of magnetically labeled cells after transplantation. J Cereb Blood Flow Metab 2002; 22:899–907.

71. Lanza G, Yu X, Winter P, et al. Targeted antiproliferative drug delivery to vascular smooth muscle cells with an MRI nanoparticle contrast agent: implications for rational therapy of restenosis. Circulation 2002; 106:2842–7.

28

High-field CMR

Matthias Stuber

Introduction

In theory, signal-to-noise ratio (SNR) in magnetic resonance imaging is directly related to the strength B_0 of the static magnetic field. Thus, improved SNR can be expected by using magnets with higher field strength, of which 3 T systems have recently been approved for clinical use by the US Food and Drug Administration (FDA). A higher SNR will result in enhanced detail visibility, higher spatial and temporal resolution, abbreviated scanning times, or a combination of these. This will ultimately result in an improved diagnostic value of cardiac MRI (CMR) in general, while new areas of innovation in CMR research are likely to emerge.

However, at present, the limited availability of these higher-field systems equipped for cardiac applications together with other potential impediments,[1] including increased susceptibility artifacts, reduced T2*,[2,3] increased T1, radiofrequency (RF) field distortions,[4] and changed tissue dielectric constants or body dielectric resonances,[5,6] are limiting factors. Further, at higher field strengths, increased RF deposition may remove flexibility for general

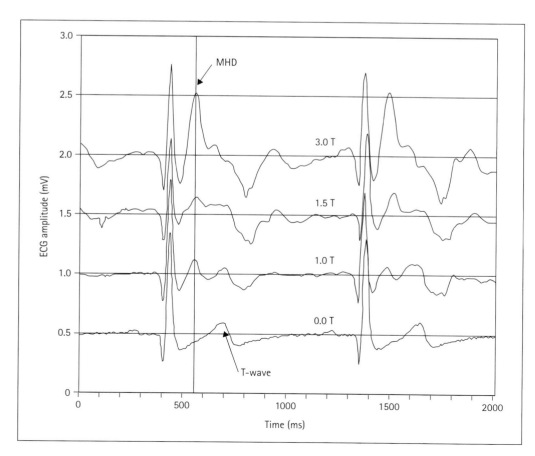

Figure 28.1
ECG traces acquired in the same individual at four different field strengths (0, 0.5, 1.5, and 3.0 T). Note the gradually increasing artifact on the T-wave of the ECG, which can be attributed to the amplified magnetohydrodynamic (MHD) effect at higher field strength. R-wave triggering is therefore one of the challenges at 3 T. This necessitates sophisticated ECG hardware and R-wave detection algorithms for successful CMR. (Reproduced from Stuber et al. Magn Res Med 2002; 48:425–9.[16])

sequence design, and reliable R-wave triggering becomes more challenging due to amplified magnetohydrodynamic (MHD) effects.[7] Figure 28.1 displays electrocardiograph (ECG) traces of the same individual recorded at four different field strengths. The gradually increasing artifact on the T-wave can readily be seen as a function of increasing B_0. Such an augmented T-wave could easily be misinterpreted as an R-wave by conventional R-wave detection algorithms, thereby compromising image quality of any segmented k-space imaging approach as utilized in the vast majority of cardiovascular applications. Therefore, adapted ECG modules and R-wave detection algorithms are a necessity for successful CMR at high field strength.

Despite the above-mentioned challenges, recent progress in hardware and the adaptation of cardiac-specific software have made it possible to implement CMR on commercial whole-body 3 T systems. The first preliminary results obtained with this new technology are discussed in this chapter.

Applications

Functional imaging

Feasibility of 3 T segmented k-space gradient-echo functional cardiac imaging using a two-element surface receive coil has already been demonstrated by Noeske and colleagues[2] (Figure 28.2).

Over the past few years, steady-state free precession (SSFP)[8] techniques have been adopted by most clinical and research MR centers for functional cardiac imaging. Hereby, local contractility of the myocardium and ventricular volume and mass are measures that are qualitatively and quantitatively assessed.[9] Using SSFP techniques at 1.5 T, a major advantage in SNR and contrast-to-noise ratio (CNR) has been obtained, and the resulting improved endocardial border definition has facilitated automated or semiautomated contouring.[10] However, a short TR is crucial to minimize flow artifacts and signal voids due to local field inhomogeneities. While these challenges have been successfully addressed by equipment manufacturers at 1.5 T, the increases in the general ΔB_0 effects and TR that may be governed by the maximum RF deposition are among the impediments for functional cardiac imaging at 3 T. However, careful adaptation of the RF excitation angles, higher-order shimming, and modifications of the imaging protocol to take account of the changed physical boundary conditions have already been successfully implemented, as displayed in Figures 28.3–28.5. In Figure 28.3, a short-axis image acquired with a body send coil and a surface receive coil using a Fiesta SSFP sequence displays high contrast between the myocardium and the blood pool in the ventricular cavities. Similarly, Figure 28.4 shows a short-axis image (A) and a long-axis image (B) (acquired with a True-FISP

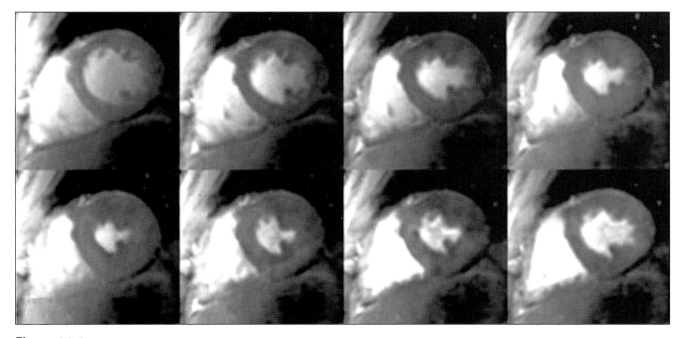

Figure 28.2
Segmented k-space gradient-echo functional short-axis cardiac images acquired with a prototype two-element cardiac surface coil and a body send coil. (Reproduced from Noeske et al. Magn Res Med 2000; 44:978–82.[2])

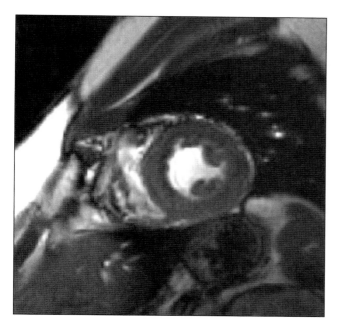

Figure 28.3
Fiesta (SSFP) functional short-axis image acquired at 3 T with a body send and a surface receive coil. Note the high contrast between the blood pool and the myocardium. (Courtesy of Bob Greenman and David Alsop, BIDMC, Boston.)

SSFP sequence and a body send/receive coil. Note the relatively high SNR despite the use of the body coil for signal reception. In Figure 28.5, SENSE short-axis functional images acquired with an acceleration factor of 2 (B) and 3 (C) using a Balanced FFE SSFP sequence are displayed adjacent to the reference image acquired without parallel imaging (A). These images were obtained with a body send and a six-element prototype synergy cardiac receive coil. Consistent with the findings in Figures 28.3 and 28.4, a high contrast between the ventricular cavities and the myocardium is observed, and high image quality can even be observed with a threefold acceleration and a breathhold of 5 s only.

Myocardial tagging

MR myocardial tagging has shown to be a useful tool for the assessment of local myocardial motion in healthy and diseased states.[11] While fading of the tags limits access to diastolic myocardial motion for most contemporary tagging sequences, this fading of the tags is T1-dependent. However, at higher field strength, T1 of myocardium is increased, resulting in a reduced fading

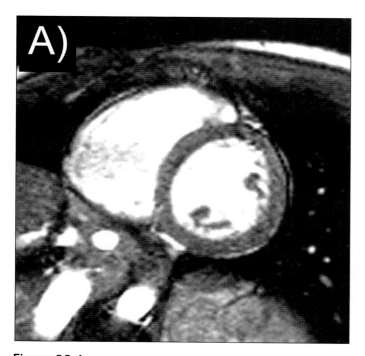
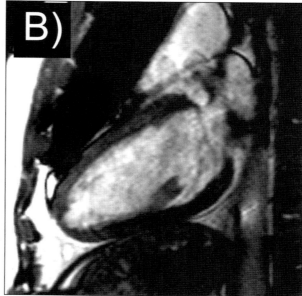

Figure 28.4
TrueFISP (SSFP) functional short-axis (A) and long-axis (B) images acquired with a body send/receive coil. The contrast between the blood pool and myocardium is high, while a substantial SNR is obtained despite the use of a body receive coil. (Courtesy of Christine Lorenz, Siemens Medical, Erlangen.)

No SENSE
15 s

SENSE 2 ×
7 s

SENSE 3 ×
5 s

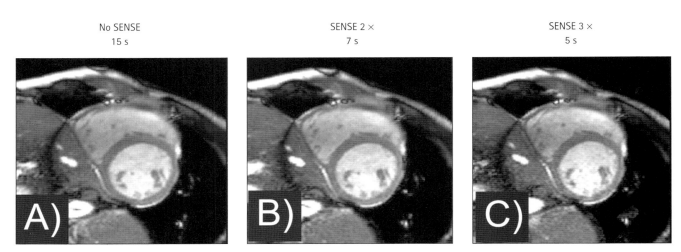

Figure 28.5
Balanced-FFE (SSFP) functional short-axis images acquired with (B,C) and without (A) parallel imaging (SENSE). Parallel imaging with an acceleration factor of 2 (B) or 3 (C) was employed, leading to abbreviated scanning times: 15 s conventional (A), 7 s with acceleration factor 2 (B), and 5 s with acceleration factor 3 (C). The images were acquired with a body send coil and a prototype six-element synergy surface receive coil. Consistent with the theory, image quality decreases as a function of the increased acceleration factor. (Courtesy of Sebastian Kozerke and Michael Schaer, IBT ETH Zürich.)

of the tags throughout the cardiac cycle. Together with the expected increase in SNR at higher field strength, this attenuated fading may result in higher temporal resolution and more accurate identification of the tags, which will facilitate access to subtle changes in myocardial motion throughout the cardiac cycle. In Figure 28.6, three CSPAMM[12] line-tagged cine frames out of a series with a temporal resolution of 70 frames per RR interval are displayed. These images were acquired using a segmented k-space echo-planar imaging (EPI) sequence together with ramped RF excitation angles that compensate for both T1 relaxation and M_z reduction due to preceding RF excitations. Quantitative preliminary findings in two subjects include an approximately twofold increase in tagging CNR at 3 T when compared with 1.5 T.[13]

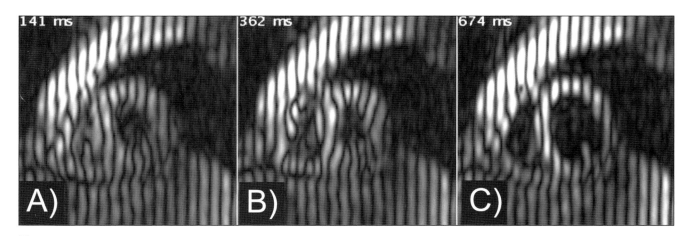

Figure 28.6
Short-axis CSPAMM myocardial tagging images acquired at 3 T. Myocardial tagging supports the quantification of local myocardial motion, including stress, strain, rotation shear, etc. Consistent with the increased muscle T1 at 3 T, the persistence of the tags is prolonged, facilitating an accurate determination of wall motion for systole and diastole. The images were acquired with a body send coil and a prototype six-element synergy surface receive coil. An almost twofold tagging CNR was found when comparing 1.5 T and 3 T data. (Courtesy of Salome Ryf, IBT ETH Zürich.)

Coronary MRA

The first international multicenter trial on coronary magnetic resonance angiography (MRA) suggests that non-endogenous contrast-enhanced navigator-gated and corrected free-breathing coronary MRA is a valuable tool for the noninvasive assessment of significant proximal coronary artery disease.[14] However, reading of distal segments and branching vessels was not included in this study, and the overall specificity and detail visibility of the method remain to be improved. Therefore, a higher spatial resolution approaching that of X-ray angiographic standards (<300 μm) may be required. Isotropic spatial resolution[15] may also enable the more accurate identification of eccentric coronary artery stenoses. It is expected that the higher SNR secondary to a higher field strength would allow for a further improved spatial resolution, which will support isotropic resolution and access to more distal or branching vessels. However, not only advantages but also potential challenges (see Introduction) have to be considered at higher field strength. Therefore, a first study investigating the feasibility of in vivo human coronary MRA at higher field strength was performed.[16] In this, the 1.5 T technique used in the multicenter trial[17] was adopted, and only minor adaptations were made to account for the changed physical boundary conditions at 3 T. Vector ECG (VECG) technology was used,[7] and a body send coil together with a prototype six-element cardiac synergy surface receive coil was employed. Nine consecutive healthy adult human subjects (age 37 ± 8) were included in this study. High-resolution imaging was performed with a three-dimensional (3D) segmented k-space gradient-echo imaging sequence using a T2Prep and fat saturation for endogenous contrast enhancement[18] and a 2D selective real-time navigator for respiratory motion suppression during free breathing.[19]

To minimize the sensitivity of the navigator 2D selective RF pulse to ΔB_0 and T2* effects, the number of turns in k-space was reduced (from $N = 12$ at 1.5 T[17] to $N = 8$ to shorten the excitation duration. To suppress contamination of the navigator with spurious signal originating from higher-order components (aliasing) concentric with the central 2D selective excitation, a local receive coil positioned over the sternum was selectively employed for navigator signal reception.

Ten RF excitations (TR = 8.2 ms, TE = 2.4 ms) were performed for imaging during each RR interval (acquisition window 82 ms). The RF excitation angles were constant (25°) and adapted to account for the prolonged blood T1 at 3.0 T (~1600 ms).[2] A heart-rate-specific individual diastolic trigger delay[20] was used to minimize intrinsic myocardial motion during the acquisition interval. The in-plane resolution was 0.6–0.7 × 0.6–1.0 mm² and the slice thickness was 3 mm.

Coronary MRA studies were completed within an hour in all subjects and without complications. Image quality was consistent and the average scan duration for each free-breathing 3D acquisition was ~7 min, with an average navigator efficiency of 55%.

In all cases, no major susceptibility artifacts were seen in the vicinity of the left or the right proximal to mid coronary arterial segments. For the left coronary system, average contiguous vessel lengths of 83 ± 9 mm for the combined left main and left anterior descending (LM + LAD), 52 ± 6 mm for the left coronary circumflex (LCX), and 122 ± 35 mm for the right coronary artery (RCA) were found. The proximal diameters of the LAD, LCX, and RCA were 2.8 ± 0.4 mm, 2.6 ± 0.2 mm, and 2.8 ± 0.3 mm, respectively ($p = $ NS).

The image of the left coronary system shown in Figure 28.7A was acquired with a voxel size of 0.6 × 0.6 × 3 mm³ and the image of the RCA displayed in Figure 28.7B with a voxel size of 0.7 × 1.0 × 3 mm³. In these images, a considerable visual contrast between the coronary blood pool and the surrounding tissue is apparent. Smaller-diameter branching vessels are seen on both images (broken arrows). In Figure 28.8, coronary MRA images of the right coronary system were acquired using a similar technique with and without parallel imaging. A conventional non-accelerated coronary MRA of an RCA is displayed in Figure 28.8A and a twofold SENSE-accelerated scan acquired in the same subject is shown in Figure 28.8B. On both acquisitions, an 8 cm segment of the RCA is displayed together with branching vessels, the LM, and a proximal segment of the LCX. Consistent with the theory of parallel imaging, the visual SNR is reduced on the twofold-accelerated images when compared with the non-accelerated images.

These preliminary data demonstrate that 3 T coronary MRA is feasible in humans. Contemporary 1.5 T methodology can easily be adopted, and the enhanced SNR facilitates acquisition with small voxel size. Extensive proximal to mid coronary segments can be displayed, together with smaller diameter branching vessels. With growing experience on higher-field systems, and in-depth analyses and new developments of pulse sequences adapted to the higher static magnetic field (e.g. fast spin-echo and spiral techniques, etc.), further improvements giving improved spatial resolution in coronary MRA are expected.

Coronary vessel wall imaging

Several studies at 1.5 T have already demonstrated the possibility of visualizing coronary vessel walls in both healthy and diseased states.[21,22] In a recent CMR study, a positive arterial remodeling of coronary artery vessel walls could already be documented in patients with suspected

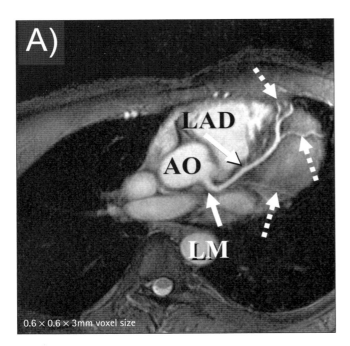
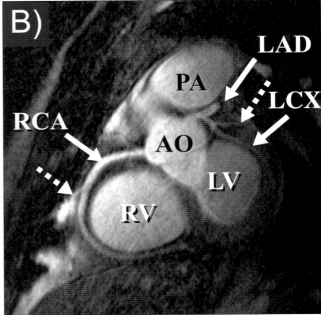

Figure 28.7
Coronary MRA of the left and right coronary arterial system acquired during free breathing using a T2Prep navigator-gated and corrected 3D segmented *k*-space gradient-echo imaging sequence (image resolution 0.6 × 0.6 × 3 mm³). The images were acquired with a body send coil and a prototype six-element synergy surface receive coil. (A) Left coronary system, including the left main (LM), 8 cm of the left anterior descending (LAD) with distal branching vessels (broken arrow), and 4 cm of the left coronary circumflex (LCX). (B) A 9 cm segment of the right coronary artery (RCA), together with the left main (LM), the left coronary circumflex (LAD), and some branching vessels (broken arrow). AO, aorta; PA, pulmonary artery; RV, right ventricle; LV, left ventricle. (Reproduced from Stuber et al. Magn Res Med 2002; 48:425–9.[16])

No SENSE   SENSE 2 x

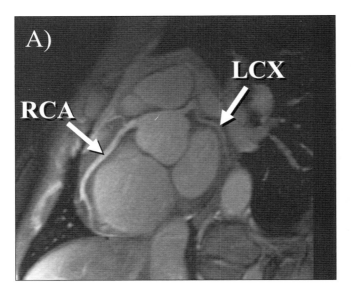
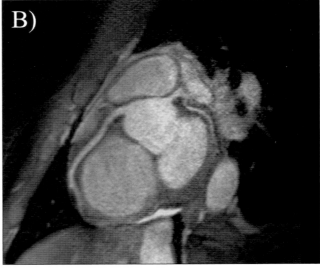

Figure 28.8
Coronary MRA images of the right coronary arterial system (RCA, solid arrow) together with the left coronary circumflex (LCX) acquired with a conventional (A) and twofold SENSE-accelerated (B) T2Prep navigator-gated and corrected 3D segmented *k*-space gradient-echo imaging sequence. The images were acquired with a body send coil and a prototype six-element synergy receive coil. (Courtesy of M Huber, IBT ETH Zürich.)

coronary artery disease at 1.5 T.[23] However, the ultimate goal is not only measurement of coronary vessel wall thickness but also differentiation between plaque components and consequently identification of vulnerable plaque.[21] This necessitates significantly improved spatial resolution. At higher field strength, a further step in this direction is expected. Due to the relatively small size of coronary vessel walls (~1 mm), their central location within the thorax, and their constant movement due to intrinsic and extrinsic myocardial motion, coronary vessel wall imaging is among the technically most challenging topics in CMR at present date.

At 3 T, navigator-gated and real-time motion-corrected (see the discussion of coronary MRA above) cross-sectional views of the RCA were obtained in six healthy adults by Botnar and colleagues.[22] The MR pulse sequence consisted of a dual-inversion black-blood prepulse with inversion delay (TI)[24] adapted for the prolonged T1 of blood (TI ~700 ms at 60 bpm, dual-inversion and data collection every other heartbeat) at 3 T. The 2D segmented k-space gradient-echo imaging sequence was immediately preceded by a 2D selective navigator pulse, a frequency-selective fat-suppression prepulse, and a

NAV-restore prepulse[25] for optimization of navigator performance in the presence of a nonselective 180° prepulse. Other imaging parameters included TE = 2.3 ms, TR = 8 ms, bandwidth 135 Hz, flip angle 30°, 10 RF excitations per shot, number of signals acquired 2, field of view 360 mm, a 512 × 512 image matrix resulting in an in-plane resolution of 0.7 × 0.7 mm², and a slice thickness of 5 mm. Adjacent to the dual-inversion fast spin-echo scout scan in parallel to the RCA shown in Figure 28.9A, an excellent depiction of the coronary vessel acquired at 3 T can be seen in Figure 28.9B. The prolonged inversion time of the dual-inversion prepulse yields an adequate suppression of the left- and right-ventricular intracavitary blood pool.

Although a relatively SNR-inefficient black-blood segmented k-space gradient-echo sequence was used, these data demonstrate the feasibility of 3 T coronary vessel wall MRI using a free-breathing black-blood 2D fast gradient-echo technique with ECG triggering and navigator gating. As for coronary MRA, a substantial further improvement in image quality and resolution is to be expected if a spiral or fast spin-echo imaging sequence is employed for coronary vessel wall imaging.

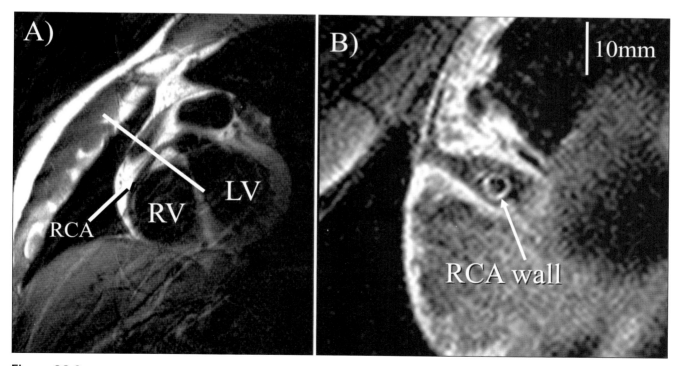

Figure 28.9
Coronary vessel wall image showing a cross-section of the proximal right coronary artery (RCA). The localizer (A) was acquired with a dual-inversion fast spin-echo sequence using navigator technology during free breathing. The coronary vessel wall image (B) was acquired during free breathing using a dual-inversion navigator-gated and corrected 2D segmented k-space gradient-echo imaging sequence. RV, right ventricle; LV, left ventricle. (Courtesy of Rene M Botnar, BIDMC Boston.)

Perfusion and late enhancement

Both perfusion imaging and late enhancement imaging require the administration of extracellular contrast agents. While enhanced efficacy of such contrast agents is expected at 3 T, the feasibility and value of both techniques remain to be evaluated at higher field strength. However, given the fact that gradient-echo techniques with short echo times have been applied successfully for both modalities at 1.5 T, no major impediments are expected from a sequence standpoint at 3 T, since gradient-echo techniques have already been successfully implemented at 3 T.

Parallel imaging

As demonstrated in Figures 28.5 and 28.8, parallel imaging at 3 T has already been performed. Parallel imaging techniques such as SMASH[26] and SENSE[27] are particularly interesting at higher field strengths and for selected applications. While the theoretically doubled SNR at 3 T necessitates an approximately fourfold signal averaging time at 1.5 T (to obtain a similar SNR), this twofold SNR at 3 T could be traded for abbreviated scanning times using parallel imaging with an acceleration factor approaching 4. In areas where SNR is not necessarily the limiting factor (e.g. functional cardiac imaging), this helps to shorten breathhold durations and will be most beneficial in patients who cannot tolerate prolonged breathholds (Figure 28.5). In coronary MRA, parallel imaging will also be useful for shortening the scanning time, which makes the technique better suited for integration as part of a comprehensive cardiac examination (Figure 28.8). However, at present, a further improvement in resolution for both coronary MRA and coronary vessel wall imaging may have a higher priority than abbreviated scanning times with subsequent SNR loss as intrinsically coupled with parallel imaging.

Shortened T2* values and an increase in ΔB_0 consistent with an increased B_0 will be among the limitations for techniques with prolonged signal readout (spiral techniques and EPI techniques).[2] However, by using parallel imaging, echo trains or readout times can be shortened, which may support optimized image quality using such techniques at higher field strength. Sodickson and colleagues[28] have also demonstrated that parallel imaging may be employed beneficially for first-pass contrast agent bolus injection techniques. Thereby, accelerated data acquisition results in more time-effective signal sampling during the first pass. This also remains to be revisited at higher field strength.

Discussion

Despite the only recent availability of high-field systems equipped for cardiovascular use, the preliminary results discussed in this chapter already demonstrate the feasibility of high-quality 3 T CMR in healthy human adult subjects.

For cardiac imaging at 3 T, the required hardware components include body send coils, surface receive coils, coil arrays for parallel imaging, higher-order shimming, and sophisticated ECG triggering hardware to avoid adverse effects of the amplified MHD effect on R-wave triggering. Cardiac-specific software with segmented k-space gradient-echo imaging sequences (including SSFP and EPI), fast spin-echo sequences, and prepulses such as fat saturation, inversion, dual inversion, and T2Prep will support the majority of contemporary cardiovascular applications. For high-resolution applications with prolonged equilibrium scanning times, navigator technology should be available. As documented in this chapter, an impressive collection of high-quality image material has already been acquired. Multiple imaging sequences, prepulses, and motion suppression strategies have been used with and without parallel imaging.

The expected theoretical SNR benefit at higher field strength and its consequences are obviously most attractive for enhanced spatial resolution, enhanced temporal resolution, and abbreviated scanning times or combinations thereof. However, potential challenges do exist, as mentioned in the Introduction, and their individual effects on image quality remain to be studied for each application.

With the higher field strength, there is increased RF deposition, and therefore certain limitations will apply for sequences with large RF excitation angles or continuous RF excitations over a prolonged period of time. Therefore, SSFP or fast spin-echo sequences need to be adapted accordingly. For coronary MRA and coronary vessel wall imaging, image data can only be acquired in a narrow time window in each cardiac cycle. On the one hand, this makes MR data acquisition rather inefficient. On the other hand, it offers more flexibility for high-field sequence design, since RF deposition is minimized for both applications.

While the increase in T1 may lead to a reduced steady-state magnetization, with subsequent relative loss in SNR, this effect could in turn also be used to boost the efficacy of myocardial tagging or spin-labeling techniques, for example, which will be able to take advantage not only of the enhanced SNR at 3 T but also of the prolonged T1.[29] Shortened T2* may be useful for blood oxygenation measurements[30] or perfusion imaging. Together with navigator technology, it may be possible to implement cardiac spectroscopy during free breathing,[31] while the enhanced

SNR will support spectroscopic data acquisition in relatively small and well-defined volumes. If extrinsic and intrinsic myocardial motions are sufficiently constrained, diffusion imaging together with fiber tracking may allow for a more detailed insight into fiber architecture and the orientation of myocytes.[32]

Conclusions

With state-of-the-art 3 T equipment, high-quality CMR images can be acquired in vivo. This applies for the majority of cardiovascular applications, except for perfusion and late enhancement, for which in vivo human data have not yet been presented.

After a further refinement of imaging sequences and adaptation of hardware components to the changed physical boundary conditions, the benefits associated with the higher field strength will have to be defined as a next step. The areas in which 3 T outperforms 1.5 T remain to be identified in direct comparisons, and the outcome of patient studies will ultimately define the value of 3 T CMR in clinical applications.

Beyond the modification and use of contemporary and already-established 1.5 T CMR methodology at 3 T, the higher field strength will open new avenues for research, development, and discoveries for many years to come.

References

1. Wen H, Denison TJ, Singerman RW, et al. The intrinsic signal-to-noise ratio in human cardiac imaging at 1.5, 3, and 4 T. J Magn Reson 1997; 125:65–71.

2. Noeske R, Seifert F, Rhein KH, et al. Human cardiac imaging at 3 T using phased array coils. Magn Reson Med 2000; 44:978–82.

3. Atalay MK, Poncelet BP, Kantor HL, et al. Cardiac susceptibility artifacts arising from the heart-lung interface. Magn Reson Med 2001; 45:341–5.

4. Dougherty L, Connick TJ, Mizsei G. Cardiac imaging at 4 tesla. Magn Reson Med 2001; 45:176–8.

5. Wen H, Jaffer FA, Denison TJ, et al. The evaluation of dielectric resonators containing H_2O or D_2O as RF coils for high-field MR imaging and spectroscopy. J Magn Reson B 1996; 110:117–23.

6. Bottomley PA, Andrew ER. RF magnetic field penetration, phase shift and power dissipation in biological tissue: implications for NMR imaging. Phys Med Biol 1978; 23:630–43.

7. Fischer SE, Wickline SA, Lorenz CH. Novel real-time R-wave detection algorithm based on the vectorcardiogram for accurate gated magnetic resonance acquisitions. Magn Reson Med 1999; 42:361–70.

8. Oppelt A, Graumann R, Barfuss H, et al. FISP – a new fast MRI sequence. Electromedica 1986; 54:15–18.

9. Salton CJ, Chuang ML, O'Donnell CJ, et al. Gender differences and normal left ventricular anatomy in an adult population free of hypertension. A cardiovascular magnetic resonance study of the Framingham Heart Study Offspring cohort. J Am Coll Cardiol 2002; 39:1055–60.

10. Heid O. True FISP cardiac fluoroscopy. In: Proceedings of the Annual Meeting of the International Society for Magnetic Resonance in Medicine 1997:320.

11. McVeigh ER. MRI of myocardial function: motion tracking techniques. Magn Reson Imaging 1996; 14:137–50.

12. Fischer SE, McKinnon GC, Scheidegger MB, et al. True myocardial motion tracking. Magn Reson Med 1994; 31:401–13.

13. Ryf S, Spiegel MA, Kozerke S, et al. CSPAMM myocardial tagging at 3 Tesla. In: Proceedings of the European Society for Magnetic Resonance in Medicine and Biology 2002.

14. Kim WY, Danias PG, Stuber M, et al. Coronary magnetic resonance angiography for the detection of coronary stenoses. N Engl J Med 2001; 345:1863–9.

15. Botnar RM, Stuber M, Kissinger KV, et al. Free-breathing 3D coronary MRA: the impact of 'isotropic' image resolution. J Magn Reson Imaging 2000; 11:389–93.

16. Stuber M, Botnar RM, Fischer SE, et al. Preliminary report on in vivo coronary MRA at 3 tesla in humans. Magn Reson Med 2002; 48:425–9.

17. Stuber M, Botnar RM, Danias PG, et al. Double oblique free-breathing high-resolution 3D coronary MRA. J Am Coll Cardiol 1999; 34:524–31.

18. Botnar RM, Stuber M, Danias PG, et al. Improved coronary artery definition with T2-weighted free-breathing 3D-coronary MRA. Circulation 1999; 99:3139–48.

19. McConnell MV, Khasgiwala VC, Savord BJ, et al. Comparison of respiratory suppression methods and navigator locations for MR coronary angiography. AJR 1997; 168:1369–75.

20. Kim WY, Stuber M, Kissinger KV, et al. Impact of bulk cardiac motion on right coronary MR angiography and vessel wall imaging. J Magn Reson Imaging 2001; 14:383–90.

21. Fayad ZA, Fuster V, Fallon JT, et al. Noninvasive in vivo human coronary artery lumen and wall imaging using black-blood magnetic resonance imaging. Circulation 2000; 102:506–10.

22. Botnar RM, Stuber M, Lamerichs R, et al. Initial experiences with coronary vessel wall imaging on a 3 T whole body system. In: Proceedings of the Annual Meeting of the International Society for Magnetic Resonance in Medicine 2002: 370.

23. Kim WY, Stuber M, Bornert P, et al. Three-dimensional black-blood cardiac magnetic resonance coronary vessel wall imaging detects positive arterial remodeling in patients with nonsignificant coronary artery disease. Circulation 2002; 106:296–9.

24. Fleckenstein JL, Archer BT, Barker BA, et al. Fast short-tau inversion-recovery MR imaging. Radiology 1991; 179:499–504.

25. Stuber M, Botnar RM, Spuentrup E, et al. Three-dimensional high-resolution fast spin-echo coronary magnetic resonance angiography. Magn Reson Med 2001; 45:206–11.

26. Sodickson DK Manning WJ. Simultaneous acquisition of spatial harmonics (SMASH): fast imaging with radiofrequency coil arrays. Magn Reson Med 1997; 38:591–603.

27. Pruessmann KP, Weiger M, Scheidegger MB, et al. SENSE: sensitivity encoding for fast MRI. Magn Reson Med 1999; 42:952–62.

28. Sodickson DK, McKenzie CA, Li W, et al. Contrast-enhanced 3D MR angiography with simultaneous acquisition of spatial harmonics: a pilot study. Radiology 2000; 217:284–9.

29. Wang J, Alsop DC, Li L, et al. Comparison of quantitative perfusion imaging using arterial spin labeling at 1.5 and 4.0 tesla. Magn Reson Med 2002; 48:242–54.

30. Li D, Waight DJ, Wang Y. In vivo correlation between blood T2* and oxygen saturation. J Magn Reson Imaging 1998; 8:1236–9.

31. Kozerke S, Schar M, Lamb HJ, et al. Volume tracking cardiac ^{31}P spectroscopy. Magn Reson Med 2002; 48:380–4.

32. Dou J, Reese TG, Tseng WY, et al. Cardiac diffusion MRI without motion effects. Magn Reson Med 2002; 48:105–14.

29

An introduction to CMR for technologists

Cindy R Comeau

Introduction

Magnetic resonance imaging (MRI) is a wonderful clinical tool for evaluating patients with heart disease. Cardiac MRI (CMR) is becoming widely available as all the major manufacturers offer capabilities that enhance the acquisition of cardiac MR images. Today, it is possible to perform a comprehensive examination within 30 minutes that includes evaluation of cardiac morphology, ventricular and valvular function, and myocardial perfusion and viability.[1] Because CMR is growing in clinical use, the demand for well-trained CMR technologists is increasing. Performing a CMR examination demands specific technical expertise and knowledge of heart anatomy and physiology. It is important that MRI technologists performing a cardiac examination obtain specialized training in this area.

Because of its motion and orientation within the chest, MRI of the heart poses special challenges as compared with MRI of other organs. Patients referred for a CMR examination may be quite ill and therefore may not tolerate a long examination. It is important to develop an imaging protocol using appropriate pulse sequences that will expedite patient throughput. Being able to recognize certain

pathology is important, as additional views may be required. The use of the electrocardiogram (ECG) in CMR allows for the suppression of motion artifacts caused by complex cardiac motion and great artery pulsation. ECG gating or cardiac triggering is important because it provides periodic timing of heart function to image acquisition. Learning the technical aspects and clinical applications of CMR can be a demanding task for technologists just entering the field.

Overview of cardiac structure and function

The human heart is a muscular organ that weighs approximately nine ounces and is about the size of a clenched fist.[2] It is a pump that is extremely durable and can be described as the 'engine' of the cardiovascular system. The heart is located in the mediastinum superior to the diaphragm and between the lungs. It is enclosed in a fibrous sac called the pericardium, which is surrounded by

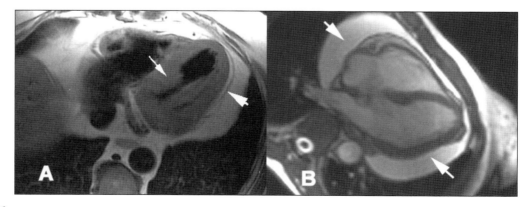

Figure 29.1

(A) Image obtained by a gated black-blood technique showing normal pericardium. The myocardium (small arrow) is abnormally thickened, consistent with left-ventricular hypertrophy. The pericardium is the low-signal-intensity line (large arrow) surrounded by fat. (B) Image obtained by a steady-state free precession bright-blood technique showing a moderately sized pericardial effusion.

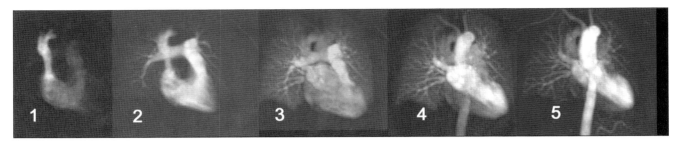

Figure 29.2
Cardiac circulation can be demonstrated by viewing a time-resolved contrast-enhanced acquisition. (1) Contrast is seen arriving in the superior vena cava, then into the right side of the heart. (2) Contrast is seen in the main pulmonary artery. (3) Contrast is circulated out to the lungs. (4) Contrast arrives back to the left side of the heart. (5) Contrast is pumped out of the aorta to the systemic circulation.

mediastinal and epicardial fat, which can be seen on an MR image (Figure 29.1).

The evaluation of pericardial disease is an important clinical indication for CMR. It is important for clinicians to be able to differentiate it from restrictive cardiomyopathy and constrictive pericarditis, an uncommon but important sequel of bypass surgery. Normal pericardial thickness is <3 mm. If the pericardium exceeds 5 mm in thickness, then constrictive pericarditis is highly suggestive.[3]

The heart consists of three layers: the epicardium is the outermost layer of the heart. The myocardium (muscle) is the thickest layer of the heart. The endocardium is the inner lining of the myocardium, and the folds of the endocardium form the cardiac valves. Usually when a clinician mentions heart disease, they are referring to the cardiac muscle tissue or the myocardium. The term 'myocardium' is often used to refer to the entire mass of the heart.

The exact orientation of the heart varies from patient to patient, since the left ventricle is ellipsoidal, with its tip (apex) usually pointing anteriorly inferiorly and to the left. A major advantage of MRI is the ability to acquire images in oblique planes. Since the axes of the heart and great vessels are not aligned with the axis of the body, electronic angulation for non-axial CMR is accomplished by varying the relative strength of gradients during slice selection.

The cardiac valves regulate the blood flow in one direction. The pathway of blood flow through the chambers starts with venous blood returning into the right atrium via the superior and inferior vena cava. The blood then passes through the tricuspid valve into the right ventricle, and travels through the pulmonic valve into the pulmonary arteries to become oxygenated. Oxygenated blood from the lungs then returns via the pulmonary veins into the left atrium. The blood in the left atrium passes through the mitral valve into the left ventricle, which pumps the blood through the aortic valve into the aorta to be circulated to the rest of the organs (Figure 29.2).

The four chambers of the heart and the cardiac valves can be viewed on a long-axis image (Figure 29.3). The right ventricle is normally the most anterior chamber of the heart; it has a thin outer wall and usually measures just a few millimeters in thickness. The tricuspid valve separates the right atrium and right ventricle, and the mitral valve separates the left atrium and left ventricle. The left atrium is normally the most posterior chamber of the heart. Because the left ventricle is designed to be a powerful muscular pump, its wall is 2–3 times thicker than that of the right ventricle. Inside the ventricles are two finger-like projections called papillary muscles. The chordae tendineae anchor valve cusps to the papillary muscles located within both ventricular chambers. The moderator bands and papillary muscles are normal structures that can be visualized on MR images (Figure 29.4).

There are two phases of the cardiac cycle: contraction (systole) and relaxation (diastole). The valves ensure that blood flows only in the forward direction. When a valve

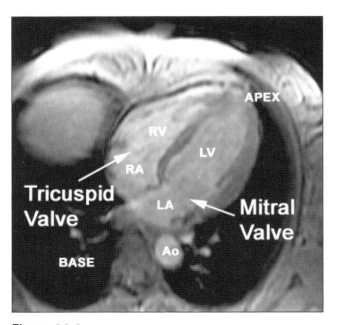

Figure 29.3
Cardiac chambers and valves: LV, left ventricle; LA, left atrium; RV, right ventricle; RA, right atrium; Ao, aorta.

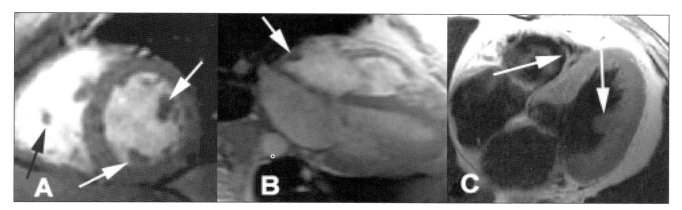

Figure 29.4
Normal cardiac structures seen by CMR include papillary muscles in both right and left ventricles (A), the crista terminalis (B), which is located in the posterior right-atrial wall, and moderator bands (C).

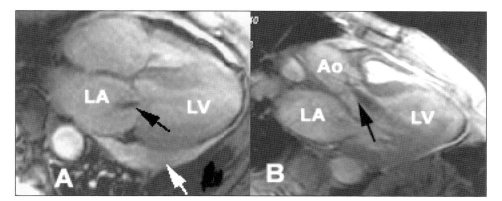

Figure 29.5
(A) Four-chamber standard fast gradient-echo cine end-systolic frame showing mitral regurgitation (black arrow) and pericardial effusion (white arrow). Mitral regurgitation occurs during systole. (B) Three-chamber view showing aortic insufficiency (arrow), which occurs in diastole.

leaks and allows blood flow backwards, the valve is termed 'regurgitant' or insufficient (Figure 29.5). When the valve restricts forward flow, it is said to be 'stenotic'. During ventricular contraction, or systole, the mitral and tricuspid valves close and the pulmonary and aortic valves open. During relaxation, or diastole, the mitral and tricuspid valves are open and the pulmonary and aortic valves are closed.

Imaging challenges related to CMR

Patient management

All patients undergoing CMR go through the same rigorous screening procedure as for any MRI examination. Patients with cardiac disease may have implantable devices such as cardiac pacemakers or automated internal cardiac defibrillators (AICDs), which are definite contraindications to CMR. Implantable devices such as coronary stents, heart valve prostheses, and annuloplasty rings are considered 'MR-safe' up to 1.5 T (Figure 29.6).[4,5]

For cardiac gating, the objective is to acquire an R-wave that is substantially larger than the T-wave of the ECG. The conduction system of the heart comprises a group of highly specialized cells. Electrical impulses cause the heart to contract and therefore blood to circulate. An ECG is a map of the electrical activity of the heart (Figure 29.7). Due to the *magnetohydrodynamic (MHD) effect*, the T-wave may become elevated when the patient is placed into the magnet.[6] This is because blood flow in the heart and great vessels generates additional voltage in the presence of a magnetic field. It is important that gating parameters be adjusted so that 'false' triggering, or triggering on the T-wave, does not occur. Using an alternative electrode placement may diminish this effect. It is recommended that the ECG leads be placed anteriorly on the patient's chest for best results. The ECG leads should be constructed in such a manner as to minimize pickup of extraneous signal induced by the applied magnetic gradients during the imaging acquisition. This effect may be minimized by placing the electrodes closer together.

Lead II is commonly used in gating, since it usually has the highest voltage. Lead II represents the voltage between the right-arm lead and the left-leg lead (Figure 29.8). If lead II is not optimal, it may be best to evaluate the other

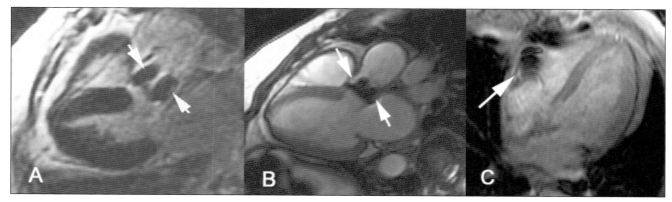

Figure 29.6
(A) Myocardial delayed enhancement long-axis view. Two sections of dark signal intensity around the aortic valve similar to the myocardium are seen. These are due to a bovine aortic valve replacement, which is confirmed on the gradient-echo image (B). (C) A susceptibility artifact (arrow) caused by a stent in the right coronary artery.

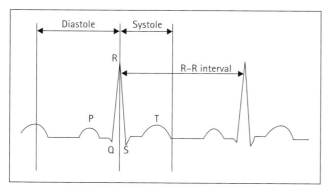

Figure 29.7
ECG components: P-wave, atrial contraction, original impulse from the sinoatrial (SA) node; PR interval, time between the onset of the P-wave and the onset of the QRS complex; QRS complex, depolarization of right and left ventricles (normal conduction); ST segment, depolarization of the ventricle and repolarization of the ventricle; T-wave, recovery after ventricular contraction.

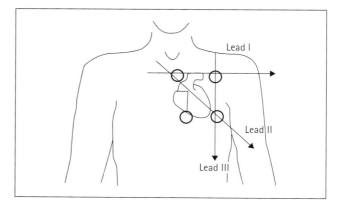

Figure 29.8
Basic ECG conventions.

lead selections prior to acquisition. Placement of the left-leg electrode should be in the vicinity of the heart's apex. However, if a robust signal is not achieved with the anterior configuration, then an alternative placement may include placing the electrodes on the lateral side of the patient's chest.

It should be noted that it is important to perform good patient preparation prior to electrode placement. This includes shaving the chest as necessary and using an abrasive gel to improve the contact between the electrode and the skin. Do not use outdated electrodes, since it is important that the electrodes have adequate conductive gel on the central portion of the electrode patch. Also, to minimize artifacts and possible heating, it is recommended that an MRI-compatible electrode be used (Figure 29.9).

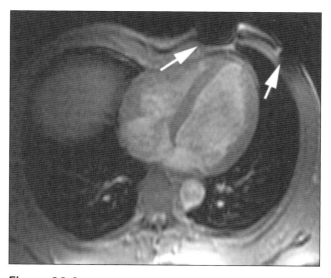

Figure 29.9
Susceptibility artifact (white arrows) from a non-MRI-compatible electrode.

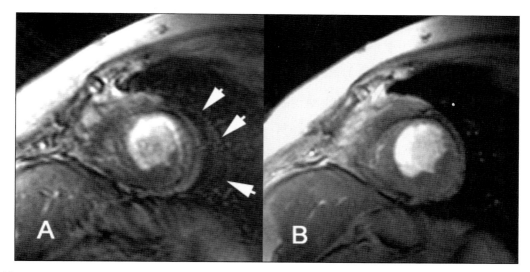

Figure 29.10
Patient referred for evaluation of left-ventricular function. The patient had a history of myocardial infarction and a left-ventricular aneurysm. Due to the patient's low voltage, a robust ECG signal could not be obtained and therefore the study had to be peripheral-pulse-gated. (A) An example of a short-axis image obtained with a breathhold. It shows phase ghosting artifacts – very poor definition of myocardial boarders. (B) The short-axis view was repeated using 2 signal averages from 0.5 signal averages (NEX) and increasing the phase matrix. The patient was free-breathing. Improved image quality was obtained with the patient free-breathing, thereby making quantification easier.

It is also important to understand a particular scanner's ECG software. Knowing how to troubleshoot and optimize key settings to obtain a robust signal will make the examination less time-consuming. There have been recent advances in ECG gating, including the use of fiberoptic technology and software enhancements that include an approach called vector ECG.[7]

Patients who have coronary artery disease, arrthythmo-genic right-ventricular dysplasia, pericardial effusion, or valvular disease may have arrhythmias. This is due to a change in the hearts conduction pattern due to disease. Arrhythmias may be benign or be related to the patient's underlying condition. Common cardiac arrhythmias that are encountered in cardiovascular patients include atrial fibrillation, bundle branch block, and premature ventricular contraction. Even though the patient may present with an arrhythmia, the examination can still be accomplished by carefully optimizing gating parameters.

The overall diagnostic quality of the CMR study relies on accurate cardiac gating. In cases in which accurate triggering cannot be achieved, an alternative technique such as gating from the peripheral pulse can be considered. The peripheral pulse can be utilized with a cine sequence that covers the full R–R interval, as featured in a pulse sequence called FastCine (GE Medical Systems, Milwaukee).[8] In our facility at the Cardiovascular Research Foundation, if we cannot easily obtain an adequate ECG signal, we switch to the peripheral pulse.

Another factor that may affect the quality of the ECG signal is the patient's breathing pattern. Sometimes, the ECG signal may become reliable enough for imaging when the patient performs the breathhold at end-expiration. Since cardiac images are best acquired on a breathhold, this situation still allows acquisition of images with excellent image quality. Breathholding on end-expiration insures the best image quality and reproducibility between views. Patients need to be instructed on how to do this prior to scanning, since it is important to explain the breathholding instructions prior to placing the patient into the magnet. The use of a cardiac or torso phased array coil is recommended to obtain images with high signal-to-noise ratio (SNR).

Assessing the patient's cooperation is important for obtaining a study that is diagnostically acceptable. Motivating the patient to follow all instructions during the study can be challenging, but this will ensure a technically good study. A very compromised patient may require a different acquisition strategy. In those circumstances, it may be necessary to adjust parameters; for example, the number of signal averages (NEX) can be increased to 'average out' breathing artifacts in patients who cannot perform the breathholds (Figure 29.10). Decreasing the phase matrix may help in reducing the scan time for patients who cannot hold their breath for a very long periods of time. Knowing which parameters to change for the acquisision is key. Real-time imaging will also play a role, since acquisitions will be able to be performed without ECG gating or breathholding. This will be advantageous when scanning patients who have arrhythmias or who cannot hold their breath.

Overview of cardiac pulse sequences

Pulse sequences utilized for imaging of the heart can be categorized as 'bright-blood' sequences and 'black-blood' sequences. Other sequences routinely utilized in CMR include flow quantification (phase-contrast) and sequences that require contrast enhancement (CE). Bright-blood techniques are used to look at function, while black-blood techniques are used to look at morphology or structural abnormalities of the heart. The latest bright-blood technique available is steady-state free precession (SSFP), which has substantially improved the ability of CMR to assess cardiac anatomic structure and function.[9,10] Sequences to assess myocardial perfusion require the use of gadolinium contrast. When contrast is used in conjunction with a pharmacological stress agent, ischemic heart disease can be further evaluated.[11,12]

A technique rapidly gaining acceptance is myocardial delayed enhancement, which can detect viable myocardium. This technique can aid cardiovascular surgeons in determining revascularization of the myocardial muscle.[13] This sequence has great utility, since it can also be used in other applications, such as evaluation of left-ventricular thrombus and myocarditis or any condition that may increase extracellular volume. Pulse sequences commonly used in clinical CMR applications are summarized in Table 29.1.

Table 29.1 Summary of CMR pulse sequences used in clinical cardiac applications

Cardiac imaging technique	Pulse sequence vendor terminology	Applications
Black-blood	• Black-blood prepulse • Double/Triple IR FSE • Dark-blood prepared • TSE • HASTE • TRIM • Black-blood prepulse • SPIR	• Morphology • Assessment of pericardium • Presence/Size tumor or mass • Assessment of valvular structure • Assessment of anomalous coronaries
Bright-blood (Cine)	• CINE • FastCard • FASTCINE • Segmented FLASH • TrueFISP Cine • FIESTA • Balanced-FFE	• Morphology • Presence of intracardiac thrombus • Cardiac dimensions and volumes • Global and regional function of left and right ventricles • Rapid imaging of great vessels
Contrast enhancement (CE)	• FastCard-ET • 2D Turbo-FLASH • 2D TFE with prepulse • SS TrueFISP (sat or IR recovery)	• Indirect assessment of coronary artery disease utilizing a first-pass approach assessing myocardial perfusion
	• IR Prep Gated FGRE • Segmented 2D Turbo-FLASH • IR TrueFISP	• Myocardial viability assessment of intracellular flow • Presence of intracardiac thrombus • Lesion characterization post gadolinium contrast (T1-weighted)
Phase-contrast	• Velocity-encoded cine GRE	Valvular function: • Quantification of regurgitation • Peak valvular gradient • Measurement of stroke volume and cardiac output of both ventricles • Quantification of shunts • Quantification of gradients or stenoses or coarctation of great arteries

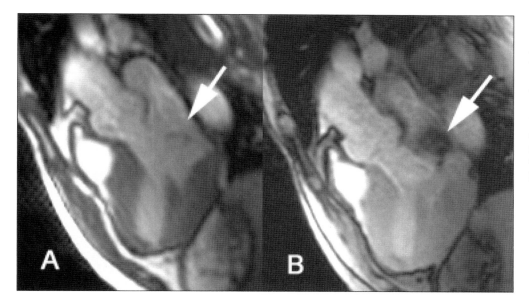

Figure 29.11
(A) Three-chamber view using a true SSFP cine end-systolic frame. (B) The same plane repeated using a standard fast gradient-echo sequence. Note the mitral regurgitation (arrow). (A) has superior contrast between the myocardium and the left-ventricular cavity, but the jet is not detected.

Bright-blood pulse sequences

Cine imaging is a technique utilized for highlighting the dynamic function of the heart. Cine imaging was introduced in the early 1980s; however, modifications made to this standard technique have greatly improved the temporal resolution of the sequence, with shorter acquisition times. In order to suspend the periodic motion of cardiac contraction, ECG gating is utilized. Spoiled gradient-echo segmented *k*-space cardiac sequences described by Atkinson and Edelman[14] allow imaging of many cardiac phases in a single breathhold with prospective cardiac gating. Prospective gating consists of initiation of the radiofrequency (RF) pulse sequences at fixed time in the cardiac cycle at each anatomic level; the data acquisition is guided by the ECG signal. Prospectively gated techniques are efficient; however, since the temporal phases are assigned on the basis of a fixed delayed time from the R-wave, the last 10–20% of diastole is not acquired. To address this issue, an improved segmented *k*-space technique is available that covers the entire R–R interval. Covering the entire R–R interval is important when evaluating diastolic function and atrial contraction.[15] Rather than reconstructing images at fixed delays from the R-wave, variable view sharing reconstructs images at different times within each cardiac cycle, depending on a temporal phase position that varies with the heart rate – otherwise known as a retrospective technique. Covering the entire cardiac cycle is essential if one wishes to use the peripheral pulse instead of the ECG for prospective gating.

With improved gradient hardware, SSFP sequences have taken the place of standard fast gradient-echo cine sequences due to higher spatial and temporal resolution, superior image contrast, and decreased artifacts from slow blood flow. These sequences offer higher contrast between the blood pool and myocardial wall, thus making them ideal for assessing cardiac function and structure. Because SSFP sequences often have very short echo times (TE), they are often less sensitive than cine techniques for detecting turbulent blood flow, such as that from valvular disease (Figure 29.11).

When utilizing any cine pulse sequence for cardiac applications, it is important to know what parameters can affect scan time and temporal resolution. The concept of views per segment (VPS), defined as the number of phase-encoding lines that are acquired as a group for each heartbeat, can affect image quality. The goal of any cine acquisition is to optimize the VPS for obtaining short scan times, while keeping in mind that the temporal resolution of an image should be ≤80 ms. For any segmented *k*-space technique, the tradeoff between scan time and temporal resolution can be achieved by adjusting the VPS accordingly. A summary of terms is listed in Table 29.2. The temporal resolution is calculated by using the repetition time (TR) × VPS. Compared with most cine pulse sequences, SSFP sequences have shorter TRs (2.0–3.5 ms). Therefore, they offer improved temporal and spatial resolution for a given breathhold. This is important when assessing structures such as the cardiac valves. When the VPS is reduced, the image will be less susceptible to blurring. However, this will increase the acquisition time of the image, thus making the breathhold time longer for the patient.

Black-blood pulse sequences

Conventional gated fast spin-echo (FSE) was the first type of pulse sequence utilized for cardiac morphology.

Table 29.2 Summary of key terms for segmented *k*-space pulse sequences

Term	Definition
TR	Repetition time: the time interval between excitations in a segment or frame
VPS	Number of phase-encoding lines acquired as a group in each defined cardiac phase
Temporal resolution	VPS × TR <80–100 ms
R–R interval	Time between heartbeats
Cine	A display of sequential images that correspond to different phases of the cardiac cycle representative of one complete heartbeat

However, even though FSE is generally thought of as a 'black-blood' pulse sequence (due to the 'wash-out' effect of flowing blood), in practice, signal from blood may not be thoroughly suppressed and related artifacts can occur. Today, this approach is hardly ever used, since improved sequences that utilize a double-inversion preparation pulse to ensure that signal from blood is adequately suppressed are now available.[16] Optimal image quality can be achieved when performed as a breathhold. It is important to notice that this technique produces images with either proton density or T2-weighted contrast. By adding a third inversion recovery preparation pulse, fat suppression can be achieved. Black-blood applications include characterization of intracardiac lesions, location of anatomic abnormalities, and defining valve leaflet morphology such as bicuspid aortic valves or valvular vegetations.[17]

General rationale for a CMR imaging protocol

A CMR examination should be tailored to achieve the proper clinical answer. In general, when acquiring oblique planes of the heart, it is best to use a standard protocol.[18] The short-axis plane is a standard oblique plane that gives the clinician a good overview view of global function. This is a standard plane that most clinicians are used to looking at from other imaging modalities. From the short-axis plane, other standard long-axis planes can be acquired. These include four-chamber (horizontal long-axis), two-chamber (vertical long-axis), and left-ventricular outflow tract (LVOT), also known as the three-chamber view.[19] These three long-axis planes allow for assessment of valvular function and wall motion. The acquisition of the short-axis and standard long-axis planes is described in Table 29.3.

Overview of clinical CMR applications

Evaluation of left-ventricular function

In our facility, we routinely quantify left-ventricular ejection fraction, end-diastolic and end-systolic volumes, stroke volume, and cardiac output as listed in Table 29.4. Left-ventricular functional parameters are normalized to body surface area. Linear measures of certain anatomic importance include left-ventricular diastolic wall thickness,[20] right-ventricular dimensions, left-atrial dimensions, and aortic root size (Figure 29.12). Normal values for cardiovascular structure and function can be found in the literature.[21,22]

To accurately quantify these parameters, a cardiac analysis software package should be used. For clinicians, global and regional ventricular performance is a very important prognostic factor in many disease states. Left-ventricular quantification and wall motion evaluation is usually performed by assessing the short-axis plane in a cine format. Patients with a history of coronary heart disease may have areas of wall motion abnormalities (Figure 29.13). The terms that describe left-ventricular wall motion are as follows:

- *hypokinesis* is characterized by decreased systolic wall motion;
- *akinesis* is characterized by absent systolic motion;
- *dyskinesis* is characterized by outward motion and thinning of the ventricular wall during systole.

Valvular function

CMR can assess most anatomic abnormalities of valve leaflets, as well as quantifying functional abnormalities

Table 29.3 Acquistion of short-axis and standard long-axis planes

	Key points	Graphic prescription of landmarks	Resulting view
1.	**Localizer plane** *Sagittal sequence* Nonsequential gradient-echo or an SSFP (TrueFISP, ungated Fiesta). *Key points:* Check coil positioning.	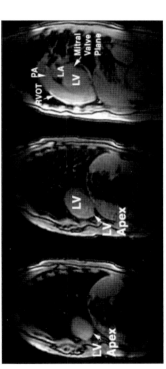 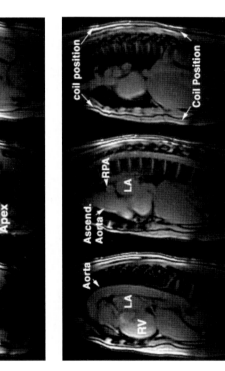	*Key:* LV, left ventricle; RV, right ventricle; RA, right atrium; LA, left atrium; AoV, aortic valve; Ao, aorta; PA/Pa, pulmonary artery; SVC, superior vena cava 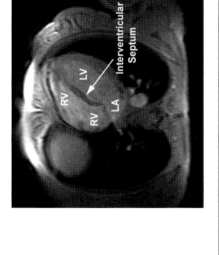
2.	**Long-axis localizer** *Sequence* Gradient-echo (GRE); segmented *k*-space sequence (FASTCINE, Fiesta). *Key points:* From a sagittal plane, prescribe a plane to the long axis of the heart, bisecting the apex and mitral valve plane.	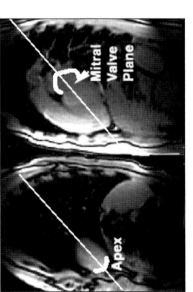	

Table 29.3 (*Continued*)

	Key points	*Graphic prescription of landmarks*	*Resulting view*

3. **Short-axis**
Sequence:
Segmented *k*-space
(GRE,
TrueFISP,
Fiesta)

Key points:
The short-axis
images cover from
base to apex. Each slice
location is typically
acquired during a
breathhold.

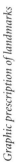

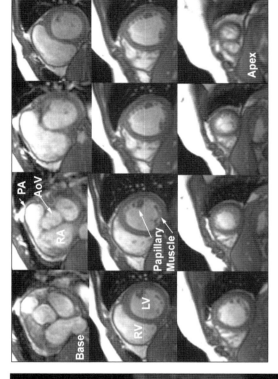

Key applications
1. Assessment of regional ventricular function.
2. Quantification of LV and RV volumes, ejection fractions and mass.

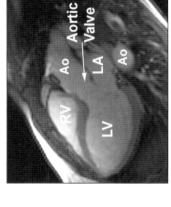

4. **Three-chamber**
(LVOT: **left-ventricular
outflow
tract,
vertical long-axis**)

Key points
Select a slice at the
level of the base of
the heart. Bisect the
aortic outflow tract
as outlined in white.

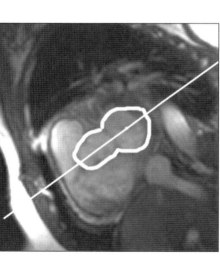
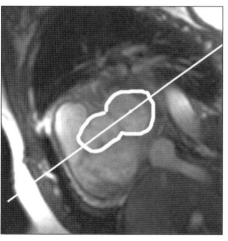

Key applications
1. Assessment of anteroseptal and inferolateral walls of the LV.
2. Assessment of mitral and aortic valves.

Table 29.3 (*Continued*)

	Key points	Graphic prescription of landmarks	Resulting view
5.	**Two-chamber (vertical long-axis)** *Key points* The two-chamber view is prescribed by bisecting the LV using the anterior and posterior papillary muscles as a guide.	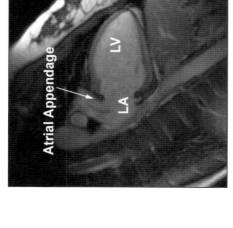	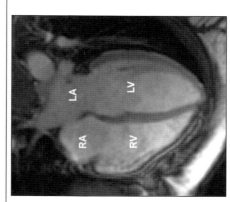 *Key applications* 1. Evaluation of anterior and inferior wall motion. 2. Assessment of LA appendage.
6.	**Four-chamber (horizontal long-axis)** *Key points* The four-chamber plane is prescribed from a mid-ventricular short-axis location bisecting the highest curvature of the RV (outlined in white)		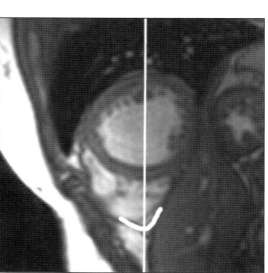 *Key applications* 1. Evaluation of septal and lateral walls of the heart. 2. Assessment of size and function of RV and tricuspid valve.

Table 29.3 (*Continued*)

Key points	*Graphic prescription of landmarks*	*Resulting view*
7. RVOT: right-ventricular outflow tract	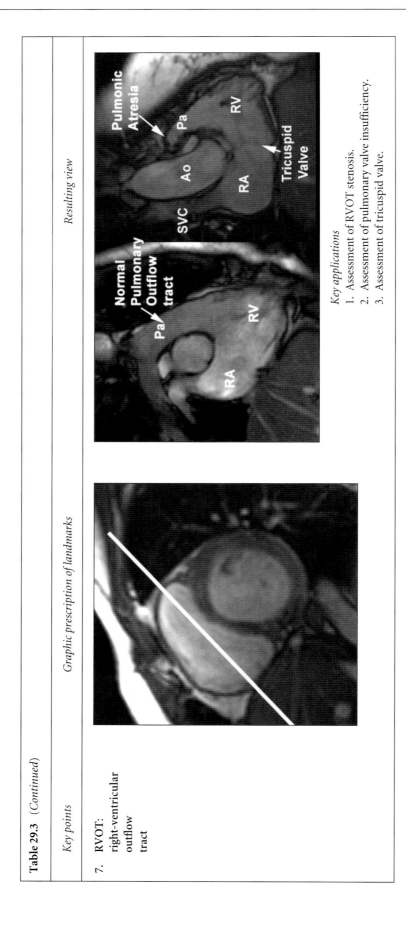	

Key applications
1. Assessment of RVOT stenosis.
2. Assessment of pulmonary valve insufficiency.
3. Assessment of tricuspid valve.

Table 29.4 Quantification of left-ventricular function

Parameter	Definition	CMR plane used for calculation
End-diastolic volume (EDV)	Largest volume of blood during left-ventricular relaxation	Multislice short-axis
End-systolic volume (ESV)	Smallest volume of blood during left-ventricular contraction	Multislice short-axis
Stroke volume (SV)	Amount of blood ejected from a ventricle with each beat. SV calculation: EDV − ESV	
Left-ventricular ejection fraction (LVEF)	Ratio of stroke volume to EDV. EF calculation: (SV/EDV) × 100	Multislice short-axis
Cardiac output (CO)	The cardiac output is the volume of blood pumped by the left ventricle per unit time, and is usually expressed in liters per minute	

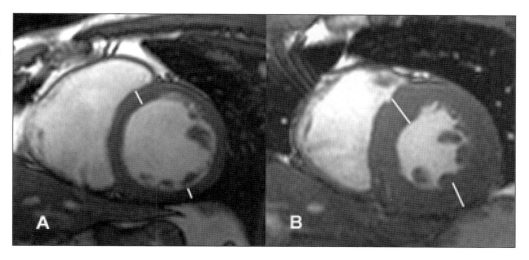

Figure 29.12
Standard measurements of wall thickness can be made on a short-axis view at the tips of the papillary muscle. (A) Normal anterior septal (1.0 cm) and posterior lateral wall (0.9 cm) thickness. (B) Left-ventricular hypertrophy; both walls measure 1.9 cm.

such as the severity of a leak. Bright-blood sequences are used to visually localize dark jets that occur with turbulent or fast flow. The appearance of fast and turbulent blood flow can be visualized on gradient-echo cine acquisitions as areas of signal void. These jets can arise at the valve leaflets, and are present in diastole or systole depending on whether the valve is stenotic (Figure 29.14) or regurgitant. To fully appreciate these jets, it is important that a long TE be used. Pulse sequence selection should also be considered, since when using an SSFP sequence, valvular regurgitation may not be as well visualized.

Introduced in the 1980s, phase-contrast imaging can quantify blood velocity (which can be used to estimate a pressure gradient) and blood flow (which can be used to quantify the regurgitant volume). The valves can be easily assessed by reviewing the three-chamber long-axis view, in which the mitral valve and the aortic valve are best seen. In the four-chamber long-axis view, both the mitral

and tricuspid valves can be assessed. If valvular disease is recognized during image acquisition, additional views may be needed to better define the abnormality. For example, if aortic insufficiency is noted, then a phase-contrast acqusition should be prescribed just above the aortic valve plane to quantify the severity of the regurgitation (Figure 29.15). The usefulness of phase-contrast imaging in the quantification of valvular regurgitation is well documented.[23–25]

Cardiac morphology and structure

Other common clinical indications for CMR include characterization of a cardiac mass,[26] arrhythmogenic right-ventricular dysplasia,[27,28] constrictive pericarditis,[29] and congenital abnormalities[30,31] (Figure 29.16). With these

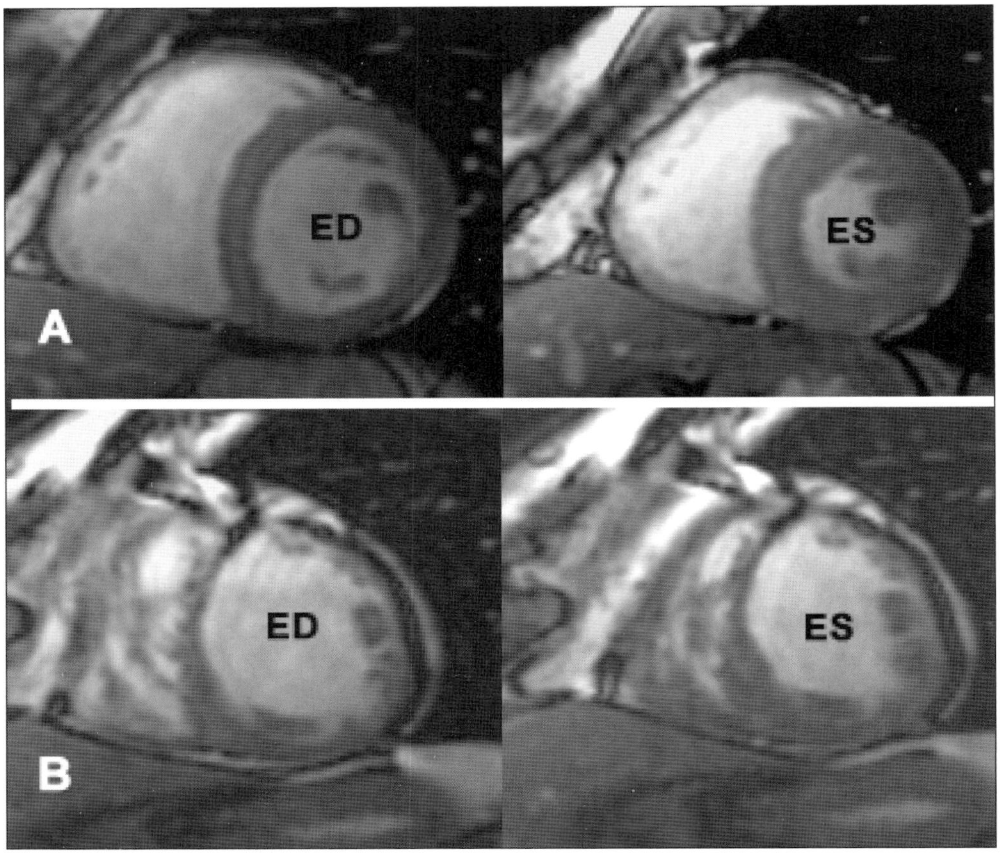

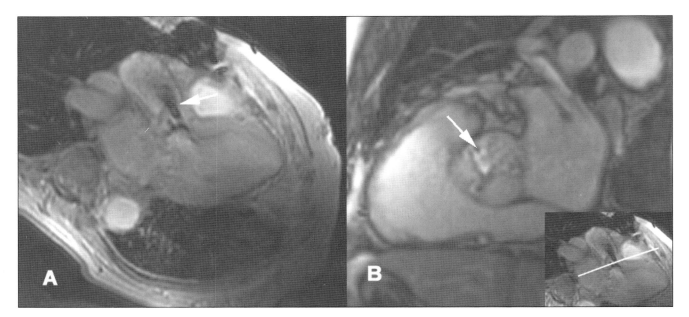

Figure 29.13
Row (A) is a short-axis plane showing normal ventricular wall thickness and normal global and regional systolic left-ventricular function. The left-ventricular ejection fraction is 75%, which is within the normal range. Row (B) is a short-axis plane showing abnormal ventricular wall thickness and wall motion. Notice how thin the anterior wall (arrow) is during end-diastole (ED) and end-systole (ES) compared with the normal heart function in (A). The anterior wall is akinetic, since systolic wall motion is absent. The left-ventricular ejection fraction is 25%, which is considered abnormally low.

Figure 29.14
(A) Three-chamber view showing a dark turbulent systolic jet. A cross-section (B) through the aortic valve shows incomplete leaflet opening in systole. Using flow analysis and obtaining the peak velocity across the valve, a pressure gradient of 40 mmHg can be calculated using the modified Bernoulli equation.

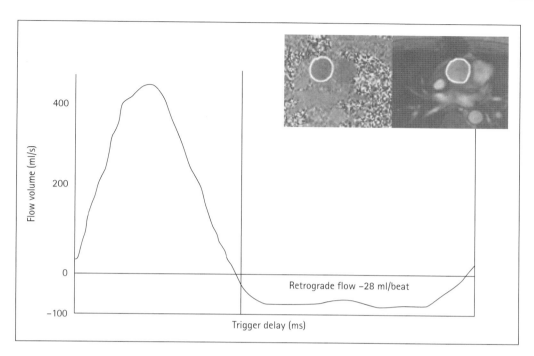

Figure 29.15
Plot of flow versus time for the ascending aorta in a patient with aortic insufficiency shows retrograde flow or a regurgitant volume of 28 ml/beat. A normal diastolic aortic curve stays at about 0 or at baseline. Using the left-ventricular stroke volume calculated from the short-axis plane of 83 ml, the regurgitant fraction is 34% (28 ml/83 ml).

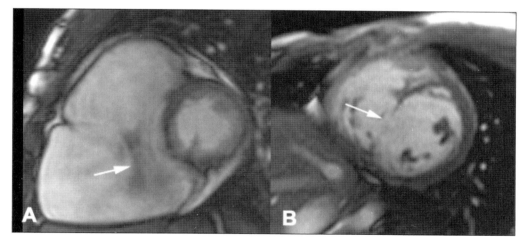

Figure 29.16
(A) A patient with Ebstein's anomaly: short-axis view showing in-plane tricuspid regurgitation. (B) A large muscular ventricular septal defect (VSD). To confirm the presence of a shunt, a phase-contrast acquisition should be performed to demonstrate the direction of flow.

types of studies, the cardiac protocol must be tailored to answer the clinical question. Besides the routine functional views, additional acquisitions may be necessary, such as using gadolinium contrast to assess for enhancement in the case of the evaluation of a cardiac mass. CMR is often the modality of choice for the evaluation of a cardiac mass.

The characterization of an apparent cardiac mass can be achieved by using different types of pulse sequences, For tissue characterization, black-blood sequences using T1 or T2 weighting can sometimes allow clinicians to be more specific in the diagnosis of an apparent cardiac mass (Figure 29.17). For patients with suspected shunts, phase-contrast imaging can be used to quantify shunt size.[32]

Evaluation of ischemic heart disease

Stress perfusion

With improved scanner hardware, faster imaging techniques can be employed to capture the first pass of gadolinium to evaluate myocardial perfusion. The detection and evaluation of patients with coronary artery disease is greatly enhanced by using MR first-pass (MRFP) perfusion with a pharmacologic stress agent such as adenosine. CMR offers improved spatial resolution compared with nuclear medicine, and therefore is the only technique that can differentiate subendocardial from

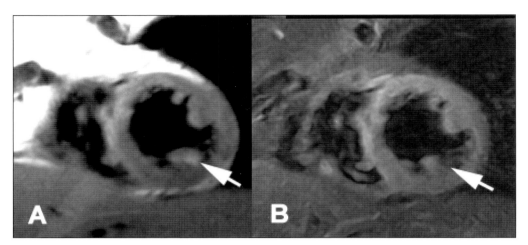

Figure 29.17
(A) Short-axis view showing a left-ventricular lipoma. Signal intensity mimics fat, which is bright on the double inversion recovery (IR) black-blood sequence. The mass is dark on the fat-suppressed double IR sequence (IB).

transmural ischemia.[33] It is important to screen patients for contraindications to the stress agent. Common side-effects from adenosine infusion include flushing, shortness of breath, and a warm feeling. Because adenosine has a very short half-life (~7 s), once the infusion is stopped, side-effects subside almost immediately.

MRFP stress perfusion is capable of assessing myocardial blood flow by observing the change in myocardial signal during the passage of a contrast agent bolus. Pulse sequences utilized for first-pass myocardial perfusion imaging include T1-weighted combined echo-planar and gradient-echo techniques.[34] Pulse sequences are designed to image the heart repeatedly and rapidly following a bolus injection of a contrast agent during the administration of a pharmacologic stress agent. Multiple slice locations to ensure entire ventricular coverage are acquired in a single acquisition. Regions of the heart with normal perfusion display a rapid and uniform enhancement, while regions with a perfusion defect enhance more slowly and to a lesser extent.

Patients who present with coronary artery disease can have a condition called ischemia in which the heart muscle is not receiving a sufficient blood supply upon demand. In order to assess for ischemic heart disease, a pharmacologic stress agent is given by intravenous administration while the patient is in the magnet. Pharmacologic stress agents should only be administered by properly trained personnel, and emergency protocols should be established. If the stress study shows a hypoenhanced defect but is normal on a resting perfusion study, then this condition is called 'ischemia' (Figure 29.18). Patients with previous myocardial infarctions have no blood supply to the muscle; therefore, the wall becomes necrotic and is hypoenhanced on both stress and resting perfusion studies. If the study includes a sequence to evaluate for viable myocardium post contrast, then a resting MRFP perfusion study is not necessary.

Stress function

Stress echocardiography can be used to evaluate for ischemic myocardium by assessing for wall motion at rest that worsens during stress. The literature shows that CMR is efficacious in this regard as well.[35,36] The stress agent typically used in this type of examination is dobutamine. The rationale behind this examination is to give dobutamine at various dose levels to be able to visualize a wall motion abnormality during stress. If the patient does not reach the maximum predicted heart rate for the age, then the agent atropine can be added. During each dobutamine dose level, cine images are acquired, usually in the short- and long-axis views. It is important that this examination be supervised by a trained physician, since the images must be reviewed while being acquired. Image interpretation during the examination is critical, because the study should be terminated once a wall motion abnormality is

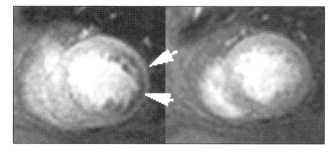

Figure 29.18
Stress myocardial perfusion short-axis view (left) shows a hypoenhanced region (arrows) in the lateral wall. The defect is subendocardial, demonstrating the ability of CMR to resolve perfusion defects within the wall of the myocardium. The rest image (right) shows the wall uniformly enhances, indicating that the patient has a flow-limiting stenosis rather than a scar from myocardial infarction. (Myocardial infarction would show hypoenhancement on both the stress and the rest images.)

Table 29.5 Comparison of stress perfusion and stress function applications		
Technical component	*Stress perfusion*	*Stress function*
Pharmacologic agent	Adenosine: • Vasodilator – very short half-life Dipyridamole: • Vasodilator – longer-lasting	Dobutamine: • Increases myocardial contractile force
Patient preparation	• Withhold caffeine (24 h prior to exam)[37] • Establish two intravenous lines	• Withhold beta-blockers (optional if low-dose study) • Establish one intravenous line
Contraindications	• Myocardial infarction <3 days • Asthma • Second- or third-degree atrioventricular block • Sick sinus syndrome or symptomatic bradycardia	• Idiopathic hypertrophic subaortic stenosis • Severe arterial hypertension • Ventricular tachyarrhythmia
Contrast requirement?	Yes: dose 0.05 mmol/kg[38]	No
Viability assessment?	Yes (when combined with a myocardial delayed enhancement sequence postcontrast)	Yes (low-dose)
Ischemic assessment?	Yes	Yes. Patient must reach maximum predicted heart rate (MPHR) for their age for accurate results.
Infarct detection?	Yes	Yes
Monitoring required	• Heart rate – continuously • Blood pressure – not required during infusion • Pulse oximetry – continuously • Symptoms – continuously	• Heart rate – continuously • Blood pressure – often • Pulse oximetry – continuously • Symptoms – continuously • Examination requires direct supervision of a qualified physician, since the images have to be reviewed while being acquired

detected. A comparison of the stress perfusion and stress function applications is summarized in Table 29.5.

Myocardial viability

All of the major manufacturers of MRI scanners have a sequence for the assessment of myocardial viability. Viability is defined as 'capability of living or of working, functioning, or developing'. The main purpose of the myocardial delayed enhancement (MDE) sequence is to determine what tissue is viable (alive) and what tissue is nonviable (infarcted). Nonviable myocardium is usually the result of a myocardial infarct. For patients facing revascularization with coronary angioplasty or coronary artery bypass, the determination of viability is an important clinical factor. Usually an inversion recovered prepped gated fast gradient-echo technique is used following gadolinium contrast administration. Early work shows

the optimal dose of gadolinium to be 0.2 mmol/kg and the optimal imaging delay time post contrast administration to be 10–20 min for this application.[39] Important scanning considerations include the selection of the inversion time (TI). If TI is selected properly, viable myocardial tissue will have no signal, whereas infarcts will be bright (Figure 29.19). This is because infarcts contain more gadolinium and have a shorter T1 than normal viable muscle. A viability study includes examination of the entire heart. Typically, short-axis images are acquired from base to apex. Sometimes, additional long-axis images are acquired to further document areas of hypenhancement.

Direct coronary artery imaging

Current proven clinical applications for coronary artery imaging include the assessment of coronary artery bypass graft patency[40] and the identification of anomalous

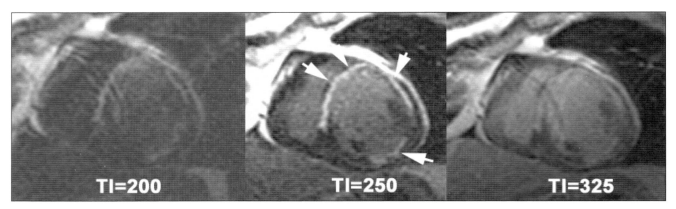

Figure 29.19
Myocardial delayed enhancement images demonstrating the proper selection of the inversion time (TI, in ms). The optimal image (center) shows an extensive transmural infarct involving the anterior and anteroseptal walls (arrows) and a small inferolateral infarct, predominantly subendocardial with bright signal intensity (hyperenhancement), with the myocardium being nulled.

coronary arteries.[41] Because of its noninvasive approach, using CMR to identify coronary stenosis is a major focus, and this application is still evolving. Techniques for images coronaries that have been described in the literature include both breathhold and non-breathhold approaches.[42]

The assessment of anomalous coronary arteries is very feasible in a clinical setting. Arteries running a course between the aorta and pulmonary artery can cause impairment of the blood flow to the heart muscle (Figure 29.20). It is important to identify these anomalies clinically, since they are associated with myocardial ischemia and sudden death. To be able to approach this application, an understanding of normal coronary artery distribution is required. The two principal vessels that supply oxygen-rich blood to the heart are the right and left main coronary arteries, which arise directly from the sinus of Valsalva.[43] The three sinuses of Valsalva are located in the most proximal portion of the aorta, just above the cusps of the aortic valve. The sinuses correspond to the individual cusps of the aortic valve. The right coronary artery, which orginates from the right sinus of Valsalva, supplies the inferior wall of the heart and runs in the atrioventricu-

lar groove. The left main coronary artery, which orginates from the left sinus of Valsalva, is usually larger than the right coronary artery. The left main divides into the left anterior descending (LAD), which feeds the anterior wall of the heart, and the left circumflex, which feeds the lateral wall of the heart muscle.

Conclusions

CMR poses a unique challenge for technologists. It can be overwhelming without specialized and dedicated training, especially given the many advances in the field. There are several ways in which MR technologists can be exposed to CMR. The major equipment manufacturers can offer specific training at facilities that have extensive experience in performing cardiovascular studies. The best environment to learn CMR is where actual clinical studies can be observed. Becoming involved in organizations such as the Section for Magnetic Resonance Technologists of the International Society for Magnetic Resonance in Medicine (www.ismrm.org/smrt) and the Technologist Section of

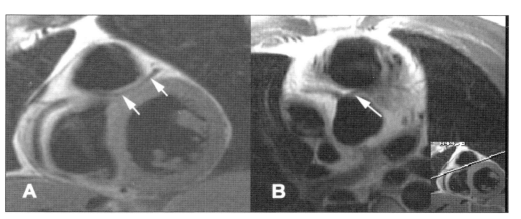

Figure 29.20
This patient was referred for CMR because the left main coronary artery could not be seen on coronary angiography. (A) An oblique view revealing an anomalous coronary artery. (B) A view parallel to the vessel showing the orgin of the left main coronary artery (arrow) from the right coronary cusp.

Table 29.6 Technical and clinical aspects of CMR: competencies required by a technologist	
Technical	*Clinical*

• MRI safety knowledge
• Good vein puncture technique
• Knowledge of intravenous contrast and power injection usage.
• Noninvasive monitoring usage (heart rate, blood pressure, etc.)
• Image artifacts and troubleshooting skills
• Basic ECG setup and interpretation
• Ability to recognize cardiac pathology during the examination and alter the examination accordingly
	• Basic cardiovascular anatomy and physiology
	• Cardiac scan plane prescription
	• Pulse sequence selection
	• Stress testing: use of pharmacologic agents
	• Good communication skills with patients
	• Cardiac analysis:
	  – Left-ventricular parameters
	  – Valvular function

the Society of Cardiovascular Magnetic Resonance (www.scmr.org) can help technologists keep current on new CMR applications. Depending on the motivation and experience of a technologist, learning many of the technical features and clinical applications of CMR listed in Table 29.6 can usually be accomplished within 3 months at a busy CMR center.

Acknowledgements

The author acknowledges Steven D Wolff MD, PhD and Lawrence G Dembo MBBS, FRACP for their review of the manuscript and Frank Macaluso RT for his assistance in image collection.

References

1. Wolff SD. Clinical cardiac MRI. Cardiovasc Rev Rep 2001; 22:305–13.

2. Introduction to Nuclear Cardiology, 3rd edn. DuPont Pharma, 1993.

3. Bogaert J. Magnetic Resonance of the Heart and Great Vessels. Berlin: Springer-Verlog, 1999.

4. Ahmed S, Shellock FG. Magnetic resonance imaging safety: implications for cardiovascular patients. J Cardiovasc Magn Reson 2001; 3:171–82.

5. Shellock FG. Prosthetic heart valves and annuloplasty rings: assessment of magnetic field interactions, heating, and artifacts at 1.5 tesla. J Cardiovasc Magn Reson 2001; 3:317–24.

6. Korcheviski EM, Marochnik LS. Magnetohydrodynamic version of movement of blood. Biofizika 1965; 10:371–3.

7. Chia JM, Fisher WE, Wickline SA, Lorenz CH. Performance of QRS detection for cardiac magnetic resonance imaging with a novel vectrocardiographic triggering method. J Magn Reson Imaging 2000; 12:678–88.

8. Feistein JA, Epstein FH, Arai AE, et al. Using cardiac phase to order resronstruction (CAPTOR): a method to improve diastolic images. J Magn Reson Imaging 1997; 7:794–8.

9. Bundy J, Simonetti O, Laub G, et al. Segmented TrueFISP imaging of the heart. In: Proceedings of the 7th Annual Meeting of the International Society for Magnetic Resonance in Medicine, 1999: 1282.

10. Barkhausen J, Ruehm SG, Goyen M, et al. MR evaluation of ventricular function: true fast imaging with steady-state precession versus fast low-angle shot cine MR imaging: feasibility study. Radiology 2001; 219:264–9.

11. Wolff SD, Comeau CR, Slavin GS, et al. Assessment of first-pass myocardial perfusion imaging using interleaved notched saturation: comparison with cardiac catheterization. In: Proceedings of the 8th Annual Meeting of the International Society for Magnetic Resonance in Medicine, 2000: 1558.

12. Schwitter J, Nanz D, Kneifel S, et al. Assessment of myocardial perfusion in coronary artery disease by magnetic resonance: a comparison with positron emission tomography and coronary angiography. Circulation 2001; 103:2230–5.

13. Kim RJ, Wu E, Rafael A, et al. The use of contrast-enhanced magnetic resonance imaging to identify reversible myocardial dysfunction. N Engl J Med 2000; 343:1445–53.

14. Atkinson DJ, Edelman RR. Cineangiography of the heart using a single breath hold with a segmented TurboFLASH sequence. Radiology 1991; 178:357–60.

15. Feistein JA, Epstein FH, Arai AE, et al. Using cardiac phase to order resronstruction (CAPTOR): a method to improve diastolic images. J Magn Reson Imaging 1997; 7:794–8.

16. Simonetti OP, Finn JP, White RD, et al. 'Black blood' T2-weighted inversion-recovery MR imaging of the heart. Radiology 1996; 199:49–57.

17. Arai AE, Epstein FH, Bove KE, Wolff SD. Visualization of aortic valve leaflets using black blood MRI. J Magn Reson Imaging 1999; 10:771–7.

18. Comeau CR. Introduction to Cardiovascular MR Imaging. GE Medical Systems Applications Guide, 1999.

19. Cerqueira MD, Weissman NJ, Dilsizian VD, et al. Standardized myocardial segmentation and nomenclature for tomographic imaging of the heart. Circulation 2002; 105:539–42.

20. Sechtem U, Sommerhoff BA, Markiewicz W, et al. Regional left ventricular wall thickening by magnetic resonance imaging: evaluation

in normal persons and patients with global and regional dysfunction. Am J Cardiol 1987; 59:145–51.

21. Lorenz CH, Walker ES, Morgan VL, et al. Normal human right and left ventricular mass, systolic function, and gender differences by cine magnetic resonance imaging. J Cardiovasc Magn Reson 1999; 1:7–21.

22. Lorenz CH. The range of normal values of cardiovascular structures in infants, children and adolescents measured by magnetic resonance imaging. Pediatr Cardiol 2000; 21:37–46.

23. Wagner S. Auffermann W, Buser P, et al. Diagnostic accuracy and estimation of the severity of valvular regurgitation from the signal void on cine magnetic resonance images. Am Heart J 1989; 118:760–7.

24. Hundley WG, Li HF, Willard JE. Magnetic resonance imaging assessment of the severity of mitral regurgitation. Comparison with invasive techniques. Circulation 1995; 92:1151–8.

25. Didier D, Ratib O, Lerch R, Friedli B. Detection and quantification of valvular heart disease with dynamic cardiac MR imaging. Radiographics 2000; 20:1279–99.

26. Martin DR, Merchant N, MacDonald C. MR imaging of cardiac masses: a review of current application and approach. Appl Radiol 2000; 29:10–20.

27. Van der Wall EE, Kayser HW, Bootsman MM. Arrthythmogenic right ventricular dysplasia: MRI findings. Hertz 2000; 25:356–64.

28. Kayser HW, de Roos A, Schalij MJ, et al. Usefulness of magnetic resonance imaging in the diagnosis of arrhythmogenic right ventricular dysplasia and agreement with electrocardiographic critera. Am J Cardiol 2003; 91:365–7.

29. Frank H, Globits S. Magnetic resonance imaging evaluation of myocardial and pericardial disease. J Magn Reson Imaging 1999; 10:617–26.

30. Nienaber CA, Rehders TC, Fratz S. Detection and assessment of congenital heart disease with magnetic resonance techniques. J Cardiovasc Magn Reson 1999; 1:164–84.

31. Chung T. Assessment of cardiovascular anatomy in patient s with congenital heart disease by magnetic resonance imaging. Pediatr Cardiol 2000; 21:18–26.

32. Beerbaum P, Korperich H, Barth P, et al. Noninvasive quantification of left-to-right shunt in pediatric patients: phase-contrast cine magnetic resonance imaging compared with invasive oximetry. Circulation 2001; 103:247–82.

33. Wolff SD. Clinical cardiac MRI. Cardiovasc Rev Rep 2001; 22:305–13.

34. Salvin GS, Wolff SD, Gupta SN, Foo TKF. First-pass myocardial perfusion imaging with interleaved notched saturation: feasibility study. Radiology 2001; 219:258–63.

35. Nagel E, Lehmkuhl HB, Bocksch W, et al. Noninvasive diagnosis of ischemia-induced wall motion abnormalities with the use of high-dose dobutamine stress MRI: comparison with dobutamine stress echocardiography. Circulation 1999; 99:763–70.

36. Hundley WG, Hamilton CA, Thomas MS, et al. Utility of fast cine magnetic resonance imaging and display for the detection of myocardial ischemia in patients not well suited for second harmonic stress echocardiography. Circulation 1999; 100:1697–702.

37. Nagel E, Lorenz C, Baer F, et al. Stress cardiovascular magnetic resonance: Consensus Panel Report. J Cardiovasc Magn Reson 2001; 3:267–81.

38. Wolff SD, Schwitter J, Coulden R, et al. Myocardial first-pass perfusion imaging: a multicenter dose ranging study. In: Proceedings of Society of Cardiovascular MR Scientific Meeting, 2002:108.

39. Comeau CR, Santiago LM, Dangas GD, et al. Myocardial delayed enhancement: determining the optimal gadolinium dose and delay time for infarct imaging. In: Proceedings of Society of Cardiovascular MR Scientific Meeting, 2002:132.

40. Bedaux WLF, Hofman MBM, Vyt SLA, et al. Assessment of coronary artery bypass graft disease using cardiovascular magnetic resonance determination of flow reserve. J Am Coll Cardiol 2002; 40:1848–55.

41. McConnell MV, Ganz P, Selwyn AP, et al. Identification of anomalous coronary arteries and their anatomic course by magnetic resonance coronary angiography. Circulation 1995; 92:3158–62.

42. Danias PG, Stuber M, Edelman RR. Coronary MRA: a clinical experience in the United States. J Magn Reson Imaging 1999; 10:713–20.

43. Green C. Coronary Cinematography. Philadelphia: Lippincott-Raven, 1996.

30

How to set up a CMR laboratory and program

Stephen Frohwein, Aysegul Yegin, Valentin Fuster, Zahi A Fayad

Introduction

Technological advances in magnetic resonance imaging (MRI) have allowed this imaging modality to come to the forefront of cardiac imaging. Advances in high-performance gradient hardware and ultrafast pulse sequence techniques that permit cine images of ventricular function, real-time imaging during pharmacological stress infusion, and the ability to evaluate the presence and degree of necrosis, fibrosis, or infiltration within the myocardium have opened this imaging modality for an array of clinical cardiovascular applications.[1–4] Unlike angiography and echocardiography, MRI is not encumbered by geometric assumptions in the calculation of geometric volumes, and has become the standard for the determination of ventricular volumes.[5–7] Cardiovascular magnetic resonance (CMR) has been shown to be an excellent modality in the determination of myocardial ischemia and viability in patients with ischemic heart disease.[2,8,9] CMR compares favorably with positron emission tomography (PET) in the evaluation of myocardial viability.[10,11] The role of CMR is rapidly expanding into visualization of atherosclerotic plaque as well as a potential role in the evaluation of coronary arterial anatomy.[12,13] For these reasons, it has become one of the fastest-growing cardiac imaging modalities. There is a need for the development of MRI centers that have the equipment, personnel and expertise to perform the full range of CMR studies. This chapter has been prepared for the benefit of clinicians or centers that wish to establish or incorporate CMR into their clinical practices. The topics covered are meant to guide the individual toward the general principles and aspects needed to establish and run an active CMR program. The common strategies necessary in establishing a CMR program either from an initial concept or from within an existing imaging center (either hospital or outpatient) will be discussed.

CMR capabilities

Prior to the start of a study, the interpreting physician and the technologist should outline the sequence strategy. Outlining a series of sequences by protocol often saves time, as well as insuring adequate image acquisition to diagnose and describe the clinical scenario. Patient preparation and study performance are different in cardiac patients compared with routine examinations performed on a daily basis in conventional imaging centers. Cardiac patients often have special needs, and may have difficulties with prolonged or repetitive breathholds. Stress imaging during CMR introduces a new paradigm in which cardiac patients with either known or unknown ventricular dysfunction, myocardial ischemia, or arrhythmias will be receiving stress agents while in the magnet. There are limitations in the ability to communicate or monitor patients when studies are being performed. Invariably, emergencies may arise during either routine or stress studies. Due to the ferromagnetic properties of required emergency equipment such as defibrillators and monitors, this equipment should be located just outside the magnet space and should be easily obtained and operated. There should be adequate space just outside the magnet for an emergency gurney and several people to perform life-sustaining procedures. Personnel working during cardiac studies should have training in basic and advanced life-support techniques such as cardiopulmonary resuscitation (CPR) or the delivery of direct current from a defibrillator. It is a good practice to have routine drills to acclimate new and current staff to emergency procedures and operation of emergency equipment.

In any high-volume MRI laboratory, time is of essence. Gone are the days when most MRI suites had the luxury of performing cardiac studies that would last an hour or longer. The mission now is to get as much information in a short time that will allow the interpreting physician to calculate ventricular volumes, mass, and ejection fraction

Table 30.1 Classification of CMR procedures	
Standard MRI procedures	*Less common procedures*
• Tomographic still-frame MRI for morphology using 'bright-blood' and/or 'dark-blood' methods with and/or without contrast agent • Cine MRI for ventricular function and other dynamic imaging studies at rest and/or stress (exercise or pharmacological) • Magnetic resonance angiography (MRA) and cine MRI of the great vessels, peripheral vessels, anomalous coronary arteries, and coronary bypass grafts	• Myocardial tagging • Phase-contrast velocity mapping for blood flow quantification • First-pass, contrast-enhanced MRI • Delayed contrast-enhanced MRI • MRA of proximal native coronary arteries • Atherosclerotic vascular wall imaging

as well as interpreting wall motion abnormalities, valvular problems, pericardial processes, and congenital abnormalities. Additional time will be necessary to perform first-pass perfusion, imaging during stress (exercise or pharmacological), tissue characterization such as delayed hyperenhancement, and evaluations of the vascular or coronary anatomy.

The radiologists and cardiologists should participate in the decision-making process and the description of each protocol and the sequences involved. However, the supervising physician should be ultimately in charge of deciding which protocols should be used on a routine basis. This will allow a rapid patient flow through the MRI department so as to accommodate as many studies as possible. CMR is a rapidly changing and dynamic imaging modality, and routine and specialized protocols will be changing frequently. Therefore, an approach that allows both the supervising and the interpreting physicians to routinely evaluate and adjust the standard and specialized protocols and sequences will keep the CMR laboratory ahead of the curve. A recent classification of standard and specialized protocols is given in Table 30.1.

Some laboratories have elected to categorize studies based on the clinical question asked so as to obtain the required information necessary to diagnose the clinical problem. The studies are commonly separated into five standard imaging protocols. Frequently different protocols are combined in one examination when clinically necessary. Each protocol described below provides only examples, and with the rapidly changing environment of CMR will need frequent modification. Advanced imaging protocols are covered in other chapters of this book.

1. *Basic functional imaging* allows calculation of ventricular volumes, masses, and ejection fractions. Regional wall motion abnormalities, valve leaflet movements, valvular regurgitation, and anatomical coronary anatomy position can also be assessed. This is accomplished using a 'bright-blood' technique. Variations on gradient-echo imaging are employed. The most

common gradient-echo technique, known as Turbo-FLASH ('fast low-angle shot'), uses a short TR and small flip angle. Steady-state free precision (SSFP) techniques, also known as TrueFISP ('true fast imaging with steady-state precession') on the Siemens platform, are variations of coherent gradient-echo sequences. Critical steps involve describing the true long axis of the left ventricle and obtaining serial short-axis slices of the left ventricle to allow for accurate measurements.

2. *First-pass perfusion imaging* allows visualization of gadolinium contrast as it initially enters the myocardial muscle. Perfusion defects related to acute and chronic obstructive coronary disease are observed. A gradient-echo Turbo-FLASH sequence is utilized along 4–6 short-axis slices. Gadolinium should be infused at 0.1–0.2 mmol/kg at 2–3 ml/s. The timing of sequence acquisition should coincide with the arrival of contrast agent within the right-ventricular cavity.

3. *Tissue characterization imaging* is a fast spin-echo (FSE) technique that visualizes the myocardium in a 'black-blood' state. Single tomographic slice images of the heart are obtained in a single breathhold. The signal of the blood in the ventricle is eliminated with a 'double inversion recovery' magnetization preparation technique. Fat saturation can be achieved by adding a nonselective fat-inversion pulse that nulls the signal from fat. This technique is useful in evaluating tissue characteristics within the myocardium as well as the pericardium.

4. *Delayed hyperenhancement (DHE) imaging* produces single-slice breathhold images, either long- or short-axis, using an inversion recovery FLASH sequence 10–30 min after a standard gadolinium bolus. Areas of DHE within the myocardium are considered to be scar tissue.

5. *Magnetic resonance phase velocity mapping (PVM)* quantifies blood flow and can be used to measure gradients across stenoses in the valves or aorta. A range (200–500 cm/s) of velocity-encoded values (VENC) is used to quantify flow.

Creating an interdisciplinary approach to the CMR center

The infiltration of cardiovascular specialists into the MRI field that heretofore has been controlled and dominated by radiology specialists has created controversies in the establishment of the CMR center. These controversies will vary in different centers and will be primarily based on which group has control over the imaging equipment. For groups of cardiologists, the creation of a freestanding CMR center is an expensive task. With low reimbursement rates and slow-rising acceptance of this imaging modality in cardiovascular disorders, the financial justification for such a venture is questionable at this time. A freestanding independent outpatient imaging center designed for both cardiac and noncardiac studies is a potential platform where either cardiologists or radiologists can either independently or jointly perform studies. The creation of a CMR center within an already-established hospital-based imaging center will require radiologists and cardiologists to work in a harmonious manner. In this type of clinical setting, each discipline brings unique attributes that when combined allow for the creation of a strong CMR program. The difficulty arises in getting these two 'competitor' groups to work together. Each situation presents its own set of difficult circumstances that will need to be sorted out and solved prior to starting a program. Since there are a number of quality control, safety, scheduling, and reimbursement-for-services issues related to the initiation of a CMR program, these problems would need to be settled to allow the smooth inception of such a program. One potential solution would be the creation of responsibilities for each member of the interdisciplinary team. Focusing specific responsibilities on each party defines the roles in the building of the program.

Examples of the cardiologist's responsibilities may include the following:

- assurance of patient safety throughout studies;
- assurance of proper clinical utility of CMR;
- education of technologists and radiologists with regard to cardiac pathophysiology;
- supervision of stress studies;
- maintenance of resuscitative equipment (stocking meds, equipment, etc.);
- education of referring physicians on clinical indications of CMR;
- quality assurance of studies along with radiologist.

Examples of the radiologist's responsibilities may include:

- assurance of patient safety throughout studies;
- assurance of proper image quality control measures;
- enforcement of safety measurements;
- supervision of noncardiac and vascular studies;
- interpretation of noncardiac abnormalities;
- quality assurance of studies along with cardiologist

Since most centers will not be performing cardiac studies exclusively, sequential scheduling of cardiac studies will allow personnel with special cardiac training such as nurses and technologists to function elsewhere when routine noncardiac studies are being performed. Scheduling of cardiac studies in this manner will allow cardiac nurses and physicians to arrange their schedules to be available during these specific times. Cost-effective utilization of these specialized individuals will allow the center to practice cost-saving measures.

Personnel and equipment

The creation of a cardiovascular laboratory requires unique equipment and personnel characteristics. If one were starting from the beginning, this list would obviously be more extensive. Building a freestanding CMR center requires a clinical setting that is uniquely able to supply a significant amount of clinical and/or research studies to generate revenue that would satisfy high operating costs. Overwhelmingly, clinical CMR centers will have to be built within existing MRI centers that are either hospital-based or within an established outpatient center. The creation of a freestanding CMR center will be limited to a few clinical settings, and each individual setting will bring a unique set of circumstances.

Whether initiating a laboratory through new construction or building it within an established hospital or outpatient imaging center, the critical initial step is to take stock of the equipment and personnel available to the program. Effective team building in the development of an active CMR laboratory is the key to success. Defining responsibilities of those involved will help create a team environment that will allow growth as well as securing safety and quality control and assurances. Members of the team should include a supervising physician, who is either a radiologist or cardiologist, interpreting physicians of both cardiology and radiology disciplines, and technologists, physicists, and nurses with CMR expertise. Administrative positions should be occupied by individuals who have the ability to work with an interdisciplinary team of physicians and allied health professionals, and if possible should be independent of the existing structure of the cardiology and radiology departments.

Creating a list of the equipment necessary to perform the full range of MRI examinations will change with the complexity of this new imaging modality. In 2003, the generation of an MR image requires at least one computer, a radio transmitter and receiver, multiple radio receiver coils, dual gradient coils, and the main magnet. A computer is necessary to generate the timing and strength of the magnetic field gradients and radio pulses that are prescribed by the operator. These instructions are sent to gradient and radiofrequency (RF) amplifiers, which create the gradient and radio pulses. The radio pulses are sent from the RF power amplifier to the transmit-and-receive driver, which triggers the generation of the radio pulses. The pulses are transmitted from an antenna coil into the body area of study. This antenna coil is utilized for both transmitting and receiving the MR signal. In the imaging of superficial body areas, a separate coil that only receives signals is preferred. The returning signal with imaging data is collected by the receiving coil. This data is then sent to the transmit-and-receive driver and subsequently to a preamplifier, which prepares the signal for analog-to-digital conversion. The initial signal is composed of nondigital radiowaves that form a composite waveform containing different frequencies, phases, and amplitudes. The conversion of this analog data to digital data is processed by the MR acquisition computer and stored in a matrix of data known as k-space. Each point in k-space contains data from all portions of an MR image. The k-space data are subsequently subjected to Fourier transform analysis, which produces pixel data with different gray-scale values that have a specific spatial location. Construction of two- or three-dimensional images can then be displayed, viewed, or subjected to further analysis.

If there is an existing magnet on site, it may be able to accept software or possibly require a hardware/software upgrade. Manufacturers will be able to assist in the evaluation of a center's current magnet. The purchase of a new system will allow incorporation of all that is needed to perform a complete CMR study. To adequately perform CMR studies, a high-field system will be required. Currently, hospitals and research facilities are routinely employing 1.5 T systems. The development of 3 T magnets has created options for research centers to explore this new exciting technology. However, the added benefit of the higher field strength is not necessary to perform routine diagnostic CMR studies, and the overall benefits of 3 T systems in cardiovascular disease have not yet been elucidated. The basic requirements of most scanners to perform CMR studies include the following:

- an actively shielded body gradient coil (preferable);
- a 1.5 T magnet;
- a minimum of 30 mT/m gradient field strength per axis to provide a minimum slew rate (SR) of 125 T/m/s per axis and with, when possible, a 100% duty cycle;
- a surface circular coil with a diameter of at least 14 cm;
- cardiac phased array surface coils;

- injector systems for the delivery of contrast material and stress agents (capable of being activated from the control desk);
- electrocardiography (ECG) monitoring equipment: each manufacturer has specific lead systems for their units that may have advantages in study performance;
- cardiac software package capable of performing the following types of studies: SSFP cine imaging, Turbo-FLASH cine imaging (TFL), black-blood inversion recovery imaging (TSE), echo-planar imaging (EPI), first-pass myocardial perfusion and DHE, MRA, and magnetic resonance spectroscopy (MRS);
- a separate workstation that allows transfer of DICOM images and is equipped with software allowing the calculation of ventricular sizes and function as well as blood flow analysis;
- a personal computer or server that will allow data storage and report generation.

The personnel required for the performance of CMR studies include a technologist and a physician who have been particularly trained to perform CMR studies. These individuals need to have knowledge of not only the physics of MRI but also an in-depth knowledge of the anatomy of complex cardiovascular disorders and a complete understanding of the safety requirements within an MRI suite. Nurses with specialized training in cardiovascular disorders and emergency situations will need to be present for stress CMR procedures.

Finally, the availability of other noninvasive methods such as nuclear imaging, echocardiography, and computed tomography (CT) should be kept in mind, since some situations they could provide necessary and complementary information for the diagnosis and follow-up of cardiovascular disease, and they should be considered if possible an integral part of the noninvasive cardiovascular imaging program.

Design and construction of the MRI laboratory

Planning

Architectural solutions that combine creativity with a knowledge of the inner workings of the healthcare industry are essential elements of financial success and marketing. Designs that are efficient, cost-effective, adaptive, and economically creative reflect the responsive solutions that are available from innovative healthcare architects.

Ideally, the facility's master plan is preceded by a strategic plan. A strategic plan defines an organization's missions, goals, programs, and services. A facility's master plan is derived from the strategic plan. The purpose of master planning is to provide a comprehensive and rational approach to the development of space. In the absence of a master plan, facilities tend to grow in a disorganized fashion. In this manner, immediate pressures take precedence over long-term considerations and the concept of planned development. Master planning takes into account the following points:[14]

- space requirements for current and future programs;
- site opportunities and constraints;
- staffing patterns;
- systems for materials handling, communications, and traffic flow;
- functional relationships among departments;
- options for the development of the site/building;
- the amount of new construction and renovation;
- the cost of development.

Master planning should emphasize operational issues that guide the architectural issues. Although design is important, it should be governed by factors such as staffing, operational efficiency, service volumes, and budgetary considerations. The implications of these factors should be evaluated for capital funding and incorporated into the functional designs. The elements of planning should include:[14]

- data collection and review;
- site analysis;
- building evaluation;
- program development;
- option analysis;
- solution recommendation;
- phasing, schedule, and budget.

The overall architectural and construction process for building of a new MRI facility includes, but is not limited to, the following stages:

- architectural drawings, including demolition plans, floor plans, reflected ceiling plans, details, and finishing plans;
- heating, ventilating, and air-conditioning design, drawings, and specifications; design of hydronic piping from the magnet chiller to the magnet;
- determination of electrical load requirements, and drawing/design/specifications for complete electrical design, including provisions for power and grounding;
- design of a complete plumbing system, including coordination of the base building system and rework of the existing MED gas piping if necessary.

Functional issues

MRI employs strong magnetic fields, and the emitted fields can affect surrounding systems such as telecommunication and information systems. Great care must be taken in selecting a site location for the MRI unit. Certain technical space requirements impose special constraints on the siting and design of MRI facilities. These may include:

- magnetic fields generated by MRI magnets;
- the sensitivity of imaging process to different radiofrequencies;
- the size and weight of the magnet;
- cryogen service;
- venting requirements.

For building systems integration, locations of depressed slabs and structures for equipment, electrical access, and magnetic and/or RF shielding should be coordinated. The size and weight of the magnet should be considered, since these could require locations on the lower or the lowest floors of the facility. Magnet installation and replacement requires crane access and a direct route for magnet passage. The radiation issue must be considered in relation to adjacent areas. Steel support structures arranged in a fashion not symmetrical to the magnetic field impose special requirements for shielding. Installation within multistory facilities may impose planning and structural restrictions on spaces above and below. A direct vent to outdoors accomplishes cryogen venting during quenching. Cryogen replenishment is accomplished via cryogen dewars, which may be stored on site. Access is required around and above the magnet for cryogen service.

The MRI reception area should be strategically located to control access to the patient areas and to secure the MRI unit from unauthorized areas. Gowning areas with secure lockers should be provided for inpatients and outpatients, and the control of ferrous materials should be rigorous. For outpatients, convenient access from patient parking should be planned. Passenger elevator access to MRI facilities should be located off main entrance levels. The MRI control area and the electronics room need to be adjacent to the MRI procedure room.

Technical issues

The standardization of all the elements built into the MRI laboratory should be optimized. Some examples of the guidelines for the construction of the MRI suite are as follows.

Partitions and doors around the MRI gantry room should provide RF shielding and be constructed of nonmagnetic materials. Floors in offices, conference rooms and waiting areas should be carpeted with a 100 mm (4 in.)-high resilient base. Floors in bathrooms should be of ceramic tiles with a ceramic tile base. Floors in other spaces should be of vinyl composition tiles with a 100 mm (4 in.)-high resilient base. Floors in MRI gantry rooms require a 40 mm (1.5 in.)-deep depression to accommodate the RF shielding. The computer/access floor system should be of nonmagnetic materials. Ceilings should be of lay-in acoustic ceiling tiles. Interior doors should be 45 mm (1.75 in.) thick, solid core, flush-panel wood doors or non-magnetic hollow metal doors with hollow metal frames.

Information management systems should include the following elements:

- image retrieval;
- processing/storage;
- treatment planning;
- patient registrations;
- patient charges;
- physician's order entry;
- patient/staff movement.

A 'life safety program' should be developed to provide a reliable system to protect the building occupants, firefighting personnel, and building contents, structure, and function. The design aspects of the facility that relate to fire and life safety include:[15]

- structural fire resistance;
- building compartmentalization;
- fire detection, alarm, and suppression;
- smoke control and exhaust;
- firefighter access and facilities;
- emergency power.

Potential problems in the CMR suite[16]

- MRI systems are still heavy, and even unshielded systems can weigh >3.5 tons, while big magnets with their shields can be >30 tons.
- Even with cryogen-recovery systems, a supply of liquid gas is still required for cryogenically cooled systems, which is a serious limitation on the scale of such systems in the developing world. Provision of the delivery of the dewars is still required, although the frequency of refill is less than it was.
- Lighting may be a problem in the examination rooms. Even with the lighting being transformed to direct current, bulbs seem to burn out with expensive regularity.

- RF doors are still heavy, with the metal tags on the door edges being prone to damage.
- RF window materials are improving, and are becoming optically much clearer.
- The price of RF rooms has stabilized and even reduced as more competing materials (copper, aluminum, and galvanized steel) and systems have entered the market.

MRI market and marketing of the CMR suite

MRI is a diagnostic technology that affords substantial advantages to physicians who treat a wide range of disorders. MRI services represent a significant improvement over older imaging technologies as well as an important market phenomenon. The market for MRI services is complex and volatile. Providers have responded to the combination of high physician demand, attractive profit margins, and substantial capital requirements by creating a number of alternative arrangements for delivering these services. As a result, many currently profitable markets are at risk of being overdeveloped as new machines are added.

It is useful to think of MRI technology as a bundle of three different attributes, each of which functions separately:[17]

- the imaging equipment itself;
- the physical facility (and its proximity to a relevant population of patients and physicians);
- the expertise of the individual cardiologists/radiologists who interpret the procedure's results.

Internal marketing

Internal marketing consists of the environment created within the center. This includes the floor plan, internal decoration, patient-friendly policies such as cleanliness of the facility, and other user-friendly policies in operating procedures for both patients and referring physicians. Some examples include flexible hours, easy scheduling, same- or next-day reporting of results, and easy payment plans.

External marketing

External marketing begins before the selection of the site for the MRI facility. Presite selection marketing is an information-gathering process. The factors to be considered when choosing a site are location, accessibility, patient population, and established referral patterns. Proximity to competitors should be evaluated when choosing a location. It should be kept in mind that there may be potential advantages to being close to a successful competitor.[18] Overall, two factors are critical to the determination of the optimal location choice for an MRI imaging center. The first factor, 1000 population machine days, incorporates the current number of MRI units in the potential location. Since there may be both fixed and mobile MRI units, the number of days that an MRI is in the market area is a useful summary measure of the availability of MRI services. As a hypothetical example, assume that one fixed MRI unit can offer seven days of service and that a mobile MRI is available on only three of seven days because it is moved to another location on the other days. Therefore, there are 10 'machine days' in a week in the market. If another fixed MRI unit were to locate in the same market, the number of machine days increases to 17. The number of potential patients served by an MRI unit is then estimated by dividing the population (in thousands) by the number of machine days. Even though the utilization rate for each machine may eventually be different from this average, for purposes of identifying a set of locations suitable for more comprehensive demand analysis, the greater the ratio of potential patients to MRI units, the more desirable is the location. A second factor is physician referrals in the market for MRI services. Referral machine days and the ratio of referrals to the number of MRI units in the area are useful information. The greater the referral machine days, the more attractive is the particular location.

Other potential providers of MRI services may also consider entry into this dynamic and profitable market, and one should take that possibility into account in the location decision. In marketing practices, the first- and second-order marginal effects are used to provide information to the decision maker. The first-order effect identifies which of the locations is the most desirable for initial entry only; the second-order effect identifies the result of physicians' competition over the referrals and patients in a given location, should a competitive response be made to the initial entry. The size of the market for a particular service that will encompass all demand for the services in a market is based on the number of firms (cardiovascular practices), the population and population density, and the land area. Not only is the potential market of interest, but the stability of that market is also a concern.

The approaches recommended for marketing investigations include the following:[17]

- Use of marginal analysis for dynamic markets, due to its value when the potential market(s) provides great opportunity and growth.

- Comparison of first-order (initial entry) with second-order (post competitive entry) conjectural variations. The information provided by these variables allows for identification of which markets are likely to be the most profitable and the impact on market share of further entry into the market.
- Careful and clear definition of the market. Given that the demand for MRI services is derived from referring physicians, the distribution of the specialists who are likely to use the service should be considered carefully. This information helps to define the market and allows for a prediction of the number of referrals in each potential market.

Postinstallation marketing

Postinstallation marketing is a process of information distribution. The information to be distributed should be chosen carefully according to what will be useful to and well accepted by the market in question. Some examples of materials are:[18]

- brochures directed toward referring physicians;
- brochures directed toward patients;
- educational conferences and lectures, advertisements in newspapers, medical journals, and magazines;
- specialty items such as posters, calendars, mugs, and candies with identifiable wrappers. Any marketing material may be distributed by mail, E-mail, or in person.

Census of MRI facilities

The March 2002 Market Summary Report (IMV Medical Information Division) of 4401 sites with fixed MRI systems revealed that MRI is experiencing an annual growth rate of 15%, resulting in 18 million procedures in 2001. Examination of the MRI procedure data illustrated emerging application trends for MRI. Vascular MRI procedures are performed in 58% of the MRI sites, growing from 1% of 1994 MRI procedures to 4% of 2001 procedures, totaling 830 000 in 2001. Breast and cardiac procedures, while constituting only 1% of procedures each, are conducted by 23% and 13% of the MRI sites, respectively.

The clinical performance of the 1.5 T and higher-field magnets continues to drive MRI purchases. Over 60% of the MRI installed base has ≥1.5 T magnets, and the reported plans for MRI purchases are consistently for high-field systems. Patient comfort and access issues made low- and mid-field open-field magnets popular in recent years, but shorter-bore 1.5 T systems for sites that want the advanced clinical capabilities of high-field systems appear to be an acceptable solution. In the late 1990s, low-field open systems expanded the MRI market, particularly in imaging centers. Going forward, nearly half of future purchase intentions are for short-bore closed systems, while the rate of acquiring regular closed-bore and open systems has declined.

The Year 2001 MRI Census represents the most comprehensive database of site-specific profiles of MRI sites in the USA. The Year 2001 MRI Market Summary Report provides a thorough overview of the MRI market in the USA, illustrating market insights that are valuable in planning for market development, product positioning, and sales strategy. The report compares nationwide trends from the 2001 census with the four prior census surveys that IMV has conducted since 1993.[19]

The adoption of MRI by individual purchasers and by the healthcare system is influenced by many factors. These influences can be incorporated into four major considerations:[20]

- MRI and its attributes – the technology, its safety and efficacy, and the benefits of acquisition;
- communication channels – commercial and professional;
- time for consideration of adoption and experimental testing;
- the medical system – including potential acquirers, health planning, and reimbursement.

Worldwide MRI equipment market

The MRI equipment market grew by 10% annually in 2000 and 2001. Annual sales reached to a total of 3.0 billion Euros, with the sales of 2400 systems. The average selling price was 1.2 million Euros per system.

Market growth has been driven by a mixed shift to systems with higher magnetic fields, new imaging procedures (in particular for the heart and for intervention), and an accelerated replacement cycle that is ~60–70% of sales. There is a very significant aftersales market, including options and upgrades (which are estimated as 3–5% per year of the initial system price) and annual maintenance contracts (>6% per year).[21]

Cost of MRI systems

In year 2002, the cost of building an MRI facility was ~$3 million, including magnets and equipment. The cost of operating an MRI suite is estimated to be around ~$500 000 a year.[22] The initial capital cost for an MRI

system, including the magnet, workstations, software, network interface kit, and injection systems, is ~$1 500 000–2 000 000. The annual maintenance service costs are estimated as between $110 000 and $200 000. These numbers are based on the information provided by major manufacturers such as GE, Phillips, and Siemens.

The cost for the construction/conversion of an MRI laboratory has a broad variability, depending on the initial space characteristics. Major additional annual cost items include maintenance (service) costs, and salary and benefits of MRI physicians and technologists, which are based on the regions, experience, and budgetary flexibility of a particular facility. MRI units typically have a useful life of 8–10 years. There are several factors that increase the overall value of a system. These include a good performance and upgrade history, a well-maintained system with service records, market demand, and configuration.

Service contract

Service contracts depend on the configuration of the system, the length of the contract, and the type of service coverage. These contracts usually include:

- principal service coverage period: Monday through Friday;
- core modality hours (hours of service support to be determined);
- emergency repair coverage (period and hours to be determined);
- engineer on-call service;
- parts, labor, and travel expenses;
- preventive maintenance inspections per year performed during service coverage hours;
- software updates;
- cryogen coverage;
- performance guarantee (for an average of 12 months);
- guaranteed on-site and telephone response times;
- guaranteed same/next-day parts delivery;
- on-site coverage (remote diagnostics);
- discounts on accessories;
- on-site applications training (limited to 5–7 days).

Running the CMR suite
Reimbursement for clinical studies

Given the fact that the field of CMR in clinical practice is in its infancy, reimbursement for professional and technological fees is being accepted slowly by insurance payers and the Medicare/Medicaid establishment in the USA.

These revenues are best collected as a global fee, which can easily be separated, into professional and technical components. According to the Center for Medicare and Medicaid Services (CMS) there are only three CPT codes for reimbursement of CMR studies: 75554, 75556, and 76375. The global reimbursement rate from CMS for CMR studies in 2002 was $432.00, with a professional component of $82.00 and a technological component of $350.00. Reimbursement rates for CMR could rise if this valuable imaging tool were demonstrated to show improved prognostic data and cost-effectiveness in utilization for the diagnosis of cardiovascular disorders. Simply put, if CMR is better at making diagnoses and can reduce the dependence on several different imaging modalities to evaluate certain disorders, physicians and centers can expect higher reimbursement rates. More details are provided in Chapter 31. Reimbursement issues for each region/country are not addressed in this text and would depend on the individual country.

Data collection and reporting/digital imaging network

Exponential advances in the technology sector and computer industry have benefited the science and practice of medical imaging. Modalities such as MRI are capable of producing DICOM-compliant images. All digital data sets can subsequently be transferred over a network between machines for display and further manipulation on workstations. Large-capacity archiving units are used to store these voluminous data sets. The enterprise components of imaging centers have undergone a transition from hardcopy to softcopy. The steps to be taken in the strategic planning process follow the formulation of responses to the following questions:

- Will this technology acquisition provide sufficient value to a particular organization to justify the expense?
- Is there a true need for the new technology?
- What issues or problems does this technology address?
- What customer needs will this technology satisfy today and tomorrow?
- How will the organization's shareholders benefit from this technology?

The answers to these questions will stimulate the strategic planning process to define demands, investigate technology and investment options, identify resources, and set goals. Important contributions must be solicited from an organization's information technology division, cardiologists, radiologists and other physicians, hospital adminis-

tration, and any other service where the use of imaging technology information is required and beneficial.

Manufacturers and consultants can be extremely valuable in generating workflow diagrams, which include imaging acquisition components and imaging display components. A detailed inventory of imaging equipment, imaging equipment locations and use, imaging equipment DICOM compatibility, imaging equipment upgrade requirements, reading locations, and user locations must be obtained and confirmed. An often-ignored issue is the human resource allocation that is required to implement, maintain and upgrade the system. These costs must be estimated and included in the financial analysis.[23]

MRI studies can produce large quantities of information, and as of yet there are no standardized reporting schemas. Poststudy image evaluation and data calculation of ventricular volumes such as ejection fraction need to be stored and reported in an organized fashion so that the information can be readily recalled and evaluated. Recently, the major societies for cardiac imaging have reported a standard method for myocardial segmentation and nomenclature for tomographic imaging of the heart.[24]

The recommendations of this collaboration are as follows:

1. All cardiac imaging modalities should define, orient, and display the heart using the long axis of the left ventricle and selected planes oriented at 90° relative to the long axis.
2. The heart should be divided into 17 segments for the assessment of the myocardium and the left-ventricular myocardium.
3. The heart should be divided into equal thirds perpendicular to the long axis, anatomical landmarks should be used to select slices, and the slice thickness should be selected on the basis of modality-specific resolution and clinical relevance
4. The names of the myocardial segments should define the location relative to the long axis of the heart and the circumferential location.
5. Individual myocardial segments can be assigned to the three major coronary arteries, with the recognition that there is anatomical variability.

Standardized reporting of cardiac studies is imperative, since different modalities are compared when addressing clinical questions such as regional myocardial function or myocardial viability. In the reporting of CMR studies, the 17-segment reporting schema would allow segmental contraction to be compared with first-pass perfusion and DHE in each of the 17 segments. Additionally, the transmural extent of the area of DHE in a particular segment may have important clinical implications with regard to the degree of myocardial viability.[8] Without software programs that allow both report generation and voluminous data storage, the task of evaluating this data is daunting. The major manufacturers of MRI scanners and workstations have not yet addressed this clinically important issue.

Safety of CMR

Precautionary safety measures for the cardiac patient start as soon as the cardiovascular physician orders a CMR study. Cardiac patients may have prosthetic materials placed to treat a number of cardiac disease processes, and the ordering physician should be aware of what is and what is not compatible in the MRI suite. Safety considerations will play an increasing role, with the expanding utilization of pharmacological stress agents during cardiac studies. CMR poses a unique set of safety precautions that are not present in the common cardiovascular studies of angiography, electrophysiology, echocardiography, and nuclear imaging modalities. In the catheterization and electrophysiology laboratories, patient exposure to iodinated compounds and invasive manipulation of catheters within the cardiac structures have fostered the development of an elaborate array of safety considerations that have limited complications to an acceptable level. The CMR suite has a number of unique characteristics for which the cardiovascular specialist needs familiarization. The development of interventional CMR procedures will bring further precautions that will combine the principles outlined here coupled with similar precautions exercised in the interventional cardiac laboratory.

The majority of the safety precautions inherent in standard CMR practice encompass the effect of ferromagnetic materials within the CMR suite, the potential effects of the magnetic field and varying RF signals on the patient, auditory considerations, and potential reactions to gadolinium contrast agents. The greatest safety concern of any MRI suite centers on the presence of ferromagnetic objects within the magnetic field. Ferromagnetic objects are capable of developing a strong intrinsic magnetic field when placed within an external magnetic field. These concerns center on objects either within the patient's body or free within the magnetic field. Any freestanding object composed of ferromagnetic material within the external magnetic field has the potential to become a projectile that can injure the patient or the staff in the CMR suite. Less importantly, these projectiles can cause considerable damage to the magnet, necessitating costly repairs.

Ferromagnetic materials that lie within the patient may be objects such as bullets or ocular metallic materials that have been introduced either knowingly or unknowingly into the patient's body, or they may be materials that have been placed in the past during a surgical procedure. Either of these types of material could have disastrous consequences, and a comprehensive review prior to placing the patient within the magnetic field is the best and easiest way of reducing this risk. A standard questionnaire filled out by the patient as well as careful questioning of the patient by the technologist can significantly reduce these possibilities. Most metallic materials that have been surgically implanted are not ferromagnetic, and are safe in the magnet. An extensive review of these materials and their effect on MRI procedures has been published by Shellock[25] and serves as an outstanding reference for any MRI laboratory. Materials composed of stainless steel are MRI-compatible simply because stainless steel is nonferromagnetic. Therefore, patients with most stainless steel implants can be imaged safely, but it should be kept in mind that the implant will cause local field incongruities that will result in artifacts. Examples of this phenomenon in cardiac imaging include the artifacts and signal loss created by stents, prosthetic valves, and sternal wires in patients who have undergone sternotomy (Figure 30.1). These metallic objects have been shown to be inherently safe in an MRI field, and there is no need to delay an MRI procedure after they have been placed.[25–27]

The ferromagnetic materials shown to be inherently unsafe in a magnetic field can be located in potentially dangerous anatomical areas where movement or dislodgement of the material due to forced rotational and/or translational motions could injure the patient. These

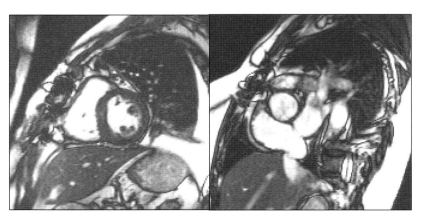

Figure 30.1
Gradient-echo image with metal artifacts from sternal wires.

materials include cerebral or vascular aneurysm clips, ocular metallic shards found in metalworkers, and implanted therapeutic equipment that could injure the patient or malfunction during the study.

Ahmed and Shellock[27] have described specific guidelines for consideration in the exposure of individuals with vascular or aneurysm clips or other implants to the MRI environment. These guidelines include the following:

1. Knowledge of specific information concerning the type, model, material, and manufacturer's serial number of a vascular clip will provide details of the degree of ferromagnetic material present that may impact the patient in the MRI suite. This information should have been placed in the patient's medical record by the implanting physician.
2. Aneurysm clips that are within their original packaging and shown to be composed of material made from phynox, elgiloy, MP35N, titanium alloy, commercially pure titanium, or other material either weakly or non-ferromagnetic in magnetic fields of ≤1.5 T are considered safe.
3. The physician performing the CMR study in consultation with the implanting physician and possibly the manufacturer of the material should take the responsibility of deciding if the study should be performed in materials in which information about the degree of ferromagnetism is either unknown or unsure. These individuals should consider the risk versus benefit of the MRI procedure.
4. A website www.MRIsafety.com now exists and provides invaluable information to MRI physicians and technologists on safety issues. On this website, there is considerable safety information, examples of screening forms, summaries of peer-reviewed articles on MRI bioeffects and safety, as well as a searchable database that contains information on implants and other objects tested for MRI safety.

Interventional cardiovascular, surgical, and radiological procedures increasingly involve the implantation of coils, stents, filters, vascular clamps, valvular prostheses, and electronic equipment. General guidelines for these passive implants that have no power associated with their operation if made from non-ferromagnetic material (e.g. elgiloy, phynox, MP35N, titanium, titanium alloy, nitinol, and tantalum) allow MRI procedures to be performed immediately after their implant. Any implant that is made of a weakly ferromagnetic material should undergo a 6–8-week waiting period after placement to allow adequate incorporation into the tissue or vessel. All heart valve prostheses that have been tested and that are well placed with no signs of dehiscence demonstrate minimal field interactions and are safe for MRI procedures. Temporary cardiovascular catheters with conductive materials, such as thermodilution accessories, should not be allowed in patients undergoing MRI procedures, but vascular access ports and catheters without conductive materials appear safe. Devices increasingly utilized for closure of patent ductus arteriosus and atrial and ventricular septal defects made from 304 V stainless steel should wait 6 weeks to allow stabilizing tissue growth, but those composed of MP35N can undergo evaluation immediately following implantation. With regard to electrically, magnetically, or mechanically activated implants and devices, of which the list is extensive, the general recommendation is that MRI examination should be avoided on patients with these materials. Examples of common implanted electronic therapeutic equipment include pacemakers and implantable defibrillators and their lead systems (temporary or permanent), cochlear implants, and insulin or pain medication pumps.[27]

The biological effects of the transient application of magnetic gradients and of the varying RF electromagnetic field impulses generated during a CMR study are generally considered safe.[28] Clinical MRI scanners have a level of field strength that appears to have no effect on cardiac contractility or ventricular arrhythmia threshold.[29,30] The effects of the magnetic fields and RF impulses on biological tissues can be characterized as either thermal or nonthermal. Thermal effects are related to the induced currents that allow power deposition within tissues. Nonthermal effects are direct effects on tissue that may cause stimulation of nerves or muscles. Nonthermal effects of varying magnetic gradients are minimal, since the threshold for nerve and muscle stimulation is much higher than those of clinical CMR conditions. The nonthermal effects of RF magnetic field impulses in clinical CMR are thought to be negligible due to the fact that these are only short-term exposures. Controversies still exist concerning RF electromagnetic fields, due to suppositions that chronic exposure may play a role in causing cancer and developmental abnormalities.[31,32] The thermal effects of the transient magnetic gradients are insignificant, but those of the varying RF impulses warrant mention and concern. Although varying RF pulses can rarely cause injury, precautions must be taken. The US Food and Drug Administration (FDA) has set certain limits on the specific absorption rates, and scanner software is set to maintain imaging sequences below those limits. Thermal injury as a result of RF magnetic field impulses can take the form of heat injuries that can occur due to the presence of loops within the field that concentrate effects locally. To eliminate the potential for these injuries, care should be taken to avoid allowing such loops within the field. This is the type of injury that occurs with pacemaker or defibrillator leads, and for that reason these are absolutely contraindicated. Retained epicardial leads after surgery also pose a potential risk, but have been shown to be safe.[33] Prevention of loops in electrocardiogram leads and running them out of the scanner parallel to the main magnetic field will prevent heat injuries, as will the use of carbon fiber electrodes instead of metallic electrodes. Finally, not allowing patients to cross their legs or hold their hands together eliminates looped currents within the patient's body.

Acoustic noise in and around the MRI suite creates a potential risk to the patient and those working in the area. Fast gradient-echo pulse sequences provide the greatest noise during studies, but acoustic noise levels have not exceeded levels deemed safe by the US Occupational Safety and Health Administration (OSHA).[34] The routine use of earplugs and active noise cancellation techniques reduce the potential for hearing loss associated with MRI procedures.[35]

The description of DHE after gadolinium contrast infusion in the determination of viable myocardial tissue will expand the utilization of this material in diagnostic CMR.[8,9,36] Gadopentatate dimeglumine (Gd-DTPA), the most popular and commonly used agent, has an excellent safety profile. Reactions to Gd-DTPA are uncommon and usually local at the site of injection; however, systemic reactions such as nausea, vomiting, and hives have been reported. Gadolinium agents do not impair renal function and are well tolerated. The incidence of anaphylactic reaction is exceedingly rare and reportedly in the range of 1 per 100 000 doses, which is much lower than that experienced with iodinated angiographic contrast agents. Newer gadolinium agents that have the ability to bind novel compounds are being developed and may have therapeutic as well as diagnostic capabilities. Iron-based compounds currently being tested may have an advantage in angiographic studies due to their ability to remain in the vascular space.

Stress CMR procedures create a unique set of safety considerations, since they combine the difficulties in monitoring cardiac patients in an MRI environment with the dangerous potential effects involved in the infusion of pharmacological stress agents. Specifically, the inability to adequately monitor ECG segment changes, arrhythmias, symptoms, and blood pressure changes in patients who are not directly in front of the observers creates a potential emergency situation. When these factors are coupled with the realization that emergency equipment and personnel are located at a distance outside the MRI suite, the performance of these studies needs to be closely watched and appropriate emergency response tactics outlined and practised. Monitoring objectives for stress studies can be found in Table 30.2 and contraindications for CMR stress testing in Table 30.3. A complete discussion of the issues regarding CMR stress testing is beyond the scope of this text and is given elsewhere in this book.

Table 30.2 Monitoring requirements for stress CMR

	Dobutamine ± atropine	*Dipyridamole/adenosine*
Heart rate/rhythm	Continuous	Continuous
Blood pressure	Minutes	Minutes
Pulse oximetry	Continuous	Continuous
Symptoms	Continuous	Continuous
Wall motion	With dose increase	At peak stress

Table 30.3 Contraindications for CMR examination and pharmacological stress testing

CMR examination: absolute contraindications	*Pharmacological stress testing*	
	Dobutamine	*Dipyridamole/adenosine*
Aneurysm clips	Severe hypertension	Acute myocardial infection <3 days
Intracranial/intraocular metals	Unstable angina	Unstable angina
Shrapnels	Severe/critical aortic stenosis	Severe hypertension
Cardiac pacemakers/AICD	Complex/frequent arrythmias	Asthma/severe chronic obstructive
Pacemaker/AICD wires	Significant hypertrophic cardiomyopathy	pulmonary disease
Cochlear implants	Myocarditis, pericarditis, endocarditis	Atrioventricular block, type IIa
	Precaution: valvular stenosis/insufficiency	
	Cardiac condition preventing supine position and breathholding	

Quality assurance

Imaging studies that provide diagnostic information to the practicing cardiovascular physician need to be precise in diagnostic accuracy. Often, decisions for interventional or surgical procedures are predicated on the results of these studies. Therefore, the performance, interpretation, and reporting of studies need to be precise and accountable and reproducible. Maintaining a regular and open quality assurance program (possibly with both internal and external observers) that reviews studies and provides feedback is a temporary solution. Certification of imaging centers by a standard independent supervising agency is probably the best solution. General principles that should be considered are stated in the American College of Radiology (ACR) 2001 MRI Quality Control Manual:[37]

- Every imaging procedure is necessary and appropriate to the clinical problem being investigated.
- Images generated contain information critical to the solution of that problem.
- The recorded information is correctly interpreted and is made available in a timely fashion to the patient's physician.
- The examination should result in the lowest possible risk, cost, and inconvenience to the patient.

Quality control

Quality control is an integral part of quality assurance. Quality control is a series of distinct technical procedures that ensure the production of satisfactory studies. The ACR has initiated a voluntary program for standard MRI studies, but quality control guidelines in the emerging technologies of EPI, MRA, CMR, and MRI-guided therapy have not as yet been addressed. General guidelines for MRI at centers are listed in Table 30.4. Additionally, there are criteria unique to cardiac studies that need to be addressed. Because the new fields of CMR and MRI-guided therapies are evolving at a rapid pace, the guidelines for quality control in these areas will be dynamic. The areas that require regular evaluation in any MRI study include maintenance of image quality, observance of supervising physicians, and interpreting physician performance. Specific areas of CMR studies that require regular evaluation include safety of CMR studies, both stress and nonstress, and adequate performance of cardiac studies.

The team member who should be placed at the direction of image quality maintenance is the technologist with the most complete knowledge and experience in running the equipment and the ability to troubleshoot technical problems. In addition, this individual should be the one who observes the performance and interpretation of a majority of the studies of the practicing physicians and has become comfortable with what each physician requests during specific types of studies. Communication with the servicing contractor allows rapid diagnosis and correction of problems when they arise, and identification of more serious problems that may require specific parts or software corrections. For this reason, most imaging centers have defined service agreements either with the manufacturer of the magnet or with a third party. Standard performance testing of all the equipment with routine preventive maintenance is provided by most service contracts. However, the responsibilities of daily maintenance and testing belong to the lead technologists or their designate. Daily responsibilities of the lead technologist include acceptance testing to detect defects in equipment that is newly installed or has undergone major repair, establishment of baseline performance of the equipment, detection and diagnosis of changes in equipment performance before they become apparent in studies, and verification

Table 30.4 Quality control issues for MRI and CMR	
MRI/Recommendations of ACR	*CMR*
Central frequency measurement (at least daily)	Defining of true long and short axes using locators
System (head/body coil) SNR measurement (daily)	Proper orientation and position of short-axis slices
Image quality and artifact assessment (daily)	Standardization of protocols for research studies
Processor sensitometric testing (weekly)	Performing the perfusion studies in a uniform manner
	Performing DHE sequences properly
Semi-annually or after major upgrade/change:	Proper monitoring of stress studies and emergency training
Review of daily quality control testing records	Physician qualifications meeting ACR/SCMR guidelines
Image quality uniformity measurement	Proper training and supervision of technologists
Spatial linearity measurement	Appropriate tagging studies performed for wall motion analysis
High-contrast spatial resolution measurement	Standardization of sequence protocols for all laboratory staff
Slice location, thickness, separation measurements	Frequent evaluation and upgrade of protocols

that the causes of deterioration in equipment performance have been corrected.

The supervising physician of a center performing CMR studies should be either a cardiologist or radiologist who has training, experience, and expertise in the practice of the full range of CMR procedures. The main duties of this individual are to maintain quality control, ensure safety measures for all studies, supervise and train the technologists, and maintain/improve sequence protocols established by the supervising physicist. The supervising physician should work closely with all the interpreting physicians to ensure that all the sequence protocols are updated on a routine practice improvement program. By far, the most important role of the supervising physician is to ensure safety measures during cardiac studies.

Interpreting physicians are cardiologists or radiologists who have demonstrated the appropriate qualifications to perform and interpret CMR studies. They must agree to adhere to the safety regulations and quality assurance and control measures established within the center. Specifically, they should also agree to follow the facility procedures for corrective action when asked to interpret images of poor quality, participate in the facility's practice improvement program, and provide documentation of their current qualifications to each MRI facility where they practice, according to ACR/Society for Cardiovascular Magnetic Resonance (SCMR) accreditation guidelines.

Performance of CMR studies creates a unique set of quality control issues that are not present in routine noncardiac studies. These issues need careful attention in a high-volume CMR center that may have a number of physicians from both cardiology and radiology disciplines performing and interpreting studies. First and foremost are the issues regarding safety of cardiac patients. These include not only patients receiving pharmacological stress agents but also patients undergoing routine study. Often, it is difficult for cardiac patients to lie still and take numerous breathholds during a CMR study. The development and utilization of real-time CMR methods will greatly overcome these difficulties. Arrhythmias that may be present can prolong each sequence and create difficulties in obtaining adequate images, as well as prolonging the study for the patient. Protocols for managing patients with potentially dangerous arrhythmias during both routine and stress CMR studies should be established and updated as necessary. Strategies in safety management as well as emergency procedures should be created and observed by all physicians.

Although standards for the performance and interpretation of CMR studies have not yet been created, certain general principles have emerged. These principles are demonstrated throughout the literature as CMR has evolved technologically. Quality control measures should be instituted that allow accurate repetitive measuring of ventricular volumes and ejection fraction so that repeat studies attempt to duplicate previously measured data. Sequence protocols that have been established should be routinely scrutinized and updated. Major quality control guidelines in the performance of CMR studies include the following:

- definition of the true long and short axes of the myocardium using locator techniques;
- gathering of short-axis slices in the proper orientation and position to allow accurate calculation of ventricular volumes;
- performance of standardized protocols for sequences and studies to allow independent interpretation and calculation of data (necessary for all centers performing research studies);
- performance of perfusion studies in a uniform manner;
- proper performance of the sequences for delayed hyperenhancement;
- appropriate monitoring of stress studies and provision of nursing staff with the proper qualifications for emergency services;
- assurance that physician qualifications meet SCMR/ACR guidelines for the performance and interpretation of studies;
- appropriate training and supervision of technologists performing cardiac studies;
- performance of appropriate tagging studies for wall motion analysis;
- agreed and established sequence protocols for all MRI laboratory physicians and technologists to utilize;
- frequent evaluation and upgrade of the protocols parallel to the progress in the field; a committee composed of technologists as well as the supervision and interpreting physicians should establish the sequence protocols on a quarterly or biannual basis.

With a quality control program in place at a center, all physicians involved in the performance and interpretation of CMR studies will be aware of the requirements necessary to participate. Although standards for the performance of CMR studies have not yet been elucidated by a certifying agency, the creation of standard quality control guidelines will allow for easier accreditation processes when such a body exists. Quality control and safety measures in the performance of CMR studies represent the most important aspects in building a successful clinical CMR program and should always be aggressively pursued.

Training in CMR

Currently, there are only a small number of training programs for physicians and technologists interested in learning CMR. Most cardiology and radiology training programs are not yet fully staffed to prepare all graduates in the interpretation and performance of CMR studies. Current training guidelines for physicians in CMR have been proposed by the SCMR. These guidelines outline several avenues of training for both cardiovascular and radiology specialists and suggest routes for training for those either still training or for those who have completed their fellowship. There is currently no certification exam for competency in CMR. The American College of Cardiology (ACC) in the most recent Core Cardiology Training in Adult Cardiovascular Medicine (COCATS)[38] has divided training in MRI for cardiology fellows into three levels. The different levels represent core competencies obtained during the training period, and vary based on the level of commitment to the field. For example, level 1 is designed to provide the trainee with a working knowledge of CMR, whereas level 3 will provide the trainee with the competency to operate a CMR facility. Training level requirements can be seen in Table 30.5. For those physicians who have completed cardiovascular and radiology training and wish to be trained for the performance of CMR studies, there are currently only a few options available. A list of training opportunities can be found in the most recent editions of the Journal of Cardiovascular Magnetic Resonance. As recommended by the SCMR, the levels for training for these individuals and their requirements mirror those seen in Table 30.5. However, attainment of these criteria is difficult for those who already have a busy clinical practice. There are additional training opportunities available from the major manufacturers of MRI scanners after the purchase and/or upgrade of a scanner. However, these training sessions generally assume that the physician or individual has a basic knowledge of not only cardiovascular anatomy and pathophysiology but also the mechanics and physics involved in the performance of MRI studies. Attendance at these training sessions will not contribute to completion of training guidelines established by the ACC or SCMR.

Summary

Establishment of an active CMR laboratory within a cardiovascular practice or hospital can be a costly and challenging undertaking in these days of declining reimbursements. In most clinical settings, the success of an active CMR program requires a workable interdisciplinary relationship amongst the cardiology and radiology departments. Most often, the administrative and financial control of the MRI center is predominantly within the radiology and/or hospital community. However, the patients requiring study as well as the knowledge of the complex pathophysiology of the cardiac system lie within the cardiovascular specialty. It is therefore crucial that these two disciplines work in collaboration to establish viable CMR laboratories. Currently there are not enough MRI-trained cardiologists or radiologists with knowledge of cardiac pathophysiology to accomplish the task of building and running a CMR laboratory at all tertiary or community-based programs with high-volume cardiovascular practices. Furthermore, within these communities, there is not a sufficient volume of CMR studies to warrant separate facilities dedicated solely for cardiac studies. At present, the prohibitive cost of not only equipment but also personnel and maintenance may preclude the development of freestanding imaging centers that offer MRI solely for cardiac studies. It is for these reasons that the establishment of a CMR program within an existing MRI radiology imaging center may offer the best opportunity for establishing a high-quality CMR program at most institutions. No matter which option is chosen, maintenance of a high level of quality control and the safest environment for all patients and healthcare workers is paramount.

References

1. Hori Y, Yamada N, Higashi M, et al. Rapid evaluation of right and left ventricular function and mass using real-time true-FISP cine MR imaging without breath-hold. Comparison with segmented true-FISP cine MR imaging with breath-hold. J Cardiovasc Magn Reson 2003; 5:439–50.

2. Hundley WG, Hamilton CA, Thomas MS, et al. Utility of fast cine magnetic resonance imaging and display for the detection of myocardial ischemia in patients not well suited for second harmonic stress echocardiography. Circulation 1999; 100:1697–1702.

3. Fieno DS, Kim RJ, Chen EL, et al. Contrast-enhanced magnetic resonance imaging of myocardium at risk: distinction between reversible and irreversible injury throughout infarct healing. J Am Coll Cardiol 2000; 36:1985–91.

4. Kim RJ, Wu E, Rafael A, et al. The use of contrast-enhanced magnetic resonance imaging to identify reversible myocardial dysfunction. N Engl J Med 2000; 343:1445–53.

5. Chuan ML, Hibberd MG, Salton CJ et al. Importance of imaging method over imaging modality in noninvasive determination of left

Table 30.5 Training levels in CMR as set forth by COCATS		
Level	*Duration of training (months)*	*No. of examinations*
1	1	50 mentored interpretations
2	3–6	100 mentored interpretations (50 as primary interpreter and operator)
3	12	≥200 mentored interpretations (100 as primary interpreter and operator)

ventricular volumes and ejection fraction; assessment by two-and three-dimensional echocardiography and magnetic resonance imaging. J Am Coll Cardiol 2000; 35:477–84.

6. Longmore DB, Klipstein RH, Underwood SR, et al. Dimensional accuracy of magnetic resonance in studies of the heart. Lancet 1985; i:1360–2.

7. Rehr RB, Malloy CR, Filipchuk NG, et al. Left ventricular volumes measured by MRI imaging. Radiology 1985; 156:717–19.

8. Choi KM, Kim RJ, Gubernikoff G, et al. Transmural extent of acute myocardial infarction predicts long-term improvement in contractile function. Circulation 2001; 104:1101–7.

9. Kim RJ, Fieno DS, Parrish TB, et al. Relationship of MRI delayed contrast enhancement to irreversible injury, infarct age, and contractile function. Circulation 1999; 100:1992–2002.

10. Klein C, Nekolla SG, Bengel FM, et al. Assessment of myocardial viability with contrast-enhanced magnetic resonance imaging: comparison with positron emission tomography. Circulation 2002; 105:162–7.

11. Schwitter JC, Nanz D, Kneifel S, et al. Assessment of myocardial perfusion in coronary artery disease by magnetic resonance: a comparison with positron emission tomography and coronary angiography. Circulation 2001; 103:2230–5.

12. Kim WY, Dania PG, Stuber M, et al. Coronary magnetic resonance angiography for the detection of coronary stenoses. N Engl J Med 2001; 345:1863–9.

13. Helft G, Worthley SG, Fuster V, et al. Progression and regression of atherosclerotic lesions: monitoring with serial noninvasive magnetic resonance imaging. Circulation 2002; 105:993–8.

14. Kenney JM, Gordon D. Facilities design in a managed care environment. Hosp Top 1996; 74:16–20.

15. Magnetic Resonance Imaging (MRI) VA Design Guide. Department of Veterans Affairs, Veterans Health Administration, Office of Facilities Management, Facilities Quality Office, Standards Service. September 1995.

16. Baker D. MRI suites update. Hosp Dev 1997; 28:18–19.

17. Colburn CB, LaTour MS, Johnson K. Locating MRIs through marginal analysis. J Healthcare Marketing 1992; 12:66–71.

18. Cox EE. MR facility organization and management. In: MRI for Technologists (Woodward P, ed). New York. McGraw-Hill, 2001; 319–49.

19. Year 2002 MRI Census of MRI Facilities. IMV Ltd, June 2002.

20. Hillman BJ, Winkler JD, Phelps CE, et al. Adoption and diffusion of a new imaging technology: a magnetic resonance imaging prospective. AJR 1984; 143:913–17.

21. Higgins C. Phillips MRI Presentation, 2001.

22. www.quitemri.com: Cross border shopping in 2002: MRI's for patients who won't wait. (Press Release) Quinte MRI Inc., 2002.

23. Ortiz AO, Luyckx MP. Preparing a business justification for going electronic. Radiol Manage 2002; 24:14–21.

24. Cerqueira MD, Weissman WK, Pennel DJ, et al. Standardized myocardial segmentation and nomenclature for tomographic imaging of the heart. Circulation 2002; 105:539–42.

25. Shellock FG. Pocket Guide of MR Procedures and Metallic Objects: Update 2000. Philadelphia: Lippincott-Raven, 2000.

26. Scott NA, Pettigrew RI. Absence or movement of coronary stents after placement in a magnetic imaging field. Am J Cardiol 1994; 73:900–1.

27. Ahmed S, Shellock FG. Magnetic resonance imaging safety: implications for cardiovascular patients. J Cardiovasc Magn Reson 2001; 3:171–82.

28. Extremely low frequency (ELF) magnetic fields. In: Health and Safety of Clinical NMR Examinations (Persson BR, Stahlberg F, eds). Boca Raton, FL: CRC Press, 1989.

29. Gulch RW, Lutz O. Influence of strong static magnetic fields on heart muscle contraction. Phys Med Biol 1986; 31:763–9.

30. Doherty JU, Whitman GJ, Robinson MD, et al. Changes in cardiac excitability and vulnerability in NMR fields. Invest Radiol 1985; 20:129–35.

31. NCRP. Biological Effects and Exposure Criteria for Radiofrequency Electromagnetic Fields. Bethesda, MD: National Council on Radiation Protection and Measurements, Report No. 86, 1986.

32. US Environmental Protection Agency. Evaluation of Potential Electromagnetic Carcinogenicity. Office of Health and Environmental Assessment, US Environmental Protection Agency, June 28, 1990 (EPA-600/6 90 005 A).

33. Hartnell GG, Spence L, Hughes LA. Safety of MR imaging in patients who have retained metallic materials after cardiac surgery. AJR 1999; 168:1157–9.

34. Shellock FG, Morisoli SM, Ziarati M. Measurement of acoustic noise during MR imaging: evaluation of six 'worst-case' pulse sequences. Radiology 1994; 191:91–3.

35. Chen CK, Chiueh TD, Chen JH. Active cancellation system of acoustic noise in MR imaging. IEEE Trans Biomed Eng 1999; 46:186–91.

36. Oshinski JN, Yang Z, Jones JR, et al. Imaging time after Gd-DTPA injection is critical in using delayed enhancement to determine infarct size accurately with magnetic resonance imaging. Circulation 2001; 104:2838–42.

37. Magnetic Resonance Imaging (MRI) Quality Control Manual. American College of Radiology, 2001.

38. Pohost GM, Kim RJ, Kramer CM, Reichek N. Task Force 12: Training in cardiovascular magnetic resonance. Core Cardiology Training in Adult Cardiovascular Medicine (COCATS). JACC (www.acc.org) March 2002:59–61.

31

Developing cost-effective strategies for CMR

Leslee J Shaw, Tracy John Robertson

Healthcare policy and the economic burden of cardiovascular disease

The economic burden of cardiovascular diseases makes up a substantial proportion of healthcare costs in most westernized societies. In the USA, diagnostic and treatment costs exceed $300 billion every year or ~15% (private sector) to ~30% (public sector – Medicare/Medicaid) of all healthcare costs.[1] Healthcare costs continue to rise, and, in the area of coronary heart disease, increased healthcare costs reflect a diversity of changes in disease prevalence, increased resource consumption levels, and the availability of new therapies and technologies for cardiovascular disease. For cardiovascular imaging, an estimated 40 million procedures are performed every year, with growth rates as high as 30%.[2] Additionally, Medicare reimbursement to cardiologists for echocardiography and nuclear imaging encompasses a large percentage of total reimbursements (i.e. 30% of all Medicare reimbursement). This would yield a total of Medicare reimbursements of $1.1 billion dollars for cardiac imaging, or ~1% of all US healthcare expenditures.[3]

Evidence-based medicine

Current efforts to contain healthcare costs in the USA and Europe have included developing evidence-based guidelines where a threshold of clinical and economic evidence is desired to support and guide reimbursement for a given clinical procedure indication. As well as the concern over excessive and rising costs of care, the current armamentarium for cardiac imaging has suffered from technical artifacts, limited resolution, and other challenges that often result in a unidimensional risk evaluation upon which patient management is based. The promise of cardiovascular magnetic resonance (CMR) is the possibility of developing a single test that may cover the gamut of risk markers from function, morphology, and perfusion to tissue characterization and metabolism. The resulting benefits to the healthcare system include not only improved diagnostic accuracy and enhanced therapeutic decision making, but also improved risk assessment, including an array of important cardiovascular outcomes. These improvements may result in decreases in overall test use, early diagnosis, reduced hospitalizations and lengths of stay, and reduced use of invasive procedures with consequent economic benefits. This chapter attempts to provide initial insight into the economic promise and current value of CMR to society, including the vast array of test techniques and add-ons to standard imaging modalities.

Economic evaluations, particularly cost-effectiveness analysis, combine information on cost with data concerning the accuracy of a screening test, the population at risk, and the therapeutic benefit of treatment. A comparative analysis of clinical and economic outcome data provides a means to evaluate new technology in relation to existing modalities. For the majority of atherosclerotic imaging techniques, there are published economic evaluations,[4–22] but many of the technological advances in cardiac imaging were introduced without undergoing rigorous scientific testing on effectiveness. Recently, in the USA and Europe, a more stringent evaluation of imaging research is consistent with a new standard of evidence-based medicine.[23] However, programs that are currently medically or economically unjustified are widespread. In many settings, the evaluation of new technology helps to assure a rigorous synthesis of clinical and cost-effectiveness data, and is used to set standards for the appropriate use of imaging modalities.

Value of CMR in drug development – impact on societal costs of care

On average, the development through final approval of a new drug costs ~$500 million.[24] Although the majority of drug development costs are in preclinical research, in the USA the average cost of Food and Drug Administration (FDA)-sponsored phase I–IIIb clinical trials ranges from $14 to $54 million dollars. There is increasing interest on the part of numerous pharmaceutical manufacturers to reduce the frequency with which large (and costly) morbidity and mortality outcome trials are utilized by refocusing resources early on in drug development to areas of distinct clinical promise. An alternative to the use of large outcome trials is to use an imaging or laboratory marker as a surrogate outcome. A surrogate outcome is, by definition, a process-of-care measure that may be used to reflect a worsening long-term outcome (e.g. worsening ejection fraction). Due to the enhanced resolution and precision (i.e. improved consistency and validity) of CMR measurements, it appears ideally suited for use as a surrogate outcome. Prior research supports the fact that CMR substantially reduces the necessary and sufficient sample sizes by as much as tenfold and thus, may decrease overall cost of clinical trials by as much as 80%.[25] For example, a 10% improvement in test reliability or precision can reduce a sample size from several thousand to several hundred patients. Further improvements in test accuracy can reduce necessary and sufficient sample sizes to elucidate changes in myocardial function or other markers to ~50 patients. Using simple cost calculations, ~5.4–10.8% of drug development costs may be saved.[26]

Defining the effectiveness of cardiovascular imaging

Requisite data for a health economic evaluation include critical information on the effect of a test on patient outcome and alterations in patient management.[5] For example, the detection of a high-risk imaging abnormality (e.g. microvascular obstruction) should result in a change in patient management and the initiation of new treatments that ultimately lead to improved survival.[27,28] The evaluation of a test's ability to risk-stratify individuals has been proposed as an alternative to the challenges involved in assessing diagnostic accuracy.[4] For any given test, risk stratification may be used as a method for defining high- and low-risk cohorts where treatment is

allocated to those in greatest need.[29] Furthermore, the intensity of management is directly proportional to the estimated risk of events, such that high-cost care is allocated to high-risk patients.[29] Of course, the economic benefit of risk stratification is that, left untreated, many of the high-risk individuals would have a cardiac event resulting in more costly care.[30] Furthermore, identification of high-risk patients before the onset of clinical cardiovascular disease may offset the significant morbidity and mortality associated with more advanced disease.[31] Conversely, low risk should equate with low cost to the healthcare system. The broad range of outcome measures that are applicable to the use of risk stratification and necessary precursors for an economic evaluation include:[5]

- intermediate clinical outcomes (e.g. disease detected and cardiac event predicted);
- major adverse cardiovascular events (e.g. survival rates);
- cumulative effects of test-driven strategy (e.g. life-years saved);
- patient assessment of a test's value (e.g. quality of life and patient preferences);
- combined quantity and quality of life-years (e.g. quality-adjusted life-years and healthy-year equivalent).

Calculating costs of care

Economic evaluations for imaging should be based on the effectiveness of subsequent treatment, accuracy of testing, cost of testing, and the direct health benefits and resource use resulting from the testing procedure.[12] The preferred method to evaluate marginal or incremental differences in clinical and economic outcomes derived from atherosclerotic imaging is to conduct randomized trials comparing different imaging modalities, as previously noted. Historically, the expense associated with this type of evaluation has been beyond the scope of available public and private funding that is allocated to diagnostic testing research. When considering testing, the recognition that randomized trials are not practical has led to the frequent use of decision-analytic methods or simulations, to try to estimate the cost for some benefit achieved. The principal advantages of modeling are that the analyses may be designed to answer a specific question, drawing available data from multiple sources. This chapter will highlight several models that have been proposed, using CMR for screening for cardiovascular disease.[32] One drawback to the use of a decision model is that data are rarely available in order to answer the specific question, and therefore numerous assumptions have to be devised using diverse evidence and/or expert opinion. Assumptions can be formally tested through sensitivity analysis, but not without interjecting bias or possibly misrepresenting a test's value.[33–36]

There are also adverse effects of imaging that have economic implications, including overdiagnosis, recall rates, and overtreatment based upon the test results. For example, the FDA's position statement on the use of whole-body scanning as a preventive measure for apparently healthy asymptomatic individuals notes that such screening provides uncertain benefit with some potential of risk, including suspicious findings requiring additional follow-up testing.[37] No test will provide perfect accuracy, and the limitations to testing, in the form of false-positive and false-negative test results, have direct economic implications. Although precise enumeration of the rates of false-positive and false-negative results are currently not available, test accuracy is affected not only by random variation but also by changes in the positivity threshold, the study population, and the completeness and duration of follow-up.[38]

For the use of atherosclerotic imaging, optimal risk detection faces challenges based upon the underlying risk in the population. In lower-disease-prevalent populations, higher rates of false positives can be expected based upon Bayesian theory. A false-positive test is documented through the use of additional downstream tests that add to the cost of a patient's workup. False-negative test results result in a downstream disease diagnosis and as a result of limitations of an imaging technique. False-negative test results are especially common in patients with mild disease or in specific population subsets. For example, for ankle-brachial index, false-negative tests are more common in patients with noncompressible arteries, in the elderly, and in diabetic patients.[39,40]

Additional adverse effects of false-negative results include the fact that patients will delay seeking medical advice or ignore symptoms, therefore presenting later on in the course of disease (i.e. with a higher cost to the healthcare system), with the possibility of an intervention, at that time, providing minimal impact on patient outcome.[41] Litigation costs that result from missed diagnoses are also rarely considered in an economic evaluation.

In estimating costs, the impact of test use on consuming additional healthcare resources should be measured comprehensively, including both downstream procedure and treatment costs.[42] For atherosclerotic imaging, the limited amounts of both clinical outcome and cost data contribute to the ensuing cost-effectiveness models being based upon insecure data from varied recruitment and selection methods, often not representative of the population being served. Despite this, the most common factors affecting the cost-effectiveness of a diagnostic test used in

imaging are (1) the sensitivity of the screening test, (2) the economic benefits of early therapy (i.e. the sum of future medical benefits, reduced suffering, and lost wages resulting from the increase in early stage disease), and (3) disease prevalence.[36]

Research on the use of atherosclerotic imaging techniques, such as CMR, has not systematically considered the management impact of testing. For cardiovascular imaging, more resource-intensive testing options are expected, with an associated higher incremental cost. It is expected that the 'frontline' lower cost test will be followed by at least one additional diagnostic test and then treatment costs (accordingly). The application of an initial imaging test does not lead directly to a diagnosis, but is preceded by an intermediate stage of additional testing.[38] This intermediate step may involve the use of one or more different tests before a definitive diagnosis is discerned (Figures 31.1 and 31.2). It is expected that, in many cases, downstream diagnostic testing would account for a greater burden of costs than that of the initial imaging procedure itself. A more sensitive, reliable, and precise imaging modality, such as CMR, is likely to require less testing in order to detect the same incident disease cases.[38] Figures 31.1 and 31.2 provide two examples of how CMR can be used in a pathway of care.[32]

The aim of economic analyses is to develop an understanding of the cost of alternative health care testing strategies. The calculation of cost-effectiveness requires one to specifically describe critical components to an economic analysis, including to:[43]

1. Define the problem.
2. Differentiate the perspective of the analysis (payer, societal, patient, etc.).
3. State explicitly the objective of analysis (guide treatment of patients, help administrators, health policy).
4. Identify alternatives for comparison.
5. State explicitly the outcome of interest: life expectancy, event averted, or functional status, to name a few.
6. State explicitly the costs of the alternatives.
7. Analyze uncertainties and biases (e.g. perform sensitivity analysis).
8. State explicitly where there is no evidence or where assumptions have been made.
9. Address any ethical issues.

(Upfront) test cost

The unit operating cost of an imaging test can be calculated using fixed and variable labor cost (e.g. supplies, equipment, and labor costs). The unit cost is largely

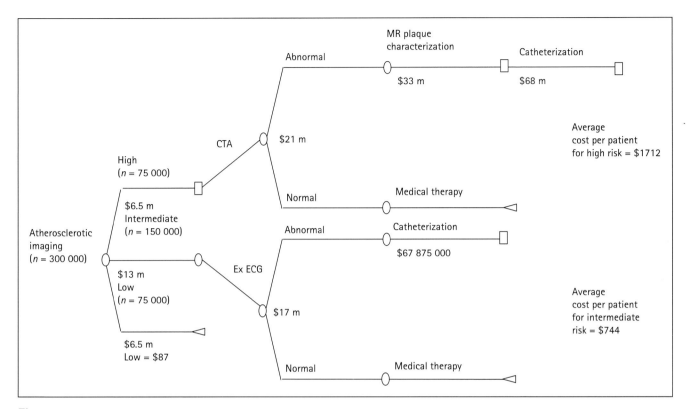

Figure 31.1

Modified testing algorithm using CMR based upon a cardiovascular risk assessment program from Mount Sinai School of Medicine that includes the use of both CMR and computed tomographic imaging. Current cardiovascular risk assessment includes referral for high-risk patients to computed tomography angiography (CTA) followed by CMR for plaque characterization and catheterization (if necessary). For intermediate-risk patients, ischemia testing includes the use of exercise electrocardiography (Ex ECG) followed by the conventional work-up of provocative ischemia. This strategy focuses higher costs of care for higher-risk patients, thereby allocating resources to those in greatest need.

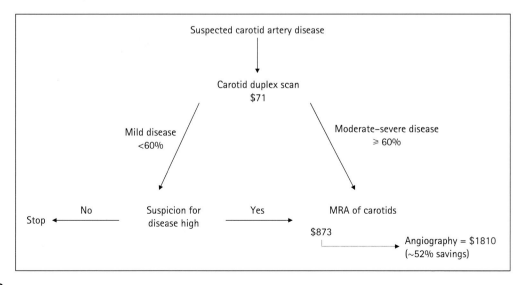

Figure 31.2

Potential cost savings with carotid MR evaluation. This includes the principle of allocative efficiency, where high-cost tests are limited to high-risk patients, thereby initiating cost savings. These results indicate that when carotid duplex scanning is selectively followed by magnetic resonance angiography (MRA) of the carotid arteries instead of angiography in all patients, a 52% cost savings could be achieved. This pathway of care was designed by Dr Edward T Martin of the Oklahoma Heart Institute.

affected by procedural volume, and is generally lower when equipment is used to image both cardiovascular and noncardiovascular systems. Imaging modalities that have quantitative scores are generally of lower cost than those requiring more technologist or physician labor components. For new technology, there are many unresolved issues that may add cost, including laboratory standards or certification, imaging protocols, and evolving equipment (e.g. 4 versus 16 multislice computed tomography (T) or 1.5 T versus 3 T CMR).[44,45] Add-on costs such as the use of intravenous contrast agents should be included in test costs. Adjusted (technical and professional) charges may also be used to reflect estimated costs. Additionally, for cost effectiveness analysis, costs should be discounted and adjusted for inflation based upon local or national rates.[46,47] Patient waiting times are also an important component of the initial test cost evaluation.[48]

Equipment costs vary, with ranges of up to $1–4 million for CMR, positron emission tomography (PET), or multislice CT scanners. New equipment prices are often cited as measures of the cost implications of test choice, but discounting and leasing options often minimize the higher upfront costs and should be considered when estimating cost. Current estimated costs of cardiac imaging modalities are reported in Table 31.1. In general, low-technology tests (e.g. treadmill exercise or ankle brachial index) are of lower cost. Recent innovations for atherosclerotic imaging include the use of multislice (e.g. 16-slice) CT, higher-strength (e.g. 3 T) magnets, and MR spectroscopic (MRS) methods; therefore, precise estimates of cost should be viewed with caution. Many of the new technologies introduced do not have widespread application in the current healthcare marketplace. Therefore, the introduction of new technology will require investment in equipment as well as extensive training of current medical personnel.[49]

Potential economic benefits and detriments of CMR: patient considerations, space and other resource requirements

Older-vintage MRI scanners were not patient-friendly in design and were burdened by relatively long examination times, causing considerable patient discomfort and anxiety. As a result, claustrophobia would occur in up to 2% of patients.[50] Current state-of-the-art scanners, however, are more spacious and can complete examinations in considerably less time than previously required. For example, a single 3D CMR scan may take as little as 15 s to acquire, and can often be done in a single breathhold. The time required for completing an examination can now be reliably estimated as <20 min.[51] This rapid imaging time may minimize loss of productivity and improve patient satisfaction when compared with other modalities.

The utility of imaging is sensitive to patient preferences that are rarely considered in most cost analyses.[52] Anxiety, inconvenience, and discomfort caused by testing are also indirect costs that are difficult to assess in terms of their monetary value. Patient satisfaction may also be improved with the use of adjustable lighting, ventilation, and music systems for patient comfort. Travel costs, family labor expenses, out-of-pocket expenses for home monitoring, and deductible rates are indirect costs that should be considered in an economic evaluation. Concomitant with greater comfort, the new MRI scanners generally have higher technical performance, lower cost, and enhanced diagnostic accuracy.[53] Additionally, when compared with older units, lower space requirements may provide for reduced overhead costs to a given department; current systems require as little as 325 square feet for an MRI system.[51] All of these factors may uniquely contribute to

Table 31.1 Average cost of common cardiac imaging procedures[7–11,13–18]

Procedure	Average cost ($)	Cost range with add-ons ($)[a]
Echocardiography	91	64–342
Computed tomography (CT)	283	90–475
Single-photon emission CT (SPECT)	296	262–574
Magnetic resonance imaging (MRI)	873	525–1220
Positron emission tomography (PET)	1272	960–1470
Right/left heart catheterization	1810	851–4741

[a] Including contrast or radiopharmaceutical use and technique add-ons (e.g. wall motion)

enhanced patient comfort and satisfaction with the procedure, and higher upfront equipment costs may be minimized by reductions in overhead and lost productivity costs.

Induced cost models

Total costs should be summed over the entire episode of care; this should also include induced downstream resource consumption as well as indirect costs. Indirect costs are those costs that can be thought of as opportunity costs, such as days missed from work (counted as wages for the patient and/or work not done for the employer) or years of wages not earned by the permanently disabled or deceased patient. Incidental findings would also drive up the downstream costs of care.[54]

For imaging, there is a directly proportional relationship between the risk and rate of abnormalities and the total costs of care.[55] That is, individuals with high-risk abnormalities will also require numerous procedures beyond the initial test, since they are at greater risk for major adverse cardiac events, including a higher rate of cardiac hospitalizations and coronary revascularization procedures. Thus, future research should focus on the downstream use of medical resources spawned by CMR and other atherosclerotic imaging modalities, as well as any hospitalizations as a result of a missed diagnosis. In a preliminary report from the Hospital Corporation of America (HCA) healthcare system, where detailed direct cost data are available, the inclusion of downstream hospitalizations and major cardiac procedures drastically changed the overall cost estimates.[55]

Cost savings models (Figures 31.2 and 31.3)

Cost savings or minimization may be defined as the lowest-cost strategy for a given equivalent choice.[13–15,19,20]

For imaging, an equivalent choice must include a similar ability to predict disease or outcome or a similar underlying risk in the referral population. Often, healthcare administrators may make choices based upon upfront test costs that rarely consider, for example, whether exercise treadmill testing without imaging is really an equivalent choice to CMR. One method of calculating a clinico-economic model for a diagnostic test includes the use of a simple cost formula where cost (loss) = waste (or false positive, FP) + retest cost (or false-negative, FN).[11] The cost of retesting is defined as false-negative tests where downstream testing is performed despite initial negative results. Conversely, cost waste is defined as false-positive tests where additional testing (e.g. cardiac catheterization) is performed where the downstream results are negative. A recent example of this type of analysis was performed on data from the Premier Hospitals, including 210 US hospitals (24 967 patients).[11] For this analysis, the episode of care included 6 months of resource consumption for the evaluation of suspected ischemic heart disease. The cost of identifying a patient with coronary disease was then calculated (Figure 31.3). From this analysis of ~25 000 cases, average costs to identify coronary disease ranged from ~$300 for CT or single-photon emission CT (SPECT) as initial testing strategies to a high of ~$1400 for PET imaging. Given a highly accurate CMR examination, the average cost of identifying coronary disease could be ~$900 (range $550–1284). An extrapolation of these results to CMR reveals that the addition of multiple risk markers (i.e. perfusion, function, metabolism, plaque characterization, etc.) could further reduce costs by minimizing redundant downstream testing.

Cost-effectiveness analysis

Cost-effectiveness is defined as the amount of added resources consumed (in an incremental comparison of test choices) in relation to any outcome (dis)advantages

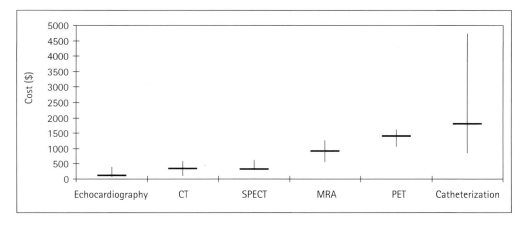

Figure 31.3
Incremental cost of identifying obstructive coronary disease: comparing magnetic resonance angiography (MRA) with other conventional strategies employing either initial noninvasive testing followed by selective angiography or direct angiography.

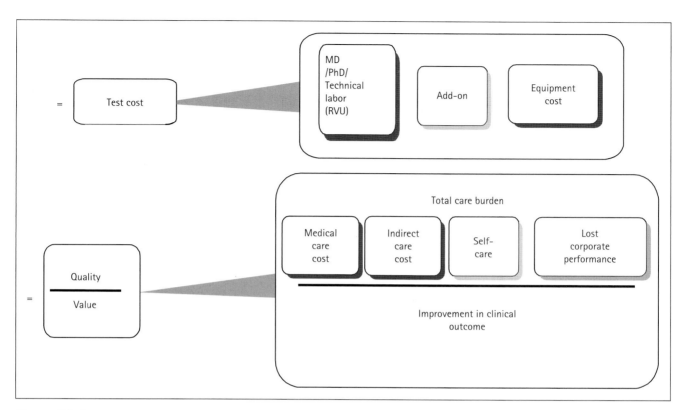

Figure 31.4
Calculating cost-effectiveness, including not only the test cost but also an integration of clinical quality in terms of some measure of economic value to the healthcare system. RVU, relative value units.

or benefits noted.[16–18,56,57] Cost-effectiveness analysis considers not only test costs but also the total care burden of a test (Figure 31.4). Cost-effectiveness analysis, although it often seems an obtuse measure, attempts to emulate physicians' decisions. That is, when physicians make decisions on what test to use, they often consider which choice is the best for any given patient. In today's healthcare environment, they also consider the cost or at least surrogates of cost (such as whether they really need an expensive invasive study where they have to miss work). These latter points are, in many ways, 'off-handed' calculation of cost-effectiveness that are employed every day in clinical practice decision making. Precisely, an incremental or marginal cost-effectiveness analysis includes a comparison of two or more tests or testing strategies with

$$\frac{\Delta \text{cost}}{\Delta \text{outcome}} = \frac{C_{\text{test 1}} - C_{\text{test 2}}}{O_{\text{test 1}} - O_{\text{test 2}}},$$

where C is cost and O is outcome. Of course, one must optimize either the numerator or the denominator in order to garner an attractive cost-effectiveness calculation. When both costs are lower and outcomes are improved, for a given comparison, this is termed a dominant strategy.

The US Public Health Service has set standards for the calculation of cost-effectiveness that include a cost per life-year saved or cost per quality-adjusted life-years saved.[56,57] The commonly applied threshold for economic efficiency has been set at $50 000 dollars per life-year saved. That is, cost-effectiveness ratios <$50 000 dollars per life-year saved are considered favorable. In many cases, European countries are setting thresholds in the range of $20 000–40 000 per life-year saved in order to reflect more stringent economic efficiency standards.

Extending the benefits of testing into life-expectancy measures appear to be more fitting of a treatment, and as such, some researchers have advocated the use of intermediate outcome measures in lieu of life-years saved.[21] For example, a diagnostic test may not save a life but rather is employed in order to estimate risk or to diagnose disease, and therefore it may be more appropriate to calculate a cost-effectiveness measure such as cost to identify a cardiac death or myocardial infarction *or* cost to identify coronary heart disease. To date, there are no differentiating standards between a diagnostic test and a therapeutic intervention. It appears, however, that the optimal strategy would be to employ a cost-effectiveness analysis that emulates how tests are being applied. That is, intermediate outcomes appear better suited for diagnostic tests. The

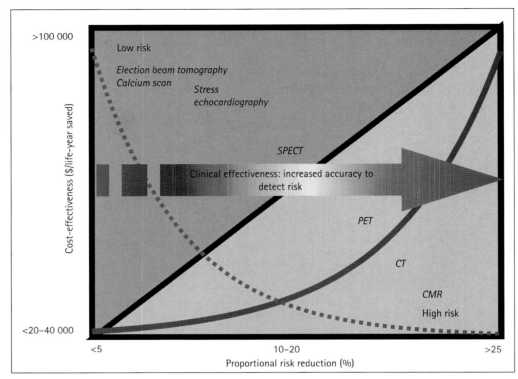

Figure 31.5
Principles of cost-effectiveness include consideration of a test's clinical effectiveness, the ensuing proportional risk reduction with treatment, and the resulting cost implications. Generally, cost-effectiveness parallels risk reduction. That is, when a greater risk reduction is noted with any given pathway of care, cost-effectiveness becomes more economically attractive. For cardiac imaging, the current evidence would suggest that lower-cost tests may be effectively applied to lower-risk populations – such as exercise echocardiography for a diagnostic population with suspected coronary disease. However, CMR and PET may become more cost-effective in higher-risk populations. When there is an increased clinical effectiveness or increased accuracy to detect risk, the ensuing cost-effectiveness will be enhanced.

challenge with this type of analysis is that there are no standards for comparing thresholds for efficiency (such as that put forth by the US Public Health Service for cost per life-year saved).

Although few analysis are available that compare CMR with other modalities, it may be helpful to explore some theoretical principles of a cost-effectiveness analysis that may provide some insight into its future value as a modality of choice (Figure 31.5). A general tenet of cost-effectiveness analysis is that as a test becomes more clinically effective, it will become more cost-effective.[20] That is, accurate tests, such as CMR, have lower rates of false-negative and false-positive tests and, thus, lowered cost, while maintaining high quality. Another trend in cost-effectiveness analysis is that when there is a greater proportional risk reduction with treatment, the cost-effectiveness is lowered. That is, as treatment becomes more effective in reducing risk in higher-risk populations, the ensuing cost-effectiveness ratios are also lowered. This can be seen in examples where secondary prevention is often more cost-effective than primary prevention. For CMR, for example, it would be more cost-effective to test

older versus younger patients, symptomatic versus asymptomatic patients, and intermediate–high pretest risk versus lower-risk patients (to name a few). This type of reasoning can be used to focus research into areas where CMR may be more clinically and cost-effective.

Comparative diagnostic imaging costs

CMR is currently under rapid development, and is one of many new or modified imaging modalities available for imaging of the cardiovascular system. The current estimated costs of cardiac imaging modalities are reported in Table 31.1. As a number of techniques for CMR are currently under development, its estimated costs should be viewed with caution. Despite this, the estimated cost of CMR, using standard techniques of adjusting Medicare charges (by a cost–charge ratio), ranges from \$525 to \$1220.[11,13] This cost is higher than the expected cost for other noninvasive imaging modalities, with the exception of PET. Further examination of estimates of physician work reveals that the estimated relative value units (RVUs, where each unit is valued in year 2001 at $38.26 with adjustments by geography and malpractice expense) are greater (on average) for MR procedures than for any other imaging modality except cardiac catheterization. The total RVUs for MR range from 13.25 to 27.64 (or estimated service payments of $507 to $1058). It should be noted that reimbursements vary by source of payment (e.g. Medicare versus Health Maintenance Organization (HMO) or Blue Cross/Blue Shield). For example, reimbursement for a CMR ventricular function study may be as low as $450 for a given HMO, but may be as high as $1000 for a Blue Cross/Blue Shield contract. Examples of the technical portion for reimbursement for CMR procedures in 2003 are reported in Table 31.2; note that these values will vary by hospital setting and geographic location, as well as teaching status and urban setting. In comparison with other techniques, there is a greater delineation in test types and procedure add-ons to augment reimbursement for other modalities, such as echocardiography and SPECT imaging. For this new technology to be assimilated into daily practice, reimbursement will have to track its expected clinical value to society in order to realize the true benefits of CMR.

Test use is guided by both economic forces (e.g. reimbursement) and information content. For CMR, the multitudes of test parameters (e.g. perfusion, function, morphology, metabolism, and tissue characterization) that may be acquired render this test unlike other noninvasive imaging modalities. Its ability to acquire diverse risk markers raises the overall test cost (as reflected above). For cardiac imaging, economic value may be achieved by developing a single, noninvasive test that assesses cardiac morphology, function, valvular disease, myocardial perfusion, and coronary arteries, as well as evaluating the anatomy of the great vessels and peripheral vasculature (Figure 31.6). CMR has the potential to provide this comprehensive examination in one sitting at considerably less risk and cost to the patient. With rapid imaging techniques, it should be possible to complete a comprehensive study in as little as 1 hour (at an estimated cost of <$1220). On the positive side, the effect of this higher initial test cost may be offset by a reduction in downstream utilization of other redundant imaging tests. Using a rudimentary cost analysis, adding CMR's ability to perform multiple test functions may provide cost savings to the healthcare system. For example, a 10% reduction in the use of other noninvasive tests could reduce by ~0.2–5% the ~$1 trillion spent on US healthcare annually.

Conversely, it appears unlikely, due to its higher initial test cost, that CMR will be applied to a wide range of patients or those at risk for cardiovascular disease. Consistent with prior research, it is more likely that it

Table 31.2 Examples of technical portion reimbursement for hospital outpatient departments for CMR procedures in 2003[a]

Current Procedural Terminology (CPT) code	Procedure	Reimbursement ($)
Head and neck		
70544	MRA: head without contrast material(s)	343.94
70545	MRA: head with contrast material(s)	377.28
70546	MRA: head without contrast material(s) followed by contrast material(s) and further sequences	481.82
70547	MRA: neck without contrast material(s)	343.94
70548	MRA: neck with contrast material(s)	377.28
70549	MRA: neck without contrast material(s), followed by contrast material(s) and further sequences	481.82
Heart		
75552	CMR for morphology, without contrast material	356.39
75553	CMR for morphology, with contrast material	390.93
75554	CMR for function, with or without morphology, complete study	340.17
75555	CMR for function, with or without morphology, limited study	340.17

[a] Note that reimbursement varies by geographic region, urban facility, and teaching status.

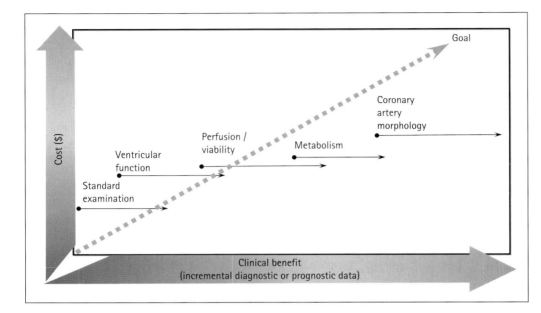

Figure 31.6
For CMR, cost-effectiveness may be visualized by exploring the intersection of cost and clinical benefit. The addition of many CMR testing parameters will add little to no cost to the clinical workup, but, in many cases, may provide substantially more diagnostic or prognostic data from which enhanced patient care may ensue. The goal of any diagnostic evaluation is to achieve the greatest magnitude of diagnostic and prognostic information while minimizing cost outlays.

will be focused as a second-line test when initial results are inconclusive or as a front-line test in high-risk subsets that benefit most from the precision and detail provided by this modality (Tables 31.3 and 31.4). This idea is consistent with an evolving paradigm in testing that includes three levels for screening (e.g. EBT), routine testing (e.g. echocardiography or SPECT), and complex procedure use (e.g. CMR or PET) that are applied from low- to higher-risk patient cohorts. As such, it seems likely that EBT, echocardiography, and SPECT imaging will remain front-line screening strategies due to the current capital equipment investment in

most hospitals, favorable reimbursement, and an abundance of supportive diagnostic and prognostic evidence.[19] The benefits of the widespread use of these tests are that they may provide a low-cost initial procedure that can be used as a gatekeeper for more expensive procedures and, particularly, to add a greater value to prognostic risk assessment. Current use of myocardial perfusion and ventricular function data provide ~20–50% incremental value over historical measures alone. It is likely that CMR could provide substantially more added information due to the array of test parameters available.

Table 31.3 Potential changes in testing patterns with CMR

CMR could become the modality of choice or a suitable replacement for many clinical indications

Example 1: CMR as a comprehensive examination could reduce the number of procedures performed by nuclear cardiology, diagnostic catheterization, or echocardiography

Example 2: CMR may be a useful and cost-competitive substitute for PET scans for myocardial perfusion and metabolism, especially when reimbursement is favorable for oncological PET (and imaging time for cardiovascular indications may be constrained). It is expected that the use of PET for oncology will continue to grow with the use of PET-CT scanners.

Example 3: CMR may become a low-cost and noninvasive option for coronary angiography to screen *certain* patients (i.e. lower-risk) suspected of having coronary disease. This could greatly reduce patient risks associated with this invasive catheterization. CMR may then become a 'feeder' to the catheterization laboratory and result in more patients sent for catheterization with disease and requiring revascularization, thus decreasing the rate of normal coronaries.

Table 31.4 Specific benefits by clinical indication for CMR

Global and regional function – improved precision and consistency with CMR
- Echocardiography is a very low-cost, portable option, and should continue to be applied in lower-risk subsets or those in intensive care situations or outpatient settings
- The result may be a tiered approach where CMR is selected for those at high risk
- Thus, CMR could become the gatekeeper to higher-cost procedures, thereby initiating cost efficiency

Perfusion and metabolism
- Very cost-competitive with PET
- The combination of physiological/anatomical assessment should result in cost-efficient care

Coronary angiography
- MRA – low-cost alternative to conventional angiography
- Gatekeeper:
  - Reduces complications, hospital costs, and overall 'workup' cost
  - ACC–NCDR: ~20–30% normal coronary rate; 1.2% in-lab complications
  - Occurrence of elevated creatinine (>2 mg/dl)
  - Outpatient procedure – lower cost versus inpatient setting

Economic benefit of CMR

The remainder of this chapter will elucidate several areas of economic advantage of CMR, including cardiac function and morphology, myocardial perfusion and metabolism, and angiography.

Cost implications of cardiac function and morphology

Precise measurements of cardiac chamber sizes and volumes may be obtained with CMR, rendering it ideally suited to detail abnormalities in chamber function and to image complex valvular and congenital heart diseases. In addition, the adjoining great vessels may be combined in this assessment. Further delineation of cardiac masses and pericardial effusions may be obtained. Imaging of tissue composition can help in the diagnosis of disorders such as amyloidosis and right-ventricular dysplasia. Thus, in patients with known cardiovascular disease or in high-risk subsets, the economic value of CMR is that high-cost care is limited to those in greatest need. This hierarchical testing approach in which lower-cost tests are applied to a greater percentage of patients (i.e. as a screening test) and higher-cost tests are limited to those high-risk patients where a greater incremental value is determined[58] is based upon a high-risk cost-effectiveness model in which economic value is greater in higher-risk populations who receive a greater proportional benefit to testing and treatment (in the form of disproportionately greater risk reduction when compared with lower-risk cohorts). By applying this principle of high-risk cost models, costs can be differentially and selectively allocated to sicker patients

and thereby result in more cost-efficient (i.e. cost-saving) care. Additionally, the upfront cost differences are minimized by the greater outcome benefit to that patient cohort, rendering the test more cost-effective.

Cost implications of perfusion and metabolism measures

CMR has the potential to provide estimates of myocardial perfusion as well as (with spectroscopy) metabolic dysfunction. Evidence in small patient samples reveals a diagnostic sensitivity and specificity in the 70–80% range, using catheterization as the gold standard.[59] A considerable amount of diagnostic and prognostic data are available with SPECT imaging, and it appears unlikely that with the current favorable reimbursement for perfusion and function and wall motion as add-ons that MR perfusion could be competitive in the near future.[19] Additionally PET, despite improved resolution, has only limited indications for reimbursement (i.e. myocardial viability). Nevertheless, with the development of MR angiography (MRA), the combined physiological and anatomical assessment may be a highly desirable and cost-efficient alternative for the assessment of ischemic heart disease.

Cost implications of MR angiography

Imaging the coronary arteries has been one of the most important advances in the management of coronary artery disease. Cardiac catheterization provides an invasive assessment of the extent and severity of coronary artery disease. Annually, ~2 million cardiac catheterizations are performed each year in the USA. Conventional X-ray angiography carries a small but noticeable risk due to the invasive nature of the procedure, the injection of radiopaque contrast media, and the radiation exposure for both patient and medical staff. Although under development, the possibility of noninvasive coronary MRA provides an opportunity to reduce the overall 1% risk of procedural complications with current catheterization-based techniques, and may serve as a lower-cost gatekeeper to this invasive procedure. It is likely that if MRA were utilized as a diagnostic test for lower-risk subsets of those patients currently referred for catherization, a 52% cost savings may be achieved for the lower risk patient. Currently, the American College of Cardiology National Cardiovascular Data Registry (ACC–NCDR) including >250 000 patients notes an average normal catheterization rate of 35%.[60] If MRA were applied initially, follow-up angiography may be averted in those patients with normal coronaries, thus reducing complication rates at a reduced 'workup' cost (i.e. 10% cost savings). Catheterization would then be limited to those patients with identifiable abnormalities noted on MRA, thereby serving as a gatekeeper to current X-ray angiography.

The UK National Health Service recently completed an economic evaluation of MRA for carotid artery stenosis and peripheral arterial disease.[6] For carotid artery disease, the review included 14 articles that examined the diagnostic performance of ultrasound versus MRA. These results reveal 93% sensitivity and 94% specificity for the detection of carotid disease. Of the 14 articles, only 1 reported a lower sensitivity to detect 70–99% stenosis with MRA than with ultrasound. The average cost per event was £204 for digital subtraction angiography (DSA) compared with £110 for MRA. These results reveal a cost-effectiveness ratio of £10 525 per disabling stroke averted per year.[6] They indicate that MRA is the lower-cost option for the evaluation of carotid artery stenosis.

For MRA versus X-ray angiography in the identification of peripheral artery disease, the data for 2D time-of-flight (TOF) and contrast-enhanced MRA had a 94% sensitivity and an 93% specificity. Unit costs were £455 for X-ray angiography, compared with £247 for MRA, including capital equipment costs. The average cost per event detected was £455 for DSA, compared with £247 for MRA, with higher costs being noted for 2D TOF MRA. These results indicate that in order to maximize 1-year outcomes, there is little difference between MRA compared with DSA. This panel suggested, however, that the optimal choice of modality would depend upon equipment availability and physician preferences. There is a notable but small complication risk with an invasive procedure, such as X-ray angiography but a slightly lower diagnostic sensi-

tivity with MRA. This balance would be influenced by the underlying risk in the patient population, with higher-risk patients going directly to X-ray angiography and MRA being applied as in Figure 31.2.

Whole-body 3D MRA

As atherosclerotic diseases affect the entire vascular system, several imaging modalities, including conventional catheter angiography, duplex ultrasound, CT, and MRA, have been proposed to provide a whole-body assessment.[61,62] Prior reports have noted a rapid assessment of the vasculature and a relatively high diagnostic accuracy and a minimal rate of false-negative or false-positive studies with MRA.[63–68] Lower rates of false-negative and false-positive studies can foster cost-efficient care for patients undergoing whole-body 3D MRA.

Using evidence to guide reimbursement: the realities of the financial perspective of healthcare for CMR

Although there were prior limitations and reports noting a cost-ineffectiveness of CMR,[69–72] a recent increase in interest coupled with a growing expansion of clinically acceptable indications has prompted a moderate growth in the field of CMR, including the addition of a scanner to most large cardiology practices in the USA. For example, in an earlier cost-effectiveness analysis that compared MRA with captopril renography and CT angiography for the diagnosis of renal artery stenosis, strategies including MRA were not cost-effective.[72] The 'realities' of today's CMR are that it may be a useful and cost-competitive substitute for PET scans for myocardial perfusion and metabolic studies – especially since many PET scanners are being optimized for use in oncology, with little imaging time available for cardiovascular indications.

Another high-impact example is the possibility of employing CMR as a low-cost and noninvasive option for coronary angiography to screen certain patients suspected of having coronary artery disease. This could greatly reduce patient complications associated with the examination.[71,72] While a certain number of *diagnostic* cardiac catheterization procedures could be replaced by CMR, this shift would create additional capacity in the catheterization laboratory for *interventional* procedures. In effect, this could reduce the rate of normal coronaries. Further, as CMR is a noninvasive approach, it could potentially

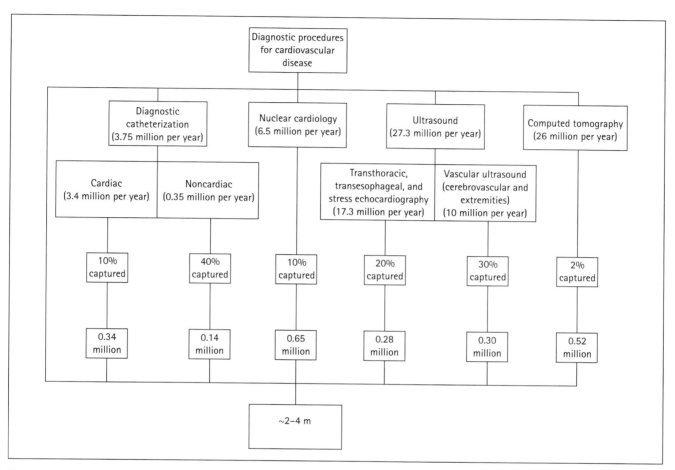

Figure 31.7
Expected migration and shifting of other procedural utilization to CMR.

screen a larger base of patients than is possible with an invasive procedure such as coronary angiography. This would inevitably result in detecting more disease. Subsequently, CMR would serve the role of 'feeding' a greater number of patients into the catheterization laboratory for therapeutic intervention (i.e. increase the number of percutaneous coronary interventions performed).

It is not expected that such changes will occur overnight or that CMR will ever completely replace other modalities. Figure 31.7 illustrates the expected migration (in number of exams per year) from current diagnostic modalities to CMR. This transfer of examination volume is based on 1999–2000 statistical data, interviews with leading industry authorities, accepted clinical indications, and trends in economic drivers, such as procedure reimbursement rates.

It does appear unlikely that CMR will replace lower-cost tests, such as echocardiography, that may be effectively used in lower-risk populations. Given this practical point, it seems likely that there will be an unfolding paradigm where lower-cost tests (e.g. echocardiography and

exercise electrocardiography) will be applied to the lower-risk subset of the population. CMR will then be used as a second tier of tests or for those higher-risk patients. Additionally, it is also unlikely that CMR will replace tests where current reimbursement is favorable (e.g. SPECT) or where there is a large capital investment (e.g. SPECT and CT). Historically, what often happens is that 'imaging begets more imaging'. Thus, the use of many conventional imaging modalities will foster the use and growth of more CMR testing (especially under the 'second tier of testing' approach). One exception is that CMR will have the ability to identify unique risk markers; such as with plaque characterization or MR spectroscopy. This could further foster testing niches where growth will be limited to CMR and not be the result of any shifting in testing patterns.

A template for a proforma model for CMR is detailed in the Appendix 1, although this must be optimized to any given setting and practice situation. Using calculations from this template, one may calculate a breakeven analysis for CMR (Table 31.5).

Table 31.5 Breakeven analysis for CMR

	Revenue per patient ($)	Breakeven daily patient load
• Total fixed expenses = $858 035	600	8.02
• Variable expenses per patient = $85	700	6.67
• Revenue per patient = $750	800	5.7
• Allowance for bad debts and free service = 20.0%	900	4.99
• Before considering impact of taxes, breakeven point for year 1 is reached at a daily patient load of 6.15 patients	1000	4.43

Conclusions

Cost-effectiveness analysis is a means to provie a rationale to allocated finite healthcare resources. This includes the integration of measures of clinical quality into terms of economic value. The calculation of cost-effective comparisons helps to educate administrators and healthcare payers as to the key considerations for evaluating CMR in relation to other noninvasive tests. One pattern is unfolding in the current research with cardiovascular imaging, namely that high-quality testing can be used to improve the allocation of ever-limited resources. The true economic value for CMR includes the minimization of its higher upfront costs by a reduction in downstream cost waste as a result of improved accuracy and evidence used to effectively guide post-test management. Increasingly, both the public and private sectors are requiring cost-effectiveness analyses when considering large purchasing decisions or for reimbursement purposes.

Rapid advances in the field of magnetic resonance imaging have occurred over the past few years, generating increased excitement about its application in routine clinical decision-making. Although rudimentary cost analyses in a variety of areas provide initial insight into the potential economic value to society, standards for evidence-based medicine require an abundance of clinical and economic data before unanimous approval by medical societies and healthcare payers (including government agencies) alike. Concomitant focus on outcomes data during technical development is critical to acquiring a body of evidence to support routine use of CMR applications. Despite these limitations, the promise of CMR affords the healthcare consumer, clinician, and society with exciting alternatives to current imaging strategies that may result in both clinically effective and cost-effective testing-based strategies.

References

1. www.americanheart.org/statistics/economic.html.

2. Levin DC, Parker L, Intenzo CM, Sunshine JH. Recent rapid increase in utilization of radionuclide myocardial perfusion imaging and related procedures: 1996–1998 practice patterns. Radiology 2002; 222:144–8.

3. http://www.acc.org/advocacy/advoc_issues/impactchart.htmwww.acc.org/advocacy/advoc_issues/impactchart.htm

4. O'Rourke RA, Brundage BH, Froelicher VF, et al. American College of Cardiology/American Heart Association Expert Consensus Document on Electron Beam Computed Tomography for the Diagnosis of Coronary Artery Disease (Committee on Electron Beam Computed Tomography). Circulation 2000; 102:126–40.

5. Berry E, Kelly S, Hutton J, et al. A systematic literature review of spiral and electron beam computed tomography: with particular reference to clinical applications in hepatic lesions, pulmonary embolus and coronary artery disease. Health Tech Assess 1999; 3:1–121.

6. Berry E, Kelly S, Westwood ME, et al. The cost-effectivenss of magnetic resonance angiography for carotid artery stenosis and peripheral vascular disease: a systematic review. Health Tech Assess 2002; 6:1–165.

7. Rumberger JA, Behrenbeck T, Breen JF, Sheedy PF. Coronary calcification by electron beam computed tomography and obstructive coronary artery disease: a model for costs and effectiveness of diagnosis as compared with conventional cardiac testing methods. J Am Coll Cardiol 1999; 33:453–62.

8. Raggi P, Callister TQ, Cooil B, et al. Evaluation of chest pain in patients with low to intermediate pretest probability of coronary artery disease by electron beam computed tomography. Am J Cardiol 2000; 85:386–7.

9. Rumberger JA. Cost effectiveness of coronary calcification scanning using electron beam tomography in intermediate and high risk asymptomatic individuals. J Cardiovasc Risk 2000; 7:113–19.

10. O'Malley PG, Greenberg B, Taylor AT. What is the marginal cost-effectiveness of EBCT in an asymptomatic screening population? Circulation 2001; 104:II-468

11. Shaw LJ, Mulvagh SL, Jacobson C, et al. Cost implications of diagnosing coronary disease. Eur Heart J 2000; 21:477.

12. Goldman L, Garber AM, Grover SA, Hlatky MA. 27th Bethesda Conference: matching the intensity of risk factor management with the hazard for CAD events. Task Force 6. Cost effectiveness of assessment and management of risk factors. J Am Coll Cardiol 1996; 27:1020–30.

13. Shaw LJ, Hachamovitch R, Berman DS, et al. for the Economics of Noninvasive Diagnosis (END) Multicenter Study Group. The economic consequences of available diagnostic and prognostic strategies for the evaluation of stable angina patients: an observational assessment of the value of pre-catheterization ischemia. J Am Coll Cardiol 1999; 33:661–9.

14. Underwood SR, Godman B, Salyani S, et al. Economics of myocardial perfusion imaging in Europe – the EMPIRE study. Eur Heart J 1999; 20:157–66.

15. Marwick TH, Shaw LJ, Case C, et al. Selection of initial investigation for risk evaluation in coronary artery disease: cost and effectiveness implications of exercise ECG and exercise echocardiography. Eur Heart J 2003; 24:1153–63.

16. Patterson RE, Eisner RL, Horowitz SF. Comparison of cost-effectiveness and utility of exercise ECG, single photon emission computed tomography, positron emission tomography, and coronary angiography for diagnosis of coronary artery disease. Circulation 1995; 91:54–65.

17. Garber AM. Cost-effectiveness of alternative test strategies for the diagnosis of coronary artery disease. Ann Intern Med 1999; 20:157.

18. Kuntz KM, Fleischmann KE, Hunink MG, Douglas PS. Cost-effectiveness of diagnostic strategies for patients with chest pain. Ann Intern Med 1999; 130:709–18.

19. Shaw LJ, Culler SD, Becker NR. Current evidence on cost effectiveness of noninvasive cardiac testing. Subsection E: Analytic approaches to cost effectiveness and outcomes measurement in cardiovascular imaging. In: Imaging in Cardiovascular Disease (Pohost G, O'Rourke R, Shah P, Berman D, eds). Philadelphia: Lippincott Williams & Wilkins, 2000; 479–500.

20. Shaw LJ, Eisenstein EL, Hachamovitch R, et al. for the Economics of Noninvasive Diagnosis Multicenter. A primer of biostatistic and economic methods for diagnostic and prognostic modeling in nuclear cardiology: Part II. J Nucl Cardiol 1997; 4:52–60.

21. Mark DB, Shaw LJ, Lauer MS, et al. Is atherosclerotic imaging cost effective? J Am Coll Cardiol 2003; 41:1906–17.

22. Krumholz HM, Weintraub WS, Bradford WD, et al. The cost of prevention: Can we afford it? Can we afford not to do it? J Am Coll Cardiol 2002; 40:603–15.

23. Sculpher M, Drummond M, Buxton M. The iterative use of economic evaluation as part of the process of health technology assessment. J Health Serv Res 1997; 2:26–30.

24. www.pharma.org.

25. Bottini PB, Carr AA, Prisant LM, et al. Magnetic resonance imaging compared to echocardiography to assess left ventricular mass in the hypertensive patient. Am J Hypertens 1995; 8:221–8.

26. www.phrma.org/publications/publications/brochure/whycostmuch.phtml.

27. He ZX, Hedrick TD, Pratt CM, et al. Severity of coronary artery calcification by electron beam computed tomography predicts silent myocardial ischemia. *Circulation* 2000; 101:244–51.

28. Wong NG, Detrano RC, Diamond G, et al. Does coronary artery screening by electron beam computed tomography motivate potentially beneficial lifestyle behaviors? Am J Cardiol 1996; 78:1220–3.

29. Califf RM, Armstrong PW, Carver JR, et al. Stratification of patients into high, medium, and low risk subgroups for purposes of risk factor management. J Am Coll Cardiol 1996; 27:964–1047.

30. Wayhs R, Zelinger A, Raggi P. High coronary artery calcium scores pose an extremely elevated risk for hard events. J Am Coll Cardiol 2002; 39:225–30.

31. Sullivan DR. Screening for cardiovascular disease with cholesterol. Clin Chim Acta 2002; 15:49–60.

32. Fayad ZA, Fuster V, Nikolaou K, Becker C. Computed tomography and magnetic resonance imaging for noninvasive coronary angiography and plaque imaging: current and potential future concepts. Circulation 2002; 106:2026–34.

33. Sheldon TA. Problems of using modelling in the economic evaluation of health care. Health Econ 1996; 5:1–11.

34. Buxton MJ, Drummond MF, Van Hout BA, et al. Modeling in economic evaluation: an unavoidable fact of life. Health Econ 1997; 6:217–27.

35. Tosteson AN, Weinstein MC, Hunink MG, et al. Cost-effectiveness of populationwide educational approaches to reduce serum cholesterol levels. Circulation 1997; 95:24–30.

36. Mowatt G, Bower DJ, Brebner JA, et al. When and how to assess fast-changing technologies: a comparative study of medical applications of four generic technologies. Health Tech Assess 1997; 1(14):1–151.

37. www.fda.gov/cdrh/CT.

38. Bell R, Petticrew M, Luengo S, Sheldon TA. Screening for ovarian cancer: a systematic review. Health Tech Assess 1998; 2(2):1–84.

39. Criqui MH, Langer RD, Fronek A, et al. Mortality over a period of 10 years in patients with peripheral arterial disease. N Engl J Med 1992; 326:381–6.

40. Criqui MH, Fronek A, Klauber MR, et al. The sensitivity, specificity, and predictive value of traditional clinical evaluation of peripheral arterial disease: results from noninvasive testing in a defined population. Circulation 1985; 71:516–22.

41. Petticrew MP, Sowden AJ, Lister-Sharp D, Wright K. False-negative results in screening programmes: systematic review of impact and implications. Health Tech Assess 2000; 4:1–60.

42. Drummond MF, Jefferson TO. Guidelines for authors and peer reviewers of economic submissions to the BMJ. The BMJ Economic Evaluation Working Party. BMJ 1996; 313:275–83.

43. Mansley EC, McKenna MT. Importance of perspective in economic analyses of cancer screening decisions. Lancet 2001; 358:1169–73.

44. Hong C, Becker CR, Schoepf UJ, et al. Coronary artery calcium: absolute quantification in nonenhanced and contrast-enhanced multi-detector row CT studies. Radiology 2002; 223:474–80.

45. Achenbach S, Ropers D, Möhlenkamp S, et al. Variability of repeated coronary artery calcium measurements by electron beam tomography. Am J Cardiol 2001; 87:210–13.

46. Smith DH, Hugh Gravelle H. The practice of discounting in economic evaluations of healthcare interventions Int J Tech Assess Health Care 2001; 17:236–43.

47. Sheldon TA. Discounting in health care decision-making: time for a change? J Pub Health Med 1992; 14:250–6.

48. Swan JS, Fryback DG, Lawrence WF, et al. A time-tradeoff method for cost-effectiveness models applied to radiology. Med Decis Making 2000; 20:79–88.

49. http://www.acc.org/clinical/training/cocats2.pdf.

50. Taskforce of the European Society of Cardiology, in collaboration with the Association of European Paediatric Cardiologists. The clinical role of magnetic resonance in cardiovascular disease. Eur Heart J 1998; 19:19–39.

51. Chien D, Oesingmann N, Laub G. New frontiers in cardiovascular magnetic resonance. Electromedica 2000; 68:11–17.

52. Gyrd-Hansen D, Sogaard J. Analysing public preferences for cancer screening programmes. Health Econ 2001; 10:617–34.

53. Merl T, Scholz M, Gerhardt P, et al. Results of a prospective multicenter study for evaluation of the diagnostic quality of an open whole-body low-field MRI unit. A comparison with high-field MRI measured by the applicable gold standard. Eur J Radiol 1999; 30:43–53.

54. Hunold P, Schmermund A, Seibel RM, et al. Prevalence and clinical significance of accidental findings in electron-beam tomographic scans for coronary artery calcification. Eur Heart J 2001; 22:1748–58.

55. Shaw LJ, Callister TQ, Raggi P. Establishing cost effective thresholds for coronary disease screening: a predictive model with risk factors and coronary calcium. Circulation 2001; 104:II-478.

56. Gold M. Cost-Effectiveness in Health and Medicine. New York: Oxford University Press, 1996.

57. Weinstein MC, Siegel JE, Gold MR, et al. Recommendations of the Panel on Cost-effectiveness in Health and Medicine. JAMA 1996; 276:1253–8.

58. Marwick TH, Anderson T, Williams MJ, et al. Exercise echocardiography is an accurate and cost-efficient technique for the detection of coronary artery disease in women. J Am Coll Cardiol 1995; 26:335–41.

59. Wilke NM, Zenovich AG, Jerosch-Herold M, Henry TD. Cardiac magnetic resonance imaging for the assessment of myocardial angiogenesis. Curr Interv Cardiol Rep 2001; 3:205–12.

60. Shaw LJ, Gibbons RJ, McCallister B, et al. Gender differences in extent and severity of coronary disease in the ACC National Cardiovascular Data Registry. J Am Coll Cardiol 2002; 39(Suppl A):851–6.

61. Shehadi WH. Contrast media adverse reactions: occurrence, recurrence, and distribution patterns. Radiology 1982; 143:11–17.

62. Shellock FG, Kanal E. Safety of magnetic resonance imaging contrast agents. J Magn Reson Imaging 1999; 10:477–84.

63. Prince MR. Gadolinium-enhanced MR aortography. Radiology 1994; 191:155–64.

64. Prince MR, Narasimham DL, Stanley JC, et al. Breath-hold gadolinium-enhanced MR angiography of the abdominal aorta and its major branches. Radiology 1995; 197:785–92.

65. Meaney JF, Weg JG, Chenevert TL, et al. Diagnosis of pulmonary embolism with magnetic resonance angiography. N Engl J Med 1997; 336:1422–7.

66. Goyen M, Debatin JF, Ruehm SG. Peripheral MR-angiography. Top Magn Reson Imaging 2001; 12:327–35.

67. Goyen M, Herborn CU, Lauenstein TC, et al. Optimization of contrast dosage For gadobenate dimeglumine-enhanced high-resolution whole body 3D MR angiography. Invest Radiol 2002; 37:263–8.

68. Goyen M, Herborn CU, Kröger K, et al. Detection of atherosclerosis: systemic imaging for a systemic disease using whole body 3D MR-angiography – initial experience. Radiology 2003; 227:277–82.

69. Ripley S. Is nuclear medicine cost-effective? Dimens Health Serv 1991; 68:21–3.

70. Durand-Zaleski I, Reizine D, Puzin D, et al. Economic assessment of magnetic resonance imaging for inpatients: Is it still too early? Int J Technol Assess Health Care 1993; 9:263–73.

71. Chissell HR, Allum RL, Keightley A. MRI of the knee: its cost-effective use in a district general hospital. Ann R Coll Surg Engl 1994; 76:26–9.

72. Nelemans PJ, Kessels AG, De Leeuw P, et al. The cost-effectiveness of the diagnosis of renal artery stenosis. Eur J Radiol 1998; 27:95–107.

Appendix: template for proforma model for CMR

PROFORMA MODEL
SUPPORT SCHEDULE A
EQUIPMENT AND FINANCING
SUMMARY

Equipment summary

Customer name	Sample
Equipment description	1.5 T CMR scanner
Sell price	$1 750 000

Financing summary

Sell price	$1 750 000
Downpayment	$0
Net financed	$1 750 000
Monthly lease payment (excludes maintenance, freight, insurance, and taxes)	$30 516.84
Useful life of equipment (months)	96

		Current estimate	Revised estimate
Other fixed asset requirements			
Room/Site Preparation		$30 000	
Useful Life in Months		60	
Furniture & Fixtures		$10 000	
Useful Life in Months		36	
Organizational costs			
Amount		$0	
Amortization period (months)		96	
Up-Front Capital Investment		$0	

Revenue summary

	Inflation/growth rate	Current estimate	Revised estimate
Charge per patient			
Year 1		$750.00	
Year 2	−5.0%	$712.50	
Year 3	−5.0%	$676.88	
Year 4	−5.0%	$643.04	
Year 5	−5.0%	$610.89	
Number of patients per day			
Year 1		12.00	
Year 2	16.7%	14.00	
Year 3	28.6%	18.00	
Year 4	11.1%	20.00	
Year 5	20.0%	24.00	
Allowance for bad debt and free service	20%		
Accounts receivable collection period (days)		60	
Operational Days			
Operational days per week		5.5	
Operational weeks per year		52	
Total operational days available		286	
Less: Holidays		10	
Less: Maintenance days		5	
Net operational days per year		271	

PROFORMA MODEL
SUPPORT SCHEDULE B
FIXED EXPENSE SUMMARY

Salary expense	No. of employees	Revised No. of employees	% age charge in salaries	Average salary per employee	Revised salary per employee
Technicians					
Year 1	3.00			$55 000	
Year 2	3.00		3.0%	$56 650	
Year 3	4.00		3.0%	$58 350	
Year 4	4.00		3.0%	$60 101	
Year 5	4.00		3.0%	$61 904	

Salary expense	No. of employees	Revised No. of employees	% age charge in salaries	Average salary per employee	Revised salary per employee
Technicians					
Year 1	3.00			$55 000	
Year 2	3.00		3.0%	$56 650	
Year 3	4.00		3.0%	$58 350	
Year 4	4.00		3.0%	$60 101	
Year 5	4.00		3.0%	$61 904	
Nurses					
Year 1	1.50			$50 000	
Year 2	1.50		3.0%	$51 500	
Year 3	2.00		3.0%	$53 045	
Year 4	2.00		3.0%	$54 636	
Year 5	2.00		3.0%	$56 275	
Other					
Year 1	3.00			$22 500	
Year 2	3.00		3.0%	$23 175	
Year 3	3.00		3.0%	$23 870	
Year 4	3.00		3.0%	$24 586	
Year 5	3.00		3.0%	$25 324	
Fringe benefits as %age of salaries				20.00%	

Other fixed expenses	Inflation/growth rate	Current estimate	Revised estimate
Service and cryogens			
Year 1		$0	
Year 2	0.0%	$135 000	
Year 3	0.0%	$135 000	
Year 4	0.0%	$135 000	
Year 5	0.0%	$135 000	
Other fixed expenses			
Year 1		$0	
Year 2	0.0%	$0	
Year 3	0.0%	$0	
Year 4	0.0%	$0	
Year 5	0.0%	$0	
Insurance			
Year 1		$30 000	
Year 2	3.0%	$30 900	
Year 3	3.0%	$31 827	
Year 4	3.0%	$32 782	
Year 5	3.0%	$33 765	

PROFORMA MODEL
SUPPORT SCHEDULE C
FIXED EXPENSE
SUMMARY

Other fixed expenses	Inflation/growth rate	Current estimate	Revised estimate
Legal and accounting			
Year 1		$10 000	
Year 2	3.0%	$10 300	
Year 3	3.0%	$10 609	
Year 4	3.0%	$10 927	
Year 5	3.0%	$11 255	
Office supplies			
Year 1		$3 000	
Year 2	3.0%	$3 090	
Year 3	3.0%	$3 183	
Year 4	3.0%	$3 278	
Year 5	3.0%	$3 376	
Rent			
Year 1		$60 000	
Year 2	0.0%	$60 000	
Year 3	0.0%	$60 000	
Year 4	0.0%	$60 000	
Year 5	0.0%	$60 000	
Utilities			
Year 1		$7 500	
Year 2	3.0%	$7 725	
Year 3	3.0%	$7 957	
Year 4	3.0%	$8 196	
Year 5	3.0%	$8 442	
Miscellaneous			
Year 1		$3 000	
Year 2	3.0%	$3 090	
Year 3	3.0%	$3 183	
Year 4	3.0%	$3 278	
Year 5	3.0%	$3 376	

PROFORMA MODEL
SUPPORT SCHEDULE D
VARIABLE EXPENSE
SUMMARY

(on a per patient basis)	*Inflation/growth rate*	*Current estimate*	*Revised estimate*
Medical supplies			
Year 1		$85.00	
Year 2	3.0%	$87.55	
Year 3	3.0%	$90.18	
Year 4	3.0%	$92.89	
Year 5	3.0%	$95.68	
Other variable expenses			
Year 1		$0.00	
Year 2	0.0%	$0.00	
Year 3	0.0%	$0.00	
Year 4	0.0%	$0.00	
Year 5	0.0%	$0.00	

TAX RATES

	Current rate	*Revised rate*
Sales tax (computed on monthly payment)	0.00%	
Personal property tax (computed on equipment sell price)	0.00%	
Income Tax	0.00%	

Index